ASCP QUICK COMPENDIUM

COMPANION

FOR

SURGICAL PATHOLOGY

including hundreds of image-based questions
and explanations keyed into the
ASCP Quick Compendium of Surgical Pathology

All *Quick Compendia* titles are available at www.ascp.org

Acknowledgments

The authors would like to thank our mentors and colleagues for their guidance and support in this project. Specifically, the following faculty members at the University of Virginia have been an invaluable resource for the completion of this book: Mark Wick, Julia Iezzoni, Robin LeGallo, Mark Stoler, Molly Galgano, Christopher Moskaluk, John Cousar, Stacey Mills, Beatriz Lopes and Kenneth Tung.

Additionally, we would like to thank our families, friends, and significant others, who supported us and allowed us to work on this project on their time. We would also like to thank the publication team at ASCP, specifically Joshua Weikersheimer for his help and support.

ASCP

Quick Compendium Companion
for Surgical Pathology

Michael W Cruise, *Editor in Chief*

William K Brix

Susanne K Jeffus

Yasmin I Lutterbie

Sarah R Nassau

Jocelyn S Posthumus

Dirk P Stanley

All of the Department of Pathology,
University of Virginia, Charlottesville

American Society for
Clinical Pathology
Press

Chicago

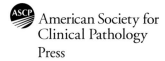 American Society for
Clinical Pathology
Press

Publishing Team

Aimee Algas (copyediting/proofreading)

Erik Tanck (production)

Joshua Weikersheimer (publishing direction)

Notice

Trade names for equipment and supplies described herein are included as suggestions only. In no way does their inclusion constitute an endorsement or preference by the American Society for Clinical Pathology. The ASCP did not test the equipment, supplies, or procedures and therefore urges all readers to read and follow all manufacturers' instructions and package insert warnings concerning the proper and safe use of products.

The views expressed in this publication are those of the author and do not reflect the official policy of the Department of the Army, Department of Defense, or United States Government.

16 15 14 12 12   5 4 3 2 1

rosebud

Printed in Hong Kong

Table of

Contents

Chapter 1

Cardiovascular System

Jocelyn S Posthumus, MD
Michael W Cruise, MD PhD

Questions 1

Answers 15

Chapter 2

Central Nervous System

Jocelyn S Posthumus, MD
Dirk P Stanley, MD

Questions 25

Answers 47

Chapter 3

Endocrine

Sarah R Nassau, MD
Dirk P Stanley, MD

Questions 61

Answers 81

Chapter 4

Breast

William K Brix, MD
Susanne K Jeffus, MS MD

Questions 95

Answers 119

Chapter 5

Female Reproductive Tract

William K Brix, MD
Sarah R Nassau, MD

Questions 129

Answers 156

Chapter 6

Ovary

William K Brix, MD
Sarah R Nassau, MD

Questions... 171

Answers.. 195

Chapter 7

Gastrointestinal Tract

Sarah R Nassau, MD
Michael W Cruise, MD PhD

Questions... 207

Answers.. 251

Chapter 8

Liver, Gallbladder, and Extrahepatic Bile Ducts

Michael W Cruise, MD PhD
Susanne K Jeffus, MS MD

Questions... 283

Answers.. 310

Chapter 9

Pancreas

Susanne K Jeffus, MS MD
Yasmin I Lutterbie, MD

Questions... 329

Answers.. 340

Chapter 10

Upper Aerodigestive Tract

Dirk P Stanley, MD
Yasmin I Lutterbie, MD

Questions... 347

Answers.. 356

Chapter 11

Lung

Susanne K Jeffus, MS MD
Yasmin I Lutterbie, MD

Questions. 363

Answers. 380

Chapter 12

Pleura and Peritoneum

Sarah R Nassau, MD
William K Brix, MD

Questions. 387

Answers. 391

Chapter 13

Mediastinum

Susanne K Jeffus, MS MD
Yasmin I Lutterbie, MD

Questions. 393

Answers. 406

Chapter 14

Lymph Node

Michael W Cruise, MD PhD
William K Brix, MD

Questions. 413

Answers. 447

Chapter 15

Male Reproductive System

Yasmin I Lutterbie, MD
Jocelyn S Posthumus, MD

Questions. 471

Answers. 480

Chapter 16

Urinary Tract

Yasmin I Lutterbie, MD
Jocelyn S Posthumus, MD

Questions 487

Answers 505

Chapter 17

Mandible and Maxilla

Dirk P Stanley, MD
Jocelyn S Posthumus, MD

Questions 517

Answers 525

Chapter 18

Salivary Glands

Dirk P Stanley, MD
William K Brix, MD

Questions 533

Answers 545

Chapter 19

Bone and Joints

Michael W Cruise, MD PhD
Susanne K Jeffus, MS MD

Questions 555

Answers 582

Chapter 20

Soft Tissue

Yasmin I Lutterbie, MD
Sarah R Nassau, MD

Questions 599

Answers 642

Author List

Editor in Chief
Michael W Cruise, MD PhD
Department of Pathology
University of Virginia
Charlottesville, VA

Authors
William K Brix, MD
Department of Pathology
University of Virginia
Charlottesville, VA

Michael W Cruise, MD PhD
Department of Pathology
University of Virginia
Charlottesville, VA

Susanne K Jeffus, MS MD
Department of Pathology
University of Virginia
Charlottesville, VA

Yasmin I Lutterbie, MD
Department of Pathology
University of Virginia
Charlottesville, VA

Sarah R Nassau, MD
Department of Pathology
University of Virginia
Charlottesville, VA

Jocelyn S Posthumus, MD
Department of Pathology
University of Virginia
Charlottesville, VA

Dirk P Stanley, MD
Department of Pathology
University of Virginia
Charlottesville, VA

Additional Contributors
Mark R Wick, MD
Department of Pathology
University of Virginia
Charlottesville, VA

Julia C Iezzoni, MD
Department of Pathology
University of Virginia
Charlottesville, VA

Christopher A Moskaluk, MD PhD
Department of Pathology
University of Virginia
Charlottesville, VA

Mark H Stoler, MD
Department of Pathology
University of Virginia
Charlottesville, VA

Robin D LeGallo, MD
Department of Pathology
University of Virginia
Charlottesville, VA

ASCP Quick Compendium Companion
Series Editor
George Leonard, MD PhD
MAJ, MC, USA
Chief, Anatomic Pathology
Madigan Army Medical Center
Tacoma, WA

Preface

This text was designed as a companion to the ASCP's *Quick Compendium of Surgical Pathology*. This is not an exhaustive review of all of surgical pathology, but we attempt to use questions and explanations to highlight important areas within surgical pathology. Specifically, we focused on important points and challenging differential diagnoses. Additionally, we utilized the questions and explanations to supplement and update some of the information in the ASCP *Quick Compendium of Surgical Pathology*. You will come across some questions that could be interpreted as "picky" or may highlight some obscure facts. These questions were written to highlight material that has appeared in standardized exams such as the ASCP RISE and the board exams. We have also included images that demonstrate some or most of the diagnostic and morphologic characteristics of the lesion and, where necessary, included ancillary information needed to make the diagnosis. The image questions also often highlight the common presentation, patient characteristics, immunohistochemical and other findings.

We are grateful to George Leonard, *ASCP Quick Compendium Companion* Series Editor for sharing *Making Things Memorable* (p xi), which discusses techniques useful for retention of this material, as well as preparation for standardized exams and clinical practice. These techniques have been used with success by the authors of this text, and we believe they are worth a review for this volume as well.

Overall, we hope that residents, fellows, and those studying for Maintenance of Certification exams find this text useful. If you have any questions or recommendations, feel free to email us at QCCSPBook@gmail.com, or contact the ASCP directly at joshua.weikersheimer@ascp.org.

Making Things Memorable

Pathology residency training is notoriously sparse in the teaching of pathology. Many times it is relegated to self-directed instruction. In addition the pathology board exam is a formidable foe. Diverse subjects are lumped together in what many consider the single most difficult exam of their lives. For these reasons and many others the *ASCP Quick Compendia* series has enjoyed great success. A lean epitome of a protean collection of information is much appreciated by residents as they try to prepare for the board exam. And the need for a text such as the *Quick Compendium* will only grow as all newly-minted pathologists and many practicing pathologists will be required to pass the Maintenance of Certification exam every 10 years.

However, with a subject so vast and a book so small the value of each word skyrockets. Space is a premium, and text is worth gold. For this reason it becomes important that the reader absorb each word. There is no filler material to skip over. How does one remember it all?

We all have our different styles of learning. For me the 3 most helpful techniques are flashcards, mnemonics, and question writing/answering. I will discuss in turn each of these techniques and explain how to get them to work for you. In addition I hope to offer examples of each of these on the website for your download and review.

Flashcards

For the purposes of discussion, a flashcard is defined as a 2-sided card with information on one side of the card that the learner is trying to associate with information on the other side of the card. For years, these have been used to learn simple associative facts. Building foreign language vocabulary is one popular example. The use of spaced repetition of flash cards was popularized by an Austrian educator named Sebastian Leitner. His text "How to Learn to Learn" (I love that title) first described the use of interval repetition as a means of increasing the efficiency of learning. His technique involves the use of categories or boxes into which one sorts "cards" of information. Each box is defined by the degree to which the student rates their own knowledge of the information on the card. If the student knows the information on the card well, the card is placed in a higher box; if the student does not know the information, it is placed in a lower box. An algorithm then presents the well-known cards at a longer-spaced interval than the less well-known cards. Several popular foreign language courses use this technology to great effect. Flashcards are an extraordinarily effective means of learning, but there are limitations and rules to be followed:

1. **The cards must be made properly.** They must be simple and not overloaded with information. For example, on one side of the card one could write, "Preferred growth medium for *Bordetella*," and on the other side "Regan-Lowe medium" (I do realize there are other suitable media, but it's just an example). An example of a poorly written card would be to have "*Bordetella*" on one side and a slew of facts, such as media, Gram stain, species, diseases, antibiotic sensitivities, etc on the other. Cards must be simple to be effective.

2. **Certain types of information are not "flashable."** There is information that does not lend itself to flashcards. For this reason it is important to be selective in the construction of flashcards. I would find it difficult to learn syndromic associations with flash cards. It would be too difficult to keep these cards simple, thus violating our 1st rule.

3. One must honestly grade his or her own performance. You aren't doing anyone any favors by upgrading or downgrading your ability to remember a card. For spaced repetition to work, there must be an accurate accounting of whether you know the information or not.

If one follows these rules, flashcards are an efficient means to learn vast amounts of information, at least in the short term. For longer-term memorization, a technique involving deep association is necessary. Which brings me to the next technique, mnemonics.

Mnemonics

Named after Mnemosyne, the Greek mother of the Muses and the personification of memory, mnemonics involve the association of a fact or concept with which one is already familiar with another to be learned. This is the key of using mnemonics—one must associate the unknown quantity with a known one. The Roman orator, Cicero, described the method of loci as a means to remember long speeches. With this technique one imagines walking around a familiar location, such as one's home. With each part of the home, one associates a portion of the speech. For example the front door is visualized as the opening of the speech. This is followed by the front hallway, perhaps the hall closet, the kitchen, the living room, the dining room, etc. There are numerous mnemonic techniques, and the discussion of each is beyond the scope of this text. The publication of this book will be supported by an online adjunct where I will be able to discuss mnemonics in more depth. One technique, however, does deserve a brief introduction because I will use it throughout the text. You can learn the technique, but it takes practice to make it work well. The technique has

many names: phonetic numbers, sound numbers, the major system, and number words, among others. The basic premise is simple: we can remember words better than numbers. Additionally, there are 10 basic consonantal sounds in the English language, which helps with the assignation of one number to one sound for numbers 0 through 9. Arbitrarily, I use the most popular mapping scheme as demonstrated below:

Number	Sound
0	S or Z
1	T or D
2	N
3	M
4	R
5	L
6	SH, TH, CH
7	K
8	F or V
9	P or B

Since the technique is based on the sounds rather than actual letters, there is leeway in creating words. Once you create a word (or words) from the number (or numbers), it is a simple task to use another mnemonic technique to memorize the words. A simple associative technique is useful to link 2 sets of numbers together. For example, I imagine a tot in a tire of a bicycle weighed down with a heavy chain on the mantel of a fireplace. To translate: tot = 11, tire = 14; bicycle = the cyclin D1 gene, the heavy chain is the immunoglobulin heavy chain gene, mantel = mantle cell lymphoma. This is how I remember that the t(11;14) translocation of cyclin D1 and Ig heavy chain is associated with mantle cell lymphoma. I have subsequently further expanded the image by placing a fishing pole hanging from the mantel to remind me that the FISH assay is the preferred molecular technique for diagnosis.

Question Writing/Answering

While I was in graduate school, a friend noticed my tendency to sleep in lecture. He taught me the trick of actively listening to the lecture and formulating 2 questions to ask the speaker. That trick is applicable to reading, with the added benefit of increasing retention of the material. When I read, I write questions to review later. Repetition is an effective means of reinforcing memories. Repetition is an effective means of reinforcing memories. Try this: read the material, come up with a question, write down the question, type up the question and answer, then later review. This cycle of repetition wears a rut in your mind and aids in "knee-jerk" responses (similar to flash cards). I have found a variety of technologies to use when typing up the questions; making an electronic presentation or a web page helps. From time to time I will post more information on the online forum for this book on newer technologies and potential applications.

Suggestions for Reading This Book

When reading this book, I encourage you to choose a single answer for each question. The action of making a decision will reinforce the information whether you are correct or not. Narrow down choices, then choose a single best answer (if applicable). If you get it correct, you are reinforcing it in your mind. If you do not get it correct you are indexing it for further study. There are a lot of questions in this book. That is by design. It can be picked up at random and reviewed, or you can go over the book from cover to cover. Do not get discouraged if you are getting questions wrong; this isn't a real test! Hopefully, it will point out areas for further study, and you can come back later and try again. A review technique that I recommend is the one put forth by SuperMemo creator, Piotr Wozniak on his website (http://www.supermemo.com/articles/paper.htm). Starting with the preformed questions in this book, utilize the algorithmic approach to maximize retention.

Summary

I hope the information presented in this introduction will help you to best utilize the resources presented both in the text and online. In addition I hope that you use these techniques to create your own unique means of studying for the boards or the Maintenance of Certification exam. The more you practice and the more personal your study routines are, the more success you will enjoy! A special thanks to Joshua Weikersheimer for pushing when he knew he could.

George Leonard, MD PhD
MAJ, MC, USA
ASCP Quick Compendium Companion Series Editor

CHALLENGE QUESTIONS
IN
SURGICAL PATHOLOGY

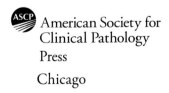

American Society for
Clinical Pathology
Press

Chicago

Chapter 1

Cardiovascular System

1. Which of the following is not a part of Carney syndrome?
    A. Cardiac myxomas
    B. Breast myxomas
    C. Spitz nevi
    D. Leydig cell tumor
    E. Psammomatous melanotic schwannomas

2. In order to differentiate a cardiac myxoma from a primary cardiac sarcoma, which of the following immunohistochemical panels would be most helpful?
    A. Vimentin and CD68
    B. Calretinin and CD31
    C. Vimentin and smooth muscle actin
    D. CD68 and smooth muscle actin
    E. None of the above

3. Which cardiac tumor has Gamna-Gandy bodies?
    A. Myxoma
    B. Papillary fibroelastoma
    C. Rhabdomyoma
    D. Angiosarcoma
    E. Epithelioid hemangioendothelioma

4. Which tumor is associated with extramedullary hematopoiesis?
    A. Myxoma
    B. Papillary fibroelastoma
    C. Rhabdomyoma
    D. Angiosarcoma
    E. Epithelioid hemangioendothelioma

5. Which tumor most commonly occurs on the valve surface?
    A. Rhabdomyoma
    B. Fibrosarcoma
    C. Myxoma
    D. Papillary fibroelastoma
    E. Synovial sarcoma

6. Rhabdomyomas are associated with which structural abnormality of the heart?
    A. Hypoplastic left heart syndrome
    B. Transposition of the great arteries
    C. Pulmonary atresia
    D. All of the above
    E. None of the above

1: Cardiovascular System Questions

7. Which of the following is not associated with tuberous sclerosis?
   A. Adenoma sebaceum
   B. Cutaneous angiomas
   C. White matter hamartoma
   D. Cardiac rhabdomyoma
   E. Retinoblastoma

8. Ultrastructural examination of a cardiac neoplasm shows tumor cells with peripheral cellular junctions that resemble intercalated disks and a cytoplasm distended by glycogen. Based on these features the diagnosis is:
   A. Myxoma
   B. Papillary fibroelastoma
   C. Rhabdomyoma
   D. Epithelioid hemangioendothelioma
   E. Fibrosarcoma

9. Which of the following statements regarding cardiac rhabdomyomas is TRUE?
   A. They are associated with a gene mutation on chromosome 17p13.
   B. They have 100% myogenin immunoreactivity.
   C. Spontaneous regression is possible.
   D. Prognosis is determined by embolic sequelae.
   E. Sporadic lesions do not occur.

10. Choose the correct sequence of prevalence of primary malignant cardiac sarcomas in adults.
    A. Fibrosarcoma > angiosarcoma > undifferentiated pleomorphic sarcoma
    B. Angiosarcoma > undifferentiated pleomorphic sarcoma > leiomyosarcoma
    C. Angiosarcoma > fibrosarcoma > synovial sarcoma
    D. Synovial sarcoma > angiosarcoma > fibrosarcoma
    E. Fibrosarcoma > synovial sarcoma > leiomyosarcoma

11. Which primary cardiac sarcoma may mimic a mesothelioma?
    A. Fibrosarcoma
    B. Synovial sarcoma
    C. Angiosarcoma
    D. All of the above
    E. None of the above

12. Primary cardiac sarcomas often clinically mimic which other cardiac tumor?
    A. Myxoma
    B. Papillary fibroelastoma
    C. Rhabdomyoma
    D. Both A and B
    E. Both B and C

13. Which immunohistochemical stain is most sensitive for angiosarcoma?
    A. Cytokeratin
    B. Epithelial membrane antigen (EMA)
    C. CD31
    D. CD34
    E. Factor VIII

1: Cardiovascular System Questions

14. Which primary cardiac sarcoma has been associated with asbestos exposure?
    A. Angiosarcoma
    B. Epithelioid hemangioendothelioma
    C. Fibrosarcoma
    D. Synovial sarcoma
    E. Leiomyosarcoma

15. Which primary cardiac sarcoma has the best prognosis?
    A. Leiomyosarcoma
    B. Synovial sarcoma
    C. Fibrosarcoma
    D. Pleomorphic malignant fibrous histiocytoma
    E. None of the above

16. Ehlers-Danlos syndrome is associated with which gene mutation?
    A. Type III collagen (COL3A1)
    B. Type V collagen (COL5A1 and COL5A2)
    C. Lysyl hydroxylase
    D. All of the above
    E. None of the above

17. Which of the following symptoms is essentially pathognomonic of Marfan syndrome?
    A. Ectopia lentis
    B. Long tapering fingers and toes
    C. Decreased ratio of the upper portion of the body to the lower portion of the body
    D. Lax joint ligaments
    E. Dolichocephalism

18. Which of the following statements regarding both Marfan and Ehlers-Danlos syndrome is TRUE?
    A. It has an autosomal recessive pattern of inheritance.
    B. It is associated with defects in synthesis or structure of collagen.
    C. Approximately 50% of deaths are due to infective endocarditis.
    D. There are no characteristic gross or microscopic findings.
    E. Electron microscopy is diagnostic.

19. A 50-year-old Mexican immigrant presents with dyspnea and chest pain. A heart biopsy shows a prominent myocardial mixed inflammatory infiltrate comprised of lymphocytes, neutrophils, macrophages, and eosinophils. Which special stain would be most helpful to prove your suspected diagnosis based on history and the hematoxylin and eosin-stained image?
    A. Gram stain
    B. Giemsa
    C. Silver
    D. Warthin-Starry
    E. Ziehl-Neelsen

20. Which of the following histologic features is necessary to make a diagnosis of myocarditis?
    A. Myocyte necrosis
    B. Lymphocytic infiltrate
    C. Interstitial fibrosis
    D. Hemosiderin
    E. Sparing of subendocardium

1: Cardiovascular System Questions

21. Which myocarditis listed below has the poorest prognosis?
     A. Idiopathic
     B. Hypersensitivity
     C. Viral
     D. Giant cell
     E. Chagas disease

22. Which of the following is not a small vessel vasculitis?
     A. Henoch-Schönlein purpura
     B. Thromboangiitis obliterans
     C. Wegener granulomatosis
     D. Churg-Strauss syndrome
     E. None of the above

23. Which vasculitis is associated with polymyalgia rheumatica?
     A. Giant cell arteritis
     B. Takayasu arteritis
     C. Polyarteritis nodosa
     D. Kawasaki disease
     E. Thromboangiitis obliterans

24. A 30-year-old female presents with decreased vision and numbness in her fingers. Physical exam is notable for hypertension and decreased pulses in the upper extremities. A subclavian biopsy shows marked mononuclear infiltrate in the adventitia with perivascular cuffing of the vasa vasorum. Based on the clinical history and histology, which of the following statements regarding the disease is TRUE?
     A. There is increased risk of aortic stenosis.
     B. There is increased risk of development of cor pulmonale.
     C. It is associated with hepatitis B antigen.
     D. It is associated with antiproteinase 3.
     E. There is no increased risk of blindness.

25. Which organ is most commonly affected in polyarteritis nodosa?
     A. Skin
     B. Liver
     C. Kidney
     D. Gastrointestinal tract
     E. Heart

26. Which vasculitis is characterized by fibrinoid necrosis of muscular arteries?
     A. Wegner granulomatosis
     B. Churg-Strauss syndrome
     C. Microscopic polyangiitis
     D. Takayasu arteritis
     E. Polyarteritis nodosa

27. The cervical lymph node of a patient with Kawasaki disease would show which of the following features?
     A. Normal architecture
     B. Zonal necrosis
     C. Follicular hyperplasia
     D. Obliteration of nodal architecture with lymphocyte depletion
     E. None of the above

1: Cardiovascular System Questions

28. A 70-year-old female with aortic root dilation undergoes aortic aneurysm repair, and biopsy shows chronic aortitis. What is the diagnosis?
    A. Giant cell arteritis
    B. Takayasu arteritis
    C. Polyarteritis nodosa
    D. Infection
    E. None of the above

29. Which vasculitis is treated with intravenous gamma globulin?
    A. Kawasaki disease
    B. Churg-Strauss syndrome
    C. Wegner granulomatosis
    D. All of the above
    E. None of the above

30. Which vasculitis is associated with recent herpes infection or history of lymphoma?
    A. Cutaneous leukocytoclastic
    B. Kawasaki disease
    C. Henoch-Schönlein purpura
    D. Microscopic polyangiitis
    E. None of the above

31. Which is the pathognomonic feature of thromboangiitis obliterans?
    A. Fibrinoid necrosis of the media
    B. Intraluminal thrombi with granulomatous inflammation
    C. Diffuse destruction of the internal elastic lamina
    D. Superimposed atherosclerosis
    E. Involvement of veins

32. In a suspected Wegner granulomatosis patient, the lung biopsy is notable only for capillaritis. Which of the following is the best diagnosis?
    A. Wegner granulomatosis
    B. Churg-Strauss syndrome
    C. Polyarteritis nodosa
    D. Microscopic polyangiitis
    E. None of the above

1: Cardiovascular System Questions

33. The atrial lesion depicted in the gross photograph was excised from a 50-year-old male. Which statement regarding this neoplasm is CORRECT?

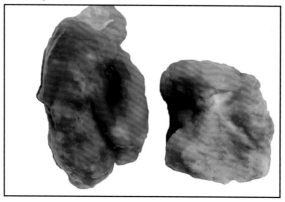

    A. There is increased incidence in men.
    B. It represents 90% of all primary cardiac tumors.
    C. It most commonly occurs in the right atrium.
    D. The majority of tumors is sporadic.
    E. It commonly presents with tricuspid stenosis.

34. A 25-year-old female presents with multiple right atrial lesions. Based on the H&E-stained image depicted below, what is the most likely genetic defect that this woman carries?

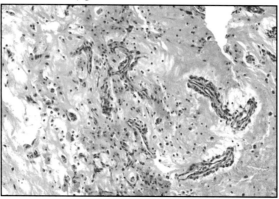

    A. Autosomal dominant mutation of PRKAR1A
    B. Autosomal recessive mutation of PRKAR1A
    C. Autosomal dominant mutation of TSC1
    D. Autosomal recessive mutation of TSC1
    E. TLS(FUS)-CHOP translocation

1: Cardiovascular System Questions

35. A 62-year-old male presents with chest pain and an EKG shows ST- elevation consistent with an acute myocardial infarction. After stabilization he is found on work-up to have an aortic valve mass, which is biopsied and shown below. Which statement regarding this lesion is TRUE?

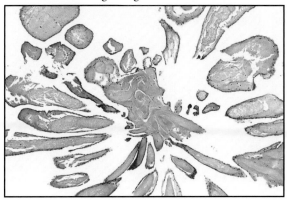

 A. Most patients are symptomatic.
 B. It is the most common cardiac tumor.
 C. It may be associated with rheumatic valvular disease.
 D. Death usually occurs due to aortic insufficiency.
 E. It is a highly vascular tumor with propensity to bleed.

36. Based on the H&E-stained image below, where was this tumor most likely excised from?

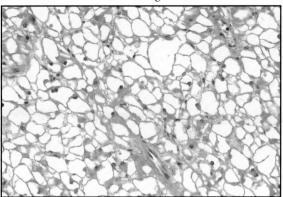

 A. Right atrium
 B. Left atrium
 C. Right ventricle
 D. Left ventricle
 E. Aortic valve

1: Cardiovascular System Questions

37. The tumor depicted below in the photomicrograph is characterized by factor VIII immunoreactivity and focal areas demonstrate tumor cells infiltrating into the muscular walls of vessels. What is the diagnosis?

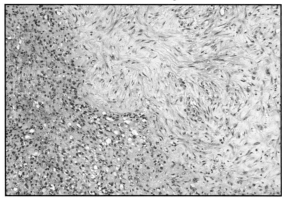 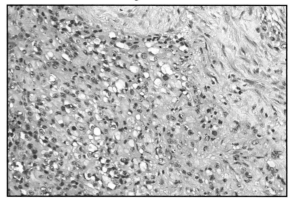

    A.   Angiosarcoma
    B.   Epithelioid hemangioendothelioma
    C.   Synovial sarcoma
    D.   Rhabdomyosarcoma
    E.   Undifferentiated pleomorphic sarcoma

38. The tumor depicted below was excised from the left atrium. Ultrastructural examination showed scattered cells with microvilli. Based on the H&E-stained image and ultrastructural characteristics, what is the diagnosis?

 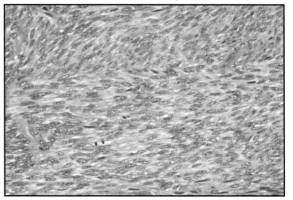

    A.   Epithelioid hemangioendothelioma
    B.   Pleomorphic malignant fibrous histiocytoma
    C.   Fibrosarcoma
    D.   Synovial sarcoma
    E.   Leiomyosarcoma

1: Cardiovascular System Questions

39. The tumor depicted below in the H&E-stained image was excised from the left atrium and was involving the mitral valve. The tumor cells are immunoreactive for myogenin. Which molecular alteration characterizes this neoplasm?

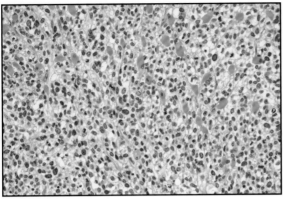

A. TP53 mutation
B. K-ras mutation
C. RB1 mutation
D. t(X;18)(p11.2;q11.2)
E. TSC1 mutation

40. The following lesion was excised from the right atrium of a 40-year-old male. Which statement regarding the neoplasm is TRUE?

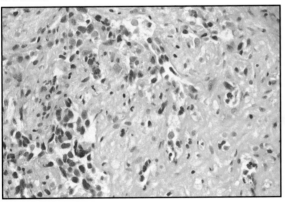 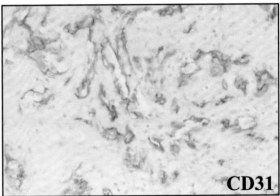

A. It is more common in men.
B. Left atrium is the most common site of involvement.
C. There are no known associated molecular alterations.
D. Weibel-Palade bodies are usually not demonstrable on electron microscopy.
E. Cytokeratin is immunonegative.

1: Cardiovascular System Questions

41. The left atrial lesion depicted below is immunoreactive for vimentin and immunonegative for smooth muscle actin, CD31, CD34, and CD99. Based on the H&E-stained image and immunohistochemical profile, the diagnosis is?

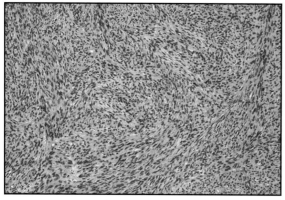

     A.   Leiomyosarcoma
     B.   Synovial sarcoma
     C.   Fibrosarcoma
     D.   Pleomorphic malignant fibrous histiocytoma
     E.   Angiosarcoma

42. A 40-year-old male presents with ascending aortic aneurysm, which is repaired. Based on the image below which of the following statements is CORRECT?

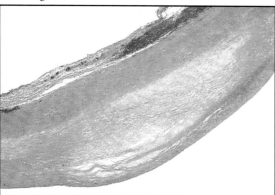

     A.   Immediate treatment with corticosteroids is required.
     B.   Labs are notable for elevated BUN and creatinine.
     C.   Physical exam is notable for a midsystolic click, followed by a late systolic murmur.
     D.   There is a history of recent motor vehicle accident.
     E.   There are positive serologies for VDRL.

1: Cardiovascular System Questions

43. A 43-year-old African American female presents with fatigue, dyspnea, palpitations, and fever. Review of systems is notable for a recent flulike illness. She has an abnormal EKG. Based on the H&E-stained heart biopsy, which of the following is the LEAST likely etiology?

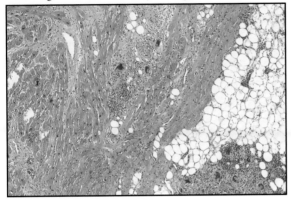

    A.   Sarcoidosis
    B.   Viral
    C.   Hypersensitivity reaction
    D.   Rheumatic fever
    E.   Idiopathic

44. Based on the image below what is the most likely etiology?

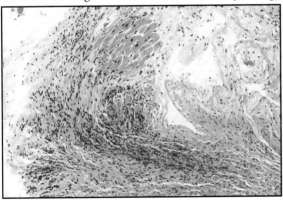

    A.   Sulfonamide toxicity
    B.   Chagas disease
    C.   Cytomegalovirus myocarditis
    D.   *Neisseria meningococcus* myocarditis
    E.   Coxsackievirus A myocarditis

1: Cardiovascular System Questions

45. A temporal artery biopsy is depicted below. Based on the H&E-stained image, which of the following statements regarding the disease is INCORRECT?

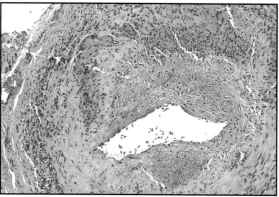

    A.   It is the most common of the vasculitides.

    B.   It may involve the vertebral arteries.

    C.   It may present with diminished pulses and intermittent claudication.

    D.   Granulomas are not required for a diagnosis.

    E.   There is no association with HLA-DR antigens.

46. Which of the following statement regarding the disease process depicted in the sinonasal biopsy below is FALSE?

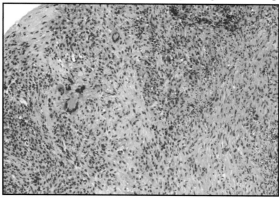

    A.   It involves necrotizing vasculitis of small vessels.

    B.   It is associated with antineutrophil cytoplasmic antibody.

    C.   Men are more commonly affected than women.

    D.   It is treated with cyclophosphamide and prednisone.

    E.   It is associated with HLA-A9 and HLA-B5.

1: Cardiovascular System Questions

47. Based on the skin biopsy depicted in the image below, which statement regarding the diagnosis is CORRECT?

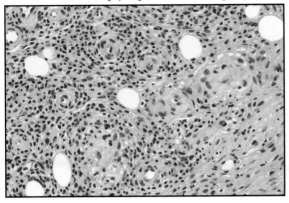

    A.   It is associated with vascular IgA immune deposits.
    B.   Kidneys are notable for crescentic glomerulonephritis.
    C.   Bronchi are notable for mucous cell hyperplasia.
    D.   Pulmonary infiltrates are uncommon.
    E.   Ulcerating destructive upper airway lesions are commonly observed.

48. A 30-year-old male presents with peripheral neuropathy and diffuse muscular pain. A skin biopsy of his calf is shown below. An elastic stain highlights the presence of an internal elastic lamina within the vessel wall. Which of the following statements regarding the most likely depicted disease process is INCORRECT?

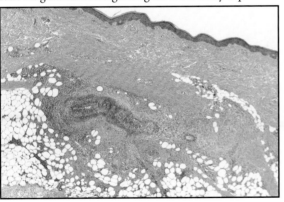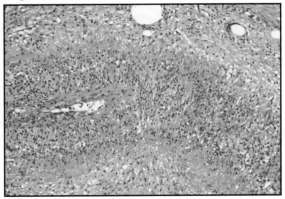

    A.   Pulmonary vasculature is usually spared.
    B.   Involvement tends to occur at branching points.
    C.   All stages of activity may coexist in the same vessel.
    D.   Acute disease is characterized by adventitial mononuclear infiltrate.
    E.   It is characterized by necrotizing inflammation of medium-sized arteries.

1: Cardiovascular System Questions

49. A 4-year-old female develops a skin rash after an upper respiratory infection. One of the lesions is biopsied and shown below. Based on the biopsy and clinical history, which of the following statements regarding the disease is TRUE?

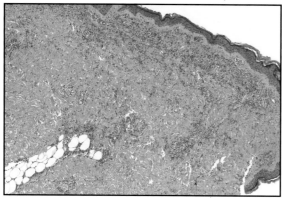 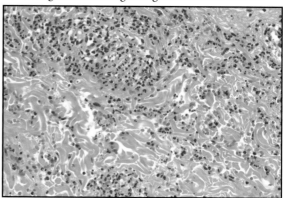

    A. Immune complexes are deposited in the subepithelium along the glomerular basement membrane.
    B. There are IgG immune deposits in small vessels.
    C. Children have a poor prognosis.
    D. Occasionally adults will develop rapidly progressive crescentic glomerulonephritis.
    E. It is associated with antimyeloperoxidase.

50. A 40-year-old male presents with diffuse palpable purpura over the lower extremity after being treated with penicillin. One of the lesions is biopsied and shown below. Which statement regarding the disease is INCORRECT?

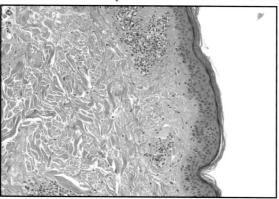 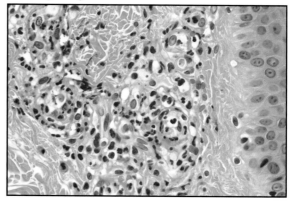

    A. It is associated with history of drug exposure.
    B. It is associated with history of infection.
    C. It is associated with history of cancer.
    D. It is not associated with immune deposits.
    E. It is associated with systemic vasculitis.

1: Cardiovascular System Answers

1. **C.   SPITZ NEVI**
    Carney syndrome is an autosomal dominant disorder involving a mutated protein kinase (*PRKAR1A*) that acts on a tumor suppressor gene on chromosome 17q22-24. Cardiac myxomas (choice A) are present in 65% of patients and are often multiple and the most serious component of the disorder, causing death in 20% of patients. 25% of women with the syndrome have breast myxomas (choice B). Carney syndrome is associated with endocrine tumors involving the adrenal gland, pituitary, and testis. Both Sertoli cell tumors and steroid-type tumors, including Leydig cell tumors (choice D), occur in the testis. An uncommon schwannoma variant (choice E), psammomatous melanotic, is seen in the disorder. Carney syndrome is associated with skin pathology including myxomas and lentiginous and blue nevi, not spitz nevi (choice C).
    QCSP, **Cardiac Myxoma and Carney Syndrome,** p 9-10.

2. **B.   CALRETININ AND CD31**
    Myxomas are typically positive for the vascular markers CD31 and CD34, with 80% reactive for vimentin and 20% reactive for cytokeratin. The myxoma tumor cells stain variably for muscle markers including smooth muscle actin and will be positive for nonspecific histiocytic markers (lysozyme, α_1-antichymotrypsin, and α_1-antitrypsin), but negative for the specific histiocytic marker CD68. Recent studies have shown that the most helpful immunohistochemical stain to differentiate myxomas from primary cardiac sarcomas is calretinin, which will be positive in the former and negative in the latter. Therefore the best answer is B.
    QCSP, **Cardiac Myxoma,** p 9.

3. **A.   MYXOMA**
    Gamna-Gandy bodies are formed by calcific elastic fiber degeneration with hemosiderosis and are seen in cardiac myxomas (choice A). These Gamna-Gandy bodies are also seen in the spleen, associated with cardiac congestion and sickle cell anemia.
    QCSP, **Cardiac Myxoma,** p 8.

4. **A.   MYXOMA**
    Foci of extramedullary hematopoiesis are present in 5%-10% of myxomas.
    QCSP, **Cardiac Myxoma,** p 8.

5. **D.   PAPILLARY FIBROELASTOMA**
    90% of papillary fibroelastomas occur on the valve surfaces, usually away from the lines of closure. The aortic valve is most frequently involved. Rhabdomyomas (choice A) are most commonly located in the left ventricle and the ventricular septum. Myxomas (choice C) and primary cardiac sarcomas (choices B and E) most commonly involve the endocardial surface of the left atrium.
    QCSP, **Papillary Fibroelastoma,** p 10.

6. **D.   ALL OF THE ABOVE**
    Cardiac rhabdomyomas are hamartomatous lesions that may occur sporadically or in association with tuberous sclerosis or structural congenital heart disease. All of the listed structural abnormalities are associated with rhabdomyomas, and therefore the correct answer is all of the above (choice D). Other abnormalities associated with this tumor include ventricular septal defect, endocardial fibroelastosis, subaortic stenosis, Ebstein anomaly, hypoplastic tricuspid valve, and double outlet right ventricle.
    QCSP, **Rhabdomyoma,** p 11-12.

7. **E.   RETINOBLASTOMA**
    Tuberous sclerosis is a neurocutaneous syndrome characterized by cutaneous and neurologic manifestations and tumors. The cutaneous manifestations include adenoma sebaceum (choice A, 80%), angiomas (choice B), ash-leaf spots (90%), shagreen patches (35%), fibromas, and café-au-lait spots (7%-16%). 90% of patients have seizures

and 60%-70% have mental retardation. There are numerous tumors associated with the syndrome, including white matter hamartomas (choice C) and cardiac rhabdomyomas (choice D, 50%). The eye is involved by retinal hamartomas, retinal giant cell astrocytomas, and hypopigmented iris spot, not by retinoblastoma (choice E). *QCSP*, **Rhabdomyoma and Tuberous Sclerosis**, p 12; WHO, p 220.

8.   C.   **RHABDOMYOMA**

The tumor cells of rhabdomyoma are altered myocytes that contain abundant glycogen. Unlike differentiated myocytes that have intercalated disks located exclusively at the poles of the cell, the tumor cells of rhabdomyoma (choice C) have intercalated disks that surround the entire periphery of the cell. Ultrastructural examination of a myxoma (choice A) would show intermediate filaments, primitive tight intercellular junctions, and variable amounts of desmosomes and villi depending on the presence or absence of a glandular component. Papillary fibroelastomas (choice B) on ultrastructural examination are characterized by mature collagen, longitudinally oriented irregular elastic fibers, and fibroblasts. Fibroblasts with prominent rough endoplasmic reticulum and no myofilaments is characteristic of fibrosarcoma (choice E). Basal lamina, pinocytotic vesicles, and occasional Weibel-Palade bodies are seen in the endothelial cells of epithelioid hemangioendothelioma (choice D). *QCSP*, **Rhabdomyoma**, p 11-12; QCSP, Primary Cardiac Sarcoma, p 15.

9.   C.   **SPONTANEOUS REGRESSION IS POSSIBLE.**

Cardiac rhabdomyomas are associated with tuberous sclerosis and mutations on chromosomes 9q34 and 16p; however, sporadic lesions do occur (choice E). The *TP53* tumor suppressor gene is located on chromosome 17p13 (choice A) and is associated with Li-Fraumeni syndrome, which is associated with numerous tumors affecting different organ systems but is not associated with cardiac rhabdomyoma. Rhabdomyomas are extremely rare in patients older than 10-years of age; however, when they occur in adults, they lose myogenin immunoreactivity (choice B). Tumor embolism (choice D) is common in myxomas not rhabdomyomas, which can cause arrhythmias and left ventricular outflow tract obstruction. The correct answer is that spontaneous regression is possible (choice C) and occurs in patients with tuberous sclerosis. *QCSP*, **Rhabdomyoma**, p 12.

10.   B.   **ANGIOSARCOMA > UNDIFFERENTIATED PLEOMORPHIC SARCOMA > LEIOMYOSARCOMA**

Angiosarcoma and undifferentiated pleomorphic sarcoma (pleomorphic malignant fibrous histiocytoma) are the most and second most common malignant cardiac sarcoma in adults, respectively. Knowing this eliminates all possible choices except B. The remaining entities each comprise 10% or less of all primary malignant cardiac sarcomas in adults. *QCSP*, **Primary Cardiac Sarcoma**, p 13-16.

11.   D.   **ALL OF THE ABOVE**

Fibrosarcoma (choice A) is the most likely cardiac sarcoma to infiltrate the pericardial space, thus mimicking a mesothelioma; however, both angiosarcoma and synovial sarcoma can also involve the pericardium with a mesothelioma-like picture. *QCSP*, **Primary Cardiac Sarcoma**, p 13-16.

12.   A.   **MYXOMA**

If one remembers the most common location of all the cardiac tumors, one can logically assume that if the tumors occupy the same location they will have similar clinical manifestations. This is indeed the case and both myxoma (choice A), and primary cardiac sarcomas most frequently arise from the left atrium. Patients present with dyspnea secondary to venous obstruction or mitral stenosis. *QCSP*, **Primary Cardiac Sarcoma**, p 13-16.

1: Cardiovascular System Answers

13.   C.   **CD31**

All of the listed immunohistochemical stains may be reactive in angiosarcoma. CD31 (choice C) is the most sensitive, with 90% of tumors reactive. Additional markers shown to be reactive in angiosarcoma are Fli-1 and *Ulex europaeus* lectin. Cytokeratin (choice A) and EMA (choice B) are usually only focally positive in angiosarcoma, unlike in epithelioid angiosarcoma, which tends to be diffusely positive.

QCSP, **Primary Cardiac Sarcoma,** p 13-16.

14.   D.   **SYNOVIAL SARCOMA**

An association between cardiac synovial sarcoma (choice D) and asbestos exposure has been reported.

QCSP, **Primary Cardiac Sarcoma,** p 13-16.

15.   E.   **NONE OF THE ABOVE**

This is somewhat of a trick question because the prognosis of all primary cardiac sarcomas is dismal, with overall survival typically <1 year. The exception to this is the extremely rare primary cardiac sarcoma epithelioid hemangioendothelioma where the behavior is unknown. Features associated with increased survival include location (left-side), lower mitotic rate (<10/hpf), and the absence of necrosis.

QCSP, **Primary Cardiac Sarcoma,** p 13-16.

16.   D.   **ALL OF THE ABOVE**

Ehlers-Danlos syndrome is a heterogeneous group of disorders resulting from defects in the synthesis or structure of collagen. There are 6 variants of the syndrome, including autosomal dominant mutations of type I, III, and V collagen and autosomal recessive mutations of lysyl hydroxylase (enzyme required during collagen synthesis) and procollagen-N-peptidase (enzyme essential for the cleavage of collagens).

QCSP, **Ehlers-Danlos Syndrome,** p 17-18.

17.   A.   **ECTOPIA LENTIS**

Bilateral subluxation or dislocation of the lens of the eye (choice A) is essentially pathognomonic of Marfan syndrome. The remaining choices are all associated with Marfan syndrome but are not pathognomonic. Dolichocephalism (choice E) is a long head with bossing of the frontal eminences and prominent supraorbital ridges.

QCSP, **Marfan Syndrome,** p 18-19.

18.   D.   **THERE ARE NO CHARACTERISTIC GROSS OR MICROSCOPIC FINDINGS.**

Although the clinical presentation of Marfan and Ehlers-Danlos syndrome can appear similar, the molecular alterations are different. Marfan syndrome is characterized by an autosomal dominant mutation of the extracellular glycoprotein, fibrillin 1. Ehlers-Danlos syndrome is a heterogenous group of disorders with both autosomal dominant and recessive (choice A) patterns of inheritance associated with genes involved in the synthesis or structure of collagen (choice B). Although Marfan syndrome has an increased risk of infective endocarditis due to mitral valve prolapse (choice C), approximately 50% of all deaths result from a ruptured aortic dissection. Electron microscopy can be helpful in Marfan syndrome to highlight the presence of fragmented elastin (choice E), but it is not diagnostic and is not helpful in Ehlers-Danlos syndrome. The best answer is choice D. Although cystic medial necrosis or degeneration is associated with Marfan syndrome, it is not pathognomonic as it is also seen in hypertension albeit to a lesser degree. There are no characteristic microscopic findings in Ehlers-Danlos syndrome.

QCSP, **Ehlers-Danlos and Marfan Syndromes,** p 17-19.

19. **B.** **GIEMSA**

The presence of eosinophils narrows the differential diagnosis to include hypersensitivity reaction, parasitic infestation, hypereosinophilic syndromes, and idiopathic. Due to the fact that he emigrated from Mexico, Chagas disease is on the top of the differential and the trypanosomes are highlighted on a Giemsa stain (choice B). *QCSP*, **Myocarditis**, p 19-21.

20. **A.** **MYOCYTE NECROSIS**

The presence of inflammatory cells (choice B) in the myocardium without associated myocyte damage is not sufficient for a diagnosis as it is also a feature of ischemia. The presence of hemosiderin deposits (choice D) and sparing of the subendocardium (choice E) are more characteristic of a myocardial infarction. In myocarditis both the endocardium and adjacent myocardium are involved. Interstitial fibrosis (choice C) is nonspecific and can develop with persistent disease. Myocyte damage as evidenced by either necrosis (choice A) or myocyte vacuolization is required to make the diagnosis of myocarditis. *QCSP*, **Myocarditis**, p 19-21.

21. **D.** **GIANT CELL**

Both idiopathic (choice A) and viral (choice C) myocarditis may spontaneously resolve. Although 10% of patients with Chagas myocarditis (choice E) die during the acute attack, patients with giant cell myocarditis (choice D) have the poorest prognosis. *QCSP*, **Myocarditis**, p 19-21.

22. **B.** **THROMBOANGIITIS OBLITERANS**

Thromboangiitis obliterans (Buerger disease) is a medium-sized vessel vasculitis. All of the remaining choices are small vessel vasculitides as well as microscopic polyangiitis and cutaneous leukocytoclastic vasculitis. *QCSP*, **Vasculitis**, p 21-30.

23. **A.** **GIANT CELL ARTERITIS**

Polymyalgia rheumatica is an inflammatory disorder of the muscles, with patients classically complaining of muscle pains involving proximal muscle groups in the morning just after waking. It is associated with giant cell or temporal arteritis (choice A). Polyarteritis nodosa (choice C) is a medium-sized vessel vasculitis associated with hepatitis B antigen. Kawasaki disease (choice D) is a medium-sized vessel vasculitis associated with mucocutaneous syndrome. Thromboangiitis obliterans (choice E) is a medium-sized vessel vasculitis associated with cigarette smoking. Like giant cell arteritis, Takayasu arteritis (choice B) is a large vessel vasculitis; however, it has no known associations. *QCSP*, **Giant Cell Arteritis**, p 21-22.

24. **B.** **THERE IS INCREASED RISK OF DEVELOPMENT OF COR PULMONALE.**

The history and histology are classic for Takayasu arteritis, which is a large vessel vasculitis which typically involves the aortic arch. Involvement of the aortic root may lead to dilation of the aortic valve with subsequent aortic insufficiency, not aortic stenosis (choice A). Takayasu arteritis has no known associations. Polyarteritis nodosa is associated with hepatitis B antigen (choice C) and antiproteinase 3 (choice D) or c-ANCA is associated with Wegener granulomatosis. Although ocular symptoms are more classically associated with giant cell arteritis, there is considerable overlap between these 2 entities, and Takayasu arteritis also has an increased risk of blindness (choice E). Pulmonary arteries are involved in 50% of the patients and can lead to pulmonary hypertension and subsequent cor pulmonale (choice B). *QCSP*, **Takayasu Arteritis**, p 22-23.

1: Cardiovascular System Answers

25. C. **KIDNEY**
Polyarteritis nodosa is a medium-sized vessel necrotizing vasculitis, which most commonly affects the kidneys (choice C), then the heart (choice E), liver (choice B), gastrointestinal tract (choice D), pancreas, testes, skeletal muscle, nervous system, and skin (choice A), in decreasing order of frequency.
QCSP, **Polyarteritis Nodosa,** p 23-24.

26. E. **POLYARTERITIS NODOSA**
Polyarteritis nodosa (choice E) affects muscular arteries and is characterized by fibrinoid necrosis. Wegner granulomatosis (choice A), Churg-Strauss syndrome (choice B), and microscopic polyangiitis (choice C) are all small vessel vasculitis with ANCA association (pauci-immune). Takayasu arteritis (choice D) also shows fibrinoid necrosis but involves elastic arteries.
QCSP, **Polyarteritis Nodosa,** p 23-24.

27. D. **OBLITERATION OF NODAL ARCHITECTURE WITH LYMPHOCYTE DEPLETION**
Kawasaki disease is a medium-sized vessel vasculitis involving muscular arteries. Patients present with fever, conjunctival and oral erythema and ulceration, edema and erythema of the hands and feet, skin rash with desquamation, and enlargement of cervical lymph nodes. Biopsy of an involved cervical lymph node would show obliteration of the nodal architecture (choice D) with depletion of lymphocytes, loss of follicular centers, and vascular proliferation with thrombi in small vessels. Small foci of necrosis not zonal necrosis (choice B) can be seen in both the interfollicular and follicular centers.
QCSP, **Kawasaki Disease,** p 24-25.

28. E. **NONE OF THE ABOVE**
An important concept in blood vessel pathology is to recognize that not every vasculitis is a result of a systemic vasculitis. The differential includes infection, infarction, and self-limited benign vasculitis. In the absence of clinical information and serologies, the specific diagnosis of a systemic vasculitis syndrome should be withheld. Although aortic root dilation is most commonly associated with Takayasu arteritis (choice B), the age is atypical as it most commonly presents in women younger than 40 years. The best answer is choice E (none of the above) and the report should be signed out descriptively with a note giving the differential diagnosis and a recommendation for rheumatologic evaluation.
QCSP, **Vasculitis,** p 21-30.

29. A. **KAWASAKI DISEASE**
Kawasaki disease is an inflammatory disease of the large, medium, and small arteries and affects children younger than 4 years of age. The major risk is the development of coronary artery aneurysm formation with subsequent rupture or thrombosis and possible sudden death. Intravenous gamma globulin is the treatment of choice for preventing coronary artery aneurysm formation and is used in conjunction with aspirin. Churg-Strauss (choice B) and Wegner granulomatosis (choice D) are both treated with corticosteroids and cytotoxic drugs.
QCSP, **Kawasaki Disease,** p 24-25.

30. E. **NONE OF THE ABOVE**
Granulomatous angiitis of the CNS is associated with recent herpes infection or history of lymphoma as well as amyloid angiopathy. The disease is characterized by a marked mononuclear and giant cell infiltrate in the arteries, arterioles, and veins of the meninges and cerebrum.
QCSP, **Granulomatous Angitis of the CNS,** p 25.

31. B. **INTRALUMINAL THROMBI WITH GRANULOMATOUS INFLAMMATION**
Thromboangiitis obliterans is linked to cigarette smoking and is an inflammatory disease of medium-sized and small arteries, which may extend into adjacent veins (choice E) and nerves. The internal elastic lamina is

usually preserved but may have focal destruction but not diffuse (choice C). Although the disease presents with symptoms of vascular insufficiency with the possibility of progression to gangrene, there is no evidence of atherosclerosis (choice D). The vessels are notable for an acute and chronic infiltrate and are characterized by intraluminal thrombi with granulomatous inflammation (choice B). Fibrinoid necrosis of the media (choice A) is characteristic of polyarteritis nodosa and Kawasaki disease.

QCSP, **Thromboangiitis Obliterans**, p 26.

32. D. **MICROSCOPIC POLYANGIITIS**

Microscopic polyangiitis (choice D) is an ANCA-related small vessel vasculitis involving vessels of the skin, mucous membranes, lungs, brain, heart, gastrointestinal tract, kidneys, and muscle. Pulmonary involvement in the form of capillaritis is common and can be mistaken for either Wegner granulomatosis or Churg-Strauss syndrome. In the absence of necrotizing parenchymal lesions, the best diagnosis is microscopic polyangiitis. The necrotizing arteritis of Wegner granulomatosis is indistinguishable from polyarteritis nodosa (choice C).

QCSP, **Microscopic Polyangiitis**, p 27-28.

33. D. **THE MAJORITY OF TUMORS IS SPORADIC.**

The gross image depicts a gelatinous mass consistent with a cardiac myxoma. Although these tumors are the most common primary cardiac tumors, they represent 50%, not 90% of all primary cardiac tumors (choice B). They are more frequent in women than men (choice A). Although these tumors can arise in the right atrium (choice C), they are more common in the left atrium near the fossa ovalis. Left atrial lesions commonly present with embolic events, and right atrial lesions are less frequently symptomatic but can present with syncope and/or ankle edema. The correct answer is choice D as 95% of the tumors are sporadic.

QCSP, **Cardiac Myxoma**, p 8.

34. A. **AUTOSOMAL DOMINANT MUTATION OF PRKAR1A**

The image depicts tumor cells in a myxoid background forming rings surrounding blood vessels and infiltrated by mononuclear inflammatory cells characteristic of a cardiac myxoma. Her young age in conjunction with multiple tumors and location in the right atrium is suggestive of a familial lesion. Cardiac myxomas are a part of Carney syndrome, which is characterized by an autosomal dominant mutation of *PRKAR1A* (choice A). Mutation of *TSC1* (choice C) on chromosome 9q is associated with tuberous sclerosis and follows an autosomal dominant not autosomal recessive (choice D) pattern of inheritance. The characteristic cardiac lesion of tuberous sclerosis is rhabdomyoma. The FUS-CHOP (choice E) translocation is characteristic of myxoid liposarcoma.

QCSP, **Cardiac Myxoma**, p 8.

35. C. **IT MAY BE ASSOCIATED WITH RHEUMATIC VALVULAR DISEASE.**

The H&E-stained image shows branching papillary fronds in a mucopolysaccharide matrix consistent with a papillary fibroelastoma. These tumors are benign, and death usually results from embolization into the coronary arteries, cerebral vasculature, or peripheral arterial tree, not from aortic insufficiency (choice D). Most patients are asymptomatic (choice A), but the tumor has the potential to embolize and become symptomatic. Cardiac myxoma is the most common primary cardiac tumor (choice B). By definition these tumors are avascular (choice E), which is a helpful feature in distinguishing these tumors from myxomas, which are highly vascular. Interestingly, these tumors may be found in the setting of preexisting heart disease such as rheumatic valvular disease (choice C).

QCSP, **Papillary Fibroelastoma**, p 10-11.

36. D. **LEFT VENTRICLE**

The H&E-stained image shows vacuolated tumor cells consistent with rhabdomyoma. Although rhabdomyomas can occur anywhere in the heart, they are most commonly located in the left ventricle (choice D) and the ventricular septum. Myxomas and primary cardiac sarcomas most commonly occur in the left atrium (choice B)

and papillary fibroelastomas most commonly involve the aortic valve (choice E). Angiosarcomas commonly occur in the right atrium (choice A).
QCSP, **Rhabdomyoma**, p 11-12.

37.　B.　**Epithelioid hemangioendothelioma**
The H&E-stained images show sheets of tumor cells with large vacuoles in a sclerotic background. The endothelial nature is suggested by the identification of red blood cells within the vacuoles and is confirmed with factor VII immunoreactivity. Epithelioid hemangioendothelioma (choice B) is a vascular tumor composed of epithelioid cells arranged in short strands or solid nests, and the tumor cells frequently infiltrate into the muscular walls of vessels. Angiosarcomas (choice A) are characterized by irregular vascular channels lined by pleomorphic and atypical cells. Synovial sarcoma (choice C), rhabdomyosarcoma (choice D), and undifferentiated pleomorphic sarcoma (choice E) are all factor VII immunonegative and are not endothelial tumors.
QCSP, **Primary Cardiac Sarcoma**, p 13-16.

38.　D.　**Synovial sarcoma**
The H&E-stained images are nonspecific and show a high-grade spindle cell tumor. This image is inconsistent with a diagnosis of epithelioid hemangioendothelioma (choice A), which is a vascular tumor composed of epithelioid, not spindled cells. The presence of fascicles intersecting at 90-degree angles or cigar-shaped nuclei would suggest leiomyosarcoma (choice E). A herringbone pattern with sweeping fascicles arranged at acute angles to one another would be suggestive of fibrosarcoma (choice C). A storiform arrangement of spindled or epithelioid pleomorphic cells may suggest pleomorphic malignant fibrous histiocytoma (choice B). Synovial sarcoma is easiest to recognize in the biphasic form with alternating spindled and epithelial components; however, the monomorphic, spindled variant is especially common in the heart. Similar to extracardiac soft tissue tumors, poorly differentiated sarcomas are almost impossible to differentiate based on H&E-stained images alone. Ancillary studies are needed, including immunohistochemistry, electron microscopy, and molecular studies. The identification of microvilli on ultrastructural examination is indicative of synovial sarcoma (choice D). Monophasic spindled synovial sarcomas will have areas of epithelial differentiation on ultrastructural examination as evidenced by slit-like glandular space and microvilli. Epithelioid hemangioendotheliomas (choice A) would show Weibel-Palade bodies. Electron microscopy would confirm the presence of undifferentiated, nonspecific mesenchymal cells in pleomorphic malignant fibrous histiocytoma (choice B). A prominent rough endoplasmic reticulum and absence of myofilaments would be supportive of a fibrosarcoma (choice C), and prominent pinocytotic vesicles and basal lamina would suggest leiomyosarcoma (choice E).
QCSP, **Primary Cardiac Sarcoma**, p 13-16.

39.　B.　**K-ras mutation**
The image shows a small round blue cell tumor with scant clear to eosinophilic cytoplasm. A helpful feature is the identification of an eccentric nucleus. The morphologic image and immunoreactivity for myogenin are diagnostic of rhabdomyosarcoma, which is associated with a mutation of *K-ras* (choice B). Rhabdomyosarcomas are the most likely of all cardiac sarcomas to involve cardiac valves. Mutation of the tumor suppressor gene TP53 (choice A) is associated with angiosarcoma (50%). RB1 mutation has been implicated in pleomorphic malignant fibrous histiocytoma. The t(X;18) translocation (choice D) is diagnostic of synovial sarcoma, and mutations involving TSC1 gene are seen in cardiac rhabdomyomas.
QCSP, **Primary Cardiac Sarcoma**, p 13-16.

40.　D.　**Weibel-Palade bodies are usually not demonstrable on electron microscopy.**
The image shows a moderately differentiated angiosarcoma as evidenced by irregular vascular channels lined by pleomorphic and atypical cells which are immunoreactive for the vascular marker CD31. Angiosarcoma is the most common primary cardiac sarcoma and affects men and women equally (choice A). The majority of primary cardiac sarcomas involve the left atrium; however, angiosarcoma typically arise in the right atrium (80%) near the atrioventricular groove. 50% of angiosarcomas are associated with TP53 mutations (choice C). The tumor cells of

angiosarcoma are immunoreactive for endothelial markers (factor VIII, CD34, and CD31) and may be focally or diffusely reactive for cytokeratin (choice E) and/or epithelial membrane antigen. Ultrastructural examination may show pinocytic vesicles and intermediate filaments; however, Weibel-Palade bodies are usually not demonstrable (choice D). The primary components of Weibel-Palade bodies are von Willebrand factor and P-selectin. They are typically seen in nonneoplastic endothelial cells.

QCSP, **Primary Cardiac Sarcoma,** p 13-16.

41. C. **FIBROSARCOMA**

The image depicts a spindled cell tumor with a vague herringbone pattern highly suggestive of a fibrosarcoma. The immunohistochemical profile is consistent with a fibrosarcoma, which would be immunoreactive for vimentin and immunonegative for the remaining markers. The main differential is with pleomorphic malignant fibrous histiocytoma (choice D), which would show a similar immunohistochemical profile; however, it would be more atypical and would not show the herringbone pattern. Smooth muscle actin reactivity would be seen in leiomyosarcoma (choice A). CD99 reactivity is observed in synovial sarcoma (choice B). Angiosarcomas (choice E) are immunoreactive for CD31 and CD34.

QCSP, **Primary Cardiac Sarcoma,** p 13-16.

42. C. **PHYSICAL EXAM IS NOTABLE FOR A MIDSYSTOLIC CLICK, FOLLOWED BY A LATE SYSTOLIC MURMUR.**

The main differential diagnosis of an ascending aortic aneurysm includes Marfan syndrome, vasculitis, trauma, syphilis, and atherosclerosis/hypertension. Importantly no inflammation is present to suggest a vasculitic process. Immediate treatment with corticosteroids (choice A) is indicated in giant cell arteritis to prevent blindness. VDRL serologies are a screening assay for syphilis (choice E); however, there is no evidence of transmural inflammation to support this diagnosis. Severe medial calcification can lead to renal failure (choice B) and is associated with hyperparathyroidism; however, there is no evidence of calcium deposition in the image. The H&E-stained image shows an artery with cystic medial necrosis and disruption of elastic fibers. Cystic medial degeneration is associated with Marfan syndrome and/or hypertension and is not trauma related (choice D). 20% of Marfan syndrome patients will have mitral valve prolapse which is characterized on auscultation by a midsystolic click and late systolic murmur (choice C). Since none of the options are related to hypertension the best answer is choice C.

QCSP, **Marfan Syndrome,** p 18-19.

43. B. **VIRAL**

The biopsy shows diffuse granulomatous inflammation with giant cell formation. The giant cell infiltrate is nonspecific and is associated with giant cell myocarditis, sarcoidosis (choice A), hypersensitivity reaction (choice C), rheumatic fever (choice D), rheumatic disease, tuberculosis, and fungal infections, or can be idiopathic (choice E). Viral myocarditis (choice B) is characterized by a lymphocytic infiltrate, and if biopsied early a neutrophilic infiltrate but not giant cells.

QCSP, **Myocarditis,** p 19-21.

44. E. **COXSACKIEVIRUS A MYOCARDITIS**

The image shows a myocarditis composed of predominantly lymphocytes. No eosinophils are seen to suggest a hypersensitivity reaction (choice A) or Chagas disease (choice B). Bacterial infections including *Neisseria meningococcus* (choice D) are often associated with a prominent neutrophilic infiltrate. The differential diagnosis of a lymphocytic myocarditis includes idiopathic, viral, toxic, collagen vascular disease, and Kawasaki disease. While both cytomegalovirus (choice C) and coxsackievirus A (choice E) are reasonable choices based on the lymphocytic infiltrate, the best answer is coxsackievirus because 50% of infectious myocarditis are due to enteroviruses.

QCSP, **Myocarditis,** p 19-21.

1: Cardiovascular System Answers

45. E. **THERE IS NO ASSOCIATION WITH HLA-DR ANTIGENS.**
The H&E-stained image shows a large vessel with marked mononuclear infiltrate and multinucleated giant cells involving the elastic lamina consistent with giant cell arteritis. Giant cell arteritis is the most common of the vasculitides (choice A), and although it has a predilection for the extracranial branches of the carotid artery, it also may involve the vertebral (choice B) and ophthalmic arteries. "Diminished pulses" (choice C) is a buzzword for Takayasu arteritis but is also present in 10%-15% of patients with giant cell arteritis. Contrary to what one might think, granulomas are not required for a diagnosis of giant cell arteritis (choice D). There are 2 histologic patterns including the well recognized granulomatous inflammation as depicted here, as well as a nonspecific panarteritis that may or may not include granulomas. Giant cell arteritis is associated with certain HLA-DR antigens, and therefore choice E is incorrect.
QCSP, **Giant Cell Arteritis,** p 21-22.

46. E. **IT IS ASSOCIATED WITH HLA-A9 AND HLA-B5.**
The H&E-stained image from the sinonasal cavity shows a mixed inflammatory infiltrate with scattered granulomas. There is no evidence of necrotizing vasculitis. The main differential is between Wegener granulomatosis and Churg-Strauss syndrome. The absence of a prominent eosinophilic infiltrate is most consistent with Wegener granulomatosis. Both Wegener granulomatosis and Churg-Strauss syndrome are necrotizing vasculitides (choice A) involving arteries, arterioles, capillaries, and venules associated with antineutrophil cytoplasmic antibody (choice B). Patients with Wegener granulomatous are typically positive for c-ANCA (antiproteinase 3), while Churg-Strauss syndrome patients are typically positive for p-ANCA (antimyeloperoxidase). Men are more commonly affected than women (choice C) in Wegner granulomatosis, and the treatment is immunosuppressive therapy with cyclophosphamide and prednisone (choice D). Thromboangiitis obliterans is associated with HLA-A9 and HLA-B5 (choice E), not the pauci-immune small vessel vasculitides as depicted in the image.
QCSP, **Wegener Granulomatosis,** p 26-27.

47. C. **BRONCHI ARE NOTABLE FOR MUCOUS CELL HYPERPLASIA.**
The H&E-stained image shows a prominent eosinophilic infiltrate with sarcoid-like granulomas consistent with Churg-Strauss syndrome. The most characteristic histologic feature not depicted in this image is a microgranuloma composed of a bright red central body of necrosis containing eosinophilic granular debris with palisading histiocytes. Renal disease in Churg-Strauss tends to be mild without crescents in the glomeruli (choice B). Pulmonary infiltrates are very common (90%) in the later stages of the disease (choice D). Ulcerating destructive upper airway lesions (choice E) are more characteristic of Wegner granulomatosis and are seen rarely in Churg-Strauss. For the diagnosis of Churg-Strauss syndrome, asthma is among the 6 clinical features required for diagnosis, and therefore the bronchi may show changes consistent with asthma including mucous cell hyperplasia (choice C) as well as eosinophils and a prominent eosinophilic basement membrane. Vascular IgA immune deposits (choice A) are associated with Henoch-Schönlein purpura.
QCSP, **Churg-Strauss Syndrome,** p 27-28.

48. D. **ACUTE DISEASE IS CHARACTERIZED BY ADVENTITIAL MONONUCLEAR INFILTRATE.**
The image shows a medium-sized artery as confirmed by the presence of an internal elastic lamina with marked destruction of the vascular wall by a mixed infiltrate of lymphocytes, neutrophils, and histiocytes. There is extensive fibrin deposition diagnostic of polyarteritis nodosa, which is a necrotizing vasculitis of medium-sized arteries (choice E). The acute disease is characterized by transmural inflammation of the arterial wall. An adventitial mononuclear infiltrate (choice D) with perivascular cuffing of the vasa vasorum is characteristic of the acute phase of Takayasu arteritis or syphilis. The remaining choices (A-C) are all characteristic of polyarteritis nodosa.
QCSP, **Polyarteritis Nodosa,** p 23-24.

2: Central Nervous System Questions

7. All of the following intracranial lesions are associated with tuberous sclerosis EXCEPT:
   A. Meningioma
   B. Cortical tuber
   C. Subependymal hamartoma
   D. Subependymal giant cell astrocytoma
   E. Retinal astrocytic hamartoma

8. Flexner-Wintersteiner rosettes are seen in:
   A. Retinoblastoma
   B. Pineoblastoma
   C. Medulloepithelioma
   D. All of the above
   E. None of the above

9. Which of the following statements is CORRECT regarding unilateral retinoblastoma?
   A. The familial form is transmitted in an autosomal dominant pattern.
   B. Mitotic figures are infrequent.
   C. Tumor cells are reactive for cytokeratin.
   D. All lesions are treated with enucleation.
   E. 5-year survival is poor.

10. Which of the following immunohistochemical stains would be the most helpful in proving that a CNS germ cell tumor contains an embryonal carcinoma component?
    A. CAM 5.2
    B. Placental alkaline phosphatase (PLAP)
    C. CD30
    D. OCT4
    E. CD117 (c-Kit)

11. Which of the following statements concerning CNS germ cell tumors is CORRECT?
    A. Teratomas are the most frequent intracranial germ cell tumors.
    B. CNS germinomas are not radiosensitive.
    C. β-hCG reactivity is seen only in choriocarcinomas.
    D. Tumor cells of germinomas are PAS positive.
    E. Yolk sac tumors are often associated with precocious puberty.

12. Central neurocytomas are characterized by all of the following statements EXCEPT:
    A. Cerebral spinal fluid spread is common.
    B. Anterior portion of the lateral ventricle is the most frequent site of involvement.
    C. They typically occur in young to middle-aged adults.
    D. Tumor cells are diffusely immunoreactive for synaptophysin.
    E. Structures resembling Homer-Wright rosettes and ganglion cells are rare.

13. Which of the following statements regarding dysembryoplastic neuroepithelial tumor is INCORRECT?
    A. These tumors usually become symptomatic during the first 2 decades of life.
    B. The temporal lobe is the most common site of involvement.
    C. Cortical dysplasia is often identified adjacent to the tumor.
    D. The tumor nodules contain abundant acid mucopolysaccharide.
    E. Malignant transformation is common.

2: Central Nervous System Questions

14. Characteristic morphologic features of oligodendrogliomas include:
    A. Secondary structures of Scherer
    B. Microcystic change
    C. "Chicken-wire" vasculature
    D. Both B and C
    E. All of the above

15. According to the 2007 World Health Organization, which of the following criteria raises a WHO grade I meningioma to an atypical WHO grade II tumor?
    A. Increased nuclear to cytoplasmic ratio
    B. Prominent nucleoli
    C. Necrosis
    D. Loss of pattern
    E. None of the above

16. Meningiomas are always positive for which of the following immunohistochemical stains?
    A. Pancytokeratin
    B. Vimentin
    C. Glial fibrillary acidic protein (GFAP)
    D. CD34
    E. CD68

17. Which of the following statements regarding meningiomas is FALSE?
    A. There is increased incidence in women.
    B. Optic nerve is the most common extracranial site.
    C. They are associated with neurofibromatosis type 1.
    D. Monosomy 22 is the most common cytogenetic finding.
    E. Prognosis depends on location.

18. Of the following meningioma variants, which is most aggressive?
    A. Secretory
    B. Microcystic
    C. Lymphoplasmacytic
    D. Transitional
    E. Papillary

19. Which of the following is NOT a feature of Gorlin syndrome?
    A. Craniopharyngiomas
    B. Meningiomas
    C. Medulloblastomas
    D. All of the above
    E. Both B and C

20. A 60-year-old male has a past medical history of tuberous sclerosis, epilepsy, prostate cancer, and peripheral neuropathy leading to multiple ground level-falls. What is this patient's biggest risk factor for developing a meningioma?
    A. Male sex
    B. Tuberous sclerosis
    C. History of head trauma
    D. Seizure disorder
    E. Prostate cancer

2: Central Nervous System Questions

21. Which neoplasm forms large and irregular rosettes of tumor cells surrounding delicate, fibrillary, and acellular zones?
    A. Neuroblastoma
    B. Medulloblastoma
    C. Ependymoma
    D. Pineocytoma
    E. CNS primitive neuroectodermal tumor

22. Which of the following statements regarding pineocytomas is INCORRECT?
    A. Tumor cells are modified neurons related to retinal photoreceptors.
    B. Tumor cells are immunoreactive for neurofilament.
    C. Reticulin will highlight the "clublike" processes that project into the rosettes.
    D. Tumor cells displace rather than infiltrate surrounding structures.
    E. Electron microscopy shows small intertwined filaments.

23. Which is the best feature/method for distinguishing a pineocytoma from normal pineal gland on a surgical biopsy?
    A. Immunohistochemistry
    B. Architectural pattern
    C. Electron microscopy
    D. Mitotic activity
    E. Presence of necrosis

24. Which of the following statements regarding pineoblastomas is TRUE?
    A. Large rosettes characteristic of pineocytomas are not present.
    B. Fibrillar zones in rosette-like structures typically are reactive for glial fibrillary acidic protein.
    C. They are not associated with any known molecular alterations.
    D. Treatment is chemotherapy.
    E. Survival rate is 10 years.

25. Which tumor is associated with polycythemia?
    A. Angiomatous meningioma
    B. Choroid plexus papilloma
    C. Hemangiopericytoma
    D. Solitary fibrous tumor
    E. Hemangioblastoma

26. What is the main role of the neuropathologist during intraoperative consultation?
    A. Provide a specific diagnosis
    B. Evaluate surgical margins
    C. Confirm that sufficient diagnostic tissue has been obtained
    D. All of the above
    E. None of the above

27. Which of the following lesions requires a more definitive diagnosis during intraoperative consultation?
    A. Pilocytic astrocytoma
    B. Fibrillary astrocytoma
    C. Glioblastoma
    D. Oligodendroglioma
    E. Mixed glioma

2: Central Nervous System Questions

28. What are the 2 most common lesions to occur at the cerebellopontine angle in children?
    A. Schwannoma and meningioma
    B. Schwannoma and ependymoma
    C. Schwannoma and choroid plexus papilloma
    D. Ependymoma and choroid plexus papilloma
    E. Ependymoma and epidermoid cyst

29. Which of the following is the most common tumor of the brainstem?
    A. Astrocytoma
    B. Ependymoma
    C. Oligodendroglioma
    D. Hemangioblastoma
    E. Medulloblastoma

30. A 14-year-old female with a long-standing history of seizures undergoes magnetic resonance imaging, which shows a large, superficial, well-circumscribed nodule overlying a cyst in the right temporal lobe. The lesion is excised, and based on the representative section shown below, the diagnosis is:

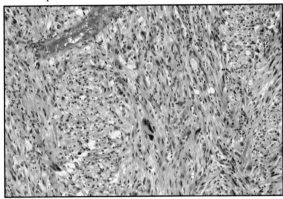

    A. Glioblastoma with giant cells
    B. Gliosarcoma
    C. Ganglioglioma
    D. Pleomorphic xanthoastrocytoma
    E. Dysembryoplastic neuroepithelial tumor

2: Central Nervous System Questions

31. The following finding (arrowhead) is consistent with all of the following diagnoses EXCEPT:

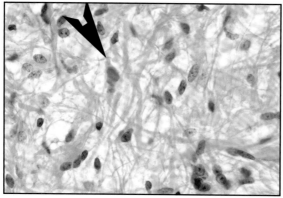

    A. Pilocytic astrocytoma
    B. Gangliocytoma
    C. Ganglioglioma
    D. Glioblastoma
    E. Pleomorphic xanthoastrocytoma

32. A 43-year-old female presents with a headache and focal neurological defects. Magnetic resonance imaging shows a diffuse nonenhancing lesion involving the right frontal, parietal, and temporal lobes as well as the left frontal lobe. Based on the following H&E-stained and KI-67-stained microscopic images the diagnosis is:

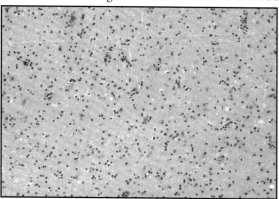 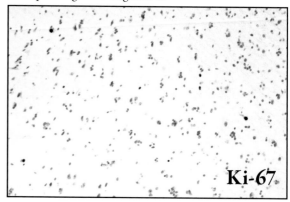

    A. Pilocytic astrocytoma, WHO grade I
    B. Diffuse astrocytoma, WHO grade II
    C. Anaplastic astrocytoma, WHO grade III
    D. Oligodendroglioma, WHO grade II
    E. Gliomatosis cerebri

2: Central Nervous System Questions

33. The tumor in the image below would be immunoreactive for all of the following immunohistochemical stains EXCEPT:

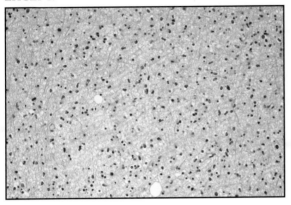

    A.   S100
    B.   Vimentin
    C.   Glial fibrillary acidic protein (GFAP)
    D.   p53
    E.   EMA

34. A 71-year-old female presents with an abrupt onset of lower extremity weakness, and magnetic resonance imaging is notable for an enhancing ring lesion shown below in the right frontoparietal cortex. Which of the following stains would be the most helpful in establishing the diagnosis?

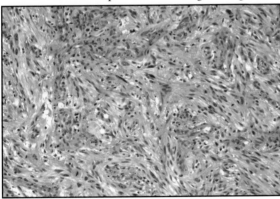

    A.   Cytokeratin
    B.   S100
    C.   Reticulin
    D.   Neu-N
    E.   None of the above

2: Central Nervous System Questions

35. A 14-year-old female presents with visual field defects, and magnetic resonance imaging is notable for a right optic nerve mass. She is taken to surgery, and a gross total resection of the lesion shows the following histologic findings. What syndrome is associated with the following lesion?

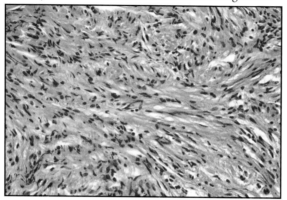

    A. Neurofibromatosis type 1
    B. Neurofibromatosis type 2
    C. Tuberous sclerosis
    D. von Hippel-Lindau
    E. Li-Fraumeni

36. A 24-year-old male presents with lower extremity weakness. Magnetic resonance imaging of the spine reveals a nonenhancing well-circumscribed lumbar lesion. The patient is taken to surgery, and a photomicrograph of the resected lesion is depicted below. What is the diagnosis?

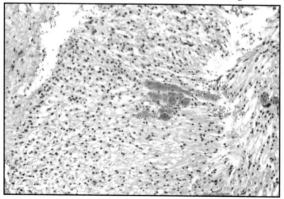

    A. Oligodendroglioma, WHO grade II
    B. Oligodendroglioma, WHO grade III
    C. Pilocytic astrocytoma, WHO grade I
    D. Clear cell ependymoma, WHO grade II
    E. Myxopapillary ependymoma, WHO grade I

2: Central Nervous System Questions

37. A 12-year-old male with a past medical history of café-au-lait spots, subungual fibromas, and renal cysts presents to the emergency department with sudden onset of headache and vomiting. Magnetic resonance imaging of the brain shows a large exophytic, broad-based, lateral ventricular mass which crosses the midline. The patient is taken to surgery, and a photomicrograph of the resected lesion is depicted below. Which of the following statements regarding this lesion is FALSE?

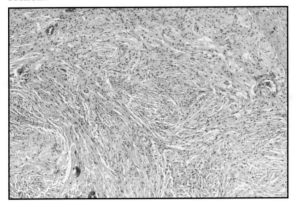

    A. It is usually seen in patients with tuberous sclerosis.
    B. It typically arises in the wall of the lateral ventricle.
    C. Malignant transformation is common.
    D. Tumor cells are immunoreactive for αβ-crystallin.
    E. Tumor cells are focally immunoreactive for GFAP.

38. A 1-year-old boy presents with vomiting and lethargy. Magnetic resonance imaging of the brain shows hydrocephalus with a large left ventricular mass. The patient is taken to surgery and a biopsy is performed, which is shown below. Immunohistochemistry for transthyretin is diffusely positive. The diagnosis is:

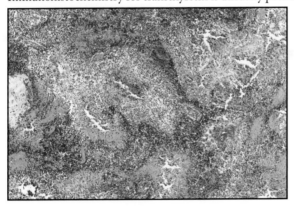

    A. Embryonal carcinoma
    B. Immature teratoma
    C. Anaplastic ependymoma, WHO grade III
    D. Choroid plexus carcinoma
    E. Atypical teratoid/ rhabdoid tumor

2: Central Nervous System Questions

39. A 3-year-old female presents with failure to thrive and vomiting. Neuroimaging is notable for a large, contrast-enhancing cerebellar tumor with cystic and necrotic areas. The lesion is excised and depicted below. Which of the following statements regarding the diagnosis is CORRECT?

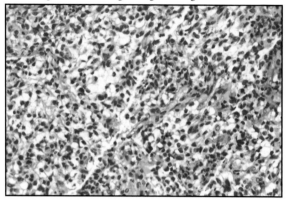

   A.   90% have INI1 mutation.
   B.   36% show EGFR amplification.
   C.   65% show TP53 mutation.
   D.   50% have isochromosome 17q.
   E.   25% have PTEN mutation.

40. A 7-year-old male presents with disturbed gait, and neuroimaging is notable for a well-circumscribed contrast-enhancing nodule of the cerebellar vermis. The lesion is excised and depicted below. Which immunohistochemical stain will be most useful in making the diagnosis of the suspected lesion?

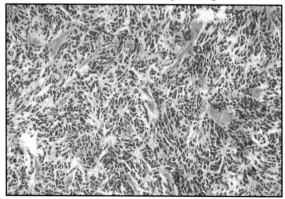

   A.   GFAP
   B.   INI1
   C.   Cytokeratin
   D.   Synaptophysin
   E.   EMA

2: Central Nervous System Questions

41. A 31-year-old male presents with disturbed gait. Neuroimaging shows a solid, intensely contrast-enhancing right cerebellar hemispheric lesion. The lesion is excised and depicted below. Based on the histopathology, which statement regarding the depicted tumor is INCORRECT?

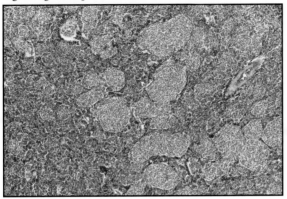

A. In children this tumor most commonly occurs in the vermis of the cerebellum.
B. Terminal neuroaxis dissemination is uncommon.
C. *c-myc* oncogene amplification is associated with aggressive behavior.
D. It is associated with Wilms tumor.
E. There is a prominent intercellular reticulin fiber network.

42. Which statement is TRUE regarding the tumor depicted in the image below?

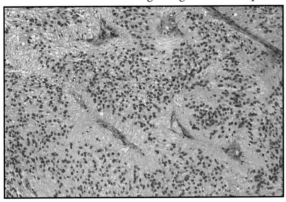

A. The tumor is immunoreactive for neurofilament.
B. Electron microscopy would show tumor cells with microvilli and scattered cilia.
C. Intramedullary tumors have the worst prognosis.
D. Patients younger than 5 years of age have the best prognosis.
E. >60% of tumors show EGFR amplification.

2: Central Nervous System Questions

43. The fourth ventricular lesion depicted below was discovered incidentally at autopsy in a 56-year-old male who was the unrestrained passenger in a motor vehicle accident. What is the diagnosis?

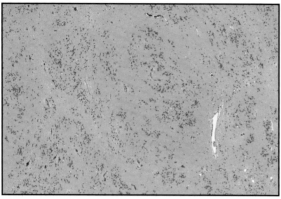

    A.   Pilocytic astrocytoma, WHO grade I
    B.   Diffuse astrocytoma, WHO grade II
    C.   Subependymoma, WHO grade I
    D.   Ependymoma, WHO grade II
    E.   Subependymal giant cell astrocytoma, WHO grade I

44. A 36-year-old male presents with back pain. Neuroimaging reveals a well-circumscribed enhancing intramedullary mass in the filum terminale. The patient is brought to the operating room and the surgeon requests an intraoperative consultation. The surgeon informs you that the tumor is well-encapsulated. A smear is prepared and shows tumor cells embedded in a conspicuous mucin background. Below are representative images from smear and the permanent section. The tumor cells are immunoreactive for S100 and immunonegative for pancytokeratin. What is the diagnosis?

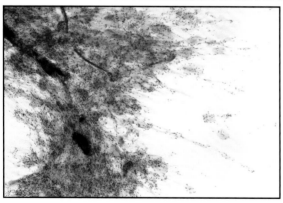 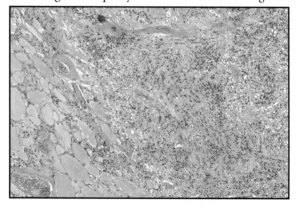

    A.   Chordoma
    B.   Schwannoma
    C.   Paraganglioma
    D.   Myxopapillary ependymoma, WHO grade I
    E.   Diffuse astrocytoma, WHO grade II

2: Central Nervous System Questions

45. An 8-year-old boy presents with headache and vomiting. Magnetic resonance imaging shows hydrocephalus with a large mass filling the fourth ventricle. Based on the image below, which of the following statements is INCORRECT?

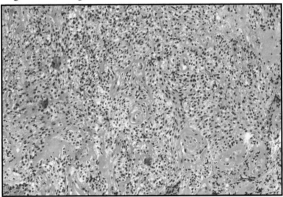

    A.   The genetic hallmark is 1p/19q co-deletion.
    B.   These tumors may follow a more aggressive course.
    C.   The tumor cells are immunoreactive for GFAP.
    D.   Perivascular rosettes are often present.
    E.   These tumors can arise throughout the neuroaxis.

46. What is the WHO grade of the following tumor (the H&E-stained and Ki-67-stained sections are shown below)?

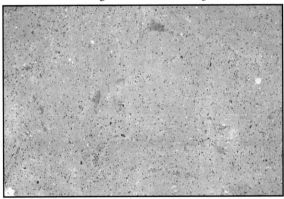 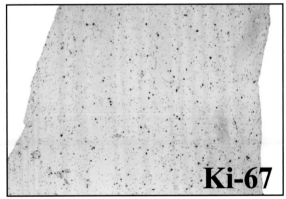

    A.   Pilocytic astrocytoma, WHO grade I
    B.   Pleomorphic xanthoastrocytoma, WHO grade II
    C.   Diffuse astrocytoma, WHO grade II
    D.   Anaplastic astrocytoma, WHO grade III
    E.   Glioblastoma, WHO grade IV

2: Central Nervous System Questions

47.   Based on the smear below from a 52-year-old male with a right temporal lobe lesion, what is the diagnosis?

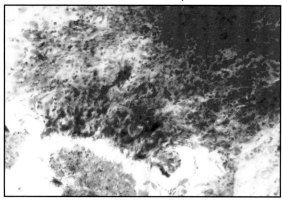

    A.   Gliosis
    B.   Demyelinating disease
    C.   Infarct
    D.   Anaplastic astrocytoma, WHO grade III
    E.   Glioblastoma, WHO grade IV

48.   A 19-year-old male presents with a headache, and neuroimaging reveals a large mass filling the third ventricle. Based on the image below, what is the diagnosis?

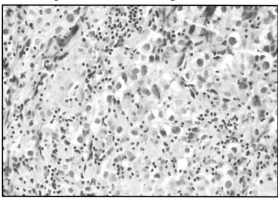

    A.   Central neurocytoma, WHO grade II
    B.   Germinoma
    C.   Choroid plexus carcinoma, WHO grade III
    D.   Pineocytoma, WHO grade I
    E.   Oligodendroglioma, WHO grade II

2: Central Nervous System Questions

49. A 28-year-old female presents with a headache. Magnetic resonance imaging is notable for a large well-circumscribed mass in the lateral ventricle. Based on the image below, what is the diagnosis?

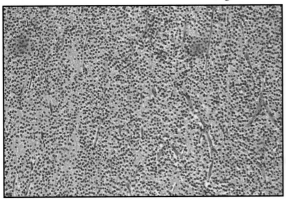

    A.   Oligodendroglioma, WHO grade II
    B.   Central neurocytoma, WHO grade II
    C.   Ependymoma, WHO grade II
    D.   Pineocytoma, WHO grade I
    E.   Choroid plexus carcinoma, WHO grade III

50. A 21-year-old male has a history of drug-resistant partial complex seizures. Magnetic resonance imaging shows a superficial well-circumscribed multicystic mass in the right temporal lobe with deformation of the overlying calvarium. Based on the history, neuroimaging, and images depicted below, the diagnosis is:

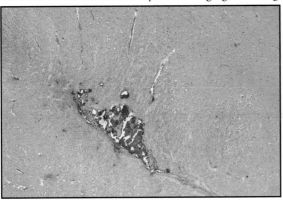 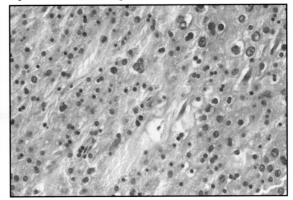

    A.   Oligodendroglioma, WHO grade II
    B.   Dysembryoplastic neuroepithelial tumor, WHO grade I
    C.   Extraventricular neurocytoma, WHO grade II
    D.   Pleomorphic xanthoastrocytoma, WHO grade II
    E.   Ganglioglioma, WHO grade I

2: Central Nervous System Questions

51. Based on the cerebellar tumor depicted below, which gene is likely mutated?

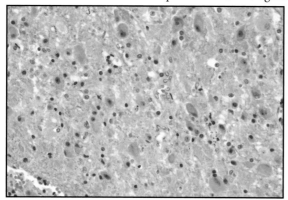

   A. NF1
   B. VHL
   C. PTEN
   D. TSC1
   E. INI1

52. Which of the following statements is TRUE regarding the tumor depicted below?

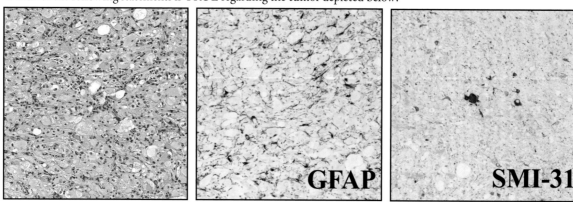

   A. The tumor cells are immunoreactive for CD34.
   B. Malignant change is common and involves the neuronal component.
   C. Perivascular lymphocytic infiltrate is rarely seen.
   D. The parietal lobe is the most common site of involvement.
   E. The tumor is seen in adults only.

2: Central Nervous System Questions

53. The BEST prognostic factor for the tumor depicted below is?

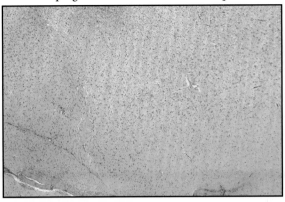 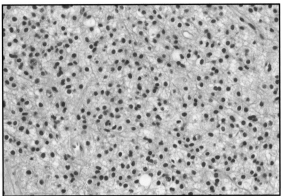

    A.   Younger age at operation
    B.   Gross total resection
    C.   Frontal lobe location
    D.   1p/19q co-deletion
    E.   Postoperative Karnofsky score

54. The tumor cells with abundant eosinophilic cytoplasm will be immunoreactive for:

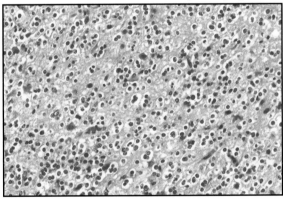

    A.   Glial fibrillary acid protein (GFAP)
    B.   S100
    C.   OLIG-1
    D.   All of the above
    E.   None of the above

2: Central Nervous System Questions

55. A 42-year-old female presents with weakness in her left arm. Neuroimaging is notable for an ill-defined lesion in the white matter of the right frontoparietal lobe. Based on the images below, what is the best diagnosis?

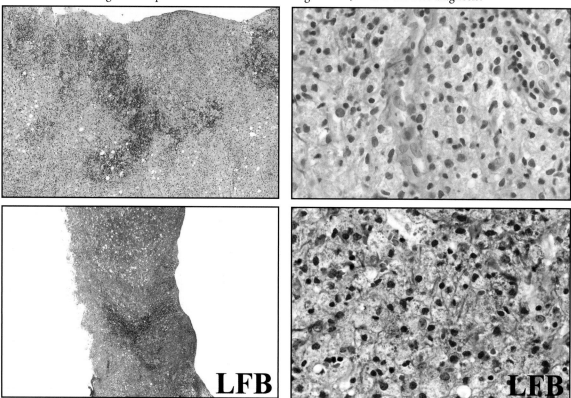

A. Oligodendroglioma, WHO grade II
B. Oligodendroglioma, WHO grade III
C. Clear cell ependymoma
D. Demyelinating disease
E. HIV encephalitis

2: Central Nervous System Questions

56. The tumor depicted below shows strong membranous reactivity for EMA. Based on the morphologic and immunohistochemical profile, the most likely genetic alteration is:

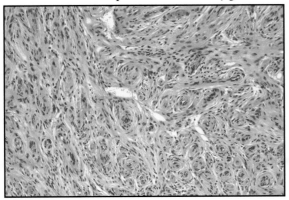

    A.   17q11
    B.   3p25
    C.   Monosomy 22
    D.   17p13
    E.   9p34

57. A 20-year-old male presents with seizures. Neuroimaging reveals a large right frontal lobe mass with possible attachment to the dura. Based on the image below, what is the diagnosis?

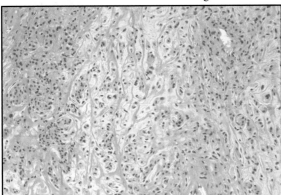

    A.   Chordoma
    B.   Chordoid meningioma, WHO grade II
    C.   Chondrosarcoma
    D.   Oligodendroglioma, WHO grade II
    E.   Microcystic meningioma, WHO grade I

2: Central Nervous System Questions

58. A 50-year-old female presents to the emergency room with a headache. Neuroimaging is notable for a well-circumscribed mass of the right frontal lobe with a dural tail and hyperostosis of the adjacent bone. The patient is taken to the operating room for a gross total resection of the tumor depicted below. What is the best diagnosis?

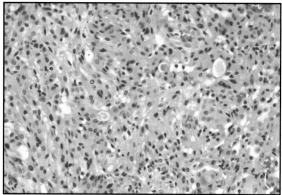 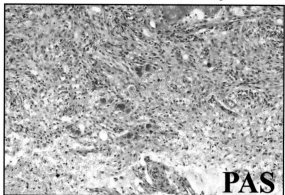

    A. Psammomatous meningioma
    B. Fibrous meningioma
    C. Secretory meningioma
    D. Solitary fibrous tumor
    E. Hemangiopericytoma

59. A 60-year-old male with von Hippel-Lindau disease presents with a cerebellar mass depicted below. To determine if the neoplasm is a primary CNS tumor or metastatic lesion, which is the best immunohistochemical panel to use?

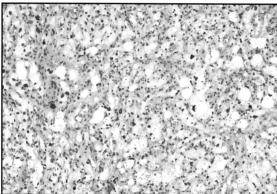

    A. GFAP, EMA, RCC
    B. S100, CD34, RCC
    C. Synaptophysin, EMA, CD10
    D. NSE, CD34, RCC
    E. S100, synaptophysin, CD10

2: Central Nervous System Questions

60. Which statement regarding the suprasellar tumor depicted below is FALSE?

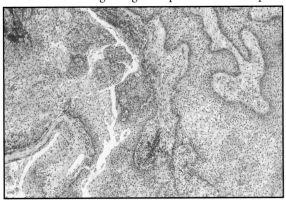

    A.   It is the most common tumor to occupy the sella turcica in a child.
    B.   Peripheral areas of the tumor show abundant Rosenthal fibers.
    C.   It may be mistaken for metastatic squamous cell carcinoma.
    D.   It is derived from Rathke pouch epithelium.
    E.   None of the above.

61. A 70-year-old female presents with a headache and neuroimaging shows a large poorly circumscribed right frontoparietal mass with focal areas of hemorrhage. Based on the images below, what is the diagnosis?

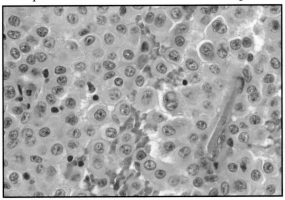 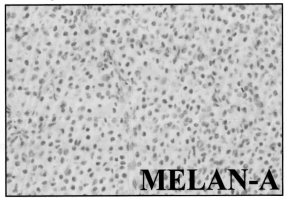

    A.   Anaplastic oligodendroglioma, WHO III
    B.   Glioblastoma, WHO IV
    C.   Anaplastic meningioma, WHO III
    D.   Ganglioglioma, WHO I
    E.   Metastatic melanoma

2: Central Nervous System Questions

62. A 35-year-old female with a history of low-grade astrocytoma status post resection and radiation presents with an enlarging and enhancing mass in the area of previous resection. She is brought back to the operating room for a biopsy, which is depicted below. What is your diagnosis?

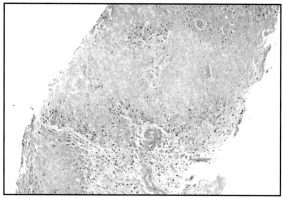

    A.   Recurrent low-grade astrocytoma
    B.   Glioblastoma
    C.   Radiation changes
    D.   Infarct
    E.   Nondiagnostic material

63. Based on the image below, what is the diagnosis?

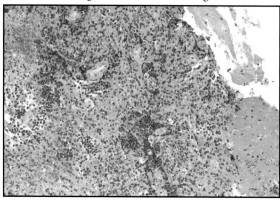 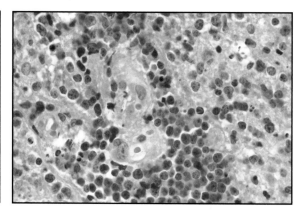

    A.   Anaplastic oligodendroglioma
    B.   Small cell glioblastoma
    C.   Lymphoma
    D.   Encephalitis
    E.   Metastatic melanoma.

2: Central Nervous System Answers

1. **A. P53 MUTATION**
    The MRI shows the so-called "butterfly-lesion" of glioblastoma. The absence of prior symptoms/lesion suggests that this is a primary or de novo glioblastoma. p53 mutations (choice A) are less common in primary glioblastomas than in secondary glioblastomas (approximately 25% vs 65%). The remaining listed molecular alterations (B-E) are all commonly seen in primary glioblastomas.
    QCSP, **Glioblastoma Multiforme,** p 37.

2. **B. >50% GEMISTOCYTIC COMPONENT**
    Favorable prognostic features include younger patients (choice A) with well-differentiated lesions. Gender (choice E) has no impact on prognosis. In terms of location, brainstem lesions frequently undergo malignant degeneration compared to cerebral hemisphere or spinal cord lesions (choices C-D). Although somewhat controversial, the presence of gemistocytes (choice B) is a poor prognostic sign, and many feel that gemistocytic astrocytomas would be better classified as anaplastic lesions.
    QCSP, **Astrocytoma,** p 36.

3. **C. MICROVASCULAR ENDOTHELIAL PROLIFERATION**
    The 2 most important histologic criteria for the diagnosis of glioblastoma are microvascular endothelial proliferation (choice C), with or without glomeruloids, and the presence of necrosis (choice A). This is somewhat of a trick question because choice E may appear to be the best answer; however, geographic necrosis is seen with radiation treatment, which would be supported by the presence of hyalinized vessels. The more characteristic necrosis of glioblastoma is the pseudopalisading pattern with small foci of necrosis surrounded by a radially-oriented collar of tumor cells that are slightly smaller than the surrounding neoplastic cells. The Ki-67 proliferative index is usually over 20%, but this is not required for a diagnosis of glioblastoma (choice B). There is a small cell variant of glioblastoma (choice D), but a small cell component is not a criteria for diagnosis.
    QCSP, **Glioblastoma Multiforme,** p 37.

4. **B. BRAINSTEM**
    In adults, glioblastoma primarily affects the cerebral hemispheres (choice D), and in children the brainstem (choice B) is a more common location. The main differential for cerebellar lesions in a child (choice A) includes embryonal tumors (medulloblastoma and atypical teratoid/rhabdoid tumor) and pilocytic astrocytomas, which are also common in the hypothalamic region (choice E).
    QCSP, **Glioblastoma Multiforme,** p 36.

5. **C. PRIMARY (DE NOVO) GLIOBLASTOMA ARISING IN AN ADULT.**
    p53 mutations are less common in primary glioblastomas with the exception of primary giant cell glioblastomas (choice D) and de novo glioblastomas arising in children (choice B). Low-grade astrocytic tumors commonly show p53 mutations (choice A) as well as glioblastomas arising from lower-grade astrocytomas (secondary glioblastomas).
    QCSP, **Glioblastoma Multiforme,** p 37.

6. **E. BRISK MITOTIC ACTIVITY**
    The vessels in pilocytic astrocytomas can be markedly hyalinized (choice B), and vascular proliferation may be quite prominent (choice A), but don't let that fool you into assigning the tumor a higher WHO grade. The presence of necrosis in the absence of a history of prior radiation should make you consider an alternative diagnosis, but microvascular endothelial proliferation is allowed and quite common in pilocytic astrocytomas. Eosinophilic granular bodies (choice C) are a hallmark of slowly growing lesions and are a helpful feature along with Rosenthal fibers, when identified to support a diagnosis of pilocytic astrocytoma. Instead of the typical biphasic appearance with prominent microcystic areas, some tumors show prominent oligodendroglial-like areas with small round hyperchromatic nuclei and perinuclear halos. These can be challenging to diagnose, but

look for the aforementioned classic features of pilocytic astrocytomas (especially eosinophilic granular bodies and Rosenthal fibers). In addition, tumor location can also be helpful (most neuropathologists do not believe that oligodendrogliomas occur in the spinal cord). Mitotic figures are usually very difficult to find in pilocytic astrocytomas and are never brisk (choice E).

QCSP, **Pilocytic Astrocytoma**, p 40.

7.　　A.　**MENINGIOMA**

Intracranial lesions associated with tuberous sclerosis include tubers (choice B), subependymal hamartomas (choice C), subependymal giant cell astrocytomas (choice D), and retinal astrocytic hamartomas (choice E). Tubers are firm, pale, raised cortical lesions characterized by scattered large cells with large nuclei, glassy eosinophilic cytoplasm, and disruption of cortical lamination. Subependymal hamartomas are likely precursor lesions to giant cell astrocytomas. Meningiomas (choice A) have an association with neurofibromatosis type 2, not tuberous sclerosis.

QCSP, **Subependymal Giant Cell Astrocytoma**, p 43.

8.　　D.　**ALL OF THE ABOVE**

Flexner-Wintersteiner rosettes consist of small lumina circumscribed by neoplastic cells joined at their apexes to produce a form of internal limiting (basement) membrane. They are seen in retinoblastomas (choice A), pineoblastomas (choice B), and medulloepitheliomas (choice C).

QCSP, **Retinoblastoma**, p 48.

9.　　A.　**THE FAMILIAL FORM IS TRANSMITTED IN AN AUTOSOMAL DOMINANT PATTERN.**

Mitotic figures are frequent (choice B) in retinoblastoma. Both Flexner-Wintersteiner and Homer Wright rosettes may be present. The tumor cells are immunoreactive for NSE, synaptophysin, S100 protein, GFAP, myelin basic protein, and Leu-7, not cytokeratin (choice C). Cases diagnosed early are treated conservatively in an attempt to preserve vision, while more advanced lesions are treated with enucleation (choice D). The 5-year survival for unilateral retinoblastoma is >90%, and it is only slightly less for bilateral disease (choice E). The hereditary form is caused by a germ cell mutation on chromosome 13q14, which results in the inactivation of the Rb protein. This is transmitted in an autosomal dominant pattern (choice A).

QCSP, **Retinoblastoma**, p 48.

10.　C.　**CD30**

Embryonal carcinomas are immunoreactive for CAM 5.2 (choice A), placental alkaline phosphatase (choice B), CD30 (choice C), and OCT4 (choice D); however, only CD30 is specific for embryonal carcinomas. CAM 5.2 is also reactive in a minority of germinomas, teratomas (epithelial component), yolk sac tumors, and choriocarcinomas (syncytiotrophoblastic cells). PLAP is consistently reactive in germinomas and occasionally reactive in yolk sac tumors and choriocarcinomas. Nuclear OCT4 reactivity is also seen commonly in germinomas. CD117 (choice E) reactivity is seen commonly in germinomas and occasionally in teratomas (mesenchymal and epithelioid components).

QCSP, **Embryonal Carcinoma**, p 53.

11.　D.　**TUMOR CELLS OF GERMINOMAS ARE PAS POSITIVE.**

Germinomas are the most frequent intracranial germ cell tumors (50%), and teratomas (choice A) are the second most common. Germinomas are usually curable and, like their gonadal counterparts, are quite radiosensitive (choice B). Germinomas are PAS positive (choice D) and are immunoreactive for placental alkaline phosphatase and CD117 as well as β-hCG if syncytiotrophoblastic cells are present. Choriocarcinomas (not yolk sac tumors) are often associated with precocious puberty (choice E.)

QCSP, **Germinoma**, p 52.

2: Central Nervous System Answers

12. A. **CEREBRAL SPINAL FLUID SPREAD IS COMMON.**
     Central neurocytomas typically occur in young to middle-aged adults (choice C) and usually present as an intraventricular mass near the foramen of Monro, with the anterior portion of the lateral ventricle the most common site (choice B). The tumor is characterized by a uniform, monotonous cellular proliferation with round nuclei, stippled chromatin, and small nucleoli. The tumor cells are diffusely immunoreactive for synaptophysin (choice D) as well as NSE and S100. The tumor cells are usually negative for chromogranin. Although helpful when present, structures resembling Homer Wright rosettes and ganglion cells are rare (choice E). The prognosis is excellent, and despite the intraventricular location, cerebral spinal fluid spread is very rare (choice A).
     QCSP, **Central Neurocytoma,** p 54.

13. E. **MALIGNANT TRANSFORMATION IS COMMON.**
     Dysembryoplastic neuroepithelial tumors are benign, with cure possible even after a subtotal resection. Of 700 reported cases, only 2 cases of malignant transformation have been described. The remaining statements (choices A-D) are all true.
     QCSP, **Dysembryoplastic Neuroepithelial Tumor,** p 55.

14. E. **ALL OF THE ABOVE**
     Oligodendrogliomas assume many different architectural patterns, including columnar, palisading, microcystic (choice B), and lobular. The vasculature is delicate and branched and assumes a characteristic "chicken-wire" appearance (choice C). Although nonspecific, the infiltrating tumor cells accumulate in the subpial region, around neurons (perineural satellitosis), and around blood vessels. This triad is referred to as the secondary structures of Scherer (choice A) and is very typical of oligodendrogliomas.
     QCSP, **Oligodendrioglioma,** p 57.

15. E. **NONE OF THE ABOVE**
     Atypical meningiomas are defined as having either an increased mitotic rate (defined as 4 or more mitoses/10 hpf) and/or 3 of the following features: increased nuclear to cytoplasmic ratio (choice A), prominent nucleoli (choice B), necrosis (choice C), loss of pattern (choice D), or increased cellularity. The best answer is none of the above (choice E), since each of the listed features is insufficient by itself to increase the grade of the tumor.
     QCSP, **Atypical and Anaplastic (Malignant) Meningiomas,** p 59.

16. B. **VIMENTIN**
     Without strong vimentin (choice B) immunoreactivity, one should rethink the diagnosis of meningioma as vimentin positivity is found in all meningiomas. Epithelial membrane antigen (EMA) reactivity is seen in a majority of meningiomas and should be included in any meningioma immunohistochemical panel. Cytokeratin positivity (choice A) is seen in the secretory variant. Meningiomas are not reactive for GFAP (choice C), CD34 (choice D), or CD68 (choice E), which would be positive in glial tumors, solitary fibrous tumors, and Rosai-Dorfman disease, respectively.
     QCSP, **Atypical and Anaplastic (Malignant) Meningiomas,** p 59.

17. C. **THEY ARE ASSOCIATED WITH NEUROFIBROMATOSIS TYPE 1.**
     Multiple meningiomas are seen in patients with neurofibromatosis type 2 due to loss of genetic information on chromosome 22 (choice D). Neurofibromatosis type 1 (choice C) is associated with optic gliomas. The remaining choices are all true.
     QCSP, **Meningioma,** p 60.

2: Central Nervous System Answers

18.   E.   **PAPILLARY**

Choices A-D are all WHO grade I tumors. Papillary meningiomas (choice E) are WHO grade III tumors by definition and are more aggressive, with a high rate of recurrence.

QCSP, **Meningioma**, p 60.

19.   A.   **CRANIOPHARYNGIOMAS**

Gorlin syndrome is an autosomal dominant disorder characterized by skeletal anomalies, cutaneous epidermoid cysts, pits on the palms and soles, odontogenic keratocysts, calcifying ovarian fibromas, and multifocal basal cell carcinomas. The CNS involvement is characterized by meningiomas (choice B) and medulloblastomas (choice C), not craniopharyngiomas (choice A).

QCSP, **Meningioma**, p 60.

20.   C.   **HISTORY OF HEAD TRAUMA**

Meningiomas may result from cranial irradiation or trauma (choice C). Females are more frequently affected, and meningiomas are associated with other estrogen-dependent tumors, including breast and endometrial cancers. Multiple meningiomas are associated with neurofibromatosis type 2, not tuberous sclerosis (choice B). Although seizures (choice D) can lead to head trauma, they are not an independent risk factor; therefore, the best answer is choice C.

QCSP, **Meningioma**, p 60.

21.   D.   **PINEOCYTOMA**

The key to the answer lies in the adjectives "large" and "irregular," which imply a pineocytomatous rosette rather than the smaller, more orderly Homer Wright rosette. Neuroblastomas (choice A), medulloblastomas (choice B), and CNS primitive neuroectodermal tumors (choice E) all show varying degrees of Homer Wright rosettes. The best answer is pineocytoma (choice D), where the rosettes vary from quite prominent to sparse and incomplete.

QCSP, **Pineocytoma**, p 63.

22.   C.   **RETICULIN WILL HIGHLIGHT THE CLUBLIKE PROCESSES THAT PROJECT INTO THE ROSETTES.**

Pineocytomas are related to retinal photoreceptors (choice A) and therefore will be immunoreactive for retinal S-antigen as well as neurofilament (choice B) and synaptophysin. This is a benign neoplasm with little tendency to invade adjacent structures (choice D). Electron microscopy is diagnostic and shows small, intertwined filaments (choice E) as well as neurosecretory granules, dense core vesicles, and clear vesicles. Silver carbonate (not reticulin) will highlight the processes that project into the pineocytomatous rosettes (choice C).

QCSP, **Pineocytoma**, p 63.

23.   B.   **ARCHITECTURAL PATTERN**

Pineocytoma is a well-differentiated tumor that resembles normal pineocytes with similar photosensory and neuroendocrine functions, and therefore will have similar immunohistochemical staining patterns (choice A) and ultrastructural features (choice C). Pineocytomas are not mitotically active (choice D) and areas of necrosis are rare (choice E). The most helpful feature is that pineocytomas are patternless and form sheets rather than the normal lobular pattern (choice B).

QCSP, **Pineocytoma**, p 63.

24.   A.   **LARGE ROSETTES CHARACTERISTIC OF PINEOCYTOMAS ARE NOT PRESENT.**

Pineoblastoma is a highly malignant primitive small cell neoplasm with a poor prognosis and survival rate rarely longer than 2 years (choice E). The characteristic deletion of neuroblastomas (11q13) has been identified in pineoblastomas (choice C). Although the large rosettes characteristic of pineocytomas are not present (choice A), both Flexner-Wintersteiner and Homer Wright rosettes may be seen. If rosettes are present, the fibrillar zones will be reactive for synaptophysin and not GFAP (choice B). The treatment is surgical excision rather than chemotherapy (choice D).

QCSP, **Pineoblastoma**, p 62.

25. E. **Hemangioblastoma**
10% of patients with hemangioblastomas will present with polycythemia secondary to tumor production of erythropoietin.

QCSP, **Hemangioblastoma**, p 64.

26. C. **Confirm that sufficient diagnostic tissue has been obtained**
Often during intraoperative consultation a generic diagnosis will be sufficient for the neurosurgeon to make a decision concerning the extent of resection based on the clinical and neuroimaging features. Neurosurgeons are aware of the limitations imposed on pathologists at the time of intraoperative consultation, namely small sample size and freezing artifact. The main role of the pathologist is to confirm that adequate, diagnostic, nonnecrotic tissue samples have been obtained (choice C). A more specific diagnosis can be rendered after examination of permanent sections. Unlike surgical pathology, margin status (choice B) has less importance in neuropathology because most tumors are infiltrative and a "negative margin" does not ensure against tumor recurrence.

QCSP, **Intraoperative Consultation**, p 32.

27. A. **Pilocytic astrocytoma**
In general the main role of the neuropathologist during intraoperative consultation is to confirm that sufficient diagnostic tissue has been obtained. Infiltrating gliomas are, generally speaking, treated in a similar fashion, and differentiating between astrocytoma and oligodendroglioma during an intraoperative consultation will not change the extent of resection. There are some exceptions to this rule, including a diagnosis of pilocytic astrocytoma (choice A). The goal of treatment for pilocytic astrocytomas is gross total resection; therefore, it is imperative to differentiate at the time of surgery between a pilocytic astrocytoma and low-grade infiltrating glioma. Other entities requiring specific diagnoses include ependymomas in the spinal cord and lymphomas.

QCSP, **Intraoperative Consultation**, p 32.

28. D. **Ependymoma and choroid plexus papilloma**
It is helpful for the pathologist to be aware of the incidence and location of brain tumors to narrow the differential diagnosis during intraoperative consultation when only a $0.2 \times 0.2 \times 0.2$ cm piece of tissue is available for examination. All of the listed tumors commonly occur at the cerebellopontine angle; however, schwannomas, meningiomas, and epidermoid cysts are more common in adults. Ependymomas and choroid plexus papillomas are the 2 most common lesions at this location in the pediatric population (choice D).

QCSP, **Intraoperative Consultation**, p 32.

29. A. **Astrocytoma**
You can quickly eliminate medulloblastoma (choice E) because by definition these tumors arise in the cerebellum. All of the remaining choices can occur in the brainstem, but by far the most common tumor in this location for both children and adults is astrocytoma (choice A).

QCSP, **Intraoperative Consultation**, p 32.

30. D. **Pleomorphic xanthoastrocytoma**
The clinical history of an adolescent with a long-standing history of seizures and a superficial cerebral lesion raises a short differential diagnosis including pleomorphic xanthoastrocytoma (PXA), ganglioglioma, dysembryoplastic neuroepithelial tumor (DNT), and pilocytic astrocytoma. The H&E-stained section shows a pleomorphic population of cells with abundant pink cytoplasm, xanthomatous change (intracellular accumulation of lipids), and scattered giant cells. Although the degree of pleomorphism is striking, no high-grade features, including

mitotic figures, microvascular endothelial proliferation, and/or necrosis, are present to suggest a diagnosis of a high-grade astrocytic neoplasm (choices A-B). A reticulin stain would highlight the presence of intercellular reticulin fibers, which is seen in both gliosarcomas (choice B) and PXAs (choice D), although no malignant mesenchymal component is seen on the H&E-stained section, inconsistent with the former diagnosis. No neuronal component is present to suggest a diagnosis of either a ganglioglioma (choice C) or DNT (choice E). The main differential based on the microscopic image is between PXA (choice D) and glioblastoma with giant cells (choice A), but the clinical history of longstanding seizures in conjunction with the absence of necrosis, microvascular endothelial proliferation, and mitotic figures is consistent with a diagnosis of pleomorphic xanthoastrocytoma, WHO grade II (choice D).

QCSP, **Pleomorphic Xanthoastrocytoma**, p 42.

31.   D.   **GLIOBLASTOMA**

The image depicts an eosinophilic granular body, which is a feature of slowly growing glial neoplasms (choices A-C, E). Granular bodies are intermediate, presumably glial filaments and are reactive for GFAP, $\alpha\beta$-crystallin, ubiquitin, α_1-antichymotrypsin, and α_1-antitrypsin. They are not seen in high-grade astrocytic tumors, including glioblastomas (choice D).

QCSP, **Astrocytomas and Glioblastomas**, p 41-42.

32.   E.   **GLIOMATOSIS CEREBRI**

The images depict a low-grade, paucicellular infiltrating astrocytic neoplasm. The tumor cells appear quite benign with little or no cytoplasm. Mitotic figures are not evident and the Ki-67 proliferative index is low. The infiltrative component seems out of proportion to both the degree of anaplasia of the tumor cells and the cellularity. The tumor cell nuclei are elongated and do not show the classic perinuclear halos to suggest an oligodendroglial component (choice D). The tumor cell population is monotonous and no Rosenthal fibers or eosinophilic granular bodies are identified to suggest a pilocytic astrocytoma (choice A). No anaplastic features are present to suggest a high-grade astrocytic neoplasm (choice C); therefore, we are left deciding between diffuse astrocytoma, WHO grade II, and gliomatosis cerebri. This is somewhat of a trick question because based on morphology the lesion is a diffuse astrocytoma, WHO grade II (choice B), but by definition gliomatosis cerebri involves 3 or more cerebral lobes, and choice E is therefore the best answer.

QCSP, **Gliomatosis Cerebri**, p 37.

33.   E.   **EMA**

The image shows a low-grade astrocytic tumor with minimal nuclear atypia, inconspicuous mitotic figures, and no evidence of microvascular endothelial proliferation or necrosis. Astrocytic tumors show cytoplasmic positivity for GFAP (choice C), and most tumor cells are reactive for S100 protein (choice A) and vimentin (choice B). Low-grade astrocytic tumors typically have p53 mutations (choice D). EMA reactivity (choice E) is seen in a variety of tumors, including meningiomas and ependymomas, but not astrocytic tumors.

QCSP, **Astrocytic Tumors, Ependymal Tumors, and Meningioma**, p 35, 50, 61.

34.   C.   **RETICULIN**

The image depicts a biphasic population of both malignant glial and malignant mesenchymal cells. Mesenchymal cells are topographically related to blood vessels and appear to be arising from vascular or adventitial elements. A reticulin stain (choice C) as shown below will help delineate the sarcomatous areas from the glial areas and is characteristic of gliosarcomas. The glial component is usually typical of glioblastoma and will be immunoreactive for GFAP. Although both cytokeratin (choice A) and S100 (choice B) will be reactive in the neoplastic glial component to varying degrees, reticulin (choice C) is the best answer to make a specific diagnosis of gliosarcoma. Neu-N is a neuronal marker and would not be immunoreactive.

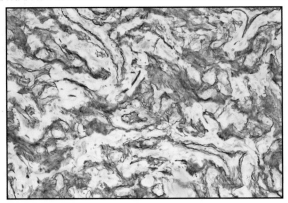

QCSP, **Gliosarcoma,** p 38.

35. A. **NEUROFIBROMATOSIS TYPE 1**
The H&E-stained image shows a pilocytic astrocytoma. 30% of patients with pilocytic astrocytomas of the optic nerve have neurofibromatosis type 1. Tuberous sclerosis (choice C) is associated with subependymal giant cell astrocytomas. von Hippel-Lindau (choice D) is associated with central nervous system hemangioblastomas. Neurofibromatosis type 2 (choice B) has an association with meningiomas. Li-Fraumeni syndrome (choice E) is characterized by p53 germline mutations, and affected family members often develop high-grade astrocytic tumors.
QCSP, **Pilocytic Astrocytoma,** p 40.

36. C. **PILOCYTIC ASTROCYTOMA, WHO GRADE I**
The H&E-stained image shows an oligodendroglial-like tumor with perinuclear halos. Although somewhat controversial, most neuropathologists believe that oligodendrogliomas (choices A-B) do not occur in the spinal cord. The main differential is between pilocytic astrocytoma (choice C) and a clear cell ependymoma (choice D). The presence of Rosenthal fibers and absence of perivascular pseudorosettes is consistent with a pilocytic astrocytoma. Myxopapillary ependymomas (choice E) characteristically occurs in the filum terminale and tends to have a pseudopapillary architecture with perivascular and intercellular mucin deposition.
QCSP, **Pilocytic Astrocytoma,** p 40l; WHO, p 40-42, 50.

37. C. **MALIGNANT TRANSFORMATION IS COMMON.**
The image depicts a subependymal giant cell astrocytoma, which is usually seen in patients with tuberous sclerosis (choice A), a syndrome that includes cutaneous lesions (including café-au-lait spots and subungual fibromas), epilepsy, and mental retardation. Tuberous sclerosis is also associated with visceral abnormalities, including renal cortical cysts, renal angiomyolipoma, cardiac rhabdomyoma, pulmonary lymphangiomatosis, renal cell carcinoma, splenic and hepatic angiomas, and fibrous dysplasia of the bone. Subependymal giant cell astrocytomas are limited to the region of the foramen of Monro and typically arise in the wall of the lateral ventricle (choice B) as a bulky, exophytic, smooth, domelike, broad-based mass that may cross the midline and produce marked dilation of the lateral ventricles. The tumor cells have abundant glassy eosinophilic cytoplasm with eccentric nuclei, and they are usually diffusely positive for S100 protein and focally or weakly positive for GFAP (choice E). The giant cell astrocytes are positive for $\alpha\beta$-crystallin (choice D). Malignant transformation (choice C) to glioblastoma is rare and long-term survival is excellent, although recurrence can occur, especially when the lesion is not amenable to gross total resection.
QCSP, **Subependymal Giant Cell Astrocytoma,** p 43.

2: Central Nervous System Answers

38.   D.   **CHOROID PLEXUS CARCINOMA**

The 2 most common tumors arising from the lateral ventricle of a young child are choroid plexus tumors (choice D) and ependymomas (choice C). Although less common, atypical teratoid/rhabdoid tumors (choice E) and germ cell tumors (choice A-B) can also present as a ventricular mass. The H&E-stained image shows large atypical cells with frank nuclear pleomorphism and high mitotic rate. The overall architecture of the lesion demonstrates a sheet-like growth pattern. Choroid plexus carcinoma (choice D) is immunoreactive for cytokeratin, S100, transthyretin, and occasionally GFAP. Embryonal carcinoma (choice A) will also be positive for cytokeratin but will be immunonegative for transthyretin and immunoreactive for CD30 and PLAP. AT/RTs (choice E) show a variable staining pattern based on the different epithelial, mesenchymal, and embryonal components present but characteristically have absent nuclear INI1 staining in tumor cells. Anaplastic ependymoma (choice C) will be immunoreactive for cytokeratins and EMA. Tissue from each of the 3 germ cell layers is not identified to suggest an immature teratoma (choice B). Therefore, based on the transthyretin immunoreactivity, choroid plexus carcinoma (choice D) is the best answer.

QCSP, **Choroid Plexus Papilloma and Carcinoma,** p 44-45, 53.

39.   A.   **90% HAVE INI1 MUTATION.**

The image shows a high-grade pleomorphic tumor with scattered rhabdoid cells as evidenced by cells with eccentric nuclei and prominent nucleoli and abundant eosinophilic cytoplasm. The image and history is consistent with an atypical teratoid/rhabdoid tumor. The characteristic molecular alteration is monosomy or deletion of chromosome 22 (choice A) with inactivation of the INI1 gene. EGFR amplification (choice B) and PTEN mutation (choice E) are characteristic of primary glioblastomas, and TP53 mutation (choice C) is seen in secondary glioblastomas. Isochromosome 17q (choice D) is common in medulloblastomas.

QCSP, **Atypical Teratoid/Rhabdoid Tumor,** p 45.

40.   D.   **SYNAPTOPHYSIN**

The image depicts sheets of large undifferentiated tumor cells with vague areas of Homer Wright (neuroblastic) rosettes suggestive of medulloblastoma. Medulloblastoma tumor cells, regardless of pattern, exhibit some degree of immunoreactivity for synaptophysin and neuron-specific enolase, and therefore choice D (synaptophysin) is the best answer. Glial differentiation with GFAP positivity (choice A) is present in only approximately 10% of cases of classic medulloblastoma. Absent INI1 staining (choice B) is seen in atypical teratoid/rhabdoid tumors. Cytokeratin staining (choice C) is seen in ependymomas and choroid plexus tumors. EMA staining (choice E) is seen in a wide variety of tumors including ependymomas, atypical teratoid/rhabdoid tumors, and meningiomas.

QCSP, **Medulloblastoma,** p 46.

41.   B.   **TERMINAL NEURAXIS DISSEMINATION IS UNCOMMON.**

The image depicts a desmoplastic medulloblastoma as seen by pale nodular islands surrounded by highly proliferative cells in a dense intercellular reticulin network (choice E), which would be highlighted on a reticulin stain. Desmoplastic medulloblastoma is more frequent in adults and is typically located in the cerebellar hemisphere, while in children medulloblastomas are more common in the vermis (choice A). There are multiple variants of medulloblastoma (classic, desmoplastic, extensive nodularity, anaplastic, and large cell). The desmoplastic and extensive nodularity variants are associated with a better prognosis, while the large cell and anaplastic medulloblastoma variants are associated with a poorer prognosis. Additional adverse prognostic factors include age <3 years, incomplete surgical resection, metastatic disease at presentation, high mitotic index, c-myc oncogene amplification (choice C), isochromosome 17q, and loss of 17p. Medulloblastomas are associated with multiple syndromes including Gorlin, Turcot, and Coffin-Sinus, and are also associated with Wilms tumor of the kidney (choice D). In all cases of suspected medulloblastoma the entire neuroaxis should be imaged preoperatively because CNS dissemination is very common and assessment will be confounded postoperatively by iatrogenic drop metastases. This is often not done in adults when the diagnosis of medulloblastoma is not entertained.

QCSP, **Medulloblastoma,** p 46.

2: Central Nervous System Answers

42.   B.   **ELECTRON MICROSCOPY WOULD SHOW TUMOR CELLS WITH MICROVILLI AND SCATTERED CILIA.**
The H&E-stained image shows a monomorphic population of tumor cells with minimal cytoplasm and round nuclei with a salt-and-pepper chromatin pattern. Perivascular pseudorosettes are seen, as evidenced by perivascular zones in which tumor cell processes approach vessel walls. Not seen in this image are true ependymal rosettes which are composed of small gland-like structures with clearly defined central lumina. The morphologic image is diagnostic of ependymoma. Immunohistochemistry for EMA would show characteristic dot-like cytoplasmic immunoreactivity. The diagnosis would be confirmed on ultrastructural examination, as ependymal cells have intermediate filaments, luminal microvilli, and cilia in a 9+2 arrangement, and have complex intercellular junctions (choice B). Ependymomas show glial differentiation and therefore will be immunoreactive for GFAP and not neurofilament (choice A). Intramedullary tumors have the best prognosis (choice C) and tend to occur more commonly in adults, while younger patients tend to have infratentorial lesions with a poorer prognosis (choice D). Primary glioblastomas are associated with EGFR amplifications (choice E). The most frequent molecular alteration in ependymomas is the loss of chromosome 22.
QCSP, **Ependymoma,** p 49.

43.   C.   **SUBEPENDYMOMA, WHO GRADE I**
The H&E-stained section shows a uniform population of tumor cells in a fibrillary background with a vague lobular architecture. Mitoses are inconspicuous and there is no evidence of necrosis. The morphologic image is consistent with a subependymoma (choice C), which are often discovered incidentally at autopsy. This tumor is often mistaken for an ependymoma (choice D), and clues to the correct diagnosis include the low cellularity, lobular architecture, and absence of true rosettes, or ependymal canals. It is important to note that perivascular pseudorosettes are occasionally identified in subependymomas. The prominent fibrillary processes bring to mind pilocytic astrocytomas (choice A); however, the overall architecture and lack of both a biphasic component and Rosenthal fibers are helpful clues. Microcyst formation is often seen in subependymomas and may lead to confusion with fibrillary astrocytomas (choice B); however, the minimal nuclear atypia and lobular architecture are inconsistent with the latter diagnosis. There is no evidence of large ganglioid astrocytes to suggest a diagnosis of subependymal giant cell astrocytomas (choice E).
QCSP, **Subependymoma,** p 51.

44.   D.   **MYXOPAPILLARY EPENDYMOMA, WHO GRADE I**
The tumor is composed of elongated, fibrillary cells with nuclei with homogeneously dispersed chromatin and small nucleoli. The tumor cells are arranged in fascicles and papillary formations, with the presence of lakes of mucinous material. While all of the listed tumors can have mucinous features with the exception of paragangliomas (choice C), the degree of mucin deposition is most suggestive of either a myxopapillary ependymoma (choice D) or chordoma (choice A). Although the characteristic physaliphorous cells with vacuolated cytoplasm of chordomas are not identified, these cells are not always prominent. The differentiation between these 2 lesions (which are both found in the cauda equina region) is made based on morphology and immunohistochemistry. Chordomas will show anastomosing chords and nests of tumor cells with immunoreactivity for S100 and pancytokeratin, while myxopapillary ependymomas will show tumor cells encircling vessels with mucoid degeneration and immunoreactivity for S100 and GFAP. Paragangliomas (choice C) are usually present as spinal intradural tumors in the cauda equina region, and intraspinal schwannomas (choice B) show a strong predilection for sensory nerve roots; however, there have been reported cases of intramedullary schwannomas. Focal mucin deposition is seen in schwannomas in the hypocellular Antoni B areas; however, the more hypercellular Antoni A areas are usually identified and the tumor is composed of cells with spindled nuclei. Fibrillary astrocytomas (choice E) can show microcystic degeneration; however, the amount of mucin deposition seen in this case exceeds what would be expected for fibrillary astrocytomas. By definition, fibrillary astrocytomas are diffusely infiltrative and would not be well-encapsulated as noted by the surgeon. Therefore, based on the location, abundant mucin, and immunohistochemical profile, the best answer is myxopapillary ependymoma (choice D).
QCSP, **Ependymoma,** p 50.

2: Central Nervous System Answers

45. A. **THE GENETIC HALLMARK IS 1p/19q CO-DELETION.**

The image shows a clear cell ependymoma with microvascular endothelial proliferation. The clear cells resemble oligodendroglial tumor cells; however, the identification of perivascular rosettes (choice D) is a helpful feature characteristic of ependymomas. The clear cell variant of ependymoma is reported to behave more aggressively (choice B). Ependymomas are immunoreactive for GFAP (choice C), vimentin, EMA (cytoplasmic dot-like reactivity), and cytokeratin. Helpful histologic features of ependymomas include the aforementioned perivascular pseudorosettes (choice D), ependymal rosettes, and ependymal canals. Ependymomas are found throughout the neuroaxis (choice E), with spinal lesions occurring more often in adults and intracranial tumors occurring more often in children. The 1p/19q co-deletion (choice A) is the genetic hallmark of oligodendroglioma. The most common molecular alteration in ependymoma is loss of chromosome 22.

QCSP, **Ependymoma,** p 49.

46. D. **ANAPLASTIC ASTROCYTOMA, WHO GRADE III**

The image shows a diffusely infiltrating hypercellular tumor in a fibrillary background composed of cells with minimal cytoplasm and pleomorphic nuclei with irregular nuclear contours. Mitotic figures are easily identified. There is no evidence of microvascular endothelial proliferation or necrosis. The degree of atypia and high Ki-67 proliferation index in the absence of microvascular endothelial proliferation and/or necrosis is consistent with an anaplastic astrocytoma, WHO grade III (choice D).

QCSP, **Anaplastic Astrocytoma,** p 34.

47. E. **GLIOBLASTOMA, WHO GRADE IV**

The smear shows a pleomorphic hypercellular proliferation with marked nuclear atypia. The cellularity and degree of atypia is consistent with a high-grade astrocytic tumor. In order to make a diagnosis of glioblastoma, necrosis and/or microvascular endothelial proliferation has to be identified. Necrosis is present in the smear as evidenced by acellular pink granular material; therefore, the best answer is glioblastoma, WHO grade IV (choice E).

QCSP, **Glioblastoma,** p 36.

48. B. **GERMINOMA**

The main differential diagnosis for a third ventricular tumor in an adolescent includes germ cell tumor, central neurocytoma, and tumors of the pineal gland. The image shows scattered monomorphic epithelioid cells with clear to eosinophilic cytoplasm and prominent nucleoli and a scattered lymphocytic infiltrate. The presence of the aforementioned 2 distinct cell types is consistent with a germinoma (choice B), similar to that seen in the testes (seminoma) and ovary (dysgerminoma). Other helpful features include the presence of granulomas and scattered syncytiotrophoblastic cells. The epithelioid tumor cells show variable positivity for PLAP, CD117, and OCT4 (nuclear) with scattered reactivity for β-hCG in syncytiotrophoblastic cells. The differentiation between pineocytomas (choice D) and central neurocytomas (choice A) can be extremely difficult as both tumors show a monomorphic population of small tumor cells with hyperchromatic nuclei and scant cytoplasm and rosette formation. Immunohistochemistry is also of little help as both are reactive for synaptophysin and retinal S-antigen; therefore, the distinction often relies on the surgeon/radiologist's impression of whether or not the tumor emanates from the pineal gland. Germinoma tumor cells can be mistaken for oligodendroglial-like cells due to the clear cytoplasm, but the location should prevent this misidentification as oligodendrogliomas (choice E) arise preferentially in the cortex and white matter of the cerebral hemispheres. The patient is too old for a choroid plexus carcinoma (choice C), and the degree of atypia is incompatible with a diagnosis of choroid plexus carcinoma.

QCSP, **Germinoma,** p 52.

49. B. **CENTRAL NEUROCYTOMA, WHO GRADE II**

The image depicts a uniform, monotonous population of tumor cells characterized by round nuclei with stippled chromatin, inconspicuous nucleoli, and minimal cytoplasm. The presence of perinuclear halos is suggestive of an oligodendroglial component; however, the location and presence of rosettes is inconsistent with an oligodendroglioma (choice A). The most helpful clue to the correct diagnosis is the overall monotony of the cellular proliferation and the identification of neuropil-like areas consistent with a central neurocytoma (choice B). Neuronal differentiation is confirmed with diffuse immunoreactivity to synaptophysin as well as ultrastructural examination showing dense core granules and microtubules. The neuropil-like areas can mimic the perivascular pseudorosettes commonly seen in ependymomas; however, true ependymal rosettes and ependymal canals are not identified. The differentiation from pineocytomas (choice D) is somewhat challenging as they can have a similar morphologic and immunohistochemical profile; however, the described lesion arises from the lateral ventricle and not the third ventricle where pineocytomas occur. The patient is too old for a choroid plexus carcinoma (choice E), and there are no frank signs of malignancy.

QCSP, **Central Neurocytoma**, p 54.

50.   B.   **Dysembryoplastic neuroepithelial tumor, WHO grade I**
Gangliogliomas, dysembryoplastic neuroepithelial tumors (DNTs), and pleomorphic xanthoastrocytomas (PXAs) all typically present with a history of longstanding seizures and most commonly involve the temporal lobe. The neuroimaging of the aforementioned 3 tumors can appear similar; however, PXAs and gangliogliomas are more likely to be cystic with an intramural nodule, while DNTs look like macrogyri or have a pseudopolycystic appearance. The images show a biphasic population of tumor cells with monomorphic oligodendroglial-like cells and neurons floating in a mucinous background. The absence of marked pleomorphism or vacuolated tumor cells is inconsistent with a diagnosis of PXA (choice D). The neuroimaging, clinical history, and identification of a neuronal component are all incompatible with a diagnosis of oligodendroglioma (choice A), although you can be fooled by the oligodendroglial-like cells. Extraventricular neurocytomas (choice C) are rare and tend to present as a single cyst with an intramural nodule. As the name implies, extraventricular neurocytomas look similar to central neurocytomas; however, these tumors can contain ganglion cells. If present, the ganglioid cells are mixed within the tumor and do not form the characteristic architectural pattern depicted in the image above. The main differential is between a ganglioglioma and DNT, and the imaging and low-power impression is the most helpful in distinguishing between these 2 entities. DNTs (choice B) are confined to the cortex and have a multinodular architecture with foci of cortical dysplasia, glial nodules, and glioneuronal elements which are characterized by columns of oligodendroglial-like cells with neurons "swimming" within the cystic fluid as depicted in the image above. While the neoplastic glial component in a ganglioglioma (choice E) can be comprised of oligodendrocytes, it is more commonly an astrocytic component. In addition, the neuronal component in a ganglioglioma is obviously dysplastic with scattered binucleated neurons. The best answer is dysembryoplastic neuroepithelial tumor (choice).

QCSP, **Dysembryoplastic Neuroepithelial Tumor**, p 55.

51.   C.   **PTEN**
The image depicts a proliferation of neurons with eosinophilic cytoplasm, large nuclei, and prominent nucleoli. The neurons vary in size and shape. Given the cerebellar location, the image is consistent with a dysplastic gangliocytoma of the cerebellum or Lhermitte-Duclos disease which is associated with Cowden syndrome characterized by a PTEN mutation (choice C) on chromosome 10q23. NF1 (choice A) on chromosome 17q11 is mutated in neurofibromatosis type 1 and is characterized in the nervous system by neurofibromas, malignant peripheral nerve sheath tumors, optic nerve gliomas, and astrocytomas. VHL (choice B) on chromosome 3p25 is mutated in von Hippel-Lindau disease and is characterized in the nervous system by hemangioblastomas. TSC1 (choice D) on chromosome 9p34 is mutated in tuberous sclerosis and is characterized in the nervous system by subependymal giant cell astrocytomas and cortical tubers. INI1 (choice E) on chromosome 22q11.2 is mutated in rhabdoid tumor predisposition syndrome and is characterized in the nervous system by atypical teratoid/rhabdoid tumor.

QCSP, **Ganglioglioma and Gangliocytoma**, p 56.

also occur in this location. Due to the presence of squamous nests, this tumor can be mistaken for a metastatic squamous cell carcinoma (choice C), particularly in the adult population.

QCSP, **Intraoperative Consultation,** p 32.

61.   E.   **METASTATIC MELANOMA**

Melanoma's reputation as the "great imitator" holds true in the brain. Metastatic amelanotic melanoma is often difficult to differentiate from a high-grade glioma on smear/frozen material, and both tumors can appear infiltrative on neuroimaging studies. It is helpful to have the clinical history at your disposal as well as the recognition that in the adult population the most common brain tumor is a metastatic neoplasm. Although high-grade gliomas can have areas of hemorrhage, metastatic melanomas often bleed. Other metastatic tumors that frequently bleed include renal cell carcinoma and choriocarcinoma. The H&E-stained image shows a monomorphic plasmacytoid cellular proliferation with pseudonuclear inclusions and prominent nucleoli. No pigment is identified; however, the tumor cells are weakly immunoreactive for melan-A, consistent with metastatic melanoma (choice E).

QCSP, **Intraoperative Consultation,** p 32.

62.   C.   **RADIATION CHANGES**

The image depicts large areas of geographic necrosis, gliosis, and hyalinized vessels, which are characteristic changes induced by radiation (choice C). It is imperative to know the clinical history of radiation treatment because otherwise one could interpret the necrosis as high-grade transformation and give an incorrect diagnosis of glioblastoma (choice B). Sometimes the history is not available but fortunately there are a few clues to help distinguish between radiation changes and high-grade transformation. Pseudopalisading tumor cells characteristically surround the necrosis in glioblastomas, while radiation induces geographic necrosis. The vessels can also be helpful as radiation causes hyalinization of the vasculature, while glioblastomas have microvascular endothelial proliferation with "glomeruloid" capillary structures. The material is diagnostic (choice E) even though the lesion is not a neoplasm. Although the lesion is technically infarcted tissue (choice D), the more specific answer is radiation changes (choice C). Typical infarcts are characterized by eosinophilic neurons that represent anoxic or ischemic changes and microcystic degeneration with gliosis and a variably prominent inflammatory infiltrate depending on the age of the lesion.

QCSP, **Intraoperative Consultation,** p 32.

63.   C.   **LYMPHOMA**

The key to the diagnosis is the recognition of the tumor cell propensity to "hug" the vessels. This angiocentric pattern with infiltration of the vessel walls by tumor cells is characteristic of primary CNS lymphoma (choice C). Primary CNS lymphomas are often hypercellular and infiltrative and may have foci of necrosis similar to high-grade gliomas. Immunohistochemistry for B- and T-cell markers as well as GFAP will help distinguish primary CNS lymphomas from high-grade gliomas (choices A-B). The incidence of primary CNS lymphoma is rising due to the AIDS epidemic but is also increasing in the immunocompetent population. The most common primary CNS lymphoma is diffuse large B-cell lymphoma. Be aware of the fact that steroids are often given to patients before surgery to decrease cerebral edema which also treats the lymphoma, leaving very few neoplastic cells on the biopsy. Molecular studies with gene rearrangements may be required in these circumstances to identify the neoplastic population. The lymphocytes in this case are too atypical for a diagnosis of encephalitis (choice D). Metastatic melanoma (choice E) will not have the prominent angiocentric pattern so characteristic of primary CNS lymphoma and may show melanin pigment, plasmacytoid features, and/or pseudonuclear inclusions.

QCSP, **Intraoperative Consultation,** p 32.

Chapter 3

Endocrine

1. Associations with adrenal cortical adenomas include all of the following EXCEPT:
    A. MEN1
    B. Li-Fraumeni syndrome
    C. Carney complex
    D. McCune-Albright syndrome
    E. Myelolipoma

2. Which of the following is a clinical feature more frequently associated with malignancy in adrenal cortical neoplasms?
    A. Female predominance
    B. Right > left adrenal gland
    C. Virilization and feminization
    D. Cushing syndrome
    E. Bilaterality

3. Which of the following immunohistochemical stains will likely be **negative** in adrenal cortical carcinomas?
    A. Inhibin-A
    B. Vimentin
    C. Synaptophysin
    D. Chromogranin A
    E. C and D

4. All of the following features can be seen in ganglioneuromas EXCEPT:
    A. Schwann cells
    B. Ganglion cells
    C. Homer Wright rosettes
    D. Collagen
    E. Lymphocytes

5. The most common site for neuroblastoma is:
    A. Ovary
    B. Posterior mediastinum
    C. Urinary bladder
    D. Adrenal gland
    E. Gastrointestinal tract

6. The differential diagnosis for neuroblastoma includes all of the following EXCEPT:
    A. Rhabdomyosarcoma
    B. Lymphoma
    C. Pheochromocytoma
    D. Ewing sarcoma/primitive neuroectodermal tumor
    E. Desmoplastic small round cell tumor

7. Which of the following factors does not significantly influence prognosis in neuroblastoma?
    A. Age <1 year
    B. Lymph node status at the time of diagnosis
    C. Lesions outside the adrenal gland
    D. Expression of *Trk* gene
    E. DNA hyperdiploidy

3: Endocrine Questions

8. Which of the following factors does not significantly influence prognosis in neuroblastoma?
    A. N-myc oncogene amplification
    B. Diploid karyotype
    C. Decreased ratio of VMA to homovanillic acid
    D. Cytogenetic abnormalities of chromosome 1
    E. Individual treatment modality

9. What is the single most important prognostic factor for neuroblastoma?
    A. Age
    B. Stage
    C. N-myc amplification
    D. Location
    E. Mitosis-karyorrhexis index (MKI)

10. What percentage of familial pheochromocytomas are bilateral?
    A. 5%
    B. 10%
    C. 20%
    D. 50%
    E. 80%

11. Syndromes associated with pheochromocytoma include all of the following EXCEPT:
    A. Beckwith-Wiedemann syndrome
    B. MEN type II
    C. von Hippel-Lindau disease
    D. Von Recklinghausen disease
    E. Sturge-Weber syndrome

12. All of the following are histologic features that are commonly seen with pheochromocytomas EXCEPT:
    A. Areas of hemorrhage and necrosis that disrupt architecture
    B. Prominent lymphocytic infiltrate
    C. Amyloid
    D. Prominent vascularity of the stroma
    E. Intracytoplasmic hyaline globules

13. Features that are reliably predictive of malignant pheochromocytoma include:
    A. Pleomorphism
    B. Mitotic activity
    C. Hemorrhage and necrosis
    D. A and B
    E. None of the above

14. Which variant of paraganglioma has the highest rate of malignancy?
    A. Bronchial paraganglioma
    B. Cardiac paraganglioma
    C. Intraabdominal (extraadrenal) paraganglioma
    D. Carotid body paraganglioma
    E. Jugular paraganglioma

3: Endocrine Questions

15. Which of the following variants of paraganglioma is/are more common in women?
    A. Laryngeal paraganglioma
    B. Vagal paraganglioma
    C. Jugulotympanic paraganglioma
    D. A and B
    E. All of the above

16. Carney triad is composed of which 3 of the following?
    A. Functioning extraadrenal paraganglioma
    B. Pulmonary chondroma
    C. Papillary carcinoma of the thyroid
    D. Gastric epithelioid leiomyosarcoma
    E. Hyperparathyroidism

17. What is the estimated 5-year survival of extra-adrenal paragangliomas with metastatic disease that is limited to lymph nodes?
    A. 10%
    B. 20%
    C. 50%
    D. 80%
    E. 95%

18. All of the following histologic features can be used to differentiate between parathyroid tissue and a microfollicular thyroid adenoma EXCEPT:
    A. Solid or sheet-like patterns of growth within the nodule
    B. Thick fibrous bands coursing through the gland
    C. Circumscribed foci of oxyphil cells
    D. Presence of various cell types, including chief cells, clear cells, and oxyphil cells
    E. Presence of fat within the lesion

19. Which of the following features is associated with secondary rather than primary chief cell hyperplasia?
    A. MEN, types I and IIa
    B. Chronic renal disease
    C. Symptoms identical to those of parathyroid adenoma
    D. All 4 glands variably enlarged
    E. Superior glands tend to be larger than inferior glands

20. A greater degree of pleomorphism would be expected in which of the following entities?
    A. Parathyroid adenoma
    B. Primary chief cell hyperplasia
    C. Secondary chief cell hyperplasia
    D. Tertiary chief cell hyperplasia
    E. Clear cell hyperplasia

21. Parathyroid hyperplasia is most commonly associated with which of the following?
    A. MEN I
    B. MEN IIA
    C. MEN IIB
    D. MEN I and IIA are equally associated with parathyroid hyperplasia.
    E. None of the above

3: Endocrine Questions

22. Which of the following statements regarding parathyroid adenoma is TRUE?
    A. It is the second most common cause of primary hyperthyroidism.
    B. Most occur during the 7th and 8th decades of life.
    C. Men are more commonly affected than women.
    D. It is less commonly associated with MEN syndromes than primary chief cell hyperplasia.
    E. It is more commonly seen in the superior glands.

23. Of the 10% of parathyroid adenomas found in anomalous locations, 70% occur where?
    A. Within the thyroid gland
    B. Behind the esophagus or in the esophageal wall
    C. Mediastinum
    D. Pericardium
    E. Soft tissue adjacent to the angle of the jaw

24. Histologic features of parathyroid adenomas may include all of the following EXCEPT:
    A. A rim of nonneoplastic chief cells
    B. Foci of enlarged, hyperchromatic nuclei
    C. Cystic structures, sometimes filled with eosinophilic material mimicking thyroid colloid
    D. Up to 6 mitotic figures/20 hpf
    E. Sparse stroma

25. All of the following are true regarding parathyroid carcinomas EXCEPT:
    A. They classically demonstrate a thick tumor capsule and thick fibrous bands within the tumor.
    B. Few patients present with symptoms of hyperparathyroidism and hypercalcemia.
    C. They affect men and women equally.
    D. Capsular invasion and vascular invasion are characteristic features.
    E. Nuclear pleomorphism is commonly only mild to moderate.

26. Which of the following prognostic features is true for parathyroid carcinoma?
    A. Local recurrence is common and typically occurs early (within 3 years).
    B. Metastatic disease occurs early (within 2 years).
    C. Metastatic disease is ultimately seen in the vast majority of patients (approximately 80%).
    D. The most common non-lymph node site for metastasis is liver (40% of cases).
    E. The tumor cells are very radiosensitive.

27. Adamantinomatous and papillary craniopharyngiomas differ in all respects EXCEPT:
    A. Age of affected patients
    B. Cystic vs solid nature
    C. Recurrence risk
    D. Degree of adherence to surrounding structures
    E. Treatment

28. Is a child with a pituitary adenoma more or less likely than an adult to have a functional (ie, secreting) lesion?
    A. More likely
    B. Less likely
    C. Equally likely
    D. It depends on the sex of the child.
    E. Unknown, as children are far less likely to have pituitary neoplasms

3: Endocrine Questions

29. All of the following are true regarding pituitary adenomas EXCEPT:
    A. Tumor cells differentiate towards cells of the adenohypophysis.
    B. There is equal prevalence in males and females.
    C. They have a predictably slow growth rate.
    D. They are rarely multiple.
    E. The most common variant is the prolactinoma.

30. Which of the following statements is TRUE regarding the growth pattern of pituitary adenomas?
    A. They tend to displace, rather than infiltrate the brain parenchyma, even if they are invasive.
    B. They may invade locally (usually lateral to involve the cavernous sinus or the dura).
    C. They usually grow in a glandular pattern.
    D. A and B are both true.
    E. All of the above are true.

31. How often is Cushing disease seen in patients with biochemically functioning corticotroph cell adenomas?
    A. 20%
    B. 40%
    C. 60%
    D. 80%
    E. 100%

32. Intraoperative distinction between papillary thyroid carcinoma and medullary carcinoma is essential because:
    A. Papillary thyroid carcinoma is well-differentiated and only a lobectomy is required, whereas a total thyroidectomy is required for medullary carcinoma.
    B. Only clinically suspicious nodes will be removed for papillary thyroid carcinoma, whereas a compartmental dissection is performed for medullary carcinoma.
    C. Calcitonin levels will be measured intraoperatively to direct surgical management for medullary carcinoma but not papillary thyroid carcinoma.
    D. Medullary carcinoma will receive postoperative radiation therapy and papillary thyroid carcinoma will not.
    E. The distinction is inconsequential

33. Intraoperative assessment of thyroid lesions is appropriate for which 3 of the following?
    A. To determine the presence and type of malignancy
    B. To direct lymph node sampling
    C. To determine why a thyroid gland appears unresectable
    D. To distinguish follicular adenoma from minimally invasive follicular carcinoma
    E. To distinguish between a hyperplastic nodule and an adenoma

34. Evaluation for which thyroid neoplasm is greatly aided by a touch or scrape preparation?
    A. Papillary carcinoma
    B. Follicular carcinoma
    C. Medullary carcinoma
    D. Insular carcinoma
    E. Anaplastic carcinoma

35. Which of the following neoplasms can be especially difficult to diagnose on frozen section or scrape preparation?
    A. Papillary thyroid carcinoma
    B. Lymphoma
    C. Medullary carcinoma
    D. Insular carcinoma
    E. Anaplastic carcinoma

3: Endocrine Questions

36. All of the following clinical or gross features are associated with fibrosing (Riedel) thyroiditis EXCEPT:
    A. Patients are generally hypothyroid, almost always with a history of antecedent acute inflammation of the gland.
    B. There is asymmetric involvement by fibrosis.
    C. There is involvement of surrounding soft tissue with obliteration of normal tissue planes.
    D. There is a "rock hard" gland that is difficult to section.
    E. Steroid therapy is occasionally effective.

37. Associations with fibrosing (Riedel) thyroiditis include which of the following:
    A. Hashimoto thyroiditis
    B. Granulomatous thyroiditis
    C. It may be part of a group of disorders characterized by fibrosis of the mediastinum or retroperitoneum, sclerosing cholangitis, or inflammatory pseudotumor of the orbit.
    D. Pituitary adenoma
    E. Radiation exposure

38. Serum antibodies to which of the following can be seen with Hashimoto thyroiditis?
    A. Thyroglobulin
    B. Thyroid peroxidase
    C. TSH receptors
    D. Iodine transporter
    E. All of the above

39. The inflammatory infiltrate seen in Hashimoto thyroiditis is best characterized by:
    A. Mixed acute and chronic inflammation
    B. Dense lymphoid and plasmacytic infiltrate with large follicles and prominent germinal centers
    C. Scant lymphoid infiltrate, more prominent within the interlobular fibrous bands
    D. Lymphoid infiltrate consisting primarily of B cells versus T cells
    E. Primarily IgA-containing plasma cells with lambda light chains

40. The most common malignancy associated with Hashimoto thyroiditis is:
    A. Lymphoma
    B. Plasmacytoma
    C. Mucoepidermoid carcinoma
    D. Medullary carcinoma
    E. Papillary carcinoma

41. Which form of thyroiditis is associated with postpartum women?
    A. Hashimoto thyroiditis
    B. Acute thyroiditis
    C. Granulomatous thyroiditis
    D. Subacute lymphocytic thyroiditis
    E. Both B and D

42. Which form of thyroiditis is typically PAINLESS at presentation?
    A. Hashimoto thyroiditis
    B. Acute thyroiditis
    C. Granulomatous thyroiditis
    D. Subacute lymphocytic thyroiditis
    E. Both A and D

3: Endocrine Questions

43. A useful histologic feature to distinguish Hashimoto thyroiditis from subacute lymphocytic thyroiditis is:
    A. Presence of plasma cells
    B. Presence of germinal centers
    C. Ratio of T to B cells
    D. Presence of scattered neutrophils
    E. Both A and B

44. What is the most common cause of hyperthyroidism in children?
    A. Follicular adenoma
    B. Graves disease
    C. Acute thyroiditis
    D. Iatrogenic
    E. None of the above

45. Clinical manifestations of Graves disease include all of the following EXCEPT:
    A. Strong female bias
    B. Atrial fibrillation
    C. Hyperthyroidism
    D. Hypothyroidism
    E. Pretibial myxedema and thyroid acropachy

46. Which of the following features is/are more commonly found in follicular carcinomas than follicular adenomas?
    A. Multiple lesions/nodules
    B. Thick capsule
    C. Small follicles with increased cell:lumen ratio and scant colloid
    D. Fibrous septa throughout the lesion
    E. A, B, and D

47. All of the following molecular alterations are associated with follicular adenoma EXCEPT:
    A. Expression of *ras*-oncogene p21 antigen is higher than in normal thyroid
    B. Rearrangements of the peroxisome proliferators-activated receptor (PPARγ) gene
    C. Aneuploid cell populations
    D. Gene for Cowden disease (chromosome 10q22-23)
    E. All of the above

48. Which of the following patterns are more likely to be associated with follicular carcinoma than follicular adenoma?
    A. Solid
    B. Trabecular
    C. Microfollicular
    D. All of the above
    E. None of the above

49. All of the following statements regarding the management and prognosis of follicular carcinoma are true EXCEPT:
    A. Minimally invasive carcinoma has a good prognosis, with >80% survival at 10 years.
    B. Widely invasive carcinoma has a poor prognosis, with tumor mortality approximating 50%.
    C. A compartmental lymph node dissection is indicated.
    D. Adjuvant radioactive iodine may be used to treat metastatic disease.
    E. Age affects prognosis.

3: Endocrine Questions

50. Which of the multiple endocrine neoplasia syndromes are associated with medullary thyroid carcinoma?
    A. MEN I
    B. MEN IIA
    C. MEN IIB
    D. All of the above
    E. B and C

51. What percentage of patients with medullary carcinoma have lymph node metastases at initial presentation?
    A. 10%
    B. 30%
    C. 50%
    D. 70%
    E. 90%

52. All of the following microscopic features can be seen in medullary thyroid carcinoma EXCEPT:
    A. Spindle cells
    B. Pseudoinclusions
    C. High mitotic activity
    D. Binucleate and giant cells
    E. Amyloid

53. All of the following immunohistochemical stains are typically positive in medullary thyroid carcinoma EXCEPT:
    A. NSE
    B. CEA
    C. Calcitonin
    D. Low-molecular-weight cytokeratin
    E. All of the above are typically positive.

54. Which of the following portends a worse prognosis in medullary carcinoma?
    A. Sporadic form
    B. Association with MEN IIA
    C. Association with MEN IIB
    D. Both B and C
    E. Female gender

55. Which immunohistochemical stains can help to distinguish between oncocytic adenoma and oncocytic carcinoma?
    A. Keratin
    B. Thyroglobulin
    C. Cytochrome C oxidase
    D. A and B
    E. None of the above

56. Which of the following molecular alterations is associated with oncocytic lesions of the thyroid?
    A. RET oncogene alterations
    B. Expression of p21 *ras*-oncogene
    C. p53 mutations
    D. All of the above
    E. None of the above

3: Endocrine Questions

57. All of the following molecular alterations are commonly associated with papillary thyroid carcinoma EXCEPT:
    A. Aneuploidy in 95% of cases
    B. Rearrangement of RET oncogene
    C. Rearrangement of TRK1
    D. RAS mutation in the follicular variant
    E. Point mutations of BRAF gene

58. Which of the following factors is NOT associated with a worse prognosis in papillary carcinoma?
    A. Regional lymph node metastases
    B. Tall or columnar cell variants
    C. Increasing tumor size
    D. Presence of extrathyroidal extension
    E. Presence of multiple lesions

59. All of the following are associated with papillary thyroid cancer EXCEPT:
    A. Radiation exposure
    B. Hashimoto thyroiditis
    C. MEN syndrome
    D. All are associated with papillary carcinoma.
    E. None are associated with papillary carcinoma.

60. How common are papillary microcarcinomas in autopsy series?
    A. 1%-4%
    B. 4%-20%
    C. 20%-25%
    D. 25%-40%
    E. 50%-60%

61. Which variant of papillary carcinoma is more likely to metastasize to the lungs than conventional papillary carcinoma?
    A. Follicular
    B. Solid/trabecular
    C. Diffuse sclerosing
    D. Tall cell
    E. Columnar cell

62. Which variant of papillary thyroid carcinoma may not display the typical nuclear features of papillary thyroid carcinoma?
    A. Follicular
    B. Solid/trabecular
    C. Diffuse sclerosing
    D. Tall cell
    E. Columnar cell

63. Which molecular alteration is less associated with anaplastic carcinoma than with carcinomas differentiated towards follicular cells of the thyroid?
    A. Expression of *ras*-oncogene p21 antigen
    B. Aneuploidy
    C. p53 mutations
    D. B and C
    E. None of the above

3: Endocrine Questions

64. From which of the following lesions is anaplastic thyroid carcinoma known to arise?
    A. Preexisting well-differentiated thyroid carcinomas
    B. Well-differentiated carcinomas treated with radioactive iodine
    C. Well-differentiated carcinomas treated with external radiation
    D. Longstanding goiter
    E. All of the above

65. Features of the pictured adenomatous lesion include all of the following, EXCEPT:

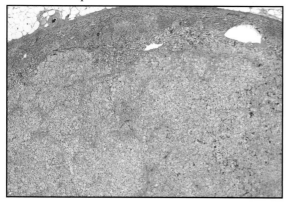 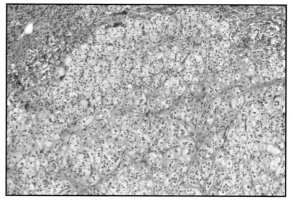

    A. It is more frequent in women than men.
    B. Its weight usually <50 gram.
    C. Its cells are larger and more pleomorphic than their normal counterparts.
    D. The most frequent endocrine abnormality is Cushing syndrome, followed by Conn syndrome.
    E. LOH at 11p15 and the P57 gene locus and IGF2 locus.

66. Criteria for malignancy for adrenal cortical carcinoma (pictured here) include all of the following, EXCEPT:

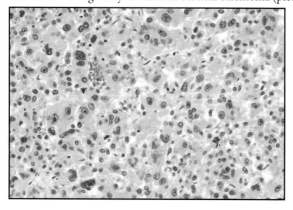

    A. Nuclear pleomorphism and hyperchromasia
    B. Mitotic rate of >5/50 hpf or atypical mitoses
    C. Diffuse architecture in >30% of the tumor
    D. Necrosis
    E. Capsular invasion

3: Endocrine Questions

67. The most common site for the lesion depicted in this image is:

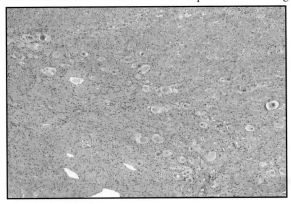

    A.   Retroperitoneum
    B.   Posterior mediastinum
    C.   Urinary bladder
    D.   Adrenal gland
    E.   Gastrointestinal tract

68. The tumor shown below arose from the adrenal gland of an 11-month-old boy and produced vanillylmandelic acid (VMA). It should be positive for all of the following immunohistochemical stains, EXCEPT:

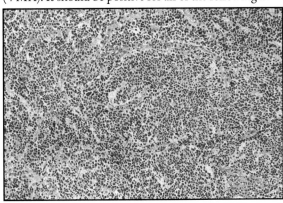 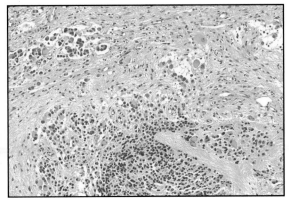

    A.   Epinephrine
    B.   Norepinephrine
    C.   NSE
    D.   Chromogranin A
    E.   S100

3: Endocrine Questions

69. A 50-year-old man presents with a mass of the right adrenal gland and a history of recent hypertension that has been difficult to control. An adrenal mass is resected with the following histology (see image). You perform immunostains to confirm your diagnosis. Which will most likely be negative?

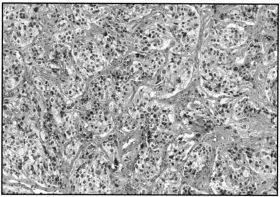

    A.   Vimentin

    B.   Chromogranin A

    C.   Synaptophysin

    D.   Inhibin

    E.   S100

70. This adrenal mass was found incidentally in a 60-year-old patient undergoing abdominal imaging following a trauma. Which of the following statements regarding this lesion are FALSE?

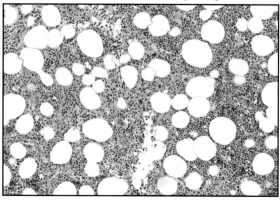

    A.   This lesion is typically bilateral.

    B.   This lesion has a higher incidence in obese patients.

    C.   This lesion is reported to occur in association with Castleman disease.

    D.   Foci of necrosis, hemorrhage, and cyst formation are commonly seen.

    E.   Symptomatic lesions may cause hematuria, hypertension, and rarely retroperitoneal hemorrhage.

3: Endocrine Questions

71. The distinction between a parathyroid adenoma and a hyperplastic parathyroid gland, pictured below, can be made on pathologic examination when which of the following conditions is/are met?

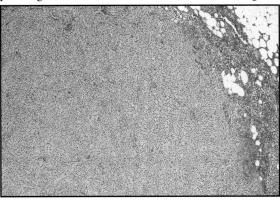 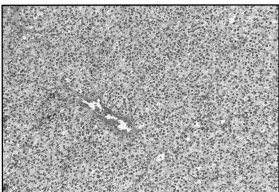

    A.   The weight of the gland is >50.0 mg.
    B.   The intraoperative PTH values decrease after removal of the tissue.
    C.   Imaging supports a predominant nodule.
    D.   All of the above
    E.   The distinction should not be attempted based solely on pathologic examination.

72. The lesion shown below is located in the suprasellar region of a 15-year-old male. The most likely diagnosis is:

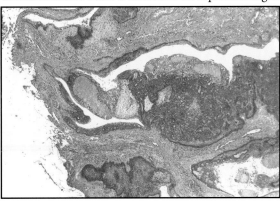 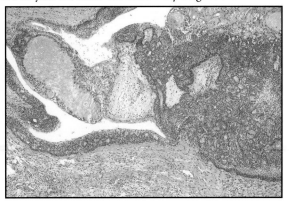

    A.   Rathke cleft cyst
    B.   Pituitary adenoma
    C.   Papillary craniopharyngioma
    D.   Adamantinomatous craniopharyngioma
    E.   Epidermoid cyst

3: Endocrine Questions

73. The following lesion was biopsied from a 45 year-old woman with a history of visual abnormalities. The lesion was found extending into the 3rd ventricle. What is the diagnosis?

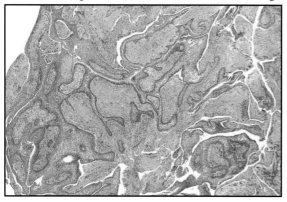 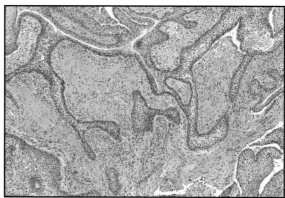

    A.   Pilocytic astrocytoma
    B.   Epidermoid cyst
    C.   Papillary craniopharyngioma
    D.   Adamantinomatous craniopharyngioma
    E.   Pituitary adenoma

74. What percentage of these sellar lesions have evidence (biochemical and/or clinical) of hormone production?

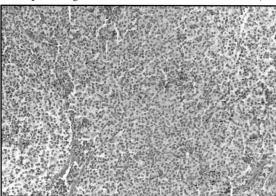

    A.   20%
    B.   30%
    C.   50%
    D.   70%
    E.   90%

3: Endocrine Questions

75. Other entities, including the one pictured here, to consider in the differential diagnosis of fibrosing (Riedel) thyroiditis include all of the following, EXCEPT:

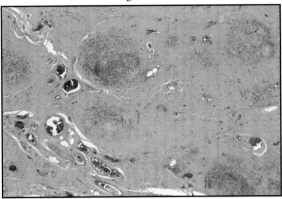 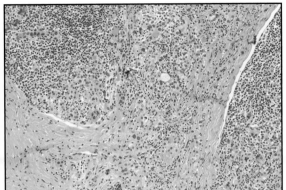

    A.   Intense desmoplastic reaction to papillary carcinoma
    B.   Prominent sclerosis of large cell lymphoma
    C.   Fibrous variant of Hashimoto thyroiditis
    D.   Spindle cell type of anaplastic carcinoma
    E.   Parathyroid carcinoma

76. Clinical features that can help to distinguish fibrosing (Riedel) thyroiditis from the entity in the image include:

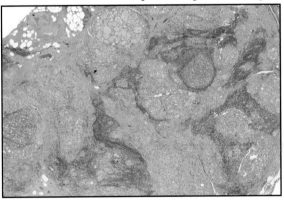

    A.   History of euthyroidism, hypothyroidism, or hyperthyroidism
    B.   Distribution of gland enlarged/affected
    C.   Age and sex of the patients typically affected
    D.   A and B
    E.   A, B, and C

3: Endocrine Questions

77.　Microscopic features of the entity pictured here commonly include all of the following, EXCEPT:

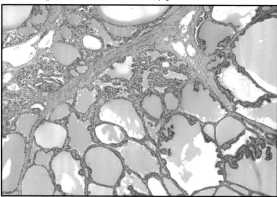 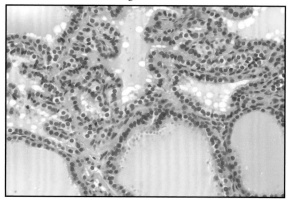

- A.　Fibrosis
- B.　Marked hypertrophy and hyperplasia of follicles with crowded epithelium
- C.　Small papillary-like projections of follicular cells without fibrovascular cores
- D.　Stromal lymphoid aggregates with germinal centers
- E.　Oncocytic cells

78.　Gross examination of the lesion pictured here often reveals all of the following EXCEPT:

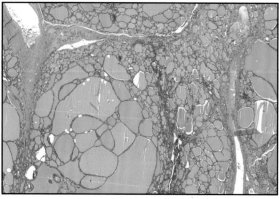

- A.　Areas of hemorrhage
- B.　Fibrotic areas
- C.　Focal calcification
- D.　Areas of cystic degeneration
- E.　All of the above can be seen.

3: Endocrine Questions

79. Which of the following findings meets the criteria for minimally invasive follicular thyroid carcinoma?

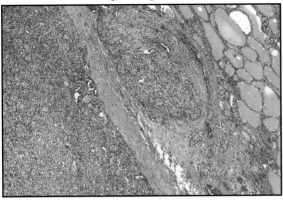 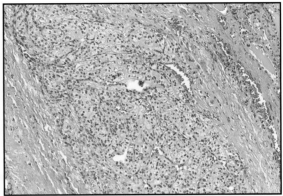

    A.   Mushroom-shaped tumor within the capsule
    B.   Sharp tumor bud into but not through the capsule
    C.   Tumor follicles completely surrounded by capsule and aligned parallel to the capsule
    D.   Tumor follicles completely surrounded by capsule and aligned perpendicular to the capsule
    E.   None of the above

80. All of the following clinical features help to distinguish the familial from sporadic form of the pictured thyroid lesion EXCEPT:

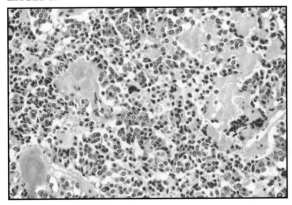

    A.   Familial lesions are more likely to be bilateral.
    B.   Familial lesions are more likely to be multiple.
    C.   Familial lesions are more likely to be seen in women than sporadic lesions.
    D.   Familial lesions tend to present at an earlier age than sporadic lesions.
    E.   All of the above are true.

3: Endocrine Questions

81. Which of the following microscopic features help to predict the clinical behavior of the pictured thyroid lesions?

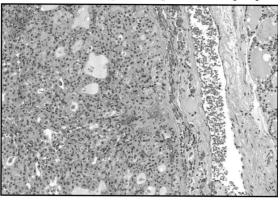 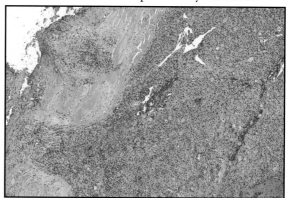

    A.   Trabecular or solid (versus follicular) growth pattern

    B.   Nuclear features, including higher N:C ratio with tall or columnar cells, scattered bizarre hyperchromatic nuclei, and cellular pleomorphism

    C.   Increased numbers of mitotic figures

    D.   All of the above

    E.   None of the above

82. All of the following are common microscopic features of the neoplasm pictured, EXCEPT:

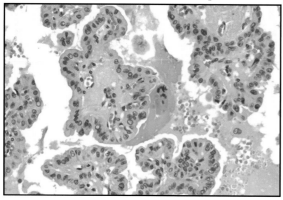

    A.   Marked irregularity of nuclear membranes

    B.   Deposition of chromatin along the inner wall of the nuclear membrane

    C.   Nucleolus pushed up against the inner wall of the nuclear membrane

    D.   Conspicuous mitotic figures

    E.   Bland cytoplasm

3: Endocrine Questions

83. Which immunohistochemical stain can help distinguish between normal follicular cells and cells of the neoplasm pictured here?

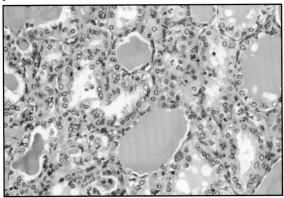

    A.   Low-molecular-weight cytokeratin
    B.   High-molecular-weight cytokeratin
    C.   Thyroglobulin
    D.   All of the above
    E.   None of the above

84. All of the following are typical microscopic features of the neoplasm pictured EXCEPT:

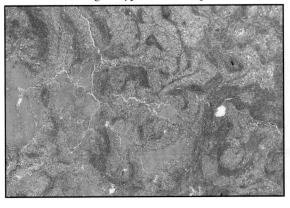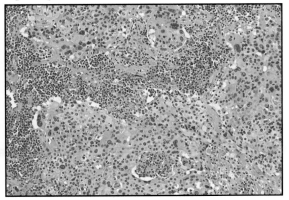

    A.   Uniform small round cells with little cytoplasm
    B.   Solid growth pattern
    C.   Conspicuous mitotic figures
    D.   Prominent vascular invasion
    E.   All are features that can be present.

3: Endocrine Questions

85. Which morphologic pattern of anaplastic carcinoma (pictured here) demonstrates the greatest degree of pleomorphism?

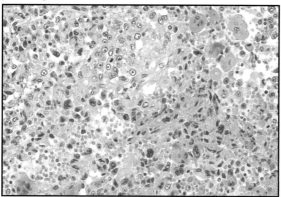

   A.   Squamoid
   B.   Spindle cell
   C.   Large cell
   D.   All of the above
   E.   None of the above

86. Which morphologic pattern of anaplastic carcinoma most commonly demonstrates foci of neoplastic cartilage and bone?

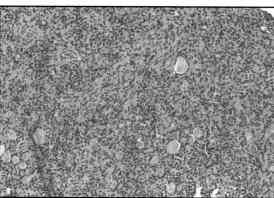

   A.   Squamoid
   B.   Spindle cell
   C.   Large cell
   D.   All of the above
   E.   None of the above

3: Endocrine Answers

1. B. **LI-FRAUMENI SYNDROME**

    Li-Fraumeni syndrome is associated with adrenal cortical carcinoma and includes kindreds predisposed to a wide variety of malignant tumors, including breast carcinoma and soft tissue sarcomas (2 most frequent), bone sarcomas, adrenal cortical carcinoma, brain tumors, and leukemia. Beckwith-Wiedemann syndrome is also associated with adrenal cortical carcinoma and is characterized by enlargement of body organs, hemihypertrophy, renal medullary cysts, adrenal cytomegaly, and an increased risk for the development of a Wilms tumor. All of the other choices are associated with adrenal cortical adenomas. MEN I (choice A) consists of parathyroid hyperplasia/adenomas, pancreatic islet cell neoplasia, and pituitary adenomas. Carney complex (choice C) is also known as "LAMB syndrome" and "NAME syndrome" and is an autosomal dominant condition with myxomas of the heart and skin, hyperpigmentation of the skin, and endocrine overactivity. McCune-Albright syndrome (choice D) is a genetic disorder of bones (polyostotic fibrous dysplasia), skin pigmentation (café-au-lait spots) and hormonal abnormalities.

    QCSP, **Adrenal Cortical Adenoma,** p 68.

2. C. **VIRILIZATION AND FEMINIZATION**

    Adrenal cortical neoplasms with associated virilization or feminization are more likely to be malignant (particularly feminization). However, 75% of adrenal cortical carcinomas are not associated with any syndrome of hormone overproduction. A female predominance is seen in both adenomas and carcinomas. No laterality predominance is seen with adenomas, but the left adrenal gland is involved more frequently than the right by carcinomas. Bilateral neoplasms are quite rare.

    QCSP, **Adrenal Cortical Adenoma,** p 68.

3. D. **CHROMOGRANIN A**

    Tumor cells are frequently positive for inhibin-A and are usually positive for vimentin. They are frequently positive for synaptophysin but are uniformly negative for chromogranin. Chromogranin A is a reliable stain to discriminate adrenal cortical carcinoma from adrenal medullary tumors. Tumor cells are also typically negative or only weakly positive for cytokeratin while normal adrenal cortical cells are uniformly keratin-positive and adrenal cortical adenomas are generally positive.

    QCSP, **Adrenal Cortical Carcinoma,** p 70.

4. C. **HOMER WRIGHT ROSETTES**

    Homer Wright rosettes are present in 25%-35% of neuroblastomas and consist of tumor cells arranged around a central area filled with neuritic fibrillary material. The Schwann cell population predominates in ganglioneuromas, which are typically arranged in small fascicles separated by a loose myxoid stroma. Mature or nearly mature ganglion cells are diffusely distributed or arranged in small clusters. Ganglion cell differentiation may be seen in neuroblastomas (< 5% in poorly-differentiated, > 5% in differentiated, and none in undifferentiated). Variable amounts of collagen are seen in ganglioneuromas, and lymphocytes are commonly present. Lymphocytes can also be seen in neuroblastomas, sometimes in clusters that may obscure the primary tumor. Mast cells can also be seen in ganglioneuromas.

    QCSP, **Neuroblastoma and Ganglioneuroblastoma,** p 72.

5. D. **ADRENAL GLAND**

    Like ganglioneuromas, neuroblastomas parallel the distribution of the sympathetic nervous system. 70% of neuroblastomas and ganglioneuroblastomas occur in the retroperitoneum and the majority of neuroblastomas involve the adrenal gland. The ratio of adrenal to extraadrenal neuroblastomas is approximately 2:1. They also occur in the head and neck region, mediastinum, and pelvis.

    QCSP, **Neuroblastoma and Ganglioneuroblastoma,** p 72.

3: Endocrine Answers

6.   C.   **PHEOCHROMOCYTOMA**

All of the other choices are in the "small round blue cell category." Renal and extrarenal malignant rhabdoid tumors would also be included in the differential with neuroblastoma. While pheochromocytomas are found in the adrenal gland, they are typically found in adults in the 5th decade of life and do not have small round blue cell morphology.

QCSP, **Neuroblastoma and Ganglioneuroblastoma,** p 72.

7.   B.   **LYMPH NODE STATUS AT THE TIME OF DIAGNOSIS**

Lymph node status at the time of diagnosis does not significantly influence prognosis. The other choices are all associated with improved prognosis. The Trk gene encodes a nerve growth factor receptor and is present in 90% of cases. Additional factors that positively influence prognosis include the presence of lymphocyte infiltration and the presence of S100 protein-positive cells.

QCSP, **Neuroblastoma and Ganglioneuroblastoma,** p 72.

8.   E.   **INDIVIDUAL TREATMENT MODALITY**

Individual treatment modality does not significantly influence prognosis. The other choices are all associated with a poor prognosis. N-myc oncogene amplification is seen in 25%-30% of patients and chromosome 1 abnormalities include deletion of 1p. Other factors associated with a poor prognosis include age greater than one year and increased serum levels of NSE, ferritin, lactate dehydrogenase, chromogranin A, and creatine kinase BB.

QCSP, **Neuroblastoma and Ganglioneuroblastoma,** p 72.

9.   B.   **STAGE**

Stage is the most important prognostic factor associated with neuroblastoma. The MKI is the number of mitotic figures and karyorrhectic nuclei per 5,000 cells in randomly selected fields. Low index = lower than 100, intermediate index = 100-200, and high index = higher than 200.

QCSP, **Neuroblastoma and Ganglioneuroblastoma,** p 72.

10.   D.   **50%**

While pheochromocytomas are known as the "10%" tumors, over 50% of these tumors are bilateral in familial cases (it is the "familial" modifier that matters here). Only 5% of sporadic cases are bilateral. The 10% rule refers to the overall incidence of bilaterality, extraadrenal location (paraganglioma), malignancy, occurrence in childhood, and percentage of cases that are familial. Sorry if that was mean and remember to read the questions carefully!

QCSP, **Pheochromocytoma,** p 75.

11.   A.   **BECKWITH-WIEDEMANN SYNDROME**

All of the other syndromes are associated with pheochromocytoma. Beckwith-Wiedemann syndrome (exomphalos, macroglossia, and gigantism) is associated with neuroblastoma. MEN IIA includes medullary thyroid carcinoma, pheochromocytoma, and parathyroid hyperplasia. MEN IIB includes medullary thyroid carcinoma, pheochromocytoma, and mucosal and gastrointestinal neuromas.

QCSP, **Pheochromocytoma,** p 75.

12.   B.   **PROMINENT LYMPHOCYTIC INFILTRATE**

A prominent lymphocytic infiltrate is not a feature associated with pheochromocytoma. Dystrophic calcifications, nuclear pseudoinclusions, pleomorphism, mitotic figures, and brown adipose tissue adjacent to the neoplasm can also be seen.

QCSP, **Pheochromocytoma,** p 75.

3: Endocrine Answers

13. E. **NONE OF THE ABOVE**
     It is notoriously difficult to predict malignant behavior based on histologic features for pheochromocytomas. While some areas of pheochromocytomas may be markedly hyperchromatic and pleomorphic, these findings do not correlate with malignant behavior. Mitotic figures may be seen but do not necessarily indicate malignancy. Areas of hemorrhage and/or necrosis may disrupt cellular architecture but are also not predictive of malignancy. Metastasis is the only definitive and agreed-upon determinant of malignancy for pheochromocytomas.
     QCSP, **Pheochromocytoma,** p 75.

14. C. **INTRAABDOMINAL (EXTRAADRENAL) PARAGANGLIOMA**
     Intraabdominal (extraadrenal) paragangliomas tend to be the most aggressive of the paragangliomas, with an incidence of malignancy (metastasis or local invasion) of 15%-50%. They are divided into superior paraaortic (45%), inferior paraaortic (30%) and urinary bladder groups and have also been reported in the kidney, urethra, prostate, spermatic cord, gallbladder, uterus, ovary, vagina, vulva, and hepatobiliary tree. Cardiac paragangliomas arise within the pericardium. Carotid body paragangliomas are seen at the angle of the mandible and can cause carotid sinus syndrome (bradycardia and syncopal episodes) and are rarely malignant. Jugular paragangliomas are also very rarely malignant but can be locally aggressive with body destruction and intracranial extension possible.
     QCSP, **Extraadrenal Paraganglioma,** p 78.

15. E. **ALL OF THE ABOVE**
     There is an increased occurrence of laryngeal paraganglioma, vagal paraganglioma, and jugulotympanic paraganglioma in women.
     QCSP, **Extraadrenal Paraganglioma,** p 78.

16. A, B, AND D
     Not to be confused with Carney *syndrome*, which has myxomas of cardiac, skin and breast origin, lentiginosis and blue nevi, and endocrine tumors involving the adrenal gland, testis, and pituitary glands as well as schwannomas.
     QCSP, **Extraadrenal Paraganglioma,** p 78.

17. D. **80%**
     The 5-year survival is as high as 80% even with metastatic disease in the lymph nodes. If distant metastases are present, the 5-year survival is only approximately 10%.
     QCSP, **Extraadrenal Paraganglioma,** p 78.

18. B. **THICK FIBROUS BANDS COURSING THROUGH THE GLAND**
     The presence of thick fibrous bands coursing through the lesion is somewhat helpful for differentiating between a parathyroid carcinoma and a parathyroid adenoma. Foci of necrosis, mitotic activity, diffuse nuclear atypia, and invasion into adjacent soft tissue are additional features of parathyroid carcinoma. The rest of the choices (A, C-E) are features that can be present in parathyroid tissue that are not expected in microfollicular thyroid adenomas. Intrathyroidal parathyroid glands can further complicate this diagnostic challenge.
     QCSP, **Parathyroid Gland,** Intraoperative Consultation, p 82.

19. B. **CHRONIC RENAL DISEASE**
     Secondary chief cell hyperplasia is typically seen in patients with chronic renal disease whose parathyroid glands are chronically stimulated due to persistent low levels of ionized calcium in the blood. It is also associated with dietary deficiency of vitamin D, abnormal vitamin D metabolism, and pseudohypoparathyroidism (target organ unresponsiveness to PTH, as seen in Albright hereditary osteodystrophy). The remaining choices are all related to primary chief cell hyperplasia.
     QCSP, **Parathyroid Hyperplasia,** p 82.

3: Endocrine Answers

20. **A.** **PARATHYROID ADENOMA**

Primary chief cell hyperplasia can demonstrate slight pleomorphism, but it is usually not as extensive as that seen in a typical adenoma. The characteristic cell seen in secondary chief cell hyperplasia is large and vacuolated with a small, dense eccentric nucleus. Clear cell hyperplasia is very rare and demonstrates cells that are polygonal with clear cytoplasm (filled with small vacuoles of glycogen) and distinct cell membranes.

QCSP, **Parathyroid Hyperplasia,** p 82.

21. **A.** **MEN I**

Approximately 20% of patients with primary chief cell hyperplasia have one of the MEN syndromes. 90% of patients with MEN I, 30%-40% with MEN IIA, and very few with MEN IIB will have parathyroid hyperplasia. Recall that MEN I is characterized by synchronous or metachronous hyperplasias, tumors, or both involving parathyroid glands, pancreatic islets, and the anterior pituitary gland (the 3 "P"s). These patients also have an increased incidence of bronchogenic and gastrointestinal carcinoids, adrenal cortical adenomas, and thyroid follicular neoplasms. MEN IIA is characterized by medullary carcinoma of the thyroid, pheochromocytoma, and parathyroid hyperplasia. MEN IIB includes pheochromocytoma, medullary carcinoma of the thyroid, and ocular, oral, and gastrointestinal ganglioneuromatosis, megacolon, marfanoid habitus, pes cavus, and other skeletal abnormalities.

QCSP, **Parathyroid Hyperplasia,** p 82.

22. **D.** **IT IS LESS COMMONLY ASSOCIATED WITH MEN SYNDROMES THAN PRIMARY CHIEF CELL HYPERPLASIA.**

Most parathyroid lesions in the MEN syndromes represent chief cell hyperplasia rather than adenoma. Parathyroid adenoma is the single most common cause of primary hyperthyroidism; 80% of patients with primary hyperparathyroidism have a single adenoma. Most adenomas occur in a younger population, particularly during the 4th and 5th decades of life. Adenomas (and hyperplasia) are more common in women than men (3:1). The inferior glands are more frequently involved (75% of adenomas).

QCSP, **Parathyroid Adenoma,** p 84.

23. **C.** **MEDIASTINUM**

70% of anomalously-located parathyroid adenomas are found in the mediastinum. 20% are within the thyroid gland. The remainder occur in the soft tissue behind the esophagus or in the esophageal wall, pericardium, vagus nerve, and soft tissue adjacent to the angle of the jaw.

QCSP, **Parathyroid Adenoma,** p 84.

24. **D.** **UP TO 6 MITOTIC FIGURES/20 HPF**

Mitotic figures are typically absent in parathyroid adenomas. Malignancy should be considered if >1 mitotic figure/10 hpf is detected. A rim of nonneoplastic chief cells is commonly seen, and up to 25% of adenomas may demonstrate enlarged, hyperchromatic nuclei (not a criterion for carcinoma). If nuclear pleomorphism is present, it is generally localized. Cystic structures surrounded by chief cells may be present and may contain colloid-like eosinophilic material that is negative for thyroglobulin. Stroma is typically sparse.

QCSP, **Parathyroid Adenoma,** p 84.

25. **B.** **FEW PATIENTS PRESENT WITH SYMPTOMS OF HYPERPARATHYROIDISM AND HYPERCALCEMIA.**

Patients with parathyroid carcinoma usually have profound hyperparathyroidism and hypercalcemia, with serum calcium levels in excess of 14.0 mg/dL and markedly elevated levels of PTH. Nephrolithiasis and bone disease are common (seen in up to 65%) and some patients have a palpable neck mass. Unlike with hyperplasia and adenoma, men and women are equally affected by parathyroid carcinoma. Classic features include a thick collagenous capsule and intratumoral fibrous bands extending from the capsule into the tumor parenchyma. Capsular and vascular invasion are strongly supportive of carcinoma, although these features are only seen in 65%

and 15% of cases, respectively. Nuclear pleomorphism is commonly only mild to moderate but occasional tumors have more marked variability.

QCSP, **Parathyroid Carcinoma,** p 86.

26.   A.   **LOCAL RECURRENCE IS COMMON AND TYPICALLY OCCURS EARLY (WITHIN 3 YEARS).**
Well-performed initial en bloc resection results in a 50% cure rate but there is a high probability of local recurrence (typically seen within 3 years). Metastatic disease to regional nodes and distant sites may occur late and 35% of patients will ultimately develop metastases, most commonly to the lung (40%) followed by the cervical lymph nodes (30%) and liver (10%). The tumor cells are not radiosensitive. The 5-year survival is around 85%, and the 10-year survival is around 50%.

QCSP, **Parathyroid Carcinoma,** p 86.

27.   E.   **TREATMENT**
Adamantinomatous craniopharyngioma affects patients in the first 2 decades of life. It forms a calcified cystic suprasellar mass that frequently has an intrasellar component and adheres to structures at the base of the brain and may be locally invasive. Papillary craniopharyngioma affects adults, presenting as a solid, noncalcified mass, frequently in the 3rd ventricle and is typically an encapsulated solid mass that can be separated from surrounding brain tissue. Surgical excision is the treatment of choice for both variants, with radiation reserved for lesions that cannot be completely excised. Adamantinomatous lesions are more likely to recur than papillary lesions, usually within 5 years of surgery.

QCSP, **Craniopharyngioma,** p 87.

28.   A.   **MORE LIKELY**
Pituitary adenomas occur more frequently in adults; however, the majority of adenomas that occur in children and adolescents are functional.

QCSP, **Pituitary Adenoma,** p 89.

29.   C.   **THEY HAVE A PREDICTABLY SLOW GROWTH RATE.**
The cells of pituitary adenomas recapitulate cells of the adenohypophysis and may therefore be basophilic, acidophilic, or amphophilic. These neoplasms affect men and women equally. While the vast majority are benign, they can demonstrate a variable and unpredictable growth rate. They are very rarely multiple (about 1%). Prolactinomas are the most common neoplasm of the adenohypophysis.

QCSP, **Pituitary Adenoma,** p 89.

30.   D.   **A AND B ARE BOTH TRUE.**
20%-80% of tumors are invasive, depending on the type. Invasive tumors tend to invade local structures and infiltrate the dura, floor of the sella, and nasal sinus and will penetrate the cavernous sinus laterally. Occasionally, tumors can be "giant" with >20 mm of extension beyond the jugum sphenoidal superiorly. The tumor cells only rarely grow in glandular patterns. Diffuse (solid), sinusoidal (trabecular), or papillary (pseudopapillary) arrangements are much more common.

QCSP, **Pituitary Adenoma,** p 89.

31.   D.   **80%**
80% of ACTH-producing adenomas are associated with Cushing disease. 10% are hormonally silent. 15% are associated with Nelson syndrome, which is caused by the loss of negative corticosteroid feedback after removal of hyperplastic adrenal glands in patients with Cushing syndrome. This results in rapid enlargement of the pituitary neoplasm.

QCSP, **Pituitary Adenoma,** p 89.

32.   B.   **ONLY CLINICALLY SUSPICIOUS NODES WILL BE REMOVED FOR PAPILLARY THYROID CARCINOMA, WHEREAS A COMPARTMENTAL DISSECTION IS PERFORMED FOR MEDULLARY CARCINOMA.**
      Determining the type of malignancy is relevant to surgical management when considering papillary and medullary thyroid carcinoma. Surgical management of papillary thyroid carcinoma includes complete thyroidectomy and removal of clinically involved lymph nodes. Medullary carcinoma also warrants a complete thyroidectomy; however, a formal compartment (usually central) lymph node dissection is also completed. Intraoperative calcitonin levels are not used for surgical management and postoperative radiation planning does not hinge on intraoperative assessment.
      QCSP, **Thyroid Gland,** Intraoperative Consultation, p 91.

33.   A, B, AND C
      Unresectability due to anaplastic carcinoma, malignant lymphoma, or sclerosing thyroiditis is an important distinction for the surgeon, and if lymphoma is suspected, then the specimen should be triaged appropriately for flow cytometric analysis. Minimally invasive follicular carcinoma is distinguished from adenoma only by evaluating the entire capsule, which is not practical at the time of frozen section. Intraoperative evaluation of an area grossly suspicious for invasion would be reasonable.
      QCSP, **Thyroid Gland,** Intraoperative Consultation, p 91.

34.   A.   PAPILLARY CARCINOMA
      While cytologic evaluation is generally a quick and easy way to assess lesions intraoperatively, it is particularly useful to evaluate for papillary thyroid cancer as many of the classic features associated with this neoplasm are present on scrape preparations. Papillary structures and nuclear details such as clearing and grooves may be easier to see.
      QCSP, **Thyroid Gland,** Intraoperative Consultation, p 91.

35.   C.   MEDULLARY CARCINOMA
      Insular and anaplastic thyroid carcinomas are generally straightforward at frozen section. The diagnosis of follicular variant of papillary thyroid carcinoma can be difficult, but can be aided by a scrape or touch preparation. Medullary thyroid carcinoma can be very difficult in the absence of amyloid because it can have various atypical patterns.
      QCSP, **Thyroid Gland,** Intraoperative Consultation, p 91.

36.   A.   **PATIENTS ARE GENERALLY HYPOTHYROID, ALMOST ALWAYS WITH A HISTORY OF ANTECEDENT ACUTE INFLAMMATION OF THE GLAND.**
      Most patients are euthyroid and there is no antecedent history of acute inflammation. The other statements are true.
      QCSP, **Fibrosing (Riedel) Thyroiditis,** p 92.

37.   C.   **IT MAY BE PART OF A GROUP OF DISORDERS CHARACTERIZED BY FIBROSIS OF THE MEDIASTINUM OR RETROPERITONEUM, SCLEROSING CHOLANGITIS, OR INFLAMMATORY PSEUDOTUMOR OF THE ORBIT.**
      There is no relationship between fibrosing thyroiditis and granulomatous thyroiditis or Hashimoto thyroiditis. Additionally, there is no association with pituitary adenoma or radiation exposure. However, fibrosing thyroiditis (Riedel thyroiditis) can be associated with other fibrosing diseases such as fibrosis of the mediastinum or retroperitoneum, sclerosing cholangitis, or inflammatory pseudotumor of the orbit.
      QCSP, **Fibrosing (Riedel) Thyroiditis,** p 92.

3: Endocrine Answers

38.   E.   **ALL OF THE ABOVE**
A variety of autoantibodies are associated with Hashimoto thyroiditis including those against thyroglobulin, thyroid cell microsomal proteins (such as thyroid peroxidase), TSH receptors, and iodine transporter.
QCSP, **Hashimoto Thyroiditis**, p 93.

39.   B.   **DENSE LYMPHOID AND PLASMACYTIC INFILTRATE WITH LARGE FOLLICLES AND PROMINENT GERMINAL CENTERS**
A dense infiltrate of lymphoid and plasma cells with follicles and germinal centers is typical for Hashimoto thyroiditis (refer to the lesion in question 49). The lymphoid cells consist of a roughly equal ratio of T and B cells. In contrast to Riedel thyroiditis, plasma cells in Hashimoto thyroiditis express kappa to lambda light chains 2:1 (vs the 70% lambda expression in fibrosing thyroiditis) and only 15% of the immunocytic population consists of IgA-containing plasma cells (versus 45% in Riedel thyroiditis).
QCSP, **Hashimoto Thyroiditis**, p 93.

40.   A.   **LYMPHOMA**
Lymphoma, especially B-cell type, is the most common malignancy associated with Hashimoto thyroiditis. All of the other choices except for medullary carcinoma do have an increased risk in Hashimoto thyroiditis.
QCSP, **Hashimoto Thyroiditis**, p 93.

41.   D.   **SUBACUTE LYMPHOCYTIC THYROIDITIS**
Subacute lymphocytic thyroiditis is more common in women, especially postpartum. Acute thyroiditis is generally seen in the immunocompromised (malnourished, debilitated, and otherwise immunocompromised), and granulomatous and Hashimoto thyroiditis is usually seen in middle-aged women.
QCSP, **Thyroiditis**, p 94.

42.   E.   **BOTH A AND D**
Both acute and granulomatous thyroiditis typically cause pain. Acute thyroiditis is associated with trauma and often presents with a painful enlarged gland. Granulomatous thyroiditis presents differently, with sore throat and tenderness, and systemic symptoms such as fever and malaise are often present.
QCSP, **Thyroiditis**, p 94.

43.   E.   **BOTH A AND B**
Choices A and B are both helpful features, as the presence of plasma cells and follicles with germinal centers are rare in subacute lymphocytic thyroiditis and suggest Hashimoto thyroiditis when present.
QCSP, **Thyroiditis**, p 94.

44.   B.   **GRAVES DISEASE**
Graves disease (diffuse toxic goiter) is the most common cause of hyperthyroidism in children.
QCSP, **Graves Disease (Diffuse Toxic Goiter)**, p 96.

45.   D.   **HYPOTHYROIDISM**
Graves disease affects young adult women at a rate approximately seven times that of men. Patients can occasionally present in atrial fibrillation, but more commonly exhibit typical signs of hyperthyroidism including weight loss, increase in appetite, muscle weakness, irritability, tachycardia and exophthalmos. Longstanding disease can result in an infiltrative ophthalmopathy, pretibial myxedema (localized infiltrative dermopathy) or thyroid acropachy (periosteal new bone formation resulting in swollen extremities and clubbing of fingers and toes). Hashimoto thyroiditis can initially have hyperthyroidism followed by hypothyroidism, but hypothyroidism is not a symptom of Graves disease.
QCSP, **Graves Disease (Diffuse Toxic Goiter)**, p 96.

3: Endocrine Answers

46.   E.   **A, B, AND D**
Follicular adenomas are typically solitary nodules with a thin fibrous capsule and a distinct interface. A thick capsule is (somewhat paradoxically) more characteristic of follicular carcinoma and should be examined completely for microinvasive disease. While a central stellate fibrous scar may be seen in follicular adenoma, fibrous septa coursing through the lesion should raise the suspicion for follicular variant of papillary thyroid carcinoma. Small, uniform follicles are characteristic of the common microfollicular variant of follicular adenoma.
QCSP, **Follicular Adenoma**, p 99.

47.   B.   **REARRANGEMENTS OF THE PEROXISOME PROLIFERATORS-ACTIVATED RECEPTOR γ (PPARγ) GENE**
Rearrangements of the PPARγ gene are associated with follicular carcinoma and are seen in 25%-50% of cases. Aneuploid cell populations are seen in approximately 30% of follicular adenomas and 60% of carcinomas. Follicular adenomas are very common in patients with Cowden syndrome (follicular adenoma and carcinoma of the thyroid; GI polyps including hamartomas, lipomas, lymphoid, ganglioneuromas and inflammatory; fibrocystic disease of the breast and breast cancer; facial trichilemmomas; papillomatosis of lips and oropharynx; multiple lipomas and hemangiomas; high arched palate; hypoplasia of the jaw; central nervous system anomalies).
QCSP, **Follicular Adenoma**, p 99.

48.   D.   **ALL OF THE ABOVE**
Atypical patterns are also more commonly seen in follicular carcinoma.
QCSP, **Follicular Carcinoma**, p 100.

49.   C.   **A COMPARTMENTAL LYMPH NODE DISSECTION IS INDICATED.**
Minimally invasive follicular carcinoma has a good prognosis with a 10-year survival of 80% while widely invasive lesions have a very poor prognosis. If the patient has had a total thyroidectomy, then metastatic disease can be treated with radioactive iodine, and tumors that do not take up this iodine have a worse prognosis. Multifocal disease and age >50 years are also poor prognostic factors.
QCSP, **Follicular Carcinoma**, p 100.

50.   E.   **B AND C**
Both MEN IIA and MEN IIB are associated with medullary thyroid cancer. MEN I includes parathyroid hyperplasia and neoplasia, pancreatic islet cell tumors, and pituitary lesions (the 3 "P"s). MEN IIA includes C-cell hyperplasia and medullary thyroid carcinoma, adrenal medullary hyperplasia and pheochromocytoma, and parathyroid hyperplasia and adenoma. MEN IIB includes the same thyroid and adrenal findings but, instead of parathyroid hyperplasia, patients also have ocular, oral, and gastrointestinal ganglioneuromatosis, marfanoid habitus, and various skeletal abnormalities.
QCSP, **Medullary Carcinoma**, p 101.

51.   C.   **50%**
Approximately half of patients with medullary thyroid carcinoma have lymph node metastases when they present. The likelihood is great enough to warrant compartmental lymph node dissection as the standard of care.
QCSP, **Medullary Carcinoma**, p 101.

52.   C.   **HIGH MITOTIC ACTIVITY**
Medullary thyroid carcinoma has a variety of microscopic appearances, which can make the diagnosis more difficult. The classic growth pattern is insular, but lobular, trabecular, and solid patterns can also be present. Tumor cells can be round, polygonal, and spindle-shaped. The cytoplasm is usually eosinophilic to amphophilic, but can be clear as in the clear cell variant (which can mimic metastatic renal cell carcinoma) or contain mucin vacuoles. There is a papillary variant with papillary or pseudopapillary growth patterns and cytoplasmic pseudoinclusions, sometimes making the distinction between papillary and medullary carcinoma difficult. There

is also a giant cell variant with syncytiotrophoblastic-type cells admixed with more classic medullary cells that can be confused with anaplastic carcinoma. Amyloid is a characteristic feature of this tumor and is seen in about 80% of cases. C-cell hyperplasia is also commonly seen in familial cases. Other histologic variants of medullary carcinoma include follicular (mimicking follicular carcinoma/adenoma), encapsulated (mimicking hyalinized trabecular variant of follicular adenoma), small cell (mimicking lymphoma), oncocytic, and squamous cell.
QCSP, **Medullary Carcinoma**, p 101.

53.　E.　**ALL OF THE ABOVE ARE TYPICALLY POSITIVE.**
All 4 immunohistochemical stains are typically positive, and synaptophysin and chromogranin should be added to that list as well. Interestingly, chromogranin is both more specific and more sensitive than calcitonin (the small cell variant, in particular, can be negative for calcitonin, but amyloid is typically positive). Virtually all tumors are positive for CEA and serum levels can also be elevated and used as a marker to follow for disease recurrence. 80% of tumors are also positive for bcl-2.
QCSP, **Medullary Carcinoma**, p 101.

54.　C.　**ASSOCIATION WITH MEN IIB**
Lesions arising in the setting of MEN IIB affect younger patients (average age 15 years) and are more aggressive, with early metastases and a 5-year survival of <5%. Patients with known MEN IIB should have a prophylactic thyroidectomy in early childhood. The size of the tumor and presence of metastases (which correlates with tumor size; only 20% if <0.7 cm but 80% if >1.5 cm) is more important for sporadic lesions and those associated with MEN IIA. Younger patients and women also do better.
QCSP, **Medullary Carcinoma**, p 101.

55.　E.　**NONE OF THE ABOVE**
All 3 of these stains are generally positive in both oncocytic adenomas and carcinomas. Cytochrome C oxidase is an enzyme in the mitochondrial respiratory chain that is highly expressed in oncocytic cells.
QCSP, **Oncocytic (Hürthle Cell) Carcinoma**, p 104.

56.　B.　**EXPRESSION OF P21 *RAS*-ONCOGENE**
Expression of p21 *ras*-oncogene is typically present in both oncocytic adenoma and carcinoma. Germline mutations in the RET oncogene are associated with both familial and sporadic medullary thyroid carcinoma. Mutations in p53 are sometimes seen in both insular and anaplastic carcinomas.
QCSP, **Oncocytic (Hürthle Cell) Carcinoma**, p 104.

57.　A.　**ANEUPLOIDY IN 95% OF CASES**
Most papillary thyroid carcinomas are diploid; only 20% are aneuploid. Aneuploidy is more commonly seen in undifferentiated (anaplastic) carcinoma. The papillary thyroid carcinoma (PTC) RET oncogene is on chromosome 10q11-q12 and TRK1 is located on chromosome 1q22. RAS mutation is seen in 45% of follicular variants of papillary thyroid carcinoma. Point mutations in the BRAF gene are seen as commonly as 70% of the time.
QCSP, **Papillary Carcinoma**, p 105.

58.　A.　**REGIONAL LYMPH NODE METASTASES**
Regional lymph node metastases do not affect the long-term prognosis of patients with papillary thyroid cancer, though distant metastases do. The tall and columnar cell variants do tend to behave more aggressively. Tumors >1.5 cm in size also do worse, as do those with multiple lesions and extrathyroidal extension.
QCSP, **Papillary Carcinoma**, p 105.

59.　D.　**ALL ARE ASSOCIATED WITH PAPILLARY CARCINOMA.**

A history of radiation exposure to the neck and Hashimoto thyroiditis are both associated with papillary thyroid carcinoma. While MEN syndrome is more commonly associated with medullary thyroid carcinoma, there is a lesser association with papillary thyroid carcinoma, and papillary thyroid carcinoma can also occur in a familial setting. There is also an increased incidence seen with ataxia-telangiectasia.

QCSP, **Papillary Carcinoma**, p 105.

60.　B.　**4%-20%**

Papillary microcarcinomas are <1.0 cm in diameter and are present in 4%-20% of thyroids at autopsy.

QCSP, **Papillary Carcinoma**, p 105.

61.　C.　**DIFFUSE SCLEROSING**

The diffuse sclerosing variant of papillary thyroid carcinoma is more likely than conventional papillary thyroid carcinoma to metastasize to the lungs. It is characterized by numerous papillae within intrathyroidal lymph vessels, extensive squamous metaplasia, marked fibrosis, numerous psammoma bodies, and a lymphocytic infiltrate. There is a high incidence of cervical lymph node involvement. It may be clinically misdiagnosed as thyroiditis, resulting in delay in appropriate treatment.

QCSP, **Papillary Carcinoma**, p 105.

62.　E.　**COLUMNAR CELL**

The columnar cell variant of papillary thyroid carcinoma demonstrates prominent nuclear stratification of cells covering papillary stalks. The histology is often reminiscent of secretory endometrium, POD3, with subnuclear vacuoles and clear cytoplasm.

QCSP, **Papillary Carcinoma**, p 105.

63.　A.　**EXPRESSION OF *RAS*-ONCOGENE P21 ANTIGEN**

Expression of *ras*-oncogene p21 antigen is seen less commonly in anaplastic carcinoma than other carcinomas with differentiation towards follicular cells of the thyroid.

QCSP, **Undifferentiated (Anaplastic) Carcinoma**, p 109.

64.　E.　**ALL OF THE ABOVE**

Anaplastic thyroid carcinomas have been reported to arise in the following: preexisting well-differentiated thyroid carcinomas (papillary or follicular), well-differentiated carcinomas treated with radioactive iodine, well-differentiated carcinomas treated with external radiation, and long-standing goiter.

QCSP, **Undifferentiated (Anaplastic) Carcinoma**, p 109.

65.　D.　**THE MOST FREQUENT ENDOCRINE ABNORMALITY IS CUSHING SYNDROME, FOLLOWED BY CONN SYNDROME.**

The image depicts an adrenal cortical adenoma. Both adrenal cortical adenomas and carcinomas occur more commonly in women. Adenomas are typically <50 g, whereas carcinomas are commonly >100.0 g and 10.0 cm in size. The cells of adenomas can be larger and more pleomorphic than normal cortical cells, and the adjacent cortex, with the exception of the glomerulosa layer, is often atrophic. Cells usually demonstrate single, round nuclei with a small single nucleolus. Mitotic figures are rare. The most frequent endocrine abnormality is Conn syndrome (primary aldosteronism), followed by Cushing syndrome. Reported molecular alterations include LOH at 11p15 and the P57 and IGF2 locus as well as overexpression of IGF2 and overexpression of FGFR at 7p12.

QCSP, **Adrenal Cortical Adenoma**, p 68.

3: Endocrine Answers

66.   A.   **Nuclear pleomorphism and hyperchromasia**

While a high grade is included in histopathologic criteria for malignancy, nuclear pleomorphism and hyperchromasia, although usually present, are not diagnostic of malignancy. Criteria for malignancy include the other choices listed, as well as invasion of venous structures and eosinophilic cytoplasm in >75% of cells. Having 3 or more of these features correlates with malignant behavior (Weiss system).

QCSP, **Adrenal Cortical Carcinoma,** p 70.

67.   B.   **Posterior mediastinum**

This is an image of a ganglioneuroma. While ganglioneuromas can be seen in all of the listed sites, they are most commonly seen in the posterior mediastinum, followed by the retroperitoneum. They occasionally arise in the adrenal gland and have also been reported in the cervical and parapharyngeal areas, urinary bladder, prostate and appendix. They can also occur in the gastrointestinal tract as a polypoid lesion.

QCSP, **Ganglioneuroma,** p 71.

68.   A.   **Epinephrine**

The image on the left represents an area of tumor consistent with neuroblastoma, and the image on the right represents an area consistent with ganglioneuroblastoma (note the mature ganglion cells as well as the immature elements). Neuroblastoma and ganglioneuroblastoma are positive for NSE, chromogranin A, synaptophysin and neurofilament proteins. Tumor cells are always positive for norepinephrine and always negative for epinephrine. S100 protein will stain fibrovascular septa surrounding the nodules of tumor cells (these cells occupy the same area that sustentacular cells occupy in paragangliomas). S100-positive sustentacular cells often surround maturing ganglion cells. Neuroblastoma (NB), ganglioneuroblastoma (GNB) and ganglioneuroma (GN) represent entities along a spectrum of maturation, with neuroblastoma being the most immature. If there is <50% schwannian stroma, the tumor should be classified as NB. If there is no ganglion cell differentiation and no neuropil, then it is considered undifferentiated. A GN, on the other end of the spectrum, is composed of Schwann cells and scattered, small clusters of mature ganglion cells with no neuroblastic cells. GBN lies in the middle of the spectrum, with some foci of neuroblastic elements as well as other areas of maturation. Both GNB and GN have >50% schwannian stroma (the first step in decision-making). However, if the foci of neuroblastic elements are large enough to form a distinct nodule, then the tumor is classified as nodular ganglioneuroma and you classify the neuroblastic nodule itself as undifferentiated, poorly differentiated, or differentiating.

QCSP, **Neuroblastoma and Ganglioneuroblastoma,** p 72.

69.   D.   **Inhibin**

The pheochromocytoma tumor cells are immunoreactive for vimentin, chromogranin A and synaptophysin, while the sustentacular cells surrounding the nests of tumor cells react strongly for S100. Inhibin is negative in pheochromocytomas but is positive in adrenal cortical adenomas and in most adrenal cortical carcinomas. Therefore, inhibin may be helpful for correctly diagnosing a pheochromocytoma with extensive vacuolization that morphologically overlaps with adrenal cortical tumors. Pheochromocytomas are usually negative for cytokeratin but can be positive in up to 25% of cases.

QCSP, **Pheochromocytoma,** p 75.

70.   A.   **This lesion is typically bilateral.**

This is an image of a myelolipoma. Myelolipomas comprise <5% of primary adrenal tumors and are typically solitary and unilateral. They are usually present in patients over 30 years of age and are typically discovered incidentally. They are composed of a variable mixture of mature adipose tissue with scattered islands of hematopoietic elements demonstrating trilineage hematopoiesis. Foci of necrosis, hemorrhage, and cyst formation are not uncommon and focal areas of calcification with bony trabeculae may be present. The lesion is benign.

QCSP, **Myelolipoma,** p 81.

3: Endocrine Answers

71. E. **THE DISTINCTION SHOULD NOT BE ATTEMPTED BASED SOLELY ON PATHOLOGIC EXAMINATION.**
The distinction between a parathyroid adenoma and a hyperplastic parathyroid gland cannot be made on pathologic examination and should not be attempted. Generally, it is enough to provide the surgeon with the information that parathyroid tissue is present and whether it appears to be hypercellular (though even this distinction can be difficult given the normal range of cellularity). Weight should be obtained on any parathyroid specimen. Glands weighing >80.0-100.0 mg (generally considered a borderline weight) are often hypercellular. Intraoperative PTH is usually not available at the time of the frozen section.
QCSP, **Parathyroid Gland,** Intraoperative Consultation, p 82.

72. D. **ADAMANTINOMATOUS CRANIOPHARYNGIOMA**
The photomicrograph depicts an adamantinomatous craniopharyngioma, which is histologically characterized by lobules of squamoid epithelial cells that are grouped in a multinodular, cloverleaf pattern resembling adamantinoma of the bone. Cells at the periphery of the lesion are polygonal to columnar and palisaded, while cells in the center are more loosely textured. There may be cystic spaces filled with fluid or amorphous debris, and "wet keratin" is characteristic (nodules of plump, eosinophilic, keratinized cells that may contain dystrophic calcifications). Extensive gliosis, chronic inflammation, and cholesterol clefts are commonly present. Adamantinomatous craniopharyngiomas demonstrate cytokeratin and EMA staining in epithelial cells as well as focal staining for estrogen receptor.
QCSP, **Craniopharyngioma,** p 87.

73. C. **PAPILLARY CRANIOPHARYNGIOMA**
The lesion demonstrates a papillary craniopharyngioma. The lesion shows solid sheets of well-differentiated no-keratinizing squamous epithelial cells with prominent fibrovascular cores, which undergo dehiscence to form pseudopapilla, are characteristic of this lesion (see image). Goblet cells and ciliated cells may be present. Palisading cells and keratin pearls, chronic inflammation and cholesterol clefts are characteristic of adamantinomatous craniopharyngioma. Sometimes, it can be difficult to differentiate this lesion from an epidermoid cyst, which demonstrates a cyst wall lined by stratified squamous epithelium.
QCSP, **Craniopharyngioma,** p 87.

74. D. **70%**
The differential diagnosis of sellar lesions is limited, and the image depicts a pituitary adenoma. 70% of pituitary adenomas have either clinical or biochemical evidence of hormone secretion and 30% are endocrinologically silent. The one in the image secreted GH.
QCSP, **Pituitary Adenoma,** p 89.

75. E. **PARATHYROID CARCINOMA**
Parathyroid carcinoma is generally not included in the differential diagnosis of fibrosing (Riedel) thyroiditis. All of the other entities listed could be considered during histologic review. The lesion depicted in the image is an example of a fibrous variant of Hashimoto thyroiditis.
QCSP, **Fibrosing (Riedel) Thyroiditis,** p 92.

76. D. **A AND B**
Hashimoto thyroiditis is depicted in this image (note the dense mononuclear infiltrate and follicles with germinal centers). Patients with Riedel thyroiditis are typically euthyroid, whereas patients with Hashimoto thyroiditis may initially be hyperthyroid followed by hypothyroidism. The gland is typically diffusely enlarged with Hashimoto thyroiditis but asymmetrically enlarged/hardened in Riedel thyroiditis. Both entities tend to more commonly affect adult women.
QCSP, **Fibrosing (Riedel) Thyroiditis and Hashimoto Thyroiditis,** p 92.-93.

3: Endocrine Answers

77.   A.   **FIBROSIS**

This image depicts Graves disease. Fibrosis is unusual for Graves disease. Hypertrophy and hyperplasia of follicles with crowded columnar epithelium with basally located nuclei are characteristic. These cells may contain fat and glycogen within their cytoplasm. They may form micropapillary structures as well. The colloid is pale and finely vacuolated with characteristic scalloping where it contacts the epithelium. Aggregates of lymphoid tissue, with or without germinal centers, are commonly seen within the stroma. Oncocytic cells may be present and can sometimes indicate evolution towards Hashimoto thyroiditis.

QCSP, **Graves Disease (Diffuse Toxic Goiter)**, p 96.

78.   E.   **ALL OF THE ABOVE CAN BE SEEN.**

This is an image of multinodular goiter. Hemorrhage, calcification, focal fibrosis, and cystic degeneration are all often detected grossly and/or microscopically.

QCSP, **Nodular Hyperplasia (Multinodular Goiter)**, p 97.

79.   E.   **NONE OF THE ABOVE**

Capsular invasion requires penetration of the entire thickness of the capsule and may be covered by a new capsule at the point of penetration. Vascular invasion requires that neoplastic cells be attached to the vessel wall and cause partial or complete occlusion of a vessel that is within or near the tumor capsule. Please see the explanatory notes in the CAP checklist for thyroid carcinoma for an excellent diagram to illustrate these points. The image here depicts true invasion, qualifying as minimally invasive follicular carcinoma.

QCSP, **Follicular Carcinoma**, p 100.

80.   C.   **FAMILIAL LESIONS ARE MORE LIKELY TO BE SEEN IN WOMEN THAN SPORADIC LESIONS.**

The image depicts medullary thyroid carcinoma (note the amyloid). Familial medullary thyroid carcinomas are more likely to be bilateral and multiple, and may present with various endocrinologically-mediated symptoms, while sporadic tumors tend to be solitary. Both usually present as painless nodules. Sporadic lesions are slightly more common in women and tend to occur around middle age, whereas familial tumors arise equally in men and women and occur at an average age of 20 years or less, depending upon the familial association. Because of this, thyroids are often removed prophylactically in patients with a known familial syndrome. Medullary thyroid carcinoma accounts for 5%-10% of all thyroid malignancies. 70% occur in a sporadic setting, and 30% are familial. The familial form and the MEN2 cases are associated with mutations in the RET protooncogene.

QCSP, **Medullary Carcinoma**, p 101.

81.   E.   **NONE OF THE ABOVE**

These are oncocytic or Hürthle cell neoplasms. The image on the left is an adenoma and the image on the right depicts capsular invasion consistent with microinvasive carcinoma (which follows the same criteria as non-oncocytic lesions). None of the listed features alone or in combination can predict the biological behavior of an oncocytic neoplasm. All of these features are more commonly seen in carcinomas, but to predict malignancy, you must see either microscopic or gross evidence of invasion (no different than the requirements for usual-type follicular adenoma versus carcinoma).

QCSP, **Oncocytic (Hürthle Cell) Carcinoma**, p 104.

82.   D.   **CONSPICUOUS MITOTIC FIGURES**

This is papillary thyroid carcinoma. Mitotic figures are usually absent in this relatively well-differentiated tumor. The irregularity of nuclear membranes accounts for both the nuclear grooves commonly seen and the pseudoinclusions formed when cytoplasm invaginates into the nucleus and appears on cut section to be a sharply demarcated cytoplasm-colored round structure. The cytoplasm is typically bland. Nuclei are also enlarged and overlapping. Fibrous stroma is typically present, psammoma bodies are common (50%), and squamous metaplasia and a lymphocytic infiltrate are also not uncommon (roughly 30%).

QCSP, **Papillary Carcinoma,** p 105.

83.   B.   **HIGH-MOLECULAR-WEIGHT CYTOKERATIN**

This is the follicular variant of papillary thyroid carcinoma. The cells of papillary thyroid carcinoma are typically positive for all 3 stains, but normal thyroid follicular cells are typically negative for high-molecular-weight cytokeratin (CK19). HBME is also being used with increasing frequency to help distinguish cells of papillary thyroid cancer (positive). Both estrogen and progesterone receptors can sometimes demonstrate nuclear staining, and tumor cells are also commonly positive for S100, EMA and vimentin. Caveat of high-molecular weight cytokeratin staining is that it will also stain some reactive processes, such as in FNA sites and in degenerative areas.

QCSP, **Papillary Carcinoma,** p 105.

84.   E.   **ALL ARE FEATURES THAT CAN BE PRESENT.**

This is insular carcinoma. Insular carcinoma is somewhere along the biological spectrum between well-differentiated and undifferentiated carcinoma, making the classification of this tumor somewhat ambiguous. The uniform small round cells with little cytoplasm are suggestive of a neuroendocrine lesion, but nuclei lack the classic salt-and-pepper chromatin. A solid growth pattern is common, with small and large foci of necrosis. Mitotic figures are prominent, as is vascular invasion, consistent with a more aggressive neoplasm.

QCSP, **Poorly-Differentiated (Insular) Carcinoma,** p 108.

85.   C.   **LARGE CELL**

The large cell pattern of anaplastic thyroid carcinoma demonstrates marked pleomorphism greater than that seen in the other 2 patterns.

QCSP, **Undifferentiated (Anaplastic) Carcinoma,** p 109.

86.   B.   **SPINDLE CELL**

The spindle cell type of anaplastic thyroid carcinoma (see image) is morphologically indistinguishable from a sarcoma (often resembling malignant fibrous histiocytoma) and may have areas of myxoid change. Foci of neoplastic cartilage and bone are most commonly seen in this pattern. Scattered osteoclast multinucleated giant cells are also sometimes admixed with tumor cells (10% of cases).

QCSP, **Undifferentiated (Anaplastic) Carcinoma,** p 109.

Chapter 4

Breast

1. What is the only appropriate use for frozen section in the case of breast neoplasia?
   A. Rule out microinvasion
   B. Diagnose a malignant phyllodes tumor
   C. To confirm the surgeon's impression of a radial scar
   D. Relieve the patient of anxiety by providing a rapid diagnosis
   E. To assess suspicious lymph nodes

2. Which of the following is NOT critical when grossing a mastectomy specimen?
   A. The oriented specimen should be inked with different colors to facilitate the examination of margins
   B. Bouin solution should be used.
   C. Ideally, sections should be taken perpendicular to the nipple.
   D. Uninvolved breast parenchyma should be sampled from all quadrants.
   E. None of the above

3. Approximately what percentage of women between the ages of 20 and 45 years are affected by fibrocystic changes?
   A. 10%-15%
   B. 20%-25%
   C. 30%-35%
   D. 40%-45%
   E. Almost 80%

4. A 32-year-old woman presents with a 3-cm hard tender mass to her family physician. What is the next appropriate step?
   A. Schedule an excisional biopsy.
   B. Recommend a mammogram.
   C. Perform a fine needle aspiration.
   D. Recommend a trial of estrogen.
   E. Since this is classic Schimmelbusch disease, counsel the patient.

5. All of the following are characteristic of fibrocystic changes EXCEPT:
   A. Dilated, cystic round to oval spaces lined by slightly attenuated epithelial and myoepithelial cell layers
   B. Sclerotic interlobular stroma
   C. Nonoverlapping cells with prominent cytoplasmic membranes
   D. Increased ductules and/or acini per lobule
   E. Abundant hyperplasia

6. A suspicious (BI-RADS 4) lesion is biopsied in a 50-year-old woman. On H&E examination you suspect microglandular adenosis. Which of the following is TRUE about this entity?
   A. The epithelial cells are S100 positive and estrogen receptor negative.
   B. Positive myoepithelial markers will confirm this benign adenosis.
   C. Perineural invasion should not dissuade you from making this diagnosis.
   D. There is no need to completely excise this "lesion."
   E. This is also called sclerosing adenosis.

4: Breast Questions

7.   On review of a core needle biopsy, you suspect sclerosing adenosis. Which of the following is INCORRECT?
     A.   The differential diagnosis includes tubular carcinoma.
     B.   The differential diagnosis includes microglandular adenosis.
     C.   The differential diagnosis includes radial scar.
     D.   The relative risk for development of invasive ductal carcinoma is approximately 5.
     E.   The treatment is local excision.

8.   Which of the following is FALSE regarding radial scars?
     A.   They mimic invasive carcinoma on mammography.
     B.   Most are not visible on gross exam.
     C.   Older lesions tend to be densely hyalinized and fibroelastic centrally.
     D.   Treatment is local excision.
     E.   None of the above

9.   Which of the following is FALSE regarding the microscopic findings of a tubular adenoma of the breast?
     A.   It is well-circumscribed with a delicate fibrous capsule.
     B.   It is composed of aggregates of compact, small, round tubules lined by both epithelial and myoepithelial cell layers.
     C.   Epithelial cells are never atypical but may be mitotically active.
     D.   Epithelial cells are not vacuolated and have no evidence of intracytoplasmic secretory material, but tubular lumens may contain eosinophilic secretory material; lumens are rarely distended.
     E.   50% have lactational and secretory changes.

10. Which of the following clinical manifestations of ductal carcinoma in situ (DCIS) is TRUE?
     A.   It does not present as a palpable mass, Paget disease, or nipple discharge.
     B.   It is rarely detected on mammography, and never incidentally at microscopic examination.
     C.   Comedonecrosis is not seen on mammography as dystrophic calcifications.
     D.   The average age at diagnosis is 55 years.
     E.   Multicentric DCIS (foci of carcinoma in >1 quadrant) is present in approximately 5%-10% of cases.

11. Microscopically, ductal carcinoma in situ (DCIS) does NOT typically show:
     A.   A proliferation of epithelial cells with morphologic features of malignancy confined to the duct system and without evidence of stromal invasion
     B.   Proliferating epithelial cells that may demonstrate various cytologic appearances from minimal atypia to anaplastic; typically ductal cells have a columnar shape and are larger, have more cytoplasm, and are more cohesive than lobular cells.
     C.   Involvement of multiple terminal duct-lobular units with extension into multiple major ducts in 1 or more segments
     D.   An intact myoepithelial cell layer may be present around the duct wall; absence of a myoepithelial layer does not mean invasion has occurred (basement membrane may be intact).
     E.   Comedonecrosis

12. Clinging carcinoma is best characterized by:
     A.   The presence of necrosis, cytologic atypia, and loosely cohesive cells
     B.   A proliferation of a uniform population of cells that form round secondary lumens; the cells surrounding the lumens are columnar with basally oriented nuclei and tend to form rigid arcades or "Roman bridges."
     C.   Proliferating epithelial cells filling and occluding ductal lumens
     D.   Ducts that are lined by several layers of highly atypical cells or 1 or more layer(s) of mildly atypical cells with lumens that are either empty or contain granular secretory material
     E.   Proliferating cells that have abundant granular, eosinophilic cytoplasm with moderate to severe cytologic atypia and central necrosis

4: Breast Questions

13. Which of the following is the appropriate treatment for ductal carcinoma in situ (DCIS)?
    A. Total mastectomy
    B. Simple lumpectomy with negative margins
    C. Simple lumpectomy with 2mm negative margins
    D. Simple lumpectomy with 3mm negative margins
    E. None of the above

14. The BRCA1 gene is located on:
    A. Chromosome 14q32
    B. Chromosome 17p12-23
    C. Chromosome 3p
    D. Chromosome 11q32
    E. Chromosome 16p

15. Which of the following immunohistochemical stains can most reliably differentiate invasive ductal carcinoma from lobular carcinoma?
    A. Cytokeratin 7
    B. p63
    C. E-cadherin
    D. Cytokeratin 20
    E. Caldesmon

16. What is the incidence of invasive carcinoma in women with ductal carcinoma in situ (DCIS)?
    A. 5% or less
    B. 5%-20%
    C. 33%
    D. 40%-50%
    E. All women with ductal carcinoma in situ (DCIS) will have at least some occult invasive carcinoma.

17. What is the incidence of axillary lymph node involvement by metastatic disease in women with ductal carcinoma in situ (DCIS)?
    A. 5% or less
    B. 5%-20%
    C. 33%
    D. 40%-50%
    E. 90%-100%. By definition, intraductal carcinoma is a systemic disease. That is why every sentinel lymph node should be serially sectioned at 2mm and every level should be stained with pancytokeratin.

18. Which of the following is TRUE regarding papillomas?
    A. A myoepithelial layer is absent.
    B. True papillomas do not show evidence of apocrine change.
    C. Papillomas cannot have any solid areas of growth.
    D. Areas of cribriform hyperplasia raise the diagnosis to at least low-grade DCIS.
    E. All papillomas are monoclonal, and the same allele of the X-chromosome–linked phosphoglycerokinase (PGK) gene is inactivated

4: Breast Questions

19. Which of the following papillary lesions are NOT treated by *total* excision?
    A.   Atypical papilloma
    B.   Sclerosing papillomas
    C.   Papillomatosis
    D.   Papilloma
    E.   None of the above

20. Which of the following is/are TRUE regarding atypical papillomas?
    A.   Papillary processes contain focal areas that consist of a proliferation of monotonous cells identical to the cells of low-grade, nonnecrotic DCIS.
    B.   A myoepithelial cell layer may or may not be present.
    C.   The atypical areas of proliferation occupy <1/3 of the lesion.
    D.   S100 and muscle-specific actin will confirm presence or absence of myoepithelial cells.
    E.   All of the above.

21. Papillary carcinoma of the breast:
    A.   Represents 8% of all breast carcinomas
    B.   Does not occur in the male breast
    C.   Shares the same molecular alterations as papillary carcinoma of the thyroid, ovary and lung
    D.   Shows <25% ER positivity; most are HER-2/neu amplified
    E.   Exhibits 10%-15% p53 positivity

22. Regarding lobular carcinoma in situ (LCIS), which of the following is FALSE?
    A.   It is typically found as an incidental finding in a breast biopsy performed on a proliferative lesion.
    B.   It rarely, if ever, produces a palpable mass.
    C.   It tends to be multifocal and multicentric (45%-95%) and bilateral (50%-60%).
    D.   Patients have a significant risk of developing an invasive carcinoma (not necessarily invasive lobular carcinoma).
    E.   The average age at diagnosis is 65 years.

23. Which of the following is TRUE regarding the immunohistochemistry for lobular carcinoma in situ (LCIS)?
    A.   Neoplastic cells usually are positive for both estrogen and progesterone receptors.
    B.   Basal lamina surrounding acinar units is negative for collagen type IV.
    C.   Tumor cells typically demonstrate HER-2/neu (C-erb B-2) amplification (overexpression).
    D.   Actin will confirm the absence of myoepithelial cells.
    E.   Tumor cells are positive for E-cadherin.

24. Which of the following is NOT a biphasic tumor?
    A.   Fibroadenoma
    B.   Juvenile fibroadenoma
    C.   Phyllodes tumor
    D.   Metaplastic carcinoma
    E.   All of the above are biphasic tumors.

25. In the differential diagnosis of juvenile fibroadenoma versus phyllodes tumor, which of the following favors phyllodes tumor?
    A.   It is usually seen between ages of 20 and 30 years of age.
    B.   It is the most common breast lesion in adolescent girls.
    C.   The stroma is more cellular with leaf-like processes, and very rarely demonstrates a pericanalicular (random or concentric) growth pattern.
    D.   The ducts are engulfed by a pericanalicular (random or concentric) arrangement of cellular stroma.
    E.   The stroma is usually much more dense and cellular than that seen in the adult type fibroadenoma.

4: Breast Questions

26. Which of the following is NOT a morphologic characteristic of phyllodes tumor?
    A. High-grade tumors have a hypercellular stroma, 5 or more mitotic figures/10 hpf, moderate to severe stromal atypia, and infiltrating margins.
    B. Tumors are classified as benign, low-grade (potential for local recurrence), and high-grade (potential to metastasize).
    C. The stroma tends to be cellular and consists of spindle-shaped fibroblastic and myofibroblastic cells; the cells tend to condense around the glandular elements.
    D. The epithelial component frequently is hyperplastic with irregular tufts overlying stratified epithelium with an appearance similar to the hyperplasia seen in gynecomastia; marked atypia may be present, reminiscent of intra-ductal carcinoma.
    E. Phyllodes tumor is architecturally characterized by formation of leaf-like processes that protrude into cystic spaces.

27. Which of the following is TRUE regarding invasive ductal carcinoma?
    A. A component of ductal carcinoma in situ (DCIS) is present in 25% of cases.
    B. A dense lymphoplasmacytic infiltrate is present in approximately 20% of cases (the lymphocytic component is composed predominately of T lymphocytes, cytotoxic-suppressor type).
    C. Patients with an extensive DCIS component have a low rate of local recurrence (up to 5%) if treated with breast-conserving surgery and radiation.
    D. Abundant DCIS within the tumor is associated with a high rate of disease free survival.
    E. Tumors typically are graded on the amount of tubule formation, degree of nuclear pleomorphism, and mitotic activity (Bloom-Richardson).

28. Over-expression of the HER-2/neu oncogene is present in what percentage of invasive ductal carcinoma?
    A. 5%-10%
    B. 15%-20%
    C. 25%-30%
    D. 35%-40%
    E. 45%-50%

29. Which of the following is TRUE regarding the prognosis of invasive ductal carcinoma?
    A. Patients with tumors <1 cm without nodal metastasis have a 10-year disease-free survival rate of 90%.
    B. Patients with tumors <2 cm in diameter with negative lymph nodes have a 10-year disease-free survival rate of 50%.
    C. Patients with tumors >2 cm and <5 cm with negative nodes have a 10-year disease-free survival rate of 40%.
    D. Patients with tumors >5 cm with negative nodes have a 10-year disease-free survival rate of <30%.
    E. For tumors <2 cm with 1-3 positive axillary lymph nodes, 10-year disease-free survival rate is 50% (without adjuvant chemotherapy).

30. What is the single most important prognostic factor regarding invasive breast carcinoma?
    A. HER-2/neu expression
    B. ER expression
    C. Presence or absence of axillary lymph node metastasis
    D. Lobular carcinoma type histology (worst prognostic factor)
    E. p53 mutation

31. Which of the following is characteristic of invasive lobular carcinoma?
    A. It is the most common type of invasive breast cancer.
    B. Mitotic figures are rare.
    C. It is rarely multicentric.
    D. It commonly presents as a well-circumscribed mass on physical exam.
    E. Tumor cells are usually ER and PR negative.

4: Breast Questions

32. Tubular carcinoma:
    A. Represents 5%-10% of invasive breast carcinomas
    B. Is multicentric in <10% of cases
    C. Is composed of tubules that tend to be angulated, oval, or elongated with open lumens, and are lined by a single layer of epithelial cells
    D. Often demonstrates angiolymphatic invasion
    E. Is negative for ER by immunohistochemistry

33. Mucinous carcinoma:
    A. Is characterized by a garland-type growth pattern with dirty necrosis
    B. Never has a signet-ring morphology
    C. Often has an abundance of calcifications
    D. Is usually PR negative
    E. Is usually HER-2/neu positive/amplified

34. Medullary carcinoma:
    A. Resembles a fibroadenoma on mammography
    B. Represents <1% of breast carcinomas
    C. Consists of well differentiated tumor cells, with a prominent plasmacytic infiltrate with infiltrative margins
    D. Demonstrates basaloid metaplasia in 10%-15% of cases
    E. Should not exhibit necrosis

35. Metaplastic carcinoma is characterized by:
    A. Tumor cells that may be large and keratinizing, acantholytic, spindled, or any such combination and typically proliferate around cystic structures
    B. Tubules of adenocarcinoma that appear to transform into a spindle cell population (tubules appear to be stretching out and merging with surrounding spindle cells) giving the appearance of a predominantly spindle cell tumor with well-formed ductal structures with either open or compressed lumens
    C. An admixture of carcinoma with benign-appearing cytokeratin-positive chondrocytes; the lesion is referred to as carcinoma with chondroid metaplasia; if the carcinoma is admixed with chondrocytes that are clearly malignant and cytokeratin negative, the lesion should be called a carcinosarcoma
    D. None of the above
    E. All of the above

36. Which of the following is FALSE regarding apocrine carcinoma of the breast?
    A. It represents <1% of all mammary carcinomas.
    B. Pain and/or nipple discharge are uncommon presenting manifestations.
    C. The average age of presentation is 45 years.
    D. Nucleoli are usually large, prominent, and eosinophilic.
    E. When arranged in a glandular pattern with lumens, the tumor cells often appear to have apical cytoplasmic snouts along the luminal margin.

37. The differential diagnosis for apocrine carcinoma includes all of the following EXCEPT:
    A. Clear cell carcinoma
    B. Apocrine carcinoma of the axilla originating in axillary apocrine glands
    C. Oncocytic carcinoma
    D. Histiocytoid carcinoma
    E. Granular cell tumor

4: Breast Questions

38. A 50-year-old HIV-positive man presents with a painless, rubbery, firm unilateral breast mass. At low-power magnification, the neoplasm appears to be a complex vascular proliferation in densely collagenized intralobular stroma; empty slit-like spaces are present, and there are spindle cells at the margins of these spaces that resemble endothelial cells. What is the most likely diagnosis?
    A. Low-grade angiosarcoma
    B. High-grade angiosarcoma
    C. Kaposi carcinoma
    D. Pseudoangiomatous stromal hyperplasia (PASH)
    E. None of the above

39. A 50-year-old man presents with a mobile, solitary, palpable, firm and nontender mass. Microscopically, it has a delicate fibrous capsule. The tumor cells are fibroblast-like, uniform, bipolar, and oval to spindle-shaped. They are arranged diffusely and in short packets, admixed with broad bands and ribbons of collagen. The tumor cells do not mingle with adjacent breast parenchyma. Mitotic figures are difficult to find. By immunohistochemistry the tumor cells are negative for pancytokeratin. What is the most likely diagnosis?
    A. Fibromatosis
    B. Myxoid fibroadenoma
    C. Nodular fasciitis
    D. Metaplastic carcinoma
    E. Myofibroblastoma

40. A 45-year-old woman has a serous nipple discharge. On mammography, stippled microcalcifications are identified in a fairly discrete subareolar mass. On microscopic examination, there is a proliferation of rounded tubules lined by both epithelial and myoepithelial cells. 8 mitotic figures are identified in 10 high-power fields. What is the most likely diagnosis?
    A. Pseudoangiomatous stromal hyperplasia (PASH)
    B. Ductal carcinoma in situ (DCIS)
    C. Myofibroblastoma
    D. Simple papilloma
    E. Adenomyoepithelioma

41. Which of the following is FALSE regarding myoepithelioma?
    A. It is more common in women than men.
    B. It is benign.
    C. It may present as a hard, lobular and painful mass.
    D. Spindle cells interlace and contain epithelioid myoepithelial cells arranged in a storiform pattern and are characterized by clear cytoplasm; fibrofatty tissue and collagen are seen in the background.
    E. The neoplastic cells are generally ER and PR positive by immunohistochemistry.

42. Which of the following is TRUE regarding Paget disease?
    A. Cytokeratin 20 and high-molecular-weight cytokeratins typically are negative.
    B. Paget cells typically are negative for GCDFP-15 and estrogen receptors.
    C. Paget cells are positive for HMB-45.
    D. 90%-100% of Paget cells are mucin and PAS positive.
    E. None of the above

4: Breast Questions

43. Which of the following is FALSE regarding gynecomastia?
    A. Increased number of ducts lined by epithelial and myoepithelial cells are characteristic.
    B. The surrounding cellular stroma contains fibroblasts, myofibroblasts, admixed lymphocytes, and plasma cells.
    C. Lobular structures are very rare unless the patient is receiving exogenous estrogen.
    D. It generally involves both breasts, but usually is more pronounced in one over the other.
    E. None of the above

44. A 48-year-old woman has a hard, tender breast nodule. This is biopsied (see image). What is her increased risk of breast cancer?

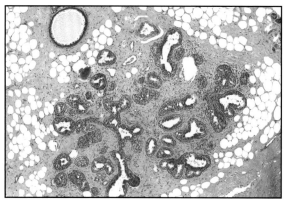

    A. 0
    B. 1.5-2 times
    C. 4-5 times
    D. 9-10 times
    E. None of the above

45. A 38 year-old woman is found to have a slight area of asymmetry on mammography. Her mother and sister both have a history of breast cancer. This image is a representative area of her biopsy. What is her increased risk of breast cancer?

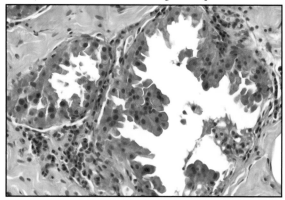

    A. 0
    B. 1.5-2 times
    C. 4-5 times
    D. 9-10 times
    E. None of the above

4: Breast Questions

46. A 55-year-old woman has a firm, tender breast nodule. This is biopsied (see image). What is her increased risk of breast cancer?

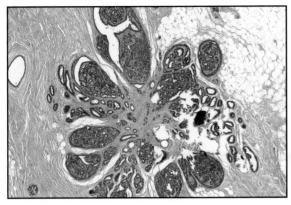

A. 0
B. 1.5-2 times
C. 4-5 times
D. 9-10 times
E. None of the above

47. The image represents a breast biopsy of a 42 year-old woman. What is your diagnosis?

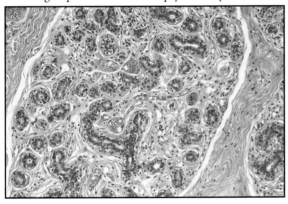

A. Tubular adenoma
B. LCIS
C. Tubular carcinoma
D. Angiosarcoma, well-differentiated
E. None of the above

4: Breast Questions

48. What is the most likely diagnosis?

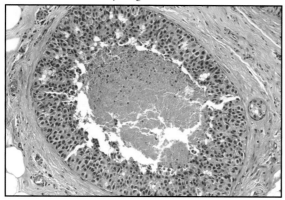

    A.   Lactational change

    B.   Apocrine change

    C.   DCIS, solid variant

    D.   DCIS with comedonecrosis

    E.   None of the above

49. The following biopsy is from the right breast of a 48-year-old woman. What is her risk of developing invasive carcinoma in her contralateral breast?

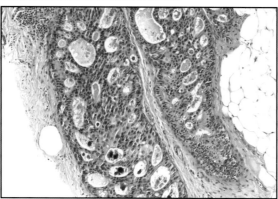

    A.   0

    B.   3%-5%

    C.   5%-10%

    D.   15%-25%

    E.   >25%

4: Breast Questions

50. What is the most likely diagnosis?

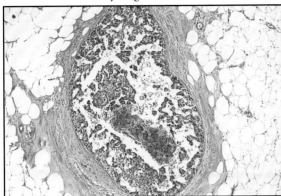 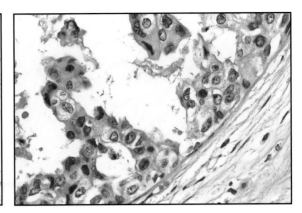

    A. Apocrine change
    B. DCIS, cribiform type
    C. DCIS, solid type
    D. Florid ductal hyperplasia
    E. Ductal carcinoma in situ, micropapillary type

51. A 45-year-old woman has a 4-cm mass in the upper, outer quadrant of her right breast. Based on the following image, what is the most likely diagnosis?

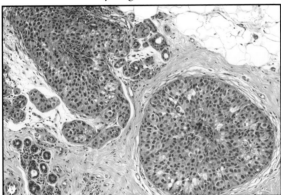

    A. Apocrine change
    B. DCIS, cribiform type
    C. DCIS, solid type
    D. Florid ductal hyperplasia
    E. Ductal carcinoma in situ, micropapillary type

4: Breast Questions

52. This variant of ductal carcinoma in situ is often multicentric.

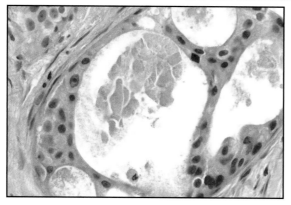

    A.   True
    B.   False

53. Which of the following statements is likely associated with the lesion shown in the image?

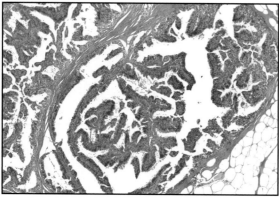

    A.   90% of patients with this lesion have a nipple discharge.
    B.   The patient is most likely in her 50s or 60s.
    C.   This does not occur in men.
    D.   A and B
    E.   A, B, and C

4: Breast Questions

54. A 40-year-old woman has a 1.5 cm breast mass and multiple calcifications on breast imaging. The mass is excised and similar lesions to what is seen in the photomicrograph are noted at multiple margins. Which of the following is/are TRUE?

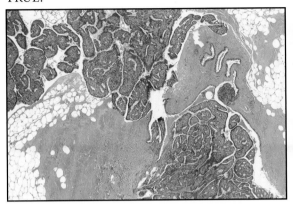
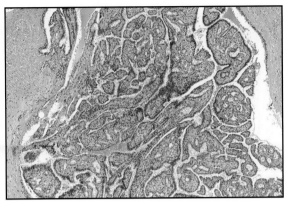

    A.   S100 and MSA will confirm the presence of a myoepithelial layer.

    B.   This is a monoclonal process.

    C.   This is due to inactivation of the phosphoglycerokinase gene.

    D.   A and B

    E.   A, B, and C

55. What is the most likely diagnosis based on the following image?

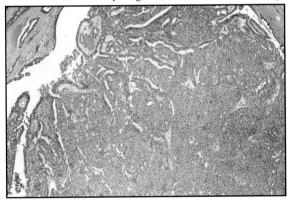
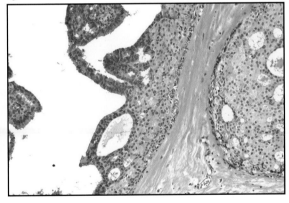

    A.   Intraductal papilloma

    B.   Sclerosing papilloma

    C.   Atypical papilloma

    D.   Carcinoma arising in a papilloma

    E.   Papillary carcinoma

4: Breast Questions

56. A 50-year-old woman has an abnormal mammogram. The following lesion is excised. What is the most likely diagnosis?

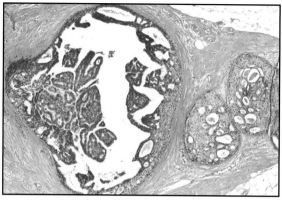

    A. Intraductal papilloma
    B. Sclerosing papilloma
    C. Atypical papilloma
    D. Carcinoma arising in a papilloma
    E. Papillary carcinoma

57. A 48-year-old woman is found to have a 2 cm subareolar, breast mass accompanied by serosanguinous discharge. Based on the following image, what is the best diagnosis?

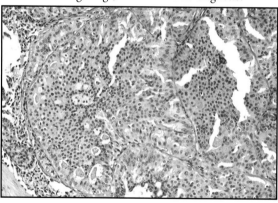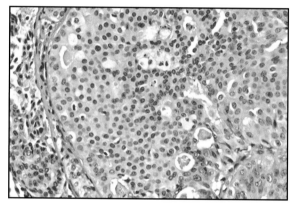

    A. Intraductal papilloma
    B. Sclerosing papilloma
    C. Atypical papilloma
    D. Carcinoma arising in a papilloma
    E. Papillary carcinoma

4: Breast Questions

58. A 48-year-old female is found to have a 5 cm right-sided breast mass. Based on the following image, what is the most likely diagnosis?

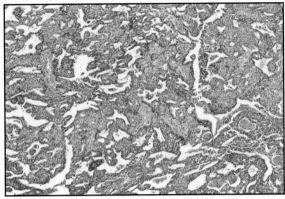 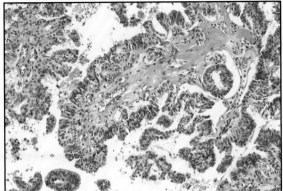

    A. Intraductal papilloma
    B. Sclerosing papilloma
    C. Atypical papilloma
    D. Carcinoma arising in a papilloma
    E. Papillary carcinoma

59. Which of the following is TRUE regarding this lesion?

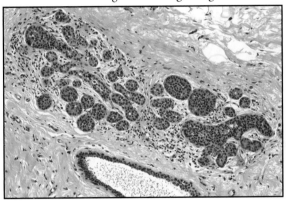 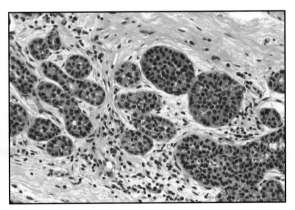

    A. The gene at 16q22 is lost.
    B. Invasive carcinoma may develop in the ipsilateral breast or contralateral breast in 20%-25% of patients.
    C. This lesion does not have to be excised.
    D. A and B
    E. A, B, and C

4: Breast Questions

60. The proliferative cells in this photomicrograph are likely positive for which of the following?

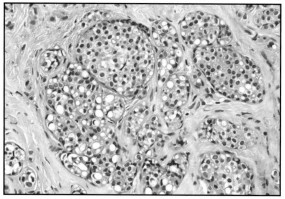

    A. Estrogen receptor
    B. Progesterone receptor
    C. E-cadherin
    D. A and B
    E. A, B, and C

61. A 45-year-old woman has a 6 cm, well-circumscribed, lobulated density on mammography. At low power, you notice a leaf-like pattern, and you count 4 mitotic figures/10 hpf in the cellular areas surrounding the ducts. Which of the following is/are TRUE regarding this lesion?

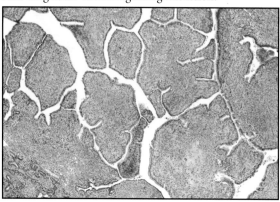 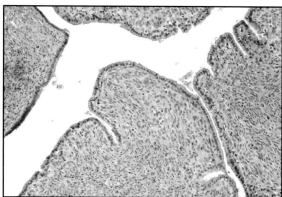

    A. 30% recur.
    B. In situ and invasive carcinomas are more likely to occur near the tumor than within this tumor.
    C. Total mastectomy with an axillary dissection is the treatment of choice
    D. A and B
    E. A, B, and C

4: Breast Questions

62. Based on the following image, what is the most likely diagnosis?

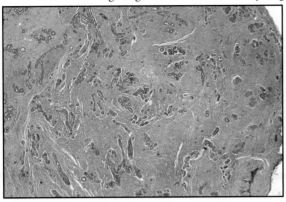

    A. Myofibroblastoma
    B. Myxoid sarcoma, low-grade
    C. Myoepithelioma
    D. Phyllodes tumor
    E. Fibroadenoma

63. This is a breast core biopsy of a 2.5 cm lesion in a 30-year-old woman. It is round rubbery and well-circumscribed on palpation. Based on the following image, what is the most likely diagnosis?

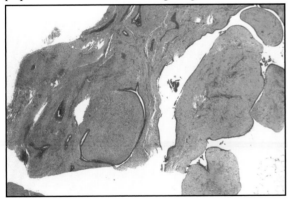

    A. Myofibroblastoma
    B. Myxoid sarcoma, low-grade
    C. Myoepithelioma
    D. Phyllodes tumor
    E. Fibroadenoma

4: Breast Questions

64. What is the most likely diagnosis?

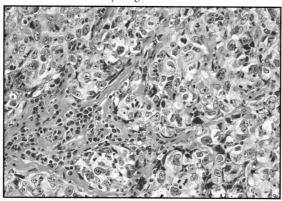 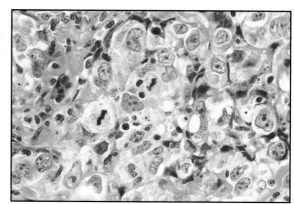

    A. Invasive lobular carcinoma
    B. Invasive ductal carcinoma, grade 1
    C. Invasive ductal carcinoma, grade 3
    D. Immunostains are required to accurately diagnose this lesion
    E. None of the above

65. A 65-year-old woman has 5 cm breast mass that was excised (see image). What is the most important prognostic factor?

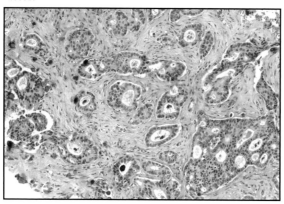

    A. Tumor size
    B. Tumor grade
    C. Estrogen receptor status
    D. HER2/neu amplification status
    E. Lymph node status

4: Breast Questions

66.   What is the most predictive factor for this lesion (see image)?

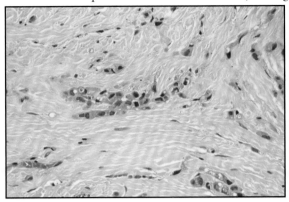

   A.   Tumor size
   B.   Tumor grade
   C.   Estrogen receptor status
   D.   E-cadherin status
   E.   Lymph node status

67.   A 43-year-old woman has a 1 cm breast mass (see image). You perform an MSA and S100, which are negative. Which of the following is/are TRUE?

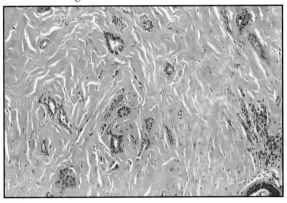 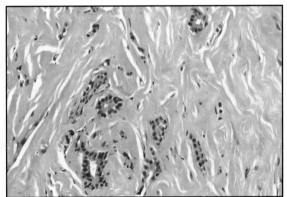

   A.   The prognosis of this lesion is excellent.
   B.   Loss of heterozygosity within the ATM gene is associated with this lesion.
   C.   LCIS is present in approximately 15% of patients.
   D.   A and B
   E.   A, B, and C

4: Breast Questions

68. A 60-year-old woman had a 1.3 cm well-circumscribed breast mass excised. The lesion is entirely submitted and a representative section is shown in the photomicrograph. What is the diagnosis?

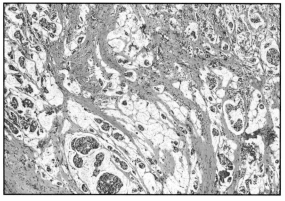

A. Mucinous carcinoma
B. Colloid carcinoma
C. Myxoid sarcoma
D. A and B
E. A, B, and C

69. These are 2 images from a well-circumscribed, 2.8 cm, unilateral breast mass from a 52-year-old woman. The tumor cells are positive for pancytokeratin, S100 and vimentin. The tumor cells are negative for ER and PR. The surrounding lymphocytes are mostly T cells. What is the most likely diagnosis?

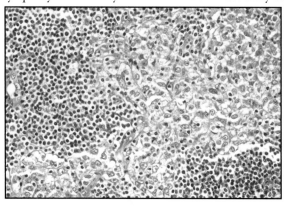 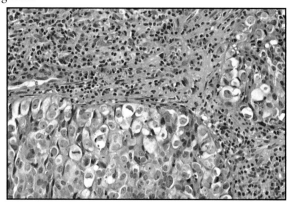

A. Metastatic melanoma
B. Metaplastic carcinoma
C. Medullary carcinoma
D. Further ancillary studies are needed.
E. None of the above

4: Breast Questions

70.   An 85-year-old woman has a 5-cm left breast mass excised. Numerous lymph nodes are involved by tumor. Every section of tissue examined looks like the below images and is strongly positive for pankeratin. What is the most likely diagnosis?

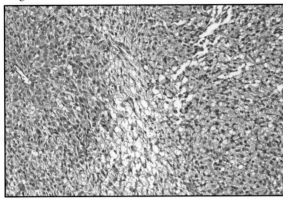 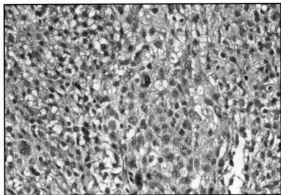

    A.   Metaplastic carcinoma
    B.   Malignant melanoma
    C.   Chondroid sarcoma
    D.   Further ancillary studies are needed.
    E.   None of the above

71.   An 80-year-old woman has this 3.7-cm mass excised. This tumor is negative for S100, c-Kit, and CD34, and positive for pancytokeratin. What is the most likely diagnosis?

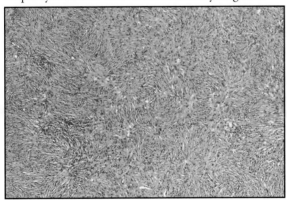

    A.   Malignant melanoma
    B.   Malignant melanoma, desmoplastic type
    C.   Metaplastic carcinoma
    D.   A and B
    E.   None of the above

4: Breast Questions

72. A 24-year-old woman has a 1.8 cm well-circumscribed breast mass excised (see image). This lesion is malignant.

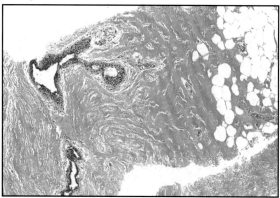 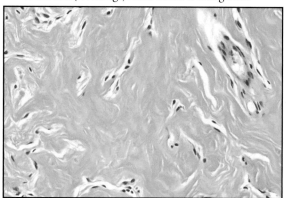

    A. True
    B. False

73. This 4.1-cm, mobile, firm and nontender mass is excised from 55-year-old woman. It is immunoreactive for CD34, desmin and vimentin. What is the most likely diagnosis?

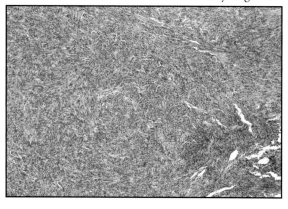 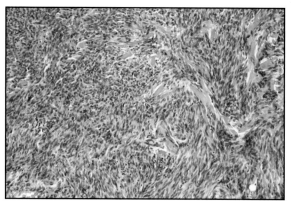

    A. Angiosarcoma
    B. Desmoplastic malignant melanoma
    C. Myofibroblastoma
    D. Pseudoangiomatous stromal hyperplasia
    E. Carcinosarcoma

4: Breast Questions

74. Based on the following image, what is the most likely diagnosis?

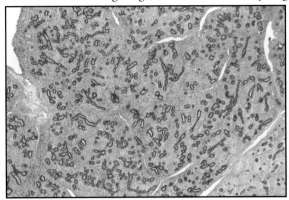

 A. Adenomyoepithelioma
 B. Fibroadenoma
 C. Phyllodes tumor
 D. Myofibroblastoma
 E. None of the above

75. This is a circumscribed, firm, painful mass (see image). It is positive for SMA and MSA, and negative for pancytokeratin. What is the most likely diagnosis?

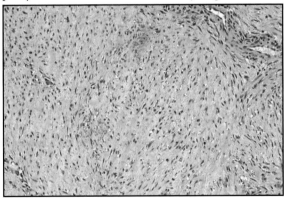

 A. Myoepithelioma
 B. Fibroadenoma
 C. Phyllodes tumor
 D. Myofibroblastoma
 E. None of the above

76. Which of the following is/are TRUE regarding the tumor cells shown in this image?

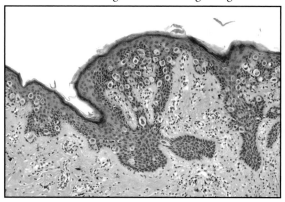 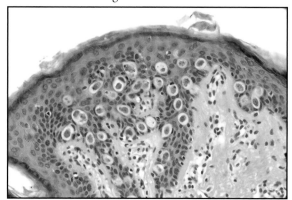

A. They are positive for CEA, CAM 5.2 and EMA.
B. They are positive for GCDFP-15 and ER.
C. They are negative for HMB-45.
D. A and B
E. A, B, and C

77. A 60-year-old man has a 3-cm breast mass (see image). What is/are TRUE for this lesion?

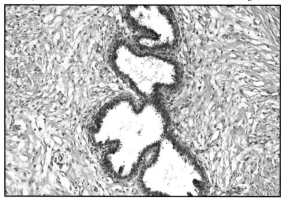

A. It is associated with Klinefelter syndrome.
B. This is not a precancerous lesion.
C. It can be positive for PSA but negative for PSAP.
D. A and B
E. A, B, and C

4: Breast Answers

1. **E.**   **TO ASSESS SUSPICIOUS LYMPH NODES**
The only reason for an intraoperative breast consultation from the above list is to confirm a positive lymph node so that the surgeon may proceed with an axillary dissection and spare the patient a second procedure.
QCSP, **Intraoperative Consultation,** p 112.

2. **E.**   **NONE OF THE ABOVE**
Everything listed is critical for grossing a mastectomy specimen. The specimen should be oriented and inked for proper examination of margins. Ink can track into breast parenchyma fissures; therefore, fixing the ink with Bouin solution (or acetic acid) is critical prior to sectioning. Uninvolved breast parenchyma should be sampled from all quadrants of the breast.
QCSP, **Specimen Handling,** p 112.

3. **C.**   **30%-35%**
Fibrocystic changes affect approximately 30%-35% of women between the ages of 20 and 45 years.
QCSP, **Benign Lesion,** p 112.

4. **E.**   **SINCE THIS IS CLASSIC SCHIMMELBUSCH DISEASE, COUNSEL THE PATIENT.**
The most likely explanation for this hard tender nodule in a young woman is fibrocystic changes. It often coincides with premenstrual pain, and the tenderness may last for 2 weeks. This has the fantastic appellation of Schimmelbusch disease! Choices A, B, and C are not indicated at this point, and a trial of estrogen would likely make her symptoms worse.
QCSP, **Benign Lesion,** p 113.

5. **C.**   **NONOVERLAPPING CELLS WITH PROMINENT CYTOPLASMIC MEMBRANES**
This is a feature of ductal carcinoma in situ (DCIS). All of the other features listed are typical of fibrocystic changes.
QCSP, **Benign Lesion,** p 113.

6. **A.**   **THE EPITHELIAL CELLS ARE S100 POSITIVE AND ESTROGEN RECEPTOR NEGATIVE.**
Microglandular adenosis for years has been considered to be a benign lesion. If not completely excised it may recur and/or develop atypia. Some consider it a form of low-grade carcinoma. The epithelial cells are characteristically S100 positive and ER negative. It does not have a myoepithelial layer and should never invade nerves.
QCSP, **Microglandular Adenosis,** p 113.

7. **D.**   **THE RELATIVE RISK FOR DEVELOPMENT OF INVASIVE DUCTAL CARCINOMA IS APPROXIMATELY 5.**
The relative risk for development of invasive ductal carcinoma is approximately 1.7. The rest of the choices are correct.
QCSP, **Sclerosing Adenosis,** p 114.

8. **E.**   **NONE OF THE ABOVE**
All of the listed choices are correct.
QCSP, **Radial Scar,** p 116.

9. **E.**   **50% HAVE LACTATIONAL AND SECRETORY CHANGES.**
20% have lactational and secretory changes. The rest of the choices are true.
QCSP, **Tubular Adenoma,** p 116.

4: Breast Answers

28.　C.　**25%-30%**
OQCSP, **Infiltrating Carcinoma,** p 130.

29.　A.　**PATIENTS WITH TUMORS <1 CM WITHOUT NODAL METASTASIS HAVE A 10-YEAR DISEASE-FREE SURVIVAL RATE OF 90%.**
Patients with tumors <2 cm in diameter with negative lymph nodes have an excellent 10-year disease-free survival rate of 80%. Patients with tumors >2 cm and <5 cm with negative nodes have a 10-year disease-free survival rate of 70%. Patients with tumors >5 cm with negative nodes have a 10-year disease-free survival rate of 60%. For tumors <2 cm with 1-3 positive axillary lymph nodes, 10-year disease-free survival rate is 75% (without adjuvant chemotherapy).
QCSP, **Infiltrating Carcinoma,** p 131.

30.　C.　**PRESENCE OR ABSENCE OF AXILLARY LYMPH NODE METASTASIS**
This is the single most important prognostic factor regarding breast cancer.
QCSP, **Infiltrating Carcinoma,** p 131.

31.　B.　**MITOTIC FIGURES ARE RARE.**
Ductal carcinoma is the most common type of invasive breast carcinoma. 15%-30% of lobular carcinoma cases are multicentric. It usually presents as an *ill-defined,* painless mass, but may present as a vague thickening or nodularity. 70%-90% are ER positive (this includes the classic form and all variants); 65% are PR positive.
QCSP, **Invasive Carcinoma,** p 131.

32.　C.　**IS COMPOSED OF TUBULES THAT TEND TO BE ANGULATED, OVAL, OR ELONGATED WITH OPEN LUMENS, AND ARE LINED BY A SINGLE LAYER OF EPITHELIAL CELLS**
Tubular carcinoma represents fewer than 2% of all breast carcinomas. 25%-30% of cases are multicentric. Angiolymphatic invasion is almost never present. It is usually ER positive.
QCSP, **Invasive Carcinoma,** p 132-133.

33.　D.　**IS USUALLY PR NEGATIVE**
Choice A describes metastatic colon cancer. Mucinous carcinoma may have signet-ring forms. Calcifications are rare and HER-2/neu is usually negative/not amplified.
QCSP, **Invasive Carcinoma,** p 134.

34.　A.　**RESEMBLES A FIBROADENOMA ON MAMMOGRAPHY**
Medullary carcinoma comprises 5%-7% of all breast carcinomas. Medullary carcinoma consists of poorly differentiated cells with scant stroma and a prominent lymphoid infiltrate that has well circumscribed margins. 10%-15% of cases demonstrate foci of squamous metaplasia. Necrosis is characteristically present.
QCSP, **Invasive Carcinoma,** p 135.

35.　E.　**ALL OF THE ABOVE**
Metaplastic carcinoma is a malignant neoplasm of the breast characterized by an admixture of adenocarcinoma with areas of benign or malignant epithelial (squamous, spindle) and mesenchymal (chondroid, osseous) differentiation. This should not be confused with *carcinosarcoma* which is defined by the presence of unequivocal carcinoma admixed with unequivocal sarcoma (sarcomatous areas must be negative for epithelial antigens).
QCSP, **Invasive Carcinoma,** p 136-139.

4: Breast Answers

36. C. **THE AVERAGE AGE OF PRESENTATION IS 45 YEARS.**
The peak age incidence 60s through 70s. The rest of the choices are correct.
QCSP, **Invasive Carcinoma,** p 139.

37. A. **CLEAR CELL CARCINOMA**
The rest of the choices are in the differential diagnosis. Of note, an oncocytic carcinoma should be negative for GCDFP-15.
QCSP, **Invasive Carcinoma,** p 140.

38. D. **PSEUDOANGIOMATOUS STROMAL HYPERPLASIA (PASH)**
The key to the diagnosis is the firm, rubbery, painless unilateral mass and the microscopic description. Particularly, the empty slit-like spaces, the lack of atypical endothelial cells, and the lack of mitotic figures are key histologic features. Kaposi carcinoma does not exist.
QCSP, **Vascular Lesions,** p 141.

39. E. **MYOFIBROBLASTOMA**
Fibromatosis is characterized by long, sweeping fascicles of thin fibroblasts. Nodular fasciitis presents rapidly and often has abundant mitotic figures. There is nothing in the description to suggest a myxoid fibroadenoma. Metaplastic carcinoma should be positive for pancytokeratin.
QCSP, **Mesenchymal Lesions,** p 141-142.

40. E. **ADENOMYOEPITHELIOMA**
QCSP, **Myoepithelial Lesions,** p 142-143.

41. E. **THE NEOPLASTIC CELLS ARE GENERALLY ER AND PR POSITIVE BY IMMUNOHISTOCHEMISTRY.**
These lesions are very rare, especially in men. They are benign, but can present as a hard, painful mass. They are muscle-specific actin positive and ER/PR negative.
QCSP, **Myoepithelial Lesions,** p 144-145.

42. A. **CYTOKERATIN 20 AND HIGH-MOLECULAR-WEIGHT CYTOKERATINS ARE TYPICALLY NEGATIVE.**
50%-60% of Paget cells are mucin and PAS positive. Paget cells are positive for CEA, most cytokeratins (especially CAM 5.2) and EMA. Paget cells are typically immunoreactive for GCDFP-15 and estrogen receptors. Paget cells are negative for HMB-45. The immunohistochemical profile for Paget cells is typically identical to that of the underlying carcinoma.
QCSP, **Diseases of the Nipple,** p 144-145.

43. E. **NONE OF THE ABOVE**
All of the choices listed are true.
QCSP, **Male Breast Lesions,** p 146-147.

44. A. **0**
This is an example of simple hyperplasia and fibrocystic changes. Fibrocystic changes with apocrine cysts and mild epithelial hyperplasia (2-4 cells thick) do not represent an increased risk for the development of carcinoma. In contrast, intraductal hyperplasia without atypia (>4 cells thick) is associated with a slightly increased risk (1.5-2 times) for the development for carcinoma. Atypical intraductal hyperplasia is associated with a moderately increased risk (4-5 times) for developing invasive carcinoma.
QCSP, **Benign Lesions,** p 112-113.

4: Breast Answers

45.   A.   **0**

This is an example of apocrine metaplasia. This by itself does not put her at increased risk for breast cancer. *QCSP*, **Benign Lesions,** p 112-113.

46.   B.   **1.5-2 TIMES**

This is a radial scar and increases a woman's risk of breast cancer by 2 times. This is the same risk as for florid hyperplasia. *QCSP*, **Benign Lesions,** p 115-116.

47.   E.   **NONE OF THE ABOVE**

This is normal breast tissue. No neoplastic proliferation is seen. *QCSP*, **Benign Lesions,** p 115-116.

48.   D.   **DCIS WITH COMEDONECROSIS**

This is DCIS with comedonecrosis. It is characterized by the presence of necrosis, cytologic atypia, and monotonous loosely cohesive cells with well-defined cell borders. *QCSP*, **Malignant Intraductal Lesion,** p 117-118.

49.   B.   **3%-5%**

This is an example of cribriform DCIS with ductal expansion by cells with neoplastic cells forming secondary lumen/punched-out spaces. The risk of subsequent invasive carcinoma in the contralateral breast is approximately 3%-5%. *QCSP*, **Malignant Intraductal Lesion,** p 118-119.

50.   E.   **DUCTAL CARCINOMA IN SITU, MICROPAPILLARY TYPE**

Epithelial cells (similar to those of cribriform DCIS) form regularly distributed papillary tufts that project into the lumen and lack a fibrovascular core. Areas of the ductal wall between the epithelial tufts have 2 cell layers. Luminal epithelial cells may be identical to those proliferating in the tufts or they may appear normal. The myoepithelial cell layer is usually intact. Neoplastic cells may have some atypia and a hobnail appearance. Occasionally, the micropapillary pattern has features of the cribriform pattern secondary to the formation of arcades and bridges. The micropapillary pattern is more frequently multicentric (>1 quadrant) than any other type of DCIS. *QCSP*, **Malignant Intraductal Lesion,** p 118.

51.   C.   **DCIS, SOLID TYPE**

The lesion demonstrates ductal carcinoma in situ. This is an example of DCIS, solid type, and also demonstrates a small focus of comedonecrosis. *QCSP*, **Malignant Intraductal Lesion,** p 118.

52.   A.   **TRUE**

This is the apocrine variant of DCIS. It also has cribriform features. The apocrine variant is usually multicentric (>1 quadrant). The proliferating cells have abundant granular, eosinophilic cytoplasm with moderate to severe atypia and central necrosis. Apical snouts are not always evident. *QCSP*, **Malignant Intraductal Lesion,** p 118.

4: Breast Answers

53. D. **A AND B**

This is an example of an intraductal papilloma. They typically are solitary and arise from a major duct in a central subareolar location. Close to 90% have a serous or serosanguinous nipple discharge. Most are diagnosed in patients age 50 to 70 years. It may occur in either men or women.

QCSP, **Papillary Lesions,** p 119-120.

54. E. **A, B, AND C**

The lesion demonstrates multiple papillary lesions with protrusion of multiple papillae into the lumen of multiple terminal ductal lobular units. This is thought to be a monoclonal process that results from inactivation of the phosphoglycerokinase gene. Additionally, the papillary lesions are mostly lined by myoepithelial, which can be highlighted by S100 and/or muscle-specific actin. As such, all of the choices are correct.

QCSP, **Papillary Lesions,** p 120-121.

55. C. **ATYPICAL PAPILLOMA**

In atypical papillomas, the papillary processes contain focal areas that consist of a proliferation of monotonous cells identical to the cells of a low-grade, nonnecrotic DCIS. A myoepithelial cell layer may or may not be present. These focal areas of proliferation occupy <1/3 of the lesion. This is a confusing area of breast pathology. The next few questions will test your diagnostic acumen.

QCSP, **Papillary Lesions,** p 122.

56. C. **ATYPICAL PAPILLOMA**

This is another example of an atypical papilloma.

QCSP, **Papillary Lesions,** p 122.

57. D. **CARCINOMA ARISING IN A PAPILLOMA**

Carefully read the difference in criteria for this lesion in contrast to an atypical papilloma (see previous question). The papillary processes consist of a proliferation of epithelial cells identical to the cells of a low-grade DCIS, occupying spaces between the papillary cores, that if seen in a single duct would qualify as DCIS. A myoepithelial cell layer may or may not present, but at least 1/3 of the papillary fronds should show an absence of the myoepithelial cell layer. In the presence of necrosis, a highly atypical cell population, or a truly anaplastic cell population, the lesion qualifies as a carcinoma arising in a papilloma (even it occupies <1/3 of the lesion).

QCSP, **Papillary Lesions,** p 122-123.

58. E. **PAPILLARY CARCINOMA**

This lesion is composed of a proliferation of papillary processes that protrude into a distended duct lumen and lack a myoepithelial cell layer. The complete absence of a myoepithelial cell layer is the single most important feature of a papillary carcinoma; its absence differentiates a carcinoma from a benign papillary lesion. Proliferating papillae may have various patterns: simple stratification of spindled epithelial cells, tufting (micropapillae), solid, or cribriform architecture. Epithelial cells, regardless of overall architectural pattern, tend to be closely packed together with hyperchromatic nuclei and a high nuclear-cytoplasmic ratio.

QCSP, **Malignant Intraductal Lesions,** p 123-124.

59. E. **A, B, AND C**

This image represents lobular carcinoma in situ. This is often an incidental finding. By itself this lesion does not need to be completely excised. If this is the only lesion identified on an excisional biopsy, then clinical follow-up on a regular basis for life is all that is absolutely necessary. The important fact is that the patient is at increased risk for developing invasive breast carcinoma compared to the general population.

QCSP, **Noninvasive Lobular Carcinoma,** p 124-126.

4: Breast Answers

60.   D.   **A AND B**

The neoplastic cells in LCIS are usually positive for both estrogen and progesterone receptors and negative for HER-2/neu (C-erb B-2) overexpression. By definition the neoplastic cells in lobular lesions are negative for E-cadherin.

QCSP, **Noninvasive Lobular Carcinoma,** p 124-126.

61.   D.   **A AND B**

The treatment of choice for this low-grade phyllodes tumor is wide local excision. Total mastectomy is reserved for large tumors, tumors with infiltrating margins, and tumors with aggressive histologic features. There is no role for axillary dissection; these neoplasms essentially never metastasize to lymph nodes.

QCSP, **Biphasic Lesions,** p 128-129.

62.   E.   **FIBROADENOMA**

Fibroadenomas can be quite variable in appearance. A few of the key characteristics include a biphasic tumor consisting of a proliferation of epithelial and mesenchymal elements; ducts usually lined by 2 cell layers: a luminal epithelial layer and an underlying or surrounding layer of myoepithelial cells; various metaplastic changes possibly seen in the epithelium (squamous, apocrine, and oncocytic). The majority have a pushing growth margin and a well-formed capsule.

QCSP, **Biphasic Lesions,** p 126-127.

63.   E.   **FIBROADENOMA**

This is another example of a fibroadenoma. The point is not to misdiagnose this common lesion of young people as a phyllodes tumor, which is an uncommon lesion. When phyllodes tumors do occur, they tend to happen in older women.

QCSP, **Biphasic Lesions,** p 126-127.

64.   C.   **INVASIVE DUCTAL CARCINOMA, GRADE 3**

This lesion has high-grade cytologic features and numerous mitotic figures, and does not show evidence of ductal formation. Therefore this cannot be a low-grade lesion. Invasive lobular carcinoma typically has much less atypia and fewer mitotic figures.

QCSP, **Infiltrating Carcinoma,** p 129-131.

65.   E.   **LYMPH NODE STATUS**

The image demonstrates a low-grade invasive ductal carcinoma. In this situation the most important prognosis factor is the status of the lymph nodes.

QCSP, **Infiltrating Carcinoma,** p 131.

66.   C.   **ESTROGEN RECEPTOR STATUS**

The image depicts an invasive lobular carcinoma. There are predictive factors and prognostic factors. Tumor size and lymph node status relate to prognosis and considered prognostic factors. Estrogen receptor status is the only predictive factor listed. It predicts the tumor's response to Tamoxifen.

QCSP, **Infiltrating Carcinoma,** p 127-128.

67.   E.   **A, B, AND C**

This is an example of tubular carcinoma. This lesion is characterized by a haphazard proliferation of tubules in a reactive-appearing fibroblastic stroma. The tubules tend to be angulated, oval, or elongated with open lumens, and are lined by a single layer of epithelial cells (no myoepithelial cell layer); the tubules may extend into adjacent adipose tissue and normal mammary structures. Epithelial cells tend to be fairly homogeneous, cuboidal, or columnar with round or oval, hyperchromatic, basally oriented nuclei; nucleoli are usually inconspicuous or

absent; the cytoplasm is typically eosinophilic or amphophilic (rarely clear). Epithelial cells are not particularly atypical and mitotic activity is rare; apical snouts may be present.
QCSP, **Infiltrating Carcinoma**, p 132-133.

68. **D.** **A AND B**
This is an example of mucinous carcinoma (aka, colloid carcinoma). It generally occurs in women in their 60s. It is often well-circumscribed and has an excellent prognosis.
QCSP, **Infiltrating Carcinoma**, p 134.

69. **C.** **MEDULLARY CARCINOMA**
In addition to the immunohistochemical profile stated in the clinical history, the following morphologic description is characteristic: it is often a well-circumscribed lesion with round tumor cells with abundant cytoplasm and round, vesicular nuclei that contain 1 or more prominent nucleoli; tumor cells grow in a syncytial pattern; the mitotic rate is often high; a prominent lymphoplasmacytic reaction accompanies the neoplasm (this lymphoplasmacytic reaction must involve at least 75% of the periphery, be present diffusely in the supporting stroma of the tumor, and/or be diffusely admixed with carcinoma cells); lastly, the nuclei are very pleomorphic.
QCSP, **Infiltrating Carcinoma**, p 134-136.

70. **A.** **METAPLASTIC CARCINOMA**
The old age and advanced stage are a tip-off to the diagnosis. The strong pankeratin positivity confirms the diagnosis. There are a number of morphologic variants to this tumor. In general, it is a malignant neoplasm of the breast characterized by an admixture of adenocarcinoma with areas of benign or malignant, epithelial (squamous, spindle) and mesenchymal (chondroid, osseous) differentiation.
QCSP, **Infiltrating Carcinoma**, p 136-139.

71. **C.** **METAPLASTIC CARCINOMA**
This is another example of metaplastic carcinoma, spindle cell type. The positive pankeratin is key to the diagnosis.
QCSP, **Infiltrating Carcinoma**, p 136-139.

72. **B.** **FALSE**
The lesion demonstrates a complex vascular proliferation in a densely collagenized stroma. The slit-like spaces are not true anastomosing vascular channels. This is an example of pseudoangiomatous stromal hyperplasia (PASH). The endothelial-like cells are never atypical and do not show mitotic activity. The lesion is benign.
QCSP, **Vascular Lesions**, p 141.

73. **C.** **MYOFIBROBLASTOMA**
This is a myofibroblastoma. In addition to the typical clinical history and immunohistochemical profile, the following are characteristic features: it usually has a delicate fibrous capsule and is rarely infiltrating; the tumor cells tend to be fibroblast-like, uniform, bipolar, and oval to spindle-shaped; it is arranged diffusely or in short packets, and admixed with broad bands and ribbons of collagen; and tumor cells do not mingle with adjacent breast parenchyma. In addition, the nuclei are oval to elongated and frequently grooved. Mitotic figures are rare.
QCSP, **Mesenchymal Lesions**, p 141-142.

74. **A.** **ADENOMYOEPITHELIOMA**
This is an adenomyoepithelioma, tubular type. The lesion demonstrates a proliferation of round tubules with both a proliferative epithelial and myoepithelial components. It is benign (with mitotic figures up to 3/10 hpfs), and local excision is adequate treatment.
QCSP, **Myoepithelial Lesions**, p 142-144.

4: Breast Answers

75.   A.   **MYOEPITHELIOMA**

This is a very uncommon benign lesion. It demonstrates spindle and epithelioid myoepithelial cells, usually in a storiform pattern. Fibrofatty tissue and collagen are often seen in the background. The cells stain for Masson trichrome. If this lesion is incompletely excised, it may recur.

QCSP, **Myoepithelial Lesions,** p 144-145.

76.   E.   **A, B, AND C**

This is an example of Paget disease of the nipple. These lesions are typically positive for carcinoma markers such as CEA, BerEP4, and EMA. They are also positive for GCDFP-15. The neoplastic cells will stain for pankeratin and low-molecular weight keratins (CAM5.2 and CK7) but are negative for CK20 and high-molecular weight keratins. The cells are negative for HMB45 and only rarely positive for S100 (few reported cases).

QCSP, **Diseases of the Nipple,** p 146.

77.   E.   **A, B, AND C**

This is an example of gynecomastia with proliferation of ductal epithelial and myoepithelial cells. It is usually seen without accompanying lobular units. Of note, if this lesion is induced by antiandrogen therapy, it may be positive for PSA, but negative for PSAP.

QCSP, **Male Breast Lesions,** p 147.

Chapter 5

Female Reproductive Tract

1. Under which scenario is an intraoperative frozen section examination appropriate for an endometrial curettage?
   A. To rule out the presence of intrauterine gestation in cases in which the distinction between an intrauterine pregnancy and an ectopic pregnancy cannot be made on clinical grounds
   B. Curetting sample obtained from a patient with massive uterine bleeding in which intraoperative diagnosis might help in the immediate clinical decision-making process
   C. As a prelude to laparoscopic hysterectomy in which the uterus will be morcellated in the peritoneal cavity
   D. A and B
   E. A, B, and C

2. Since the uterus, fallopian tube and ovary are "freely floating in the abdominal cavity," inking the specimens is unnecessary and only delays the turnaround time of a frozen section diagnosis. TRUE or FALSE?
   A. True
   B. False

3. Which of the following is/are NOT criteria of minimal deviation adenocarcinoma (MDA; adenoma malignum)?
   A. Increased mitotic activity
   B. Complex outlines and some element of desmoplasia usually present
   C. Perineural invasion
   D. Bizarre atypia
   E. All of the above

4. Which of the following is a variant of minimal deviation adenocarcinoma (MDA; adenoma malignum)?
   A. Mucinous
   B. Endometrioid
   C. Clear cell
   D. All of the above
   E. By definition, MDA looks like bland endocervical glands.

5. Which of the following techniques may aid in the diagnosis of minimal deviation adenocarcinoma (MDA; adenoma malignum)?
   A. Trichrome stain
   B. Grimelius stain
   C. Vimentin
   D. CEA
   E. AFP

6. Adenoma malignum is also associated with which of the following?
   A. Carcinoma of stomach
   B. Sex-cord tumor with annular tubules
   C. Ovarian mucinous tumors
   D. Ovarian tumors of Wolffian origin (FATWO)
   E. All of the above

5: Female Reproductive Tract Questions

7. Adenocarcinoma in situ typically:
    A. Involves surface endocervical glandular epithelium in the transitional zone
    B. Involved glands extend below the level of normal glands
    C. Demonstrates endometrioid differentiation
    D. All of the above
    E. None of the above

8. Which of the following is/are TRUE regarding adenocarcinoma in situ?
    A. CIN or invasive squamous cell carcinoma coexists with adenocarcinoma in situ in <10%-15% of cases.
    B. CIN I present in squamous epithelium adjacent to areas of adenocarcinoma in situ <5% of cases.
    C. Approximately 90% contain HPV messenger RNA, usually types 16 and 18.
    D. A and B
    E. None of the above

9. A 55-year-old woman with a history of a supracervical hysterectomy 15 years prior for benign reasons is diagnosed with adenocarcinoma on Pap smear. A loop electrosurgical excision procedure is performed and is negative. The Pap smear diagnosis is confirmed. What is the most likely explanation for this discrepancy?
    A. The patient's Pap smear sample was misidentified.
    B. The patient cleared her adenocarcinoma during the interim.
    C. The lesion was "excised" during her Pap smear.
    D. B and C
    E. None of the above

10. Which of the following is/are TRUE regarding adenocarcinoma microscopic findings?
    A. Cells may resemble normal endocervix with pale granular cytoplasm and basal nuclei (endocervical type); it may be entirely papillary or partly papillary.
    B. Cells may resemble intestinal cells and line papillae or infiltrate in a manner similar to that of adenocarcinoma of the colon (intestinal type); epithelium tends to be pseudostratified and contains only small amounts of mucin, but may include goblet cells, Paneth cells, and/or argentaffin cells.
    C. Signet-ring cell carcinoma usually represents a breast primary.
    D. A and B
    E. A, B, and C

11. After breast cancer, which of the following is the most common new cancer in women worldwide?
    A. Non-small cell lung carcinoma
    B. Breast carcinoma
    C. Ovarian carcinoma
    D. Endometrial carcinoma
    E. Cervical squamous cancer

12. Which of the following is the most common viral infection associated with cervical adenocarcinoma?
    A. Herpes simplex virus I and II
    B. HPV6
    C. HPV11
    D. HPV16
    E. HPV18

5: Female Reproductive Tract Questions

13. What is the maximum depth that cervical squamous cell carcinoma can invade and still be considered microinvasive (Stage T1A1)?
    A. <0.5 mm
    B. ≤1 mm
    C. ≤2 mm
    D. ≤3 mm
    E. ≤5 mm

14. A 44-year-old woman has invasive squamous cell carcinoma. You note mature squamous cells, with abundant keratin pearl formation and few mitotic figures. The nuclei tend to be uniform and the cells have well-developed intercellular bridges. What is the most appropriate grade for this lesion?
    A. Grade I (well-differentiated)
    B. Grade II (moderately-differentiated)
    C. Grade III (poorly-differentiated)
    D. Cervical squamous cell carcinoma is not graded.
    E. None of the above

15. What is of greatest prognostic significance regarding squamous cell carcinoma of the cervix?
    A. Tumor grade
    B. Depth of invasion
    C. Tumor size
    D. Vascular invasion
    E. Lymph node status

16. Which subtype of HPV is associated with squamous cell carcinoma?
    A. HPV6
    B. HPV11
    C. HPV13
    D. HPV16
    E. None of the above

17. Which HPV subtype is more commonly associated with metastatic lymph node involvement?
    A. HPV6
    B. HPV11
    C. HPV18
    D. HPV31
    E. HPV33

18. Your microscopic examination of an endometrial curettage specimen shows large, polygonal, intermediate trophoblasts that infiltrate the myometrium and insinuate themselves between smooth muscle fibers at the interface between tumor and myometrium. The tumor cells also invade the walls of blood vessels from the outside and are starting to replace the entire vessel wall. This most closely describes which lesion?
    A. Choriocarcinoma
    B. Epithelioid trophoblastic tumor
    C. Placental site trophoblastic tumor
    D. Partial mole
    E. Chorioadenoma destruens

5: Female Reproductive Tract Questions

19. What is the prognosis for placental site trophoblastic tumors?
    A. All are benign.
    B. Most are benign.
    C. About 50% are malignant.
    D. >75% of cases present with metastasis.
    E. None of the above

20. All of the following are malignant features of a placental site trophoblastic tumor, EXCEPT?
    A. Tumor cells with clear rather than amphophilic cytoplasm aggregating in large masses and sheets
    B. Extensive necrosis
    C. A high mitotic rate (≥5 mitotic figures/10 hpf)
    D. Atypical mitotic figures
    E. All of the above support a malignant process

21. A 20-year-old woman has a spontaneous abortion. The microscopic examination of the aborted material demonstrates some hydropic villi that contain a central, acellular cistern, while others contain capillaries with nucleated red blood cells. Some chorionic villi are enlarged and have a scalloped outline while others are small and normal in appearance. This is diagnostic of which of the following?
    A. Placental site trophoblastic tumor
    B. Epithelioid trophoblastic tumor
    C. Partial mole
    D. Complete mole
    E. Cannot be determined without further studies

22. What is the most likely karyotype of a partial mole?
    A. 69,XYY
    B. 69,XXX
    C. 69,XXY
    D. 46,XX
    E. 46,XY

23. What is the best way to differentiate a hydropic abortion from a partial mole?
    A. Flow cytometry for aneuploidy
    B. β-hCG levels
    C. Molecular karyotype
    D. Immunohistochemical stains
    E. None of the above

24. What percentage of patients with complete moles have persistent gestational trophoblastic disease?
    A. <1%
    B. 5%-10%
    C. 10%-30%
    D. By definition none of them have persistent gestational trophoblastic disease.
    E. All complete moles have persistent gestational trophoblastic disease.

25. What percentage of partial moles patients have persistent gestational trophoblastic disease?
    A. <1%
    B. 5%-10%
    C. 10%-30%
    D. By definition none of them have persistent gestational trophoblastic disease.
    E. All complete moles have persistent gestational trophoblastic disease.

5: Female Reproductive Tract Questions

26. What percentage of partial moles develop into choriocarcinoma?
    A. <1%
    B. 5%-10%
    C. 10%-30%
    D. By definition none of them have persistent gestational trophoblastic disease.
    E. All complete moles have persistent gestational trophoblastic disease.

27. What percentage of complete moles develop into choriocarcinoma?
    A. 2%-3%
    B. 5%-10%
    C. 10%-30%
    D. By definition none of them have persistent gestational trophoblastic disease.
    E. All complete moles have persistent gestational trophoblastic disease.

28. What is the most likely karyotype of a compete mole?
    A. 69,XYY
    B. 69,XXX
    C. 69,XXY
    D. 46,XX
    E. 46,XY

29. By definition, which of the following karyotypes is impossible to have in a complete mole?
    A. 46,XX
    B. All paternally derived chromosomes
    C. 46,YY
    D. 46,XY
    E. None of the above

30. A 35-year-old woman is found to have an invasive hydatidiform mole. What is/are the most likely place(s) to find extrauterine disease?
    A. Vagina
    B. Vulva
    C. Lungs
    D. A and B
    E. A, B, and C

31. In complete moles, intermediate trophoblasts are positive for which immunohistochemical stain(s)?
    A. hCG
    B. hPL
    C. PLAP
    D. None of the above
    E. A, B, and C

32. In complete moles, cytotrophoblasts are positive for which immunohistochemical stain(s)?
    A. hCG
    B. hPL
    C. PLAP
    D. None of the above
    E. A, B, and C

5: Female Reproductive Tract Questions

33. In complete moles, syncytiotrophoblasts are positive for which immunohistochemical stain(s)?
    A. hCG
    B. hPL
    C. PLAP
    D. None of the above
    E. A, B, and C

34. Which of the following has been known to be associated with choriocarcinoma?
    A. Normal pregnancy
    B. Ectopic pregnancy
    C. Spontaneous abortion
    D. Molar pregnancy
    E. All of the above

35. These cells are usually mononucleate small cells with scant pale cytoplasm that tend to be either granular or clear. They are mitotically active and cell borders are usually prominent. What cell type is most likely described?
    A. Intermediate trophoblastic cells
    B. Syncytiotrophoblastic cells
    C. Cytotrophoblastic cells
    D. Choriocarcinoma
    E. All of the above

36. In choriocarcinoma syncytiotrophoblastic cells and intermediate trophoblastic cells typically stain positively for what immunohistochemical stain(s)?
    A. β-hCG
    B. hPL
    C. PLAP
    D. A and B
    E. A, B, and C

37. Which of the following conditions typically precedes choriocarcinoma?
    A. Hydatidiform mole
    B. Abortion
    C. Normal pregnancy
    D. Ectopic pregnancy
    E. C and D

38. Which blood group is most commonly associated with choriocarcinoma?
    A. A
    B. B
    C. AB
    D. O
    E. None of the above

5: Female Reproductive Tract Questions

39. A 55-year-old woman has a hysterectomy for persistent bleeding. On gross examination you see a 2-cm polypoid mass with a villous surface. The cut surface is white, spongy and cystic. Microscopically the surface of the lesion has broad, club-shaped papillae of stroma covered by proliferative phase endometrial cells. The stroma consists of bland cells that resemble fibroblasts and benign endometrial stromal cells. What is the diagnosis?
    - A. Adenomyoma
    - B. Atypical polypoid adenoma
    - C. Adenofibroma
    - D. Benign polyp
    - E. Adenomatoid tumor

40. Which of the following is FALSE regarding adenomatoid tumors?
    - A. It is an incidental finding in 1% of hysterectomy specimens.
    - B. They typically resemble small leiomyomata but with a softer consistency, a yellow color, and ill-defined margins.
    - C. They are usually found in the myometrium near the serosal surface in the area of the cornua.
    - D. These lesions consist of anastomosing tubules or gland-like spaces of varying sizes and shapes that are lined by cells that are flattened to cuboidal and lack nuclear atypia.
    - E. They are thought to arise from invaginated fallopian tube epithelium.

41. Your microscopic examination of a fragmented polypoid lesion from an endometrial curettage specimen shows glands that exhibit architectural atypia and slight cytologic atypia. The stroma consists of interlacing fascicles of smooth muscle that are cytologically benign. Squamous metaplasia is also found. This is diagnostic of which of the following?
    - A. Adenomyoma
    - B. Atypical polypoid adenoma
    - C. Adenofibroma
    - D. Benign polyp
    - E. Adenomatoid tumor

42. Which of the following is TRUE regarding adenomyosis?
    - A. It is seen in <5% of hysterectomy specimens in the United States.
    - B. It is typically seen in women during post-menopausal years.
    - C. Diffuse involvement produces a uterus that is symmetrically enlarged and soft with a globoid shape.
    - D. Generally accepted criterion for diagnosis requires presence of endometrial glands at least 2 40× fields below the endometrial-myometrial junction.
    - E. All of the above

43. Which of the following can be seen in atypical hyperplasia?
    - A. Architectural pattern may be simple or complex.
    - B. Metaplastic changes may be present in any type of hyperplasia (particularly the morular variant of squamous metaplasia).
    - C. True nuclear stratification (2-4 cells thick) with loss of polarity usually present and often more marked than in complex hyperplasia without atypia.
    - D. Atypical cells tend to be enlarged; nuclear-cytoplasmic ratio is increased; nuclei large, hyperchromatic, and pleomorphic (tend to be more rounded than oval); nuclear membranes usually irregular and thick; nucleoli prominent.
    - E. All of the above

5: Female Reproductive Tract Questions

56. Which of the following conditions predisposes a woman to endometrial carcinoma?
    A. Polycystic ovaries
    B. Stromal hyperplasia
    C. Hyperthecosis
    D. Granulosa cell tumor
    E. All of the above

57. What percent of patients diagnosed with an adenosarcoma die from disease?
    A. <1%
    B. 5%-10%
    C. 10%-25%
    D. 25%-40%
    E. >50%

58. Which of the following features does NOT portend a worse prognosis for a malignant mixed Müllerian tumor (carcinosarcoma)?
    A. Sex-cord differentiation
    B. Homologous differentiation that typically contains a high-grade sarcomatous component that consists predominantly of spindled cells, round cells, or giant cells; may resemble a low-grade fibrosarcoma or leiomyosarcoma
    C. Heterologous differentiation that may contain foci of rhabdomyosarcoma, chondrosarcoma, osteosarcoma, liposarcoma, or any combination
    D. >10 mitotic figures/10 hpf
    E. None of the above

59. Endometrial stromal sarcomas most commonly have what staining pattern?
    A. ER+, PR–, CD10+
    B. ER+, PR+, CD10+
    C. ER–, PR–, CD10+
    D. ER–, PR–, CD10+
    E. ER–, PR–, CD10–

60. Which of the following are criteria for a leiomyosarcoma?
    A. Cytologic atypia and 2-5 mitotic figures/10 hpf
    B. Hypercellularity, no atypia, and 5-10 mitotic figures/10 hpf
    C. 10-15 mitotic figures/10 hpf, without hypercellularity or atypia
    D. Infiltrating margins and 5-9 mitotic figures/10 hpf
    E. None of the above

61. Clear cell adenocarcinoma of the vagina is most commonly seen at what age?
    A. <5 years
    B. 5-10 years
    C. 15-25 years
    D. 25-35 years
    E. >50 years

5: Female Reproductive Tract Questions

62. Which of the following statements is TRUE regarding an aggressive angiomyxoma (AA) versus an angiomyofibroblastoma (AMF)?
    A. AAs typically are well circumscribed.
    B. AAs typically have hyalinized and hypertrophied vessels.
    C. AMFs tend to have fewer stromal cells than AAs.
    D. AMFs tend to have abundant stromal mucin and extravasated erythrocytes.
    E. Electron microscopy is needed.

63. Which of the following is TRUE regarding Paget disease?
    A. It rarely presents as an intraepithelial adenocarcinoma arising from a multipotential cell in the epidermis, adnexa, or perineal mammary-like glands.
    B. It most commonly presents as invasive carcinoma arising from an intraepithelial adenocarcinoma or pagetoid extension or metastasis from a nearby carcinoma.
    C. Extramammary Paget disease only develops in the breast, axilla or perineum.
    D. It represents 10% of all vulvar neoplasms.
    E. None of the above

Questions 64-68 are based on these images:

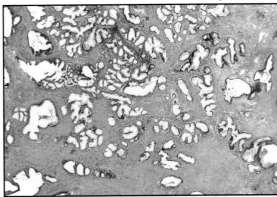 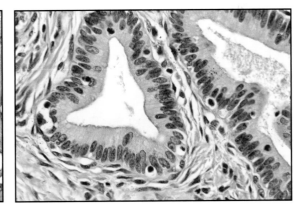

64. This lesion is characterized by which of the following?
    A. Cytologically bland, architecturally complex glands that vary in size and shape
    B. Increased mitotic activity
    C. Glands tend to be lined by a single layer of tall, columnar, cytologically bland cells that have basal nuclei that are slightly larger than normal endocervical nuclei; small nucleoli usually present
    D. A and B
    E. A, B, and C

65. Which of the following histologic variants can be seen in this lesion?
    A. Mucinous
    B. Endometrioid
    C. Clear cell
    D. A and B
    E. A, B, and C

66. This lesion is will likely show focal positivity for which of the following?
    A. CEA
    B. Vimentin
    C. ER
    D. PR
    E. All of the above

67. Which of the following is included in the differential diagnosis?
    A. Nodular clustering of endocervical glands
    B. Microglandular hyperplasia
    C. Mesonephric hyperplasia
    D. A and B
    E. A, B, and C

68. This lesion has also been associated with which of the following?
    A. Gastric adenocarcinoma
    B. SCTAT
    C. FATWO
    D. A and B
    E. A, B, and C

Questions 69-71 are based on these images:

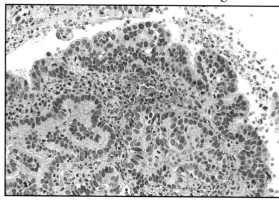 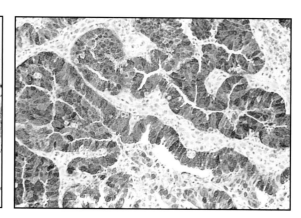

69. The cervix is biopsied from a 28-year-old woman. What is the diagnosis?
    A. Microglandular hyperplasia
    B. Mesonephric hyperplasia
    C. Adenocarcinoma in situ
    D. A and B
    E. A, B, and C

70. This lesion is stained for p16 (which is displayed above right). Which HPV type is most commonly seen with this lesion?
    A. HPV6
    B. HPV11
    C. HPV18
    D. HPV33
    E. A, B, and C

71. A Ki-67 was also performed on this lesion. Which of the following histologic features is/are seen in this type of lesion?

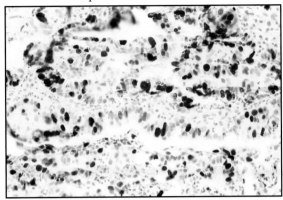

A. It frequently involves surface endocervical glandular epithelium in the transitional zone.
B. Involved glands do not extend below the level of normal glands.
C. Intestinal variants are characterized by the presence of goblet cells with or without argyrophilic cells.
D. A and B
E. A, B, and C

Questions 72 and 73 are based on this image:

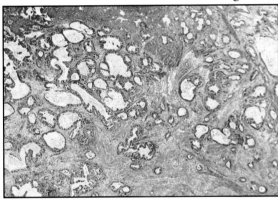

72. This lesion was biopsied from the cervix of a 31-year-old woman. It is positive for CEA. What is the diagnosis?
A. Endometrioid adenocarcinoma
B. Adenocarcinoma of the cervix
C. Squamous cell carcinoma
D. A and B
E. A, B, and C

73. What HPV type is most likely associated with this p16-positive lesion?
A. HPV6
B. HPV11
C. HPV16
D. HPV18
E. HPV33

5: Female Reproductive Tract Questions

74. This lesion is most commonly associated with which HPV type?

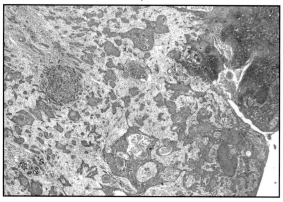

    A.   HPV6
    B.   HPV11
    C.   HPV16
    D.   HPV18
    E.   HPV33

75. Which of the following has the least prognostic significance?

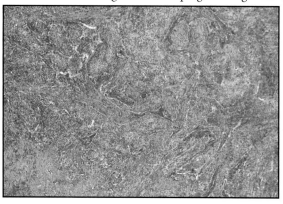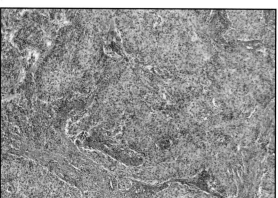

    A.   Depth of invasion
    B.   Histologic grade
    C.   Presence or absence of vascular invasion
    D.   Greatest dimension of tumor
    E.   All of the above are significant.

5: Female Reproductive Tract Questions

76. A 24-year-old woman is 6 months postpartum. She returns to her doctor for persistent vaginal bleeding. This lesion is biopsied from the uterus. What is the diagnosis?

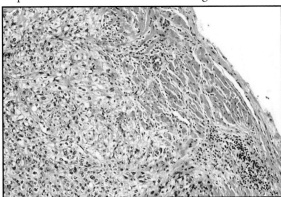 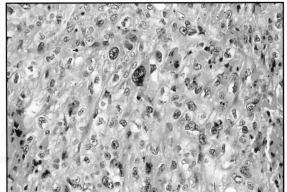

    A. Complete hydatidiform mole
    B. Partial hydatidiform mole
    C. Choriocarcinoma
    D. Placental site trophoblastic tumor

77. These are the uterine contents from a 26-year-old woman. What is the diagnosis?

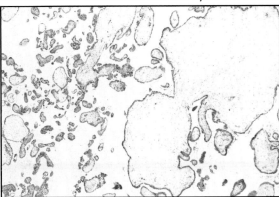

    A. Hydropic abortus
    B. Partial hydatidiform mole
    C. Complete hydatidiform mole
    D. Fetal hydrops
    E. Choriocarcinoma

78. This lesion is characterized by which of the following?

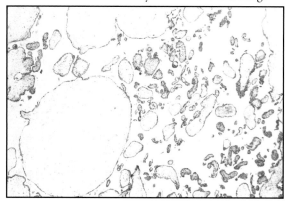

    A.   46,XX
    B.   46,XY
    C.   69,XXY
    D.   69,XXX
    E.   69,XYY

Questions 79 and 80 are based on these images:

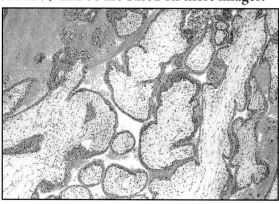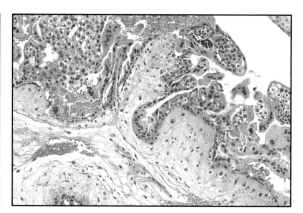

79. What is the most likely diagnosis?
    A.   Hydropic abortus
    B.   Partial hydatidiform mole
    C.   Complete hydatidiform mole
    D.   Fetal hydrops
    E.   Choriocarcinoma

80. Genetically, this lesion is characterized by which of the following?
    A.   46,XX
    B.   46,XY
    C.   69,XXY
    D.   69,XXX
    E.   69,XYY

5: Female Reproductive Tract Questions

81. Which of the following is TRUE regarding this lesion?

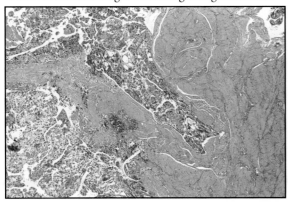 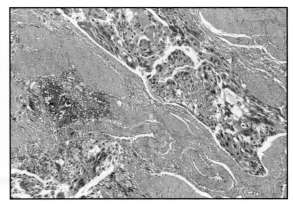

A. Treatment is cytotoxic chemotherapy followed by hysterectomy.
B. Lung metastases present in 90% of patients with extrauterine spread of disease.
C. Blood group A is more frequent; blood group O is less frequent.
D. A and B
E. A, B, and C

82. A 39-year-old woman has a hysterectomy for persistent uterine bleeding. This is found in a polyp on examination. This lesion is diagnostic of which of the following?

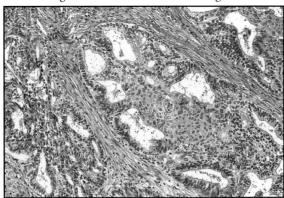

A. Endometrioid adenocarcinoma, FIGO grade 1
B. Adenofibroma
C. Adenosarcoma
D. Atypical polypoid adenomyoma
E. Adenocarcinoma of the cervix

83. A 43-year-old woman has a hysterectomy for severe monthly abdominal pain. The lesion in the image below was found in the wall of the uterus. What is the diagnosis?

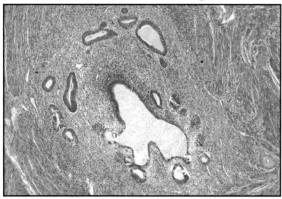

A. Endometriosis
B. Endometrioid adenocarcinoma
C. Atypical polypoid adenomyoma
D. Adenosarcoma
E. Adenomyosis

84. This is an endometrial biopsy from a 49-year-old woman with persistent uterine bleeding. What percent of patients are at risk of developing adenocarcinoma from this lesion?

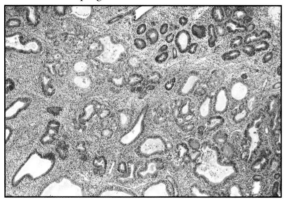

A. 0
B. <5%
C. 10%
D. 30%
E. This is an adenocarcinoma.

5: Female Reproductive Tract Questions

85. The following is noted in an endometrial curettage specimen. What is the diagnosis?

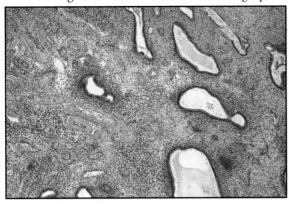

    A.   Adenosarcoma
    B.   Adenofibroma
    C.   Atypical polypoid adenomyoma
    D.   Atrophy
    E.   Endometrial polyp

86. The below image is noted in a hysterectomy specimen. What is the diagnosis?

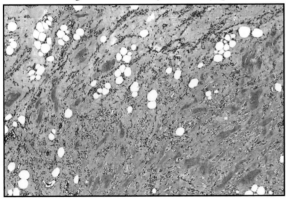

    A.   Adenomatoid tumor
    B.   Leiomyoma
    C.   Hyalinized leiomyoma
    D.   Lipoleiomyoma
    E.   Well-differentiated liposarcoma

5: Female Reproductive Tract Questions

91.   This lesion is characterized by which of the following?

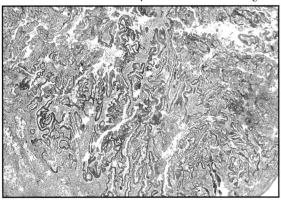 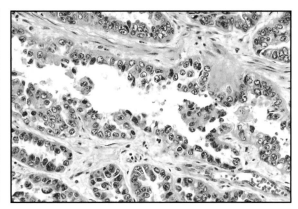

    A.   It represents 5%-10% of all endometrial carcinomas.

    B.   It is an aggressive neoplasm that tends to invade myometrium early.

    C.   Psammoma bodies present in 30%.

    D.   A and B

    E.   A, B, and C

92.   After TAH-BSO and surgical staging, this lesion is found in 2 paraortic lymph nodes. What is this woman's most likely 5-year survival rate?

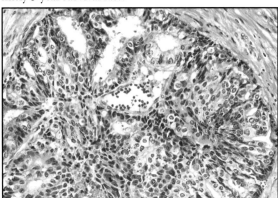

    A.   >95%

    B.   80%-95%

    C.   50%-60%

    D.   15%-25%

    E.   <5%

5: Female Reproductive Tract Questions

93. This lesion is found in a polypoid mass from a uterus of a 76-year-old woman. The surface of the polyp has broad leaflike structures. Several of these glands are identified in the lesion. The stroma surrounding these glands is noticeably condensed and a mitotic count yields >20 mitotic figures/10 hpf. What is the diagnosis?

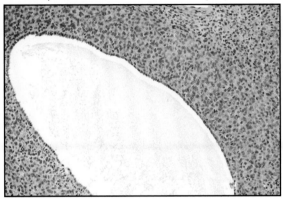

    A.   Adenofibroma
    B.   Atypical polypoid adenomyoma
    C.   Adenosarcoma
    D.   Malignant mixed Müllerian tumor
    E.   Carcinosarcoma

94. The lesion pictured below is a deeply invasive tumor, which was found in the wall of an 86-year-old woman. Pancytokeratin is positive in the tumor cells. What is the diagnosis?

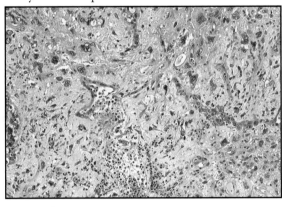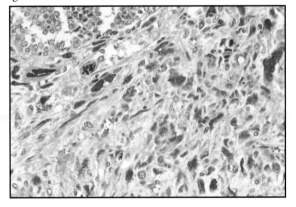

    A.   Carcinosarcoma
    B.   Hodgkin lymphoma classical type
    C.   Diffuse large B-cell lymphoma
    D.   Epithelioid leiomyosarcoma
    E.   Endometrial stromal sarcoma

95.   Upon TAH-BSO for persistent uterine bleeding, this 40-year-old woman has this deeply infiltrating tumor. What is the diagnosis?

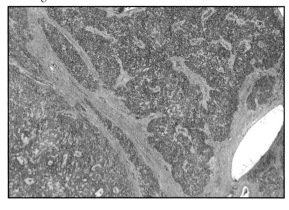 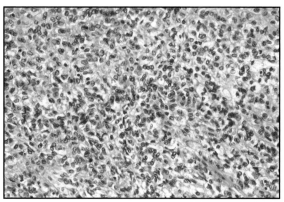

   A.   Endometrioid carcinoma, FIGO grade 1
   B.   Endometrial stromal nodule
   C.   Adenosarcoma
   D.   Endometrial stromal sarcoma
   E.   Carcinosarcoma

96.   An 88-year-old woman was found to have a rapidly enlarging uterine mass. This lesion stained strongly positive for SMA, MSA and was negative for S100, NSE, CD34 and CD10. 6 mitotic figures/10 hpf were noted. What is the most likely diagnosis?

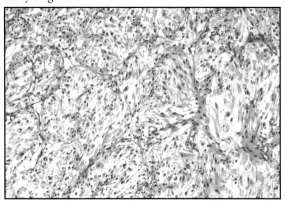

   A.   Alveolar soft part sarcoma
   B.   Malignant fibrous histiocytoma
   C.   Rhabdomyosarcoma
   D.   Epithelioid leiomyosarcoma
   E.   Myxoid leiomyosarcoma

5: Female Reproductive Tract Questions

97. A 22-year-old woman has vaginal discharge. An erythematous, 9-mm lesion is noted in the upper 1/3 of the lateral wall of her vagina. A serum β-HCG is negative. What is the most likely diagnosis?

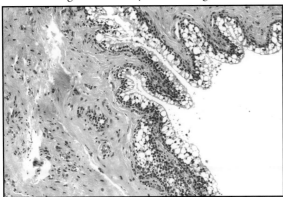

    A. Arias-Stella changes
    B. Clear cell adenocarcinoma
    C. Microglandular hyperplasia
    D. Metastatic renal cell carcinoma
    E. Endodermal sinus tumor

98. A 25-year-old woman had a 12-cm polypoid vulvar mass excised. What is the most likely diagnosis?

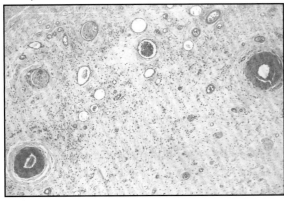 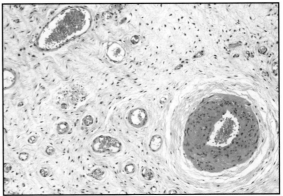

    A. Bartholin gland cyst
    B. Myxoma
    C. Myxolipoma
    D. Botryoid rhabdomyosarcoma
    E. Aggressive angiomyxoma

5: Female Reproductive Tract Questions

99. A 3-cm well-circumscribed, pink mass is easily excised from the vulva of a 28-year-old woman. What is the best diagnosis?

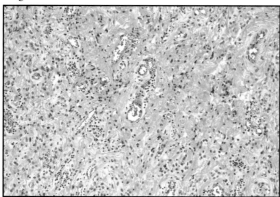 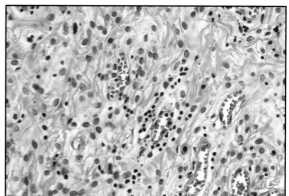

    A.   Leiomyoma
    B.   Angiomyofibroblastoma
    C.   Leiomyoma
    D.   Epithelioid hemangioendothelioma
    E.   Aggressive angiomyxoma

100. This vulvar lesion was biopsied from a 38-year-old woman. The tumor cells are positive for c-erb2. Which of the following is likely negative by immunohistochemistry?

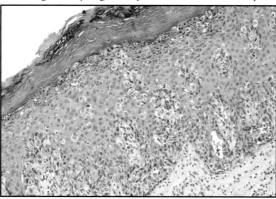

    A.   Low-molecular weight cytokeratin
    B.   CEA
    C.   EMA
    D.   S100
    E.   A, B, and C

5: Female Reproductive Tract Questions

101. A 22-year-old woman has a 5-mm nodule on her labia majora. It is completely excised. What is the most likely diagnosis?

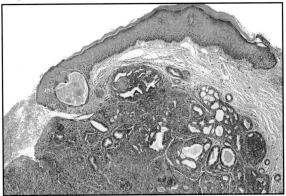

    A.   Metastatic papillary serous carcinoma

    B.   Paget disease

    C.   Microglandular hyperplasia

    D.   Papillary hidradenoma

    E.   Endometriosis

5: Female Reproductive Tract Answers

14.   A.   **GRADE I (WELL-DIFFERENTIATED)**

Microscopic grading of cervical squamous carcinoma is defined by the following criteria. Well-differentiated (grade I): mature squamous cells, with abundant keratin pearl formation and few mitotic figures; nuclei tend to be uniform and cells have well-developed intercellular bridges. Moderately differentiated (grade II): cells with less cytoplasm and more indistinct cell borders; nuclei pleomorphic and mitotic activity increased over that seen in a well-differentiated tumor. Poorly differentiated (grade III): masses and nests of small, primitive oval cells with scant cytoplasm and hyperchromatic spindle-shaped nuclei with very high mitotic rates; little or no keratinization (neoplastic cells tend to resemble those seen in high-grade CIN).

QCSP, **Cervix,** p 156.

15.   E.   **LYMPH NODE STATUS**

The presence of positive lymph nodes has a profound effect on prognosis (negative nodes associated with 95% 5-year survival; ≥2 positive nodes associated with a 17% 5-year survival). Histologic grading and classification (keratinizing versus nonkeratinizing) are not of prognostic significance. The size of the tumor is important. The 5-year survival rate for patients with tumors <2 cm is 90%; 5-year survival rate for patients with tumors ≥2 cm is 65%.

QCSP, **Cervix,** p 156-157.

16.   D.   **HPV16**

It is estimated that HPV16 infections are associated with approximately 55% of cases and HPV18 with another 16%. Additionally, HPV33, HPV45, HPV31, HPV58, HPV52, HPV35, HPV59, HPV56, HPV51, HPV39, HPV73, HPV68, and HPV82 are also associated with squamous cell carcinoma; HPV16, HPV18, HPV31, and HPV45 are associated with 80% of all cervical carcinomas.

QCSP, **Trophoblastic Disease,** p 157.

17.   C.   **HPV18**

HPV18 is associated with both adenocarcinoma and poorly differentiated carcinoma and has more frequent lymph node involvement than HPV16.

QCSP, **Trophoblastic Disease,** p 157.

18.   C.   **PLACENTAL SITE TROPHOBLASTIC TUMOR**

In addition to the microscopic findings described in the question, placental site trophoblastic tumor can demonstrate fibrinoid material that is deposited into the destroyed vessel. Chorionic villi are always absent, but the uninvolved endometrium demonstrates decidualization.

QCSP, **Trophoblastic Disease,** p 157.

19.   B.   **MOST ARE BENIGN.**

Most PSTTs are benign and adequately treated with hysterectomy; however, 10%-15% behave in a malignant fashion with rapid development of metastatic disease. Malignant disease is unresponsive to chemotherapy.

QCSP, **Trophoblastic Disease,** p 158.

20.   D.   **ATYPICAL MITOTIC FIGURES**

It should be noted that these tumors are very rare and the biology is variable. Malignant features include tumor cells with clear rather than amphophilic cytoplasm aggregating in large masses and sheets, extensive necrosis, and a high mitotic rate (≥5 mitotic figures/10 hpf). Atypical mitotic figures can be seen in either benign or malignant tumors.

QCSP, **Trophoblastic Disease,** p 157.

5: Female Reproductive Tract Answers

21. C. **PARTIAL MOLE**
Given the differential diagnosis listed, the microscopic description is diagnostic of a partial mole, characterized by a mixture of large edematous villi and normal-sized villi. Some hydropic villi contain a central, acellular cistern, but cisterns are less prominent than in complete moles. Chorionic villi frequently have a scalloped outline compared with the typically round and distended appearance of villi of a complete mole; this irregular outline of a partial mole results from infolding of trophoblasts into the villous stroma (which often appear as inclusions).
QCSP, **Trophoblastic Disease,** p 158.

22. C. **69,XXY**
Typically karyotype shows triploidy (69 chromosomes) with 2 paternal sets and 1 maternal chromosome complement. When triploidy is present, 70% have a complement that is XXY, 27% have a complement that is XXX, and 3% have a complement that is XYY. The egg is fertilized with a haploid set of chromosomes by either 2 sperms (each with a haploid set of chromosomes) or by a single sperm with a diploid 46,XY complement. 15%-20% of triploid fetuses have a diploid 46,XX maternal genome and a haploid paternal set of chromosomes (digynic conceptus).
QCSP, **Trophoblastic Disease,** p 159.

23. E. **NONE OF THE ABOVE**
Despite all of the answers providing some value, the best way to differentiate a hydropic abortion from a partial mole is by H&E examination. In a nonmolar pregnancy, especially one with hydropic changes, the trophoblastic proliferation, is typically polar and characterized by growth arising from 1 pole of the villus; trophoblastic proliferation in a mole is more haphazard and circumferential. Nonmolar pregnancies are not characterized by the formation of cisterns or the presence of atypia in the trophoblastic proliferation.
QCSP, **Trophoblastic Disease,** p 159.

24. C. **10%-30%**
Of those patients with the diagnosis of complete hydatidiform mole, approximately 10%-30% will have persistently elevated hCG levels after removal/evacuation, thus indicating persistence of a gestational trophoblastic disease.
QCSP, **Trophoblastic Disease,** p 159.

25. B. **5%-10%**
As compared with complete hydatidiform mole, only 5%-10% of patients with partial hydatidiform with have residual disease after evacuation of the lesion.
QCSP, **Trophoblastic Disease,** p 159.

26. A. **<1%**
It is rare for choriocarcinoma to develop after partial hydatidiform moles, and it only occurs in <1% of cases.
QCSP, **Trophoblastic Disease,** p 159.

27. A. **2%-3%**
While 50% of choriocarcinomas occur after a hydatidiform mole, only 2%-3% of patients with a history of a complete hydatidiform mole will progress to a choriocarcinoma.
QCSP, **Trophoblastic Disease,** p 159.

5: Female Reproductive Tract Answers

28. **D. 46,XX**

    The most common karyotype in complete moles is 46,XX. The chromosomes are all paternally derived with both sex chromosomes (XX) derived from duplication of the haploid sperm in an empty ovum. The duplication of a 23,Y yields a nonviable 46,YY cell. Occasionally, 2 sperm (23,Y and 23,X) can fertilize an empty ovum resulting in a 46,XY karyotype. Rare (extremely) cases can be triploid or tetraploid.

    QCSP, **Trophoblastic Disease,** p 160.

29. **E. NONE OF THE ABOVE**

    In fact, all of the answers listed are possible. Most are diploid with a 46,XX karyotype and rarely triploid or tetraploid. All chromosome complements are paternally derived. Both X chromosomes result from duplication of a haploid sperm pronucleus in an empty ovum (an ovum that has lost its maternal chromosomal haploid set). Duplication of a 23,Y sperm results in a nonviable 46,YY cell. 5%-15% have a 46,XY chromosome complement, probably the result of an empty ovum being fertilized by 2 sperm pronuclei, 1 with an X and 1 with a Y chromosome.

    QCSP, **Trophoblastic Disease,** p 160.

30. **E. A, B, AND C**

    Invasive hydatidiform mole typically demonstrates deportation (presence of molar villi or intermediate-type trophoblastic cells in the blood vessels without invasion) as compared to true metastasis. Approximately 20% of cases demonstrate extrauterine involvement. Interestingly, pulmonary lesions often regress after hysterectomy.

    QCSP, **Trophoblastic Disease,** p 161.

31. **B. HPL**

    Intermediate trophoblasts are positive for hPL, but negative for hCG and PLAP.

    QCSP, **Trophoblastic Disease,** p 161.

32. **D. NONE OF THE ABOVE**

    Cytotrophoblasts are generally negative for hCG, PLAP, and hPL but positive for p53.

    QCSP, **Trophoblastic Disease,** p 161.

33. **E. A, B, AND C**

    Syncytiotrophoblasts are generally positive for hCG, hPL and PLAP.

    QCSP, **Trophoblastic Disease,** p 161.

34. **E. ALL OF THE ABOVE**

    The development of choriocarcinoma may be associated with any form of gestation, but abnormal types of pregnancy are more likely to be associated with choriocarcinoma, eg, spontaneous abortion, ectopic pregnancy, and molar pregnancy.

    QCSP, **Trophoblastic Disease,** p 162.

35. **C. CYTOTROPHOBLASTIC CELLS**

    Syncytiotrophoblastic cells are multinucleate cells without mitotic activity (3-20 nuclei per cell). The cytoplasm is dense and stains deeply eosinophilic to basophilic. The cytoplasm may contain vacuoles and lacunae, some of which contain red blood cells. In contrast, intermediate trophoblastic cells share features of both cytotrophoblastic and syncytiotrophoblastic cells. They are typically large and polyhedral with 1 nucleus and abundant eosinophilic to amphophilic cytoplasm without vacuoles. The cell membranes are less distinct than cytotrophoblastic cell membranes.

    QCSP, **Trophoblastic Disease,** p 162.

5: Female Reproductive Tract Answers

36. **D. A AND B**
     Syncytiotrophoblastic cells and intermediate trophoblastic cells typically stain intensely for β-hCG and are variably positive for human placental lactogen. The hPL staining is a feature unique to a choriocarcinoma; it rarely, if ever, occurs in other tumors.
     QCSP, **Trophoblastic Disease,** p 162.

37. **A. HYDATIDIFORM MOLE**
     50% of choriocarcinomas are preceded by a hydatidiform mole, but only 2.5% of hydatidiform moles are followed by choriocarcinoma. 25% of choriocarcinomas follow an abortion, 22% follow a normal pregnancy, and 2.5% follow an ectopic pregnancy.
     QCSP, **Trophoblastic Disease,** p 163.

38. **A. A**
     Blood group A is the most frequent; blood group O is less frequent.
     QCSP, **Trophoblastic Disease,** p 163.

39. **C. ADENOFIBROMA**
     This is a typical description of an adenofibroma.
     QCSP, **Uterus,** Benign Lesions, p 164.

40. **E. THEY ARE THOUGHT TO ARISE FROM INVAGINATED FALLOPIAN TUBE EPITHELIUM**
     Adenomatoid tumors are thought to arise from serosal mesothelium, not fallopian tubal epithelium. All of the other answers are correct.
     QCSP, **Uterus,** Benign Lesions, p 151.

41. **B. ATYPICAL POLYPOID ADENOMA**
     Recurrence is common if the lesion is incompletely excised. Adenocarcinoma may arise in an atypical polypoid adenomyoma.
     QCSP, **Uterus,** Benign Lesions, p 165.

42. **C. DIFFUSE INVOLVEMENT PRODUCES A UTERUS THAT IS SYMMETRICALLY ENLARGED AND SOFT WITH A GLOBOID SHAPE.**
     Adenomyosis is seen in 10%-20% of hysterectomy specimens in the United States. It is typically seen in women during reproductive years. Generally accepted criterion for diagnosis requires presence of endometrial glands at least 0.2 cm (1/2 of a 40× field) below the endometrial-myometrial junction.
     QCSP, **Uterus,** Benign Lesions, p 166.

43. **E. ALL OF THE ABOVE**
     All of these findings can be seen in the spectrum of atypical endometrial hyperplasia. While they can demonstrate papillary infolding, a cribriform or confluent pattern is never seen. There are no characteristic stromal findings for atypical hyperplasia.
     QCSP, **Uterus,** Benign Lesions, p 167.

44. **C. 15%-25%**
     Approximately 15%-25% of uteri removed for atypical hyperplasia will contain at least a single focus of adenocarcinoma. As such, uteri removed for atypical hyperplasia are often extensively sampled.
     QCSP, **Uterus,** Benign Lesions, p 168.

5: Female Reproductive Tract Answers

45.   E.   **A, B, AND C**
      Choices A-C describe findings associated with endometrial polyps.
      QCSP, **Uterus**, Benign Lesions, p 168.

46.   D.   **NO FURTHER ACTION IS REQUIRED.**
      This is intravenous leiomyomatosis. You have documented it, and no further treatment is required. This is a benign neoplasm that can metastasize, but even then only requires simple excision and some lesions may be watched depending on location. Any of the histologic variants of leiomyoma may be present (bizarre, cellular, epithelioid, myxoid, or lipoleiomyoma), and as long as the features are benign, tumors behave in a benign fashion.
      QCSP, **Uterus**, Benign Lesions, p 169.

47.   E.   **ALL OF THE ABOVE**
      Not only are all of the choices benign, they are all synonyms for the same entity.
      QCSP, **Uterus**, Benign Lesions, p 171.

48.   D.   **CD10**
      The description is diagnostic of an endometrial stromal nodule. It is an H&E diagnosis. Immunohistochemical stains can be used to help differentiate the tumor from variants of leiomyoma. While focal staining for SMA, MSA and desmin may be seen in rare foci of the tumor; these tumors are strongly positive for CD10. This strong CD10 positivity supports their origin of endometrial stromal cells.
      QCSP, **Uterus**, Benign Lesions, p 172.

49.   B.   **BREAST FEEDING**
      Breast feeding may actually be protective as it provides a window of decreased exposure to estrogen. The rest of the answers are associated with increased exposure to estrogen.
      QCSP, **Uterus**, Malignant Lesions, p 173.

50.   A.   **STROMAL INVASION ONLY**
      The diagnosis of adenocarcinoma vs complex atypical hyperplasia is based on the presence of stromal invasion. Stromal invasion is characterized by glandular fusion (disappearance of endometrial stroma between adjacent glands), stromal fibrosis, or stromal necrosis.
      QCSP, **Uterus**, Malignant Lesions, p 173.

51.   D.   **A AND B**
      The International Federation of Gynecology and Obstetrics (FIGO) grading system grades carcinoma as 1 of 3 grades based on both architectural and nuclear features: architecture grade I: 95% of tumor forms glands ($\leq$5% solid growth pattern); architecture grade II: 6%-50% of the tumor has a solid growth pattern; architecture grade III: >50% of the neoplasm has a solid growth pattern (importantly, areas of squamous differentiation and squamous morules do not count as solid areas); nuclear grade I: oval, small, uniform nuclei with fine chromatin, small nucleoli, and few mitoses; nuclear grade II: features between grades I and III; nuclear grade III: enlarged, elongated, pleomorphic nuclei with irregular outlines, coarse chromatin, macronuclei and numerous mitoses. If the nuclear atypia is out of proportion to the architectural grade, then the architectural grade is raised by 1.
      QCSP, **Uterus**, Malignant Lesions, p 174.

52.   D.   **SEROUS ADENOCARCINOMA: TUMOR CELLS ARE LARGE AND HAVE CLEAR CYTOPLASM, AND DENSE HYALINIZED STROMA MAY BE PRESENT; CELLS MAY GROW IN A SOLID, PAPILLARY, TUBULAR, OR MIXED PATTERN**
      This is the description for clear cell carcinoma and not serous adenocarcinoma.
      QCSP, **Uterus**, Malignant Lesions, p 174.

5: Female Reproductive Tract Answers

53. **B.** **ER POSITIVE AND P16 NEGATIVE**

The other staining patterns would be confusing. Mucinous adenocarcinoma of endometrium frequently shows endocervical differentiation, but is usually ER positive and p16 negative. It can be difficult to distinguish from adenocarcinoma arising from the endocervix, which is usually ER negative and p16 positive.

QCSP, **Uterus**, Malignant Lesions, p 175.

54. **E.** **A, B, AND C**

Choices A-C are all true regarding the treatment of endometrial adenocarcinoma of the uterus. While hysterectomy is usually the first line of treatment, staging with lymph node dissections is often undertaken for high-grade lesions and myometrial invasion of >50%. Inoperable endometrial adenocarcinoma is often treated with radiation alone.

QCSP, **Uterus**, Malignant Lesions, p 176.

55. **B.** **PRESENCE OR ABSENCE OF SQUAMOUS DIFFERENTIATION**

The presence or absence of benign squamous differentiation has no effect on prognosis. However, adenosquamous carcinomas (malignant squamous differentiation) have a worse prognosis than adenocarcinomas with benign squamous differentiation.

QCSP, **Uterus**, Malignant Lesions, p 176.

56. **E.** **ALL OF THE ABOVE**

Conditions of increased estrogen production (especially in postmenopausal women) increase a woman's risk of endometrial carcinoma. Specifically, unopposed exogenous estrogen and ovarian lesions are associated with increased estrogen production: granulosa cell tumor, hyperthecosis, stromal hyperthecosis, and polycystic ovaries. Other risk factors include obesity, nulliparity, and late menopause.

QCSP, **Uterus**, Malignant Lesions, p 177.

57. **C.** **10%-25%**

Even though most patients can be successfully treated with hysterectomy, there is a high recurrence risk. Also approximately 10%-25% of patients will die from the disease. These patients demonstrate stromal overgrowth on their initial tumor, and death might occur several years after the initial diagnosis.

QCSP, **Uterus**, Malignant Lesions, p 178.

58. **E.** **NONE OF THE ABOVE**

In the past it was believed that heterologous differentiation indicated a worse prognosis; however, subsequent studies have not supported that notion.

QCSP, **Uterus**, Malignant Lesions, p 178.

59. **B.** **ER+, PR+, CD10+**

Endometrial stromal tumors are typically ER, PR, and CD10 positive. Additionally the tumors are usually BCL-2 and vimentin positive. The tumors are usually EMA negative. The neoplastic cells can focally express desmin, MSA, and cytokeratin in tumors with epithelioid differentiation.

QCSP, **Uterus**, Malignant Lesions, p 180.

60. **E.** **NONE OF THE ABOVE**

All of the choices describe smooth muscle tumors of uncertain malignant potential. The criteria for leiomyosarcoma are complex. In general, one needs coagulative necrosis, diffuse or multifocal atypia and >10 mitotic figures/10 hpf. However, an authoritative text should be referenced prior to making such a diagnosis.

QCSP, **Uterus**, Malignant Lesions, p 181-182.

5: Female Reproductive Tract Answers

61. C. **15-25 YEARS**

The age range is 5-45 years, with a peak at 20 years. It is uncommon before age 15 years and after age 30 years. *QCSP,* **Vagina,** p 182.

62. B. **AAS TYPICALLY HAVE HYALINIZED AND HYPERTROPHIED VESSELS.**

Angiomyofibroblastomas in general are more circumscribed, the blood vessels are not hyalinized or hypertrophied, plump stromal cells surround more numerous vessels, there is little stromal mucin, and extravasated erythrocytes are rare. In contrast, aggressive angiomyxomas are not circumscribed. The blood vessels tend to be hyalinized and hypertrophied. Stromal cells are fewer in number, less plump, and do not tend to surround vessels. There is usually abundant stromal mucin and extravasated erythrocytes are present. *QCSP,* **Vulva,** p 184-185.

63. E. **NONE OF THE ABOVE**

Extramammary Paget disease usually presents as an intraepithelial adenocarcinoma arising from a multipotential cell in the epidermis, adnexa, or perineal mammary-like glands. Less often it presents as an invasive carcinoma arising from an intraepithelial adenocarcinoma or pagetoid extension or metastasis from a nearby carcinoma (eg, cervix, Bartholin gland, urinary bladder, urethra). Extramammary Paget disease can develop anywhere along the milk line, from axilla to perineum. It represents 2% of all vulvar neoplasms. It most frequently is diagnosed in white, postmenopausal women around the 7th decade. *QCSP,* **Vulva,** p 186.

64. E. **A, B, AND C**

This is an example of minimal deviation adenocarcinoma (adenoma malignum). The criteria for diagnosis include cytologically bland, architecturally complex glands that vary in size and shape; increased mitotic activity; hyperplastic-appearing surface glands; an increased number of glands positioned deeper than normal in the region of the endocervix (normal glands seldom extend >5 mm below the endocervical surface); glands typically varying in size ranging from small and round to large, irregular, and distorted, with complex outlines and some element of desmoplasia usually present; perineural invasion that can be seen. Glands tend to be lined by a single layer of tall, columnar, cytologically bland cells that have basal nuclei that are slightly larger than normal endocervical nuclei; small nucleoli are usually present. *QCSP,* **Cervix,** p 151.

65. E. **A, B, AND C**

Histologic variants of minimal deviation adenocarcinoma include all of the listed types. Mucinous is the most common form and demonstrates glands lined by a single layer of columnar, mucin-producing cells that resemble the cells of the endocervix. The glands are often elongated or branching. The endometrioid variant has tumor cells that resemble those of proliferative endometrium or endometrial hyperplasia. The clear cell variant not surprisingly has tumor cells with clear cytoplasm. *QCSP,* **Cervix,** p 152.

66. A. **CEA**

Focal staining with CEA may be present (a well-differentiated cervical adenocarcinoma is more diffusely positive for CEA and all benign lesions are negative for CEA except microglandular hyperplasia). The other stains are characteristically positive in lesions primary to the endometrium and negative in the cervix. *QCSP,* **Interoperative Consultation,** p 151.

5: Female Reproductive Tract Answers

67.   E.   **A, B, AND C**
      The cytologic and histologic differential for minimal deviation adenocarcinoma includes hyperplasia, adenocarcinoma in situ, tunnel clusters of endocervical glands, deeply positioned nabothian cyst, and adenomyosis.
      QCSP, **Cervix,** p 152.

68.   E.   **A, B, AND C**
      Minimal deviation adenocarcinoma has be seen in association with Peutz-Jeghers syndrome, which is characterized by multiple (almost always <100) hamartomatous polyps scattered throughout the entire gastrointestinal tract (stomach [25%], small intestine [100%], and large intestine [30%]) with melanotic mucosal and cutaneous pigmentation of the lips, oral mucosa, face, genitalia, digits, palms, and soles; also associated with an increased incidence of other malignant neoplasms, including carcinoma of stomach, small intestine, and colon, a distinctive ovarian neoplasm (sex-cord tumor with annular tubules [SCTAT]), ovarian mucinous tumors, and female adnexal tumors of Wolffian origin (FATWO); also breast carcinoma (often bilateral).
      QCSP, **Cervix,** p 152.

69.   C.   **ADENOCARCINOMA IN SITU**
      The cervical lesion demonstrates cytologically malignant cells with prominent mitotic activity and a glandular morphology. The best diagnosis based on the image is an adenocarcinoma in situ.
      QCSP, **Cervix,** p 152.

70.   C.   **HPV18**
      >90% of adenocarcinoma in situ cases are infected with HPV. Similar to squamous cervical carcinoma, HPV16 and HPV18 are the 2 most common subtypes. However, in cases of AIS, HPV18 appears to be the dominant subtype. Additional subtypes reported in AIS include HPV45, HPV52, and HPV35.
      QCSP, **Cervix,** p 153.

71.   E.   **A, B, AND C**
      All of the answers are true. In addition, the following histologic features may be seen: the endocervical (mucinous) variant (most common) is characterized by cells that resemble those of the endocervix with basal nuclei and pale granular cytoplasm that contains mucin; tumor cells have markedly enlarged, crowded nuclei that are hyperchromatic and have coarse chromatin; prominent mitotic activity and apoptotic cells are both typical; the endometrioid variant lacks both the goblet cells of the intestinal variant and the clear light staining cytoplasm of endocervical variant; typically cells have scant cytoplasm and marked nuclear stratification (resemble malignant endometrial glands). There is also an adenosquamous variant.
      QCSP, **Cervix,** p 153.

72.   B.   **ADENOCARCINOMA OF THE CERVIX**
      The low-grade architecture, mucinous features, CEA positivity and cervical location all point to adenocarcinoma of the cervix.
      QCSP, **Cervix,** p 154.

73.   D.   **HPV18**
      Don't let the numbers confuse you. HPV types 6 and 11 are associated with low-grade squamous lesion. HPV16 is the most common cause of high-grade squamous lesions. HPV18 is the most common cause of adenocarcinoma of the cervix. HPV33 is associated with high-grade lesions, but it is less common than types 16 and 18.
      QCSP, **Cervix,** p 154.

5: Female Reproductive Tract Answers

74.   C.   **HPV16**

Sorry for the redundancy. You must have this down. See the answer to question 10. As an aside, the HPV vaccine covers HPV types 6, 11, 16 and 18. More research has demonstrated that the vaccine actually covers a broader spectrum of disease to include more of the less common carcinogenic HPV types.

QCSP, **Cervix,** p 151.

75.   B.   **Histologic grade**

Histologic grading is not of prognostic significance. All of the other listed choices affect prognosis. The most important is lymph node status and metastases.

QCSP, **Cervix,** p 157.

76.   D.   **Placental site trophoblastic tumor**

This is the rarest form of gestational trophoblastic disease. This is characterized by a predominance of intermediate trophoblasts and a smaller population of cytotrophoblastic and syncytiotrophoblastic cells. Chorionic villi are always absent. The differential diagnosis for this lesion includes choriocarcinoma, placental site nodule, exaggerated implantation site, epithelioid leiomyosarcoma, clear cell carcinoma, and hyalinized squamous cell carcinoma. Of these the only one listed was choriocarcinoma, which is characterized by a biphasic proliferation that always includes syncytiotrophoblasts and either cytotrophoblasts or intermediate trophoblasts. Choriocarcinoma is quite necrotic and angioinvasive, features not seen in this picture.

QCSP, **Trophoblastic Disease,** p 151.

77.   B.   **Partial hydatidiform mole**

This is a partial hydatidiform mole. It is characterized by a mixture of large edematous villi and normal-sized villi. The degree of hydropic swelling is less than that seen with complete moles. Some hydropic villi contain a central, acellular cistern, but cisterns are less prominent than in complete moles. Chorionic villi frequently have a scalloped outline compared with the typically round and distended appearance of villi of a complete mole; this irregular outline of a partial mole results from infoldings of trophoblasts into the villous stroma (often appear as inclusions). Villous stroma is often fibrotic and contains capillaries with fetal (nucleated) red blood cells. This is in contrast to complete moles. Fetal parts or amnion are often present and are very helpful in sorting out the differential diagnosis.

QCSP, **Trophoblastic Disease,** p 158.

78.   C.   **69,XXY**

Partial moles most commonly (70%) have a complement that is XXY. 27% have a complement that is XXX. 3% have a complement that is XYY.

QCSP, **Trophoblastic Disease,** p 159.

79.   C.   **Complete hydatidiform mole**

Complete moles are characterized by generalized hydropic villous change; almost all of the villi are edematous, but some may be small (average size 0.4 cm). Many have cisterns consisting of a central, acellular, fluid-filled space without mesenchymal cells. Villous stroma lacks both fibrosis and capillaries with fetal (nucleated) red blood cells. Villous surfaces have some degree of circumferential, haphazard trophoblastic proliferation; the trophoblastic proliferation may affect almost all the villi in the specimen or may be minimal and focal. Proliferating trophoblasts are composed of all 3 cell types (syncytiotrophoblast, cytotrophoblast, and intermediate trophoblast). Characteristically there is no evidence of the development of an embryo/fetus (no fetal parts or amnion present); villous stroma lacks the blood vessels that are a normal feature of embryogenesis.

QCSP, **Trophoblastic Disease,** p 160.

5: Female Reproductive Tract Answers

80.   A.   **46,XX**

Most complete moles are diploid with a 46,XX karyotype; rarely triploid or tetraploid. All chromosome complements are paternally derived. Both X chromosomes result from duplication of a haploid sperm pronucleus in an empty ovum (an ovum that has lost its maternal chromosomal haploid set). Duplication of a 23,Y sperm results in a nonviable 46,YY cell. 5%-15% have a 46,XY chromosome complement, probably the result of an empty ovum being fertilized by 2 sperm pronuclei, 1 with an X and 1 with a Y chromosome.

QCSP, **Trophoblastic Disease,** p 151.

81.   E.   **A, B, AND C**

This is a photo of choriocarcinoma. This is a very aggressive, but curable disease. All of the choices are correct.

QCSP, **Trophoblastic Disease,** p 162-163.

82.   D.   **ATYPICAL POLYPOID ADENOMYOMA**

It is a well-known pitfall to call this malignant. Glands in an atypical polypoid adenomyoma exhibit architectural atypia and slight cytologic atypia similar to that seen in atypical hyperplasia of the endometrium. The stromal component consists of interlacing or whorling fascicles of smooth muscle that are cytologically benign (mitotic figures are occasionally seen in the stromal component). Squamous or morular metaplasia is almost always found and may be extensive; areas of necrosis may be found in the areas of squamous or morular metaplasia but the cytology of the squamous component is always benign.

QCSP, **Uterus,** p 165.

83.   E.   **ADENOMYOSIS**

This benign lesion is characterized by small or large islands of endometrial glands and stroma (basalis-type) in the myometrium surrounded by hypertrophied bands of smooth muscle. During pregnancy, decidual change may be present. Foci of hemorrhage or hemosiderin pigment are rarely present. Generally accepted criterion for diagnosis requires the presence of endometrial glands at least 0.2 cm (1/2 of a 40× field) below the endometrial-myometrial junction.

QCSP, **Uterus,** p 166.

84.   B.   **<5%**

This is complex hyperplasia without atypia. Notice the architecturally complex glands randomly distributed and closely packed together. Some are nearly back-to-back with little intervening stroma. Cytologically, epithelium of the complex glands is identical to that of simple hyperplasia. The nuclei are uniform in size and shape, show normal polarity. Nucleoli tend to be inconspicuous. Mitotic activity is variable. The stromal component is much less prominent than in simple hyperplasia. There is no fibrosis or necrosis. Simple or complex hyperplasia without atypia is usually self-limited and spontaneously regresses (risk of progression to carcinoma 1% and 3% respectively). The risk of progression to carcinoma is 10% for simple atypical hyperplasia and 30% for complex atypical hyperplasia.

QCSP, **Uterus,** p 167-168.

85.   E.   **ENDOMETRIAL POLYP**

These are typically seen in perimenopausal women. They are typically pedunculated and extend above the endometrial surface. They will frequently be in a different phase of the menstrual cycle than surrounding nonpolypoid endometrium. Glands are often sparse, irregularly distributed, dilated, and lined by atrophic, inactive, or weakly proliferative endometrium. Stroma is either focally or diffusely fibrotic, rarely cytologically atypical. Various endometrial changes may be present: secretory changes (usually poorly developed), gestational changes, the entire spectrum of metaplastic changes, and various forms of hyperplasia, carcinoma, sarcoma, and carcinosarcoma. Large, thick-walled, coiled vessels are usually found in the center.

QCSP, **Uterus,** p 168.

5: Female Reproductive Tract Answers

100. **D.** **S100**

This is Paget disease of the vulva. One should consider the possibility of melanoma, but the c-erb2 positivity helps rule this out. Choices A, B, and C are all positive.

QCSP, **Vulva,** p 186.

101. **D.** **PAPILLARY HIDRADENOMA**

This is usually well-circumscribed with a pseudocapsule. Typically they are composed of complex tubules and acini lined by tall columnar cells that usually have basal nuclei and an apocrine appearance with an underlying layer of cuboidal cells that are smaller and lie along the basement membrane. Some degree of nuclear pleomorphism may be present as well as mitotic figures.

QCSP, **Vulva,** p 187.

Chapter 6

Ovary

1. Which of the following is FALSE regarding the proper processing of ovarian neoplasms?
   A. The external surface of every ovarian neoplasm should be inked every time without exception.
   B. Papillary areas of cystic neoplasms should be sampled.
   C. Solid areas of cystic neoplasms should be sampled.
   D. At least 1 section should be taken for each centimeter of maximal diameter.
   E. The pathologist should use his or her judgment whether to ink an ovarian neoplasm, especially during an intraoperative consultation as this adds time and is unnecessary for benign lesions.

2. Choriocarcinoma characteristically:
   A. Represents approximately 3% of all ovarian tumors
   B. Is more commonly seen in Down syndrome patients
   C. Is bilateral
   D. Tends to occur in peri-menopausal women
   E. Is solid, friable and hemorrhagic

3. Choriocarcinoma does NOT react immunohistochemically with which of the following?
   A. Inhibin
   B. hCG
   C. Human placental lactogen
   D. Pancytokeratin
   E. Placental-like alkaline phosphatase

4. Which of the following describes choriocarcinoma?
   A. Tumor cells resemble primitive germ cells and tend to be arranged in solid, insular, trabecular, cordlike, and rarely, tubular patterns.
   B. Tumor cells are relatively uniform and round with clear cytoplasm (glycogen-rich) and distinct cell membranes.
   C. Tumor cells represent a mixture of uninucleated trophoblastic cells with either scanty or abundant clear cytoplasm admixed with multinucleated cells in a background of massive hemorrhage.
   D. Syncytiotrophoblastic giant cells present in <3% of cases.
   E. Electron microscopy is diagnostic.

5. Dysgerminomas:
   A. Are among the least common malignant germ cell tumors
   B. Characteristically occur in postmenopausal women
   C. Are AFP positive
   D. May contain granulomata
   E. Are mitotically inert

6. Which of the following is TRUE about embryonal carcinomas?
   A. Serum hCG and AFP are elevated in all patients.
   B. Pure form represents fewer than 30% of malignant primitive ovarian germ cell neoplasms.
   C. They are much more common than yolk sac tumors.
   D. 90% of patients are prepubertal; median age at diagnosis is 12 years.
   E. Extraovarian spread is rarely found at initial surgery.

6: Ovary Questions

7. A 12-year-old girl is diagnosed with an embryonal carcinoma. Which of the following would you expect to see microscopically?
    A. Tumor cells typically arranged in solid sheets and nests and often with areas of central necrosis, glandlike spaces, and papillae
    B. Tumor cells tend to be large and primitive with amphophilic and occasionally clear cytoplasm with well-defined cell membranes
    C. Nuclei that tend to overlap and are round and vesicular with a coarse irregular nuclear membrane and 1 or more prominent nucleoli
    D. Mitotic figures, many of which are atypical, easily identified
    E. All of the above

8. A 9-year-old-female is brought to the operating room for what is thought to be a torsed ovary. Instead a bulky tumor with a soft, spongy, and microcystic cut surface is found. On microscopic exam, syncytiotrophoblastic giant cells and mature and immature teratomatous elements are present along with many small round structures consist of a thick germ cell disc with an amniotic cavity on one side and a yolk sac cavity on the other. This is diagnostic of which of the following?
    A. Choriocarcinoma
    B. Juvenile granulosa cell tumor
    C. Immature teratoma
    D. Polyembryoma
    E. Endodermal sinus tumor

9. A Schiller-Duval body is characterized by:
    A. Follicles that are typically separated by well-differentiated coffee bean-shaped cells growing in a diffuse pattern and filled with eosinophilic material and nuclear debris
    B. Intracellular and extracellular hyaline bodies that are often present and tend to be most numerous in reticular areas and in areas with a hepatoid pattern
    C. Round or elongated papillae with fibrovascular cores containing a single vessel; these papillae are covered with primitive columnar cells and are found in spaces lined by cuboidal, flat, or hobnail cells.
    D. Linear, extracellular accumulations of (periodic acid-Schiff positive) basement membrane material, typically in the reticular and solid areas, present in 90% and representing "parietal" differentiation
    E. None of the above

10. Which of the following tumors would be included in the differential diagnosis of a yolk sac tumor?
    A. Clear cell carcinoma
    B. Hepatocellular carcinoma
    C. Dysgerminoma
    D. Sertoli-Leydig tumor
    E. All of the above

11. When making the diagnosis of mixed malignant germ cell tumor, how many histologic types are most commonly present?
    A. 2
    B. 3
    C. 4
    D. 5
    E. By definition, all histologic types are present in each tumor.

12.　What are the 2 most common histologic types of tumor encountered in mixed malignant germ cell tumors?
    A.　Embryonal carcinoma and seminoma
    B.　Dysgerminoma and endodermal sinus tumor
    C.　Yolk sac tumor and immature teratoma
    D.　Yolk sac tumor and choriocarcinoma
    E.　Polyembryoma and embryonal carcinoma

13.　Which of the following is most consistently associated with gonadoblastoma?
    A.　Distant metastases
    B.　Bilateral involvement
    C.　Charcot-Böttcher filaments on electron microscopy
    D.　Presence of a Y chromosome
    E.　Trisomy 21

14.　Which of the following microscopic descriptions most accurately characterizes a gonadoblastoma?
    A.　Cells that are large, polygonal, and have abundant eosinophilic cytoplasm with distinct cell borders; nuclei that tend to be central with a single prominent nucleolus; hepatoid cells that tend to grow in solid masses separated by thin bands of fibrous tissue and resemble hepatocellular carcinoma; hyaline bodies that are usually very numerous.
    B.　Typically an admixture of germ cells resembling seminoma cells and small, immature Sertoli-like cells arranged in round to irregularly shaped nests that contain hyaline deposits of basement membrane that are surrounded by sex cord cells
    C.　Many small structures resembling perfect or imperfect early embryos scattered throughout a fibrous or edematous stroma
    D.　Tumor cells typically arranged in solid sheets and nests and often having areas of central necrosis, glandlike spaces, and papillae
    E.　Tumor cells that resemble primitive germ cells and tend to be arranged in solid, insular, trabecular, cordlike, and rarely, tubular patterns

15.　Which of the following is TRUE regarding Sertoli-stromal tumors?
    A.　The average age at diagnosis is 12 years.
    B.　Tumors of oxyphil cell type are seen in association with Peutz-Jeghers syndrome.
    C.　They are associated with mutations in the merlin gene on chromosome 22.
    D.　Tumor cells are typically negative for cytokeratins and inhibin and positive for EMA.
    E.　They can be seen in association with Carney syndrome.

16.　Which of the following is TRUE regarding Sertoli-Leydig cell tumors (SLCT)?
    A.　Tumor cells are negative for alpha-inhibin.
    B.　Leydig cells form tubular structures and are characterized by interdigitating cell borders, basal lamina, cell junctions, and rarely Charcot-Böttcher crystalloids.
    C.　Sertoli cells contain smooth endoplasmic reticulum, lipid, lipofuscin, mitochondria with tubular cristae, and occasional Reinke crystals.
    D.　Grimelius stain can confirm the presence of argyrophil cells and a focus of carcinoid tumor in a Sertoli cell tumor with heterologous elements.
    E.　None of the above

6: Ovary Questions

17. Which of the following is TRUE regarding sex cord tumor with annular tubules?
    A. Special stains are diagnostic.
    B. Tumors associated with Peutz-Jeghers syndrome are malignant.
    C. Tumor cells are positive for AFP.
    D. Electron microscopy is not helpful.
    E. None of the above

18. Which of the following tumors most commonly secrete estrogen?
    A. Choriocarcinomas
    B. Mucinous carcinomas
    C. Adult granulosa cell tumors
    D. Gonadoblastomas
    E. None of the above

19. Granulosa cell tumors are immunohistochemically reactive for which of the following?
    A. S100
    B. Vimentin
    C. Cytokeratin
    D. All of the above
    E. None of the above

20. Granulosa cell tumors are typically negative for which of the following?
    A. Inhibin
    B. Smooth muscle actin
    C. Cytokeratin 7
    D. >1 of the above
    E. None of the above

21. Granulosa cell tumors consistently demonstrate which of the following chromosomal abnormalities?
    A. Loss of 3q27
    B. Trisomy 12
    C. Trisomy 13
    D. Loss of 17q
    E. Trisomy 21

22. Which of the following is/are associated with juvenile granulosa cell tumors?
    A. Ollier disease
    B. Peutz-Jeghers syndrome
    C. Maffucci syndrome
    D. >1 of the above
    E. None of the above

23. Typical clinical manifestations of Leydig tumors include which of the following?
    A. Average age at diagnosis is 30 years.
    B. 75%-80% of patients will have hirsutism or virilization secondary to testosterone production.
    C. It is almost always malignant.
    D. >1 of the above
    E. None of the above

6: Ovary Questions

24. Which of the following is/are characteristic of Leydig cell tumors?
    A. Reinke crystals
    B. Call-Exner bodies
    C. Schiller-Duval bodies
    D. Hyaline globules
    E. >1 of the above

25. Which of the following characteristics is/are associated with malignancy in steroid cell tumors, not otherwise specified?
    A. Diameter >5 cm
    B. 2 or more mitoses per 10 high-powered fields
    C. Edematous and microcystic architecture
    D. Clear cytoplasm
    E. >1 of the above

26. Ovarian fibromas are associated with which of the following?
    A. Meig syndrome
    B. Ollier syndrome
    C. Gorlin syndrome
    D. Nevoid basal cell syndrome
    E. >1 of the above

27. Which of the following findings are associated with recurrence of cellular ovarian fibromas?
    A. Gorlin syndrome
    B. >4 mitotic figures/10 hpf
    C. Bilateral tumors
    D. Hemorrhagic foci
    E. Reticulin-rich mesh surrounding individual cells

28. Which of the following is TRUE regarding typical thecomas (versus luteinized)?
    A. Most occur in women in their late 50s and early 60s.
    B. 20% are bilateral.
    C. 20% are unilateral.
    D. They are rarely aneuploid.
    E. None of the above

29. Which of the following is/are associated with typical and/or luteinized thecomas?
    A. Endometrial carcinoma
    B. Mixed malignant Müllerian tumor
    C. Endometrial stromal sarcoma
    D. Sclerosing peritonitis
    E. All of the above

30. Which of the following is TRUE regarding serous tumors?
    A. Approximately 60% are benign, 30% are borderline and 10% are malignant.
    B. They represent approximately 10% of all ovarian neoplasms.
    C. Malignant tumors tend to occur in women of reproductive age.
    D. Benign tumors tend to occur in elderly women.
    E. Carcinomas are occasionally associated with paraneoplastic endocrine abnormalities and hypercalcemia.

6: Ovary Questions

31. Cystic serous tumors may contain mucoid fluid on gross examination. TRUE or FALSE?
     A.   True
     B.   False

32. Once serous borderline tumors extend beyond the ovary into the pelvis, abdomen and lymph nodes they are then classified as serous carcinoma. TRUE or FALSE?
     A.   True
     B.   False

33. What is the treatment for a stage IV serous borderline tumor in a 23-year-old woman who wants to preserve fertility?
     A.   Salpingo-oophorectomy with ovarian conservation of the opposite ovary if bilateral
     B.   Hysterectomy and bilateral salpingo-oophorectomy with surgical staging
     C.   Hysterectomy and bilateral salpingo-oophorectomy with staging to include lymph node sampling
     D.   Surgery offers no benefit for a stage IV tumor. The treatment is chemotherapy.
     E.   None of the above

34. What is the 5-year survival for patients with stage III serous borderline tumor?
     A.   10%
     B.   25%
     C.   55%
     D.   75%
     E.   >90%

35. What is the 5-year survival for patients with stage III serous carcinoma?
     A.   10%
     B.   25%
     C.   55%
     D.   75%
     E.   >90%

36. Familial ovarian cancer seen in patients with BRCA mutations is most commonly associated with which type of tumors?
     A.   Serous carcinoma
     B.   Mucinous carcinoma
     C.   Mucinous borderline tumors
     D.   Clear cell carcinoma
     E.   All of the above

37. Which of the following is/are TRUE regarding ovarian mucinous tumors?
     A.   It is typically the largest of all ovarian neoplasms.
     B.   It represents 10%-15% of all ovarian neoplasms; 75% benign, 10% borderline, and 15% carcinoma.
     C.   Benign tumors are usually diagnosed in women between 30 and 50 years.
     D.   None of the above
     E.   All of the above

38. Mucinous tumors of low malignant potential typically:
     A.   Occur in women between the ages of 50 and 55 years
     B.   Have an elevated serum CA125 in 65%-70%
     C.   Have an elevated CEA in approximately 85%
     D.   Have an elevated carbohydrate antigen (CA19-9) in 85%
     E.   None of the above

6: Ovary Questions

39. Mucinous carcinomas may have which of the following?
    A. Stromal invasion, defined as either disorderly penetration of cyst wall or stromal component by carcinoma cells, with or without a stromal reaction
    B. Endocervical-like cells, intestinal-type cells, or both, but most frequently the cells are not classically endocervical or intestinal
    C. Tumor cells that may be arranged in cysts, glands, clusters, solid sheets, and individually
    D. Resemblance to those of a well-differentiated endometrioid adenocarcinoma or a typical adenocarcinoma of the large intestine
    E. All of the above

40. Struma ovarii may be associated with which of the following tumors?
    A. Mature teratoma
    B. Mucinous tumor
    C. Carcinoid tumor
    D. Brenner tumor
    E. All of the above

41. What stage IA ovarian tumor has the worst 5-year disease-free survival?
    A. Immature teratomas
    B. Serous borderline tumors
    C. Borderline endometrioid tumor
    D. Mucinous borderline tumors
    E. Small cell carcinoma, hypercalcemic type

42. Which of the following elevations in serum markers have been associated with mucinous carcinoma?
    A. CA125
    B. CEA
    C. CA19-9
    D. A and B.
    E. A, B, and C

43. Which of the following molecular alterations is most commonly seen in mucinous carcinomas of the ovary?
    A. p53 mutation
    B. K-ras mutation
    C. BRCA1 mutation
    D. BRCA2 mutation
    E. Aneuploidy

44. All of the following IS associated with mucinous tumors of the ovary EXCEPT:
    A. Human papillomavirus types 16 and 18
    B. Endometriosis
    C. Peutz-Jeghers syndrome
    D. Pseudomyxoma peritonei
    E. Dermoid cyst

6: Ovary Questions

45. A 55-year-old woman presents with severe abdominal pain. She is brought to the operating room where she is found to have an abdomen full of mucin, a ruptured appendix, and a 30-cm mucinous right ovary. The microscopic examination shows a low-grade mucinous carcinoma of the appendix (1.5 cm in greatest dimension) and ovary (30 cm in greatest dimension). What is the most likely explanation for these findings?
    A. They are 2 independent primaries and should be staged separately.
    B. The primary tumor is ovarian with spread to the appendix.
    C. The primary tumor is from the appendix with spread to the ovary.
    D. This is classic for a lung primary mucinous carcinoma and the patient should get chest imaging.
    E. None of the above

46. Which of the following patterns can be seen in ovarian endometrioid carcinomas?
    A. A villoglandular pattern
    B. Sex-cord-like foci
    C. Areas of spindle-shaped epithelial cells
    D. Areas of neuroendocrine differentiation
    E. All of the above

47. Squamous metaplasia is noted in an ovary with endometrioid carcinoma. What is the significance of this finding?
    A. This is evidence of metastasis from the endometrium and the patient should be staged accordingly.
    B. This is evidence of metastasis from the cervix, and a review of all prior Pap smears and cervical biopsies should be performed to confirm this possibility.
    C. This can be seen, and the diagnosis is adenosquamous carcinoma.
    D. >1 of the above
    E. None of the above

48. A 60-year-old woman has a 12-cm ovarian mass with the following microscopic characteristics: the tumor cells are round with clear cytoplasm, have eccentric nuclei and indistinct nucleoli, and are hobnailed. The tumors cells are arranged in solid nests and line cysts. What is the most likely diagnosis?
    A. Clear cell carcinoma
    B. Serous carcinoma
    C. Secretory endometrioid carcinoma
    D. Metastatic renal cell carcinoma
    E. Metastatic melanoma

49. Given the findings in the above tumor, which of the following would be evidence against your diagnosis?
    A. Multiple and complex papillae that contain densely eosinophilic hyaline basement membrane material that actually expands the core of the papillae
    B. Psammoma bodies
    C. Oxyphilic cells seen lining glands or growing in nests and solid masses
    D. All of the above
    E. None of the above

50. Benign Brenner tumors can be associated with other ovarian neoplasia. What is the most common tumor identified in association with benign Brenner tumors?
    A. Serous cystadenoma
    B. Serous cystadenofibroma
    C. Serous carcinoma
    D. Mucinous cystadenoma
    E. Mucinous carcinoma

6: Ovary Questions

51. What differentiates a malignant Brenner tumor from an ovarian transitional cell tumor?
    A. History of a primary bladder tumor
    B. Mucinous metaplasia
    C. A grade III epithelial component
    D. A and C
    E. None of the above

52. What is the most common ovarian carcinoid tumor associated with an ovarian teratoma?
    A. Insular carcinoid
    B. Trabecular carcinoid
    C. Struma carcinoid
    D. Goblet cell (mucinous) carcinoid
    E. A, B, and C

53. Which of the following supports the diagnosis of an immature teratoma?
    A. Immature element of neuroectodermal tissue present
    B. Mitotically active glia, and areas that resemble glioblastoma or neuroblastoma
    C. Embryonal neural tissue in <1 low-power field (×40) on one slide
    D. A and C
    E. All of the above

54. Which of the following is the most common ovarian neoplasm?
    A. Serous cystadenoma
    B. Endometriosis
    C. Endosalpingiosis
    D. Mesothelial hyperplasia
    E. None of the above

55. Which of the following microscopic findings does not support the diagnosis of a mature cystic teratoma?
    A. Presence of neuroectodermal elements as well as foci of cerebrum, cerebellum and choroid plexus
    B. Presence of neuroendocrine cells
    C. Tissue often arranged in an organoid fashion
    D. B and C
    E. None of the above

56. Which of the following is associated with mature teratomas?
    A. Coombs positive autoimmune hemolytic anemia
    B. Erythrocytosis secondary to secretion of erythropoietin
    C. Neutropenia (resolves after removal of tumor)
    D. A and B
    E. A, B, and C

57. What portion of struma ovarii are malignant?
    A. <1%
    B. <5%
    C. 5%-10%
    D. 10%-15%
    E. Malignant foci can be seen in almost all struma ovarii, but it is only clinically significant when >10% of the tumor is malignant.

6: Ovary Questions

62. What is the most likely diagnosis?

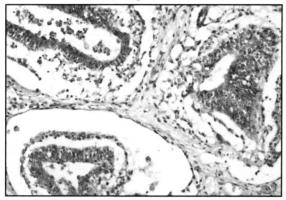

    A. Polyembryoma
    B. Choriocarcinoma
    C. Embryonal carcinoma
    D. Gonadoblastoma
    E. None of the above

63. A 2-year-old boy with ambiguous genitalia has cryptorchidism and hypospadias. His testes are prophylactically removed. On gross examination they are streaked and bilaterally enlarged. As you slice through them, you notice that they are quite gritty. You consult the patient's pediatrician, and she tells you the boy's genotype is 45X/46XY. What is the most likely diagnosis?

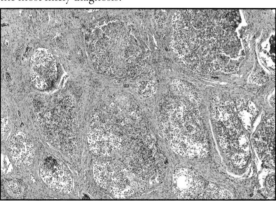 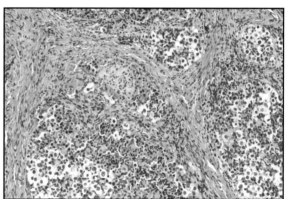

    A. Embryonal carcinoma
    B. Yolk sac tumor
    C. Sertoli-Leydig cell tumor
    D. Polyembryoma
    E. Gonadoblastoma

6: Ovary Questions

64. These tumor cells are positive for cytokeratin and inhibin, and negative for EMA. What is the most likely diagnosis?

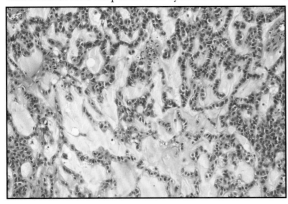

    A. Adenoid cystic carcinoma
    B. Sclerosing tumor of Medved
    C. Sertoli cell tumor
    D. Gonadoblastoma
    E. None of the above

65. A 25-year-old woman demonstrates virilism and is found to have an 8-cm, unilateral ovarian mass. What is the most likely diagnosis?

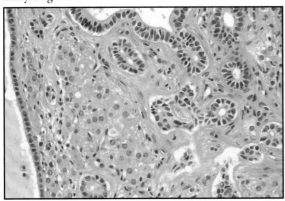

    A. Sertoli cell tumor
    B. Sertoli-Leydig cell tumor
    C. Sex cord tumor with annular tubules
    D. Granulosa cell tumor
    E. Gonadoblastoma

6: Ovary Questions

66. When this ovarian tumor is found in patients with Peutz-Jeghers syndrome, it is always?

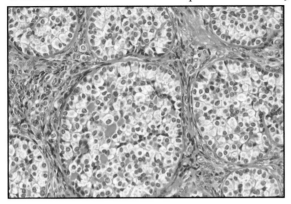

    A.   Malignant
    B.   Benign

67. A 55-year-old female presents with uterine bleeding and virilism. On exam she is found to have a 12-cm unilateral ovarian tumor. What is the most likely diagnosis?

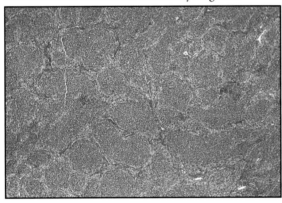 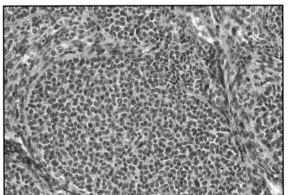

    A.   Sertoli cell tumor solid type
    B.   Juvenile granulosa cell tumor
    C.   Adult granulosa cell tumor
    D.   Small cell carcinoma
    E.   Steroid cell tumor, NOS

6: Ovary Questions

68. An 8-year-old girl presents to the emergency department with an acute abdomen. She is immediately taken to surgery and found to have a ruptured, right ovary and a subsequent hemoperitoneum. The cut-surface of the excised ovary is extensively hemorrhagic and necrotic. The tumor cells are strongly positive for inhibin and negative for EMA. What is the molecular alteration likely to be found in the tumor cells?

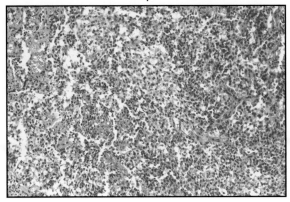

A. Trisomy 12
B. Trisomy 13
C. Trisomy 18
D. Trisomy 21
E. None of the above

69. What is the most likely diagnosis?

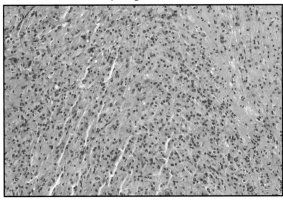 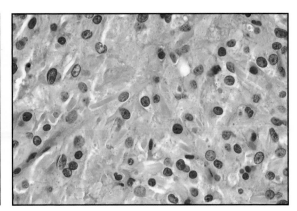

A. Steroid cell tumor
B. Sex cord tumor with annular tubules
C. Metastatic melanoma
D. Sertoli cell tumor
E. Leydig cell tumor

6: Ovary Questions

70. A 50-year-old female experienced the gradual onset of facial hair and a deeper voice. She was found to have a 6-cm unilateral ovarian tumor. An H&E slide is shown above on the left. The panel on the right is the result of α-inhibin immunohistochemical stain. What is the most likely diagnosis?

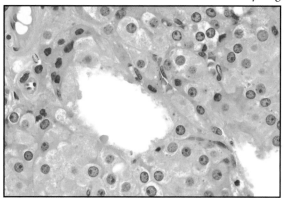 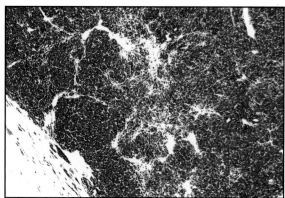

- A. Yolk sac tumor
- B. Metastatic melanoma
- C. Renal cell carcinoma
- D. Leydig cell tumor
- E. Steroid cell tumor

71. A 48-year-old woman is found to have a 20-cm unilateral ovarian mass. What of the following may be associated with this tumor?

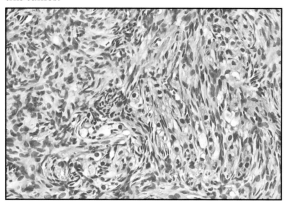

- A. Meigs syndrome
- B. Gorlin syndrome
- C. Nevoid basal cell syndrome
- D. A and B
- E. A, B, and C

6: Ovary Questions

72. A 52-year-old female is found to have a 13-cm right-sided ovarian mass, ascites and pleural effusion. What is the most likely diagnosis?

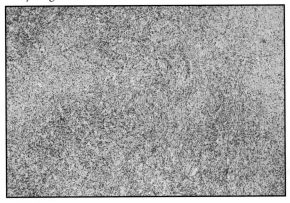

    A. Thecoma
    B. Fibroma
    C. Leiomyoma
    D. Leiomyosarcoma
    E. None of the above

73. A 55-year-old woman has a 9-cm ovarian mass. What is the most likely diagnosis?

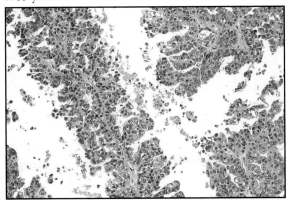

    A. Serous cystadenoma
    B. Serous borderline tumor
    C. Endometrioid carcinoma
    D. Serous carcinoma
    E. Malignant melanoma

6: Ovary Questions

74. Stage for stage, this ovarian tumor has a better prognosis than which of the following ovarian tumors?

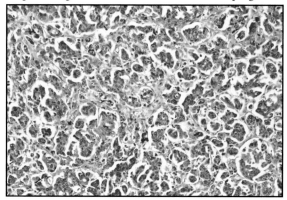

 A. Granulosa cell tumor
 B. Steroid cell tumor
 C. Fibroma
 D. All of the above
 E. None of the above

75. A 25-year-old woman has a 9-cm ovarian mass. What is the most likely diagnosis?

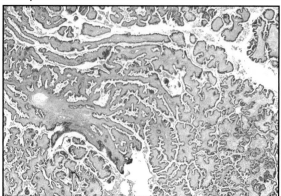

 A. Serous cystadenoma
 B. Serous borderline tumor
 C. Endometrioid carcinoma
 D. Serous carcinoma
 E. Metastatic colon carcinoma

6: Ovary Questions

76.   What is the most likely diagnosis?

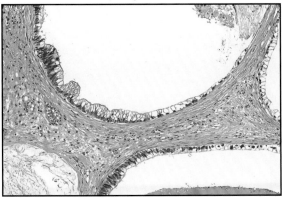

A.   Serous cystadenoma
B.   Serous borderline tumor
C.   Mucinous carcinoma
D.   Serous carcinoma
E.   Mucinous borderline tumor

77.   A 48-year-old woman has a 48-cm left ovarian mass, a right 18-cm ovarian mass and widespread peritoneal disease. What is the most likely diagnosis?

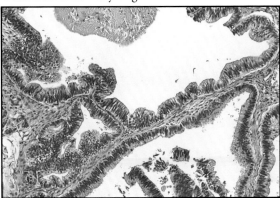

A.   Mucinous cystadenoma
B.   Serous borderline tumor
C.   Mucinous carcinoma
D.   Serous carcinoma
E.   Mucinous borderline tumor

6: Ovary Questions

78. What malignant ovarian neoplasm is most often associated with ovarian and/or pelvic endometriosis?

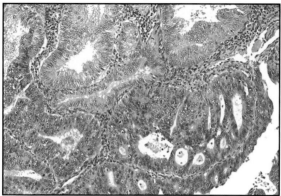

    A.   Endometrial carcinoma
    B.   Borderline endometrial tumor
    C.   Mucinous carcinoma
    D.   Serous carcinoma
    E.   Clear cell carcinoma

79. A 65-year-old woman has bilateral ovarian masses with extensive metastatic disease. What is the most likely diagnosis?

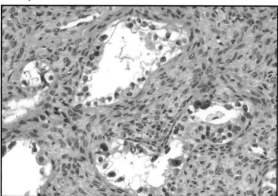

    A.   Endometrial carcinoma
    B.   Borderline endometrial tumor
    C.   Mucinous carcinoma
    D.   Serous carcinoma
    E.   Clear cell carcinoma

6: Ovary Questions

80. A 13-cm, right ovarian mass is removed from a 58-year-old woman. What is the most likely diagnosis?

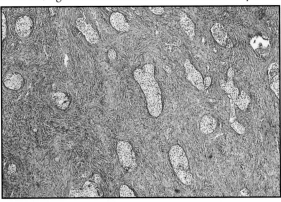 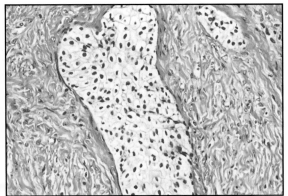

    A. Clear cell carcinoma
    B. Borderline endometrial tumor
    C. Mucinous carcinoma
    D. Granulosa cell tumor
    E. Brenner tumor

81. A 14-cm unilateral, multilocular mass is removed from a 58-year-old woman. At high magnification numerous mitotic figures and foci of atypical cells are identified. What is the most likely diagnosis?

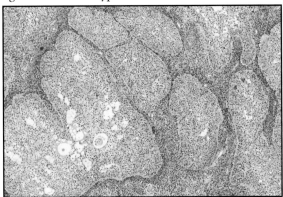 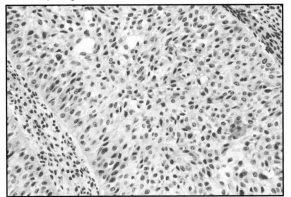

    A. Serous borderline tumor
    B. Endometrioid borderline tumor
    C. Mucinous borderline tumor
    D. Borderline Brenner tumor
    E. Clear cell borderline tumor

6: Ovary Questions

82. What is the most likely diagnosis?

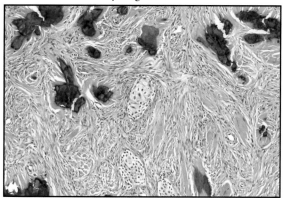

    A.   Brenner tumor
    B.   Borderline Brenner tumor
    C.   Malignant Brenner tumor
    D.   Transitional Brenner tumor
    E.   None of the above

83. What is the most likely diagnosis?

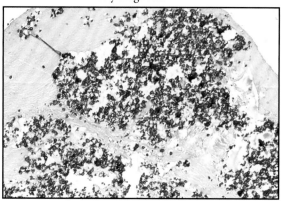

    A.   Low-grade serous carcinoma
    B.   Psammocarcinoma
    C.   Benign calcifications
    D.   A and B
    E.   A, B, and C

6: Ovary Questions

84. A 75-year-old woman has a 14-cm left ovarian mass removed. Numerous lymph nodes are involved by tumor. Every section of tissue examined looks like the above images. What is the most likely diagnosis?

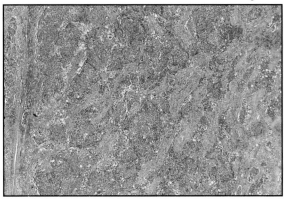 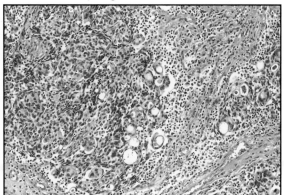

    A.   Borderline Brenner tumor
    B.   Malignant Brenner tumor
    C.   Transitional cell carcinoma
    D.   A and B
    E.   A, B, and C

85. What is the most likely diagnosis?

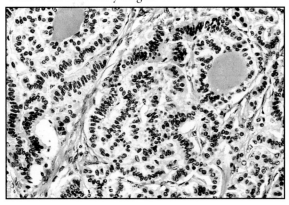

    A.   Malignant teratoma
    B.   Carcinoid tumor
    C.   Yolk sac tumor
    D.   A and B
    E.   A, B, and C

6: Ovary Questions

86.   This is an ovarian mass from 24-year-old woman. What is the most likely diagnosis?

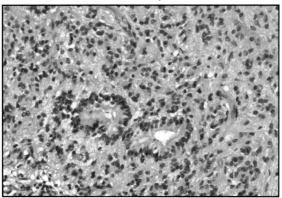

A.   Malignant epithelial tumor
B.   Malignant germ cell tumor
C.   Malignant sex-cord tumor
D.   Malignant stromal tumor
E.   None of the above

6: Ovary Answers

1. **E.** **THE PATHOLOGIST SHOULD USE HIS OR HER JUDGMENT WHETHER TO INK AN OVARIAN NEOPLASM, ESPECIALLY DURING AN INTRAOPERATIVE CONSULTATION AS THIS ADDS TIME AND IS UNNECESSARY FOR BENIGN LESIONS.**

   The external surface of all ovarian neoplasms should be inked. All neoplasms with a cystic component should be sampled in areas in which the wall of the cyst contains papillary structures or areas of thickening. Extensive sampling of all solid areas is of paramount importance, particularly in lesions that are primarily cystic. One section is customarily taken for each centimeter of maximal diameter with emphasis on obtaining most of the sections from solid and papillary areas. Sections should also document tumor to fallopian tube and presence of surface involvement.

   QCSP, **Specimen Handling**, p 190.

2. **E.** **IS SOLID, FRIABLE AND HEMORRHAGIC**

   Choriocarcinoma represents <1% of all ovarian neoplasms. Down syndrome patients are not at higher risk. The tumors tend to be unilateral. They tend to occur in children and young adults.

   QCSP, **Germ Cell Tumors**, p 190.

3. **A.** **INHIBIN**

   Inhibin most commonly reacts with sex-cord tumors.

   QCSP, **Germ Cell Tumors**, p 191.

4. **C.** **TUMOR CELLS REPRESENT A MIXTURE OF UNINUCLEATED TROPHOBLASTIC CELLS WITH EITHER SCANTY OR ABUNDANT CLEAR CYTOPLASM ADMIXED WITH MULTINUCLEATED CELLS IN A BACKGROUND OF MASSIVE HEMORRHAGE.**

   Choices A and B describe dysgerminomas. Syncytiotrophoblasts are seen in every case of choriocarcinoma and EM is not helpful.

   QCSP, **Germ Cell Tumors**, p 191.

5. **D.** **MAY CONTAIN GRANULOMATA**

   Dysgerminomas are the most common (~50%) malignant primitive germ cell tumor and typically occur in patients between the ages of 10 and 30 (rare under the age of 5 years or over the age of 50 years). They are negative for AFP and are quite mitotically active.

   QCSP, **Germ Cell Tumors**, p 191-192.

6. **A.** **SERUM hCG AND AFP ARE ELEVATED IN ALL PATIENTS.**

   Embryonal carcinomas are usually a component of a mixed germ cell tumor; the pure form represents fewer than 3% of malignant primitive ovarian germ cell neoplasms. They are much less common than yolk sac tumors. Approximately 50% of patients are prepubertal with a median age at diagnosis of 12 years. Extraovarian spread is found in 40% at initial surgery.

   QCSP, **Germ Cell Tumors**, p 193.

7. **E.** **ALL OF THE ABOVE**

   Microscopically, the tumor cells in embryonal carcinoma are typically arranged in solid sheets and nests and often have areas of central necrosis, gland-like spaces, and papillae. They tend to be large and primitive with amphophilic and occasionally clear cytoplasm with well-defined cell membranes. Nuclei tend to overlap and are round and vesicular with a coarse irregular nuclear membrane and 1 or more prominent nucleoli. Mitotic figures, many of which are atypical, are easily identified. Additionally, the neoplastic cells are usually positive for pancytokeratin, PLAP, NSE and CD30, but are negative for EMA, CEA, and vimentin.

   QCSP, **Germ Cell Tumors**, p 193.

6: Ovary Answers

---

25. **B.** **2 OR MORE MITOSES PER 10 HIGH-POWERED FIELDS**

In addition to choice B, the following features are also associated with malignancy: diameter >7 cm, necrosis and hemorrhage, grade II or III nuclear atypia.

QCSP, **Steroid Cell Tumors,** p 206.

26. **E.** **>1 OF THE ABOVE**

Most pathologists remember that Meigs syndrome can be seen with ovarian fibromas, but Gorlin syndrome (nevoid basal cell syndrome) is also associated with this tumor.

QCSP, **Stromal Tumors,** p 207.

27. **B.** **>4 MITOTIC FIGURES/10 HPF**

Fibromas are almost always benign. However, the densely cellular fibromas can recur, especially in those with >4 mitotic figures/10 hpf.

QCSP, **Stromal Tumors,** p 207.

28. **A.** **MOST OCCUR IN WOMEN IN THEIR LATE 50S AND EARLY 60S.**

95% of thecomas are unilateral, and they are usually aneuploid.

QCSP, **Stromal Tumors,** p 209.

29. **E.** **ALL OF THE ABOVE**

20% of postmenopausal women with typical thecomas have a concurrent endometrial carcinoma. Luteinized thecomas tend to occur in younger patients and may be associated with sclerosing peritonitis.

QCSP, **Stromal Tumors,** p 209.

30. **E.** **CARCINOMAS ARE OCCASIONALLY ASSOCIATED WITH PARANEOPLASTIC ENDOCRINE ABNORMALITIES AND HYPERCALCEMIA.**

Of serous tumors, 60% are benign, 10% are borderline, and 30% are carcinomas. Benign tumors most commonly occur in women during the reproductive ages, and serous carcinomas tend to occur in women over 50. Serous tumors represent approximately 30% of all ovarian neoplasms.

QCSP, **Surface Epithelial-Stromal Tumors,** p 190.

31. **A.** **TRUE**

Gross examination of an ovarian cyst fluid is notoriously deceiving. Only microscopic examination can determine the differentiation of the cystic lesion.

QCSP, **Surface Epithelial-Stromal Tumors,** p 210.

32. **B.** **FALSE**

65% of borderline serous ovarian tumors with an exophytic component will have peritoneal implants; neoplasms without an exophytic component will have peritoneal implants in <5%. There are 2 different types of implants: noninvasive (epithelial and desmoplastic type) and invasive. The microscopic features of the implant should be evaluated independent of the associated ovarian neoplasm. Peritoneal implants may appear as benign foci of serous epithelium forming glands, cysts, and occasionally papillae with psammoma bodies (endosalpingiosis), as noninvasive deposits of borderline epithelium and stroma, and as invasive implants morphologically identical to serous carcinoma.

QCSP, **Surface Epithelial-Stromal Tumors,** p 210.

6: Ovary Answers

33.   E.   **NONE OF THE ABOVE**

Young women who desire to preserve reproductive function can be treated with unilateral oophorectomy and careful follow-up with eventual likelihood of a residual salpingo-oophorectomy and hysterectomy, but only if the tumor is unilateral and low grade.

QCSP, **Surface Epithelial-Stromal Tumors,** p 212.

34.   E.   **>90%**

The 5-year survival for stage I, II, and III tumors is 90%-95%.

QCSP, **Surface Epithelial-Stromal Tumors,** p 212.

35.   B.   **25%**

The 5-year survival for serous carcinoma is as follows: 75% (stage I); 55% (stage II); 25% (stage III); 10% (stage IV). The very different survival and morphologic characteristics of serous borderline tumors vs serous carcinoma emphasizes the difference in biology and the necessity in the correct of diagnosis of these tumors.

QCSP, **Surface Epithelial-Stromal Tumors,** p 212.

36.   A.   **SEROUS CARCINOMA**

Patients with a mutated BRCA gene demonstrate an increased number of serous carcinoma as compared with those without a BRCA mutation. Specifically, >90% of ovarian tumors occurring in women with BRCA1 mutations are serous.

QCSP, **Surface Epithelial-Stromal Tumors,** p 212.

37.   E.   **ALL OF THE ABOVE**

Choices A-C all describe mucinous ovarian tumors.

QCSP, **Surface Epithelial-Stromal Tumors,** p 213.

38.   A.   **OCCUR IN WOMEN BETWEEN THE AGES OF 50 AND 55 YEARS**

Choices B through D are true about mucinous carcinoma and not necessarily mucinous tumors of low malignant potential.

QCSP, **Surface Epithelial-Stromal Tumors,** p 213.

39.   E.   **ALL OF THE ABOVE**

All the features in choices A-D describe findings in mucinous carcinomas. Additionally, these lesions can demonstrate extravasated pools of mucin in the stroma in 25%-30% often with histiocytes and foreign body giant cell reactions.

QCSP, **Surface Epithelial-Stromal Tumors,** p 213.

40.   E.   **ALL OF THE ABOVE**

Struma ovarii is an ovarian tumor defined by the presence of thyroid tissue comprising >50% of the overall mass. While this usually occurs in a pure form, it can be associated with other lesions, such as immature teratoma, as a component of strumal carcinoid, and can be found in the wall of mucinous cystadenomas or admixed with Brenner tumor.

QCSP, **Teratomas,** p 226.

41.   E.   **SMALL CELL CARCINOMA, HYPERCALCEMIC TYPE**

30% of stage IA small cell carcinoma, hypercalcemic type will have a disease-free survival of up to 6 years. The other tumors listed have an excellent disease-free survival rate.

QCSP, **Miscellaneous Tumors,** p 227.

42. E. **A, B, and C**
     Elevated CA125, CEA, and CA19-9 have been associated with mucinous carcinoma in 65%, 85%, and 85% of cases, respectively.
     QCSP, **Surface Epithelial-Stromal Tumors,** p 213.

43. B. **K-ras mutation**
     K-ras mutation is commonly seen in mucinous carcinomas (choice B). p53 mutations are more often seen in carcinomas of serous type (choice A). BRCA1 and BRCA2 mutations have both been associated with increased risk of ovarian cancer, particularly in BRCA1 mutations, although it is typically a serous carcinoma (choices C and D). Aneuploidy is a common molecular alteration in neoplasia, but has not been particularly closely associated with mucinous carcinoma of the ovary (choice E).
     QCSP, **Surface Epithelial-Stromal Tumors,** p 214.

44. A. **Human papillomavirus types 16 and 18**
     Mucinous tumors of low malignant potential in the ovary can be classified into endocervical-like and intestinal-like tumors and have correspondingly different associations. Endocervical-like tumors are associated with endometriosis (choice B), while intestinal-like tumors are more commonly associated with pseudomyxoma peritonei (choice D) and Peutz-Jeghers syndrome (choice C). These tumors are furthermore associated with mucinous tumors in other organs, particularly the appendix, and may be seen in conjunction with a dermoid cyst (choice E). An association with HPV has not been demonstrated to date (choice A).
     QCSP, **Surface Epithelial-Stromal Tumors,** p 214.

45. C. **The primary tumor is from the appendix with spread to the ovary.**
     When synchronous appendiceal and ovarian mucinous tumors are present, are they independent primaries or is one the primary (either ovarian or appendiceal) and the other a metastasis? Clinicopathologic studies favor intestinal (appendiceal) origin in most cases.
     QCSP, **Surface Epithelial-Stromal Tumors,** p 214.

46. E. **All of the above**
     Various uncommon patterns may be present and represent pitfalls in the differential diagnosis; a villoglandular pattern, sex-cord-like foci, focal to abundant areas of spindle-shaped epithelial cells, tumor cells with oxyphilic cytoplasm (may represent clear cell carcinoma), glands that resemble 16-day secretory endometrium, neuroendocrine (argyrophil cells) (present in 10%), clear cell component (present in 20%-25%), epithelial islands and trabeculae reminiscent of a granulosa cell tumor, and luteinized cells throughout stroma can all be seen.
     QCSP, **Surface Epithelial-Stromal Tumors,** p 215.

47. E. **None of the above**
     30%-50% will have foci of squamous differentiation; the squamous component may be either benign or malignant (adenoacanthoma or adenosquamous carcinoma respectively).
     QCSP, **Surface Epithelial-Stromal Tumors,** p 215.

48. A. **Clear cell carcinoma**
     Clear cell carcinomas most frequently have a complex papillary pattern, but may be solid; tumor cells are usually round with clear cytoplasm, have eccentric nuclei and indistinct nucleoli, and are usually hobnailed; the cells may be arranged in solid nests or line cysts, tubules and papillae—all patterns may be present in same tumor.
     QCSP, **Surface Epithelial-Stromal Tumors,** p 217.

6: Ovary Answers

49. E. **NONE OF THE ABOVE**

Choices A, B, and C all represent histologic findings in clear cell carcinomas.

QCSP, **Surface Epithelial-Stromal Tumors,** p 217.

50. D. **MUCINOUS CYSTADENOMA**

In approximately 25% of benign Brenner tumors, another ovarian neoplasm may be present. 65% are mucinous tumors (almost always benign), and the remainder tends to be serous cystadenomas and dermoid cysts.

QCSP, **Surface Epithelial-Stromal Tumors,** p 218.

51. E. **NONE OF THE ABOVE**

A malignant Brenner tumor has malignant-appearing transitional cells or squamous cells, with or without the presence of mucinous cells, which clearly invade the cyst wall and/or adjacent stroma, with a background of benign or borderline Brenner tumor. Transitional cell carcinomas tumor cells have the characteristics of malignant transitional cells (in most cases at least grade II and usually grade III), with no evidence of a benign or borderline Brenner tumor. In most cases, the transitional cell elements will be mixed with other types of surface epithelial carcinoma (typically serous type).

QCSP, **Surface Epithelial-Stromal Tumors,** p 219.

52. A. **INSULAR CARCINOID**

The most common carcinoid tumor associated with an ovarian teratoma is insular carcinoid. It is also the only type associated with carcinoid syndrome. Goblet cell carcinoid is a subclass of carcinoid tumors that is often seen in the appendix. Microscopically, goblet cell carcinoid demonstrates goblet/signet ring cells and can demonstrate cells floating in mucin pools. Struma carcinoid (2nd most common type) is an admixture of carcinoid and struma ovarii. Trabecular subtype is characterized by the absence of carcinoid syndrome and resembles hindgut carcinoids.

QCSP, **Teratomas,** p 220.

53. E. **ALL OF THE ABOVE**

The differential between mature and immature teratomas includes the presence of immature elements of neuroectodermal tissue in immature teratomas. This includes mitotically active glia and areas resembling glioblastoma or neuroblastoma. Additionally, there can be immature elements of epithelium and mesenchymal tissue; however "immature" requires the presence of embryonic tissue and not just fetal-type tissue.

QCSP, **Teratomas,** p 223.

54. E. **NONE OF THE ABOVE**

The most common ovarian neoplasm is a mature cystic teratoma (dermoid cyst). They represent 50% of ovarian neoplasms in women under the age of 20 years and 65% of ovarian neoplasms in children under the age of 15 years.

QCSP, **Teratomas,** p 223.

55. E. **NONE OF THE ABOVE**

All of the listed findings are common in mature cystic teratomas.

QCSP, **Teratomas,** p 224.

56. D. **A AND B**

There are many interesting associations with mature teratomas. Coombs positive autoimmune hemolytic anemia will disappear with removal of the tumor. Erythrocytosis is secondary to the secretion of erythropoietin (very rare). A ruptured dermoid can be associated with peritoneal melanosis (focal or diffuse peritoneal tan to black staining) or tumor-like nodules. 1%-2% of mature teratomas will contain an adult-type cancer; in patients

older than 70 years, the incidence is 15%. Grossly malignant areas usually appear as a cauliflower-like mass that protrudes into a cystic cavity, and 80% are squamous cell carcinomas (the remainder are adenocarcinoma and variants or various sarcomas).
QCSP, **Teratomas,** p 225.

57. C. **5%-10%**

Approximately 5%-10% of struma ovarii are malignant. Theses lesions demonstrate typical features of thyroid carcinoma (including overlapping "ground glass" nuclei lining papillary formations and vascular space invasion by follicular cells).
QCSP, **Teratomas,** p 225.

58. C. ELEVATED CALCIUM

Small cell carcinoma, hypercalcemic type, typically presents in young women at an advanced stage. It is an aggressive tumor. Patients characteristically have hypercalcemia. Morphologically they most commonly have a diffuse arrangement (occasionally insular, nested, cords, or trabeculae) of small, closely packed epithelial cells with scant cytoplasm and small, round, or oval nuclei with a single small nucleolus. 50% of neoplasms will have foci in which the neoplastic cells have abundant eosinophilic cytoplasm; these larger cells have a larger and less hyperchromatic nucleus with a more prominent nucleolus.
QCSP, **Miscellaneous Tumors,** p 226-228.

59. B. CHORIOCARCINOMA

The tumor cells represent a mixture of mononucleated trophoblastic cells with either scanty or abundant clear cytoplasm (cytotrophoblastic or intermediate trophoblastic cells, respectively) admixed with syncytiotrophoblastic cells in a background of massive hemorrhage. Syncytiotrophoblastic cells typically contain eosinophilic cytoplasm with vacuoles and many dark nuclei and may form syncytial knots. Foci may be poorly differentiated. Neoplastic cells often aggregate around dilated vascular spaces; vascular invasion is often prominent. The young age, high-β-hCG and widespread metastases are more clues to the answer. (Photo courtesy of Mark R Wick, MD, University of Virginia)
QCSP, **Germ Cell Tumors,** p 191.

60. A. TUMOR CELLS ARE IMMUNOREACTIVE FOR PLAP AND VIMENTIN.

This is a dysgerminoma. The tumor cells are immunoreactive for PLAP and vimentin. The tumor cells are variably positive for lactic dehydrogenase, NSE, Leu-7, cytokeratin, desmin, and glial fibrillary acidic protein (GFAP). The tumor cells are almost always negative for EMA and CEA. If syncytiotrophoblastic giant cells are present, they are typically positive for both hCG and cytokeratin.
QCSP, **Germ Cell Tumors,** p 192.

61. D. EMBRYONAL CARCINOMA

This is a classic presentation for embryonal carcinoma. The following is a typical staining pattern: cytoplasm of tumor cells are positive for pancytokeratin, PLAP, and NSE; 80% are positive for CD30 (Ber-H2, Ki-1); 30%-50% are positive for AFP; tumor cells are typically negative for EMA, CEA, and vimentin. Syncytiotrophoblastic giant cells stain with β-hCG
QCSP, **Germ Cell Tumors,** p 192.

62. A. POLYEMBRYOMA

This is an extremely rare tumor, but it has a very characteristic appearance. Many small structures resembling perfect or imperfect early embryos (embryoid bodies) are scattered throughout a fibrous or edematous stroma. Embryoid bodies typically consist of a thick germ cell disc with an amniotic cavity on 1 side and a yolk sac cavity on the other. Syncytiotrophoblastic giant cells and mature and immature teratomatous elements (usually intestinal tissue or adult or embryonal hepatic tissue) are usually present. (Photo courtesy of Mark R. Wick, MD, University of Virginia)

QCSP, **Germ Cell Tumors,** p 193-194.

63. E. **GONADOBLASTOMA**

The clue here is the dysgenic gonads and the mosaicism. One could also consider seminoma/dysgerminoma, but that choice was not offered.

QCSP, **Germ Cell Tumors,** p 196-197.

64. C. **SERTOLI CELL TUMOR**

From the choices given, morphologically and immunophenotypically this must be a Sertoli cell tumor. Sclerosing tumor of Medved is made up.

QCSP, **Sertoli-Stroma Cell Tumors,** p 197-198.

65. B. **SERTOLI-LEYDIG CELL TUMOR**

The cells that comprise the tubules tend to be cuboidal or columnar and have moderate to large amounts of cytoplasm that may be densely eosinophilic or vacuolated and lipid-rich. The nuclei of tumor cells are round or oblong without prominent nucleoli; nuclear atypia and mitotic figures are rare. The stromal component consists of bands of fibrous tissue with variably conspicuous clusters of Leydig cells.

QCSP, **Sertoli-Stroma Cell Tumors,** p 199.

66. B. **BENIGN**

This is a sex cord stromal tumor with annular tubules (SCTAT). 20% of tumors unassociated with Peutz-Jeghers syndrome are clinically malignant and metastasize by way of lymphatics; occurrences are usually late. All tumors associated with Peutz-Jeghers syndrome are benign.

QCSP, **Sertoli-Stroma Cell Tumors,** p 201-202.

67. C. **ADULT GRANULOSA CELL TUMOR**

This is one of the more common sex cord-stromal tumors. Granulosa cells grow in solid (diffuse), trabecular, insular, and microfollicular patterns; less frequent architectural patterns include macrofollicular, watered silk (undulating parallel rows of granulosa cells), and gyriform (zigzag arrangement of cords of granulosa cells); an admixture of patterns is frequently present.

QCSP, **Germ Cell Tumors,** p 202-203.

68. A. **TRISOMY 12**

This is a juvenile granulosa cell tumor. These tumors cells are positive for α-inhibin and negative for EMA, and consistently demonstrate trisomy 12.

QCSP, **Germ Cell Tumors,** p 204.

69. E. **LEYDIG CELL TUMOR**

The cells of Leydig tumors typically have round, hyperchromatic nuclei with a single nucleolus and abundant eosinophilic cytoplasm. Elongated eosinophilic crystals of Reinke can be seen in the cytoplasm or nucleus of tumor cells and, while these inclusions are often difficult to find, once you notice them there can be only one diagnosis.

QCSP, **Sertoli-Stroma Cell Tumors,** p 199-201.

70.   E.   **STEROID CELL TUMOR**
        Given the clinical and immunohistochemical features, the most likely diagnosis is a steroid cell tumor. Leydig cell tumor is not favored as Reinke crystals are absent.
        QCSP, **Steroid Cell Tumors**, p 205-206.

71.   E.   **A, B, AND C**
        This is a fibroma/fibrothecoma. It can be associated with all of the above. Actually choices B and C refer to the same entity. Meigs syndrome (seen in 1%): ascites and pleural effusion accompanying an ovarian fibroma; the ascites and pleural effusion disappear on removal of the tumor. Gorlin syndrome (nevoid basal cell syndrome): multiple nevoid basal cell carcinomas, multiple jaw keratocysts, developmental defects of skeletal system (rib, vertebral and craniofacial), palmar and plantar pits (defective keratin production), epidermal inclusion cysts, ectopic calcification (falx cerebri, diaphragma sella), ovarian fibromas, medulloblastoma, meningioma and cardiac fibroma.
        QCSP, **Stromal Tumors**, p 206-207.

72.   B.   **FIBROMA**
        The low-magnification examination of this specimen demonstrates intersecting bundles of spindle cells with little cytoplasm. A pure thecoma would have sheets of ill-defined round or oval cells with abundant vacuolated cytoplasm, which is due to lipid. A leiomyoma of the ovary would be uncommon and a leiomyosarcoma would be exceptionally uncommon.
        QCSP, **Stromal Tumors**, p 206-208.

73.   D.   **SEROUS CARCINOMA**
        This is the most common malignant ovarian carcinoma. It is characterized by high cellularity, nuclear atypia, cellular budding, and obvious stromal invasion. Neoplastic cells almost invariably have more pronounced nuclear atypia than is seen in borderline tumors. Papillae are present with areas of solid proliferation of tumor cells with irregular slit-like spaces, which is evidence of invasion.
        QCSP, **Surface Epithelial Stromal Tumors**, p 209-211.

74.   E.   **NONE OF THE ABOVE**
        This is a high-grade serous papillary tumor. Stage for stage, it is much more aggressive than any of the tumors listed.
        QCSP, **Surface Epithelial Stromal Tumors**, p 226-227.

75.   B.   **SEROUS BORDERLINE TUMOR**
        This is a tumor that can be seen with some frequency in younger women. It is important to recognize in order to not overcall this carcinoma. The diagnosis of "borderline" tumor is typically based on 4 rather characteristic features: formation of cellular buds that appear to float in the intracystic fluid, cells with at least some degree of nuclear atypia, absence of "obvious" invasion of the stromal component of the ovary, and hierarchical branching. Tumor cells usually have little cytoplasm, although the cells in the papillary buds may have prominent eosinophilic cytoplasm. Psammoma bodies may be present.
        QCSP, **Surface Epithelial Stromal Tumors**, p 209-211.

76.   E.   **MUCINOUS BORDERLINE TUMOR**
        The glandular epithelium lining the cysts on the left side of the photograph demonstrate stratified epithelium; some nuclei have prominent nucleoli, and a few mitotic figures are seen in the upper gland. In contrast, the epithelium on the right maintains polarity and resembles benign endocervical glands. >50% of this tumor

demonstrated epithelium characteristic of the glands on the left. One could argue that this may be a benign mucinous cystadenoma; however, that was not a choice.

QCSP, **Surface Epithelial Stromal Tumors**, p 212-214.

77.　C.　**MUCINOUS CARCINOMA**

Make sure you examine the entire photograph. The question implies a malignant high-stage neoplasm. The photo demonstrates a mucinous neoplasm with invasion in the lower left-hand corner with small clusters of neoplastic cells.

QCSP, **Surface Epithelial Stromal Tumors**, p 212-214.

78.　E.　**CLEAR CELL CARCINOMA**

Did you read the question carefully? This picture has nothing to do with the question. This is a favorite board question. Clear cell carcinoma is the most common malignant neoplasm associated with endometriosis.

QCSP, **Surface Epithelial Stromal Tumors**, p 216-217.

79.　E.　**CLEAR CELL CARCINOMA**

Oxyphilic cells may be a major component of a clear cell carcinoma and are typically seen lining glands or growing in nests and solid masses. Clear cell carcinomas often have a complex papillary architecture but can be solid or be arranged in solid nests or line cysts, tubules, and papillae, all within the same tumor. This image demonstrates the hobnail appearance of cells lining tubules.

QCSP, **Surface Epithelial Stromal Tumors**, p 216-217.

80.　E.　**BRENNER TUMOR**

This is a benign Brenner tumor. Notice the focus of mucinous differentiation in the upper right corner. Transitional cells are arranged in round or oval nests (occasionally trabeculae) in a prominent fibrous stroma. The tumor cells have pale cytoplasm and oval nuclei that are frequently grooved. Nests of tumor cells may be either solid or have a central cavity filled with dense eosinophilic material; occasionally a transitional cell nest with a cavity will be lined by mucinous, ciliated, serous or undifferentiated glandular epithelium. Pure mucinous glands and cysts may be present (metaplastic Brenner). 30% will have spicula of calcification that tend to be located near nests of transitional cells. Foci of squamous differentiation may be present in transitional cell nests.

QCSP, **Surface Epithelial Stromal Tumors**, p 218-219.

81.　D.　**BRENNER BORDERLINE TUMOR**

This tumor is characterized by papillae lined by proliferating transitional-type cells that protrude into the lumen of a cyst. Mucin-containing cells may be present. Criteria for this diagnosis include the presence of atypical or frankly carcinomatous transitional cells *without* stromal invasion.

QCSP, **Surface Epithelial Stromal Tumors**, p 218-219.

82.　A.　**BRENNER TUMOR**

This represents another example of a benign Brenner tumor. Extensive calcifications may be present.

QCSP, **Surface Epithelial Stromal Tumors**, p 218-219.

83.　D.　**A AND B**

This is an example of psammocarcinoma. It is a low-grade variant of serous carcinoma. It has a more favorable prognosis than typical serous carcinoma.

QCSP, **Surface Epithelial Stromal Tumors**, p 211.

6: Ovary Answers

84.   C.   **TRANSITIONAL CELL CARCINOMA**
The images are diagnostic and there are clues to the answer in the history. It is a high-grade lesion that is invasive and metastatic. This eliminates a borderline tumor. Since there is no evidence of a benign Brenner tumor in any of the sections, the answer must be transitional cell carcinoma.
QCSP, **Germ Cell Tumors**, p 219.

85.   B.   **CARCINOID TUMOR**
This is a carcinoid tumor found in a teratoma. (Photo courtesy of Mark R Wick, MD, University of Virginia)
QCSP, **Germ Cell Tumors**, p 219-222.

86.   B.   **MALIGNANT GERM CELL TUMOR**
This is an immature teratoma. Notice the immature neural tissue; this can be a focal finding.
QCSP, **Germ Cell Tumors**, p 222-226.

Chapter 7

Gastrointestinal Tract

1. Which of the following are features that favor radiation atypia over dysplasia/carcinoma in situ in a post-treatment surgical specimen of the GI tract?
   A. Enlarged cells with a low N:C ratio
   B. Absence of full thickness changes
   C. Mitotic figures /lack of it)
   D. Both A and B
   E. All of the above

2. Which of the following scenarios does NOT warrant an intraoperative consultation with frozen section analysis?
   A. Emergent resection of a newly diagnosed gastric ulcer
   B. Margins for ischemic enteritis involving the small intestine
   C. Appendectomy on a 55-year-old with a lumen distended by mucus
   D. Colonic resection for Hirschsprung disease
   E. All of the above warrant intraoperative frozen section consultation.

3. Which metastatic neoplasm can mimic signet ring carcinoma of the stomach, causing significant consternation at the time of frozen section?
   A. Metastatic lobular carcinoma of the breast
   B. Metastatic endometrioid adenocarcinoma
   C. Mucinous carcinoma of the ovary
   D. Lymphoma
   E. None of the above is likely to mimic signet ring adenocarcinoma of the stomach.

4. What is the most common site in the gastrointestinal tract to be involved by endometriosis?
   A. Terminal ileum
   B. Right colon
   C. Left colon
   D. Rectosigmoid colon
   E. Both B and C

5. Why might a surgeon care at the time of colonic resection whether the patient has Crohn disease or ulcerative colitis?
   A. Crohn colitis is much more likely to be associated with a malignancy and the surgeon will look harder if that is the case.
   B. The surgeon will create an ileal pouch only if the patient has ulcerative colitis vs Crohn colitis.
   C. Immediate postoperative treatment differs for the 2 forms of inflammatory bowel disease.
   D. All of the above
   E. None of the above

6. What percentage of neoplasms in the lower 1/3 of the esophagus are adenocarcinomas vs other carcinomas?
   A. 20%
   B. 40%
   C. 60%
   D. 80%
   E. 95%

7: Gastrointestinal Tract Questions

7.   All of the following clinical features increase the risk for esophageal adenocarcinoma EXCEPT:
     A.   Tobacco and alcohol use
     B.   Males
     C.   Blacks
     D.   Reflux disease
     E.   All of the above

8.   What minimum percentage of an esophageal adenocarcinoma must be mucinous to be considered a mucinous adenocarcinoma?
     A.   Any mucinous portion
     B.   10%
     C.   25%
     D.   50%
     E.   75%

9.   Which of the following molecular alterations are commonly seen in esophageal adenocarcinoma?
     A.   C-myc expression
     B.   *H-ras* gene expression
     C.   TP53 mutations
     D.   Both a and b
     E.   All of the above

10.   What survival is expected with esophageal adenocarcinomas that penetrate **into** and **beyond** the muscularis propria, respectively?
     A.   80% and 50%
     B.   45% and 15%-25%
     C.   35% and 5%
     D.   80% and 20%
     E.   75% and 25%

11.   Esophageal adenocarcinoma without accompanying Barrett metaplasia can be explained by:
     A.   Replacement of Barrett mucosa by invasive cancer
     B.   Adenocarcinoma arising in a focus of heterotopic gastric mucosa (inlet patch)
     C.   Adenocarcinoma arising in a submucosal esophageal gland or their ducts
     D.   Both choice A and C
     E.   All of the above

12.   What is the incidence of Barrett esophagus in patients with prolonged GERD?
     A.   5%-10%
     B.   10%-20%
     C.   35%-40%
     D.   55%-60%
     E.   80%-85%

13.   What is the incidence of dysplasia in patients who have Barrett mucosa?
     A.   5%-10%
     B.   15%-20%
     C.   35%-40%
     D.   55%-60%
     E.   80%-85%

7: Gastrointestinal Tract Questions

14. Microscopically, Barrett esophagus is distinguished by:
    A. Replacement of the esophageal squamous lining by gastric mucosa
    B. Presence of purple mucin, identified by staining with PAS-Alcian blue at pH 2.5
    C. Goblet cells
    D. All of the above
    E. None of the above

15. The typical staining pattern of PAS-Alcian blue is:
    A. Acid mucin stains blue; neutral mucins do not stain
    B. Acid mucin stains red-purple; neutral mucins do not stain
    C. Acid mucin stains blue; neutral mucins stain red-purple
    D. Acid mucins do not stain; neutral mucins stain blue
    E. Acid mucins do not stain; neutral mucins stain red-purple

16. All of the following are factors that may contribute to the transformation of squamous mucosa to Barrett mucosa to dysplasia to carcinoma, EXCEPT:
    A. Hereditary factors
    B. p53 mutations
    C. Reflux disease
    D. B and C
    E. A, B, and C

17. What is the incidence of carcinoma developing during the lifetime of a patient with Barrett mucosa who is older than 50 years of age?
    A. <5%
    B. 5%-10%
    C. 20%-25%
    D. 50%
    E. 75%

18. What percentage of esophagectomy specimens removed for biopsy-proven high-grade dysplasia have carcinoma?
    A. 5%-10%
    B. 15%-25%
    C. 35%-50%
    D. 60%-70%
    E. 80%

19. All of the following are features of low-grade gastroesophageal reflux, EXCEPT:
    A. Widening of the basal zone of epithelium
    B. Increased numbers and elongation of vascular papillae with dilated vessels ("lakes") at the top of papillae
    C. Loss of longitudinal orientation of the superficial epithelial cells due to immature cells at the surface
    D. Increased mitotic figures
    E. All of the above are features of low-grade GERD

20. All of the following are features of high-grade gastroesophageal reflux disease sans Barrett mucosa EXCEPT:
    A. Marked neutrophilia and/or eosinophilia
    B. Dysplasia
    C. Edema
    D. Ulceration
    E. Inflammatory polyps

7: Gastrointestinal Tract Questions

21. Worldwide, which region has the highest incidence of squamous cell carcinoma of the esophagus?
    A. North America
    B. Northern China
    C. South America
    D. Europe
    E. Australia

22. Risk factors for squamous cell carcinoma include all of the following, EXCEPT:
    A. Pickled and dried vegetables
    B. N-nitrosamines
    C. GERD
    D. Alcohol and tobacco
    E. Radiation

23. In which portion of the esophagus do most squamous cell carcinomas arise?
    A. Proximal/upper 1/3
    B. Middle 1/3
    C. Distal/lower 1/3
    D. A and B equally
    E. All portions equally

24. Which type of early (vs advanced) squamous cell carcinoma is most likely to present as a submucosal lesion?
    A. Plaque type
    B. Erosive type
    C. Papillary type
    D. Occult type
    E. None of the above

25. Which of the following histologic features can be seen in esophageal squamous cell carcinoma?
    A. Koilocytes
    B. Foci of glandular differentiation
    C. Foci morphologically similar to small cell undifferentiated carcinoma
    D. All of the above
    E. None of the above

26. Which variant of advanced squamous cell carcinoma is typically admixed with and/or surrounded by an inflammatory infiltrate?
    A. Verrucous carcinoma
    B. Basaloid squamous cell carcinoma
    C. Spindle cell carcinoma/carcinosarcoma
    D. All of the above
    E. None of the above

27. The 2 groups of spindle cell carcinoma/carcinosarcoma can be distinguished based on which of the following features:
    A. Careful morphologic evaluation of multiple tumor sections
    B. Immunohistochemical stains
    C. Electron microscopy
    D. Molecular alterations
    E. There is no reliable way to distinguish

7: Gastrointestinal Tract Questions

28. Tumors associated with squamous cell carcinoma of the esophagus include:
     A.   Synchronous tumors of the esophagus
     B.   Squamous cell carcinoma of the head and neck
     C.   Gastric carcinoma
     D.   Primary lung cancer
     E.   All of the above

29. Autoimmune gastritis primarily involves which portion of the stomach:
     A.   Corpus-fundic region
     B.   Antrum
     C.   Pylorus
     D.   Both B and C
     E.   All of the above

30. Changes seen in the body of the stomach in patients with autoimmune gastritis include, which of the following?
     A.   Mononuclear infiltrate of lamina propria and mucosa with destruction of fundic glands
     B.   Intestinal and pyloric metaplasia
     C.   Enterochromaffin cell hyperplasia positive for chromogranin
     D.   Both A and C
     E.   All of the above

31. Which of the following is NOT associated with autoimmune gastritis?
     A.   Adenocarcinoma
     B.   Hypothyroidism
     C.   Myasthenia gravis
     D.   Immunodeficiency disorders
     E.   Dermatitis herpetiformis

32. Which special stain is useful to facilitate the identification of *H pylori* organisms in a stomach biopsy?
     A.   Warthin-Starry
     B.   Giemsa
     C.   Dieterle
     D.   All of the above
     E.   None of the above; you should really use an immunohistochemical stain

33. Which of the following organisms would be considered in the differential diagnosis of *H pylori* organisms?
     A.   Oral contaminants, including *Actinomyces israelii*
     B.   *Amoeba*
     C.   *Gastrospirillum hominis*
     D.   *Treponema pallidum*
     E.   None of the above

34. Which of the following are associated with complete (mature) intestinal metaplasia (type I) and not incomplete (immature) intestinal metaplasia (type II)?
     A.   Irregular crypts
     B.   Paneth cells
     C.   Adenocarcinoma
     D.   Both A and C
     E.   All of the above

7: Gastrointestinal Tract Questions

35. In which area of the stomach is adenocarcinoma most likely to arise:
    A. Pyloric area
    B. Cardia
    C. Fundic area
    D. Both fundic and pyloric involved
    E. All areas are affected equally

36. Which subtype of gastric adenocarcinoma is associated with *Helicobacter pylori* infection?
    A. Diffuse type
    B. Intestinal type
    C. Mucinous adenocarcinoma
    D. Adenosquamous carcinoma
    E. Small cell carcinoma

37. How much mucin is necessary to diagnose a mucinous adenocarcinoma of the stomach:
    A. >5% of the tumor area is occupied by mucin
    B. >15% of the tumor area is occupied by mucin
    C. >30% of the tumor area is occupied by mucin
    D. >50% of the tumor area is occupied by mucin
    E. >70% of the tumor area is occupied by mucin

38. Which type of gastric carcinoma may be related to Epstein-Barr virus:
    A. Mucinous adenocarcinoma
    B. Signet-ring cell carcinoma
    C. Adenosquamous carcinoma
    D. Small cell carcinoma
    E. Undifferentiated carcinoma

39. Germline mutations in which genes have been documented in familial gastric cancer:
    A. p53
    B. c-myc
    C. E-cadherin/CDH1
    D. C-erbB-2
    E. Ras

40. How often is "surgical resection for cure" possible in patients with gastric carcinoma?
    A. <10%
    B. <25%
    C. <50%
    D. <75%
    E. <90%

41. All of the following are either considered precancerous conditions or associated with gastric cancer, EXCEPT:
    A. Adenoma
    B. Hyperplastic polyp
    C. Chronic gastric ulceration due to *H pylori* infection
    D. Chronic atrophic gastritis
    E. All of the above

7: Gastrointestinal Tract Questions

42. Which of the following clinical features is associated with the development of gastric carcinoma?
    A. Gastric remnants (after Billroth I and II procedures)
    B. Immunodeficiency disorders
    C. Hereditary tumor syndromes
    D. Both A and C
    E. All of the above

43. Which of the following features is commonly seen in sporadic fundic gland polyps?
    A. Dysplasia
    B. Disordered glandular architecture and microcysts
    C. Features overlapping with changes induced by proton pump inhibitors
    D. Inflammation, sometimes associated with *H pylori* infection
    E. Both B and C

44. How often are GISTs of the stomach malignant?
    A. 10%
    B. 30%
    C. 50%
    D. 70%
    E. 90%

45. Which variant of GISTs is most common in the stomach?
    A. Spindled
    B. Epithelioid
    C. Sarcomatous
    D. Both A and B equally
    E. All equally

46. Which of the following morphologic features do spindle cell and epithelioid variants of gastric GISTs share?
    A. Perinuclear vacuoles that indent the nucleus
    B. Skeinoid fibers
    C. Generally low mitotic count
    D. Cellular pleomorphism
    E. Both B and C

47. The 2 most important prognostic factors for GISTs are:
    A. Tumor size
    B. Depth of invasion
    C. Mitotic rate
    D. Pleomorphism
    E. Cellularity

48. All of the following stains have been known to, at least rarely, stain positive in GISTs. Order them from MOST commonly positive to LEAST commonly positive in stomach GISTs?
    A. CD34
    B. CD117 (c-Kit)
    C. Desmin
    D. S100
    E. Smooth muscle actin

7: Gastrointestinal Tract Questions

49. Which of the following would NOT be part of the differential diagnosis of spindled GIST based on H&E morphology?
    A. Leiomyoma and leiomyosarcoma
    B. Schwannoma
    C. Fibromatosis
    D. Solitary fibrous tumor/hemangiopericytoma
    E. All of the above are on the differential diagnosis

50. What is the treatment of choice for unresectable GISTs?
    A. R-CHOP chemotherapy regimen
    B. Radiation
    C. Combination chemo and radiation therapy
    D. Tyrosine kinase inhibitors
    E. Palliative care only

51. Genetic syndromes associated with GISTs include:
    A. Neurofibromatosis type 1
    B. Neurofibromatosis type 2
    C. Carney triad
    D. Both A and B
    E. Both A and C

52. The glomus cells of the glomus tumor are:
    A. Modified histiocytes
    B. Modified glandular cells
    C. Modified smooth muscle cells
    D. All of the above
    E. None of the above

53. Gastric hyperplastic polyps are generally associated with which of the following:
    A. Dysplasia
    B. Damage/inflammation
    C. Underlying malignancy of various organs
    D. ECL hyperplasia
    E. None of the above

54. All of the following are common histologic features of hyperplastic polyps, EXCEPT:
    A. Cystic dilation in the deeper parts of the polyp
    B. Bundles of smooth muscle fibers extending into the polyp from the muscularis mucosa
    C. Edematous lamina propria with mixed inflammatory infiltrate
    D. Lymphoid aggregates
    E. All of the above are features of hyperplastic polyps

55. Patients with a hyperplastic polyp are more likely to have which of the following?
    A. Autoimmune gastritis
    B. *H pylori* infection
    C. Synchronous or metachronous adenocarcinoma
    D. Both A and B
    E. All of the above

7: Gastrointestinal Tract Questions

56. In which of the following locations does inflammatory fibroid polyps most often occur?
    A. Stomach and terminal ileum
    B. Esophagus and stomach
    C. Stomach and proximal small intestine
    D. Esophagus and colon
    E. Terminal ileum and colon

57. Which of the following features are shared by inflammatory fibroid polyps of the stomach and terminal ileum?
    A. Slight predilection for men over women
    B. Tendency to affect adults, typically diagnosed in the 6th decade
    C. Tend to be small in size and asymptomatic
    D. Both A and B
    E. All of the above

58. All of the following are features of gastric inflammatory fibroid polyps vs ileal inflammatory fibroid polyps, EXCEPT:
    A. Composed of plump spindle cells
    B. Eosinophils commonly dominate the inflammatory infiltrate
    C. Tend to involve the muscularis propria
    D. Demonstrate a perivascular orientation of neoplastic cells
    E. All of the above are features of inflammatory fibroid polyps of the stomach vs the ileum

59. Commonly seen microscopic features of gastric MALTomas include all of the following EXCEPT:
    A. Lymphoepithelial lesions
    B. Background of *H pylori* gastritis
    C. Plasmacytoid features
    D. A single lesion
    E. Reactive lymphoid follicles with germinal centers with interspersed sheets of marginal zone cells

60. It is sometimes difficult to distinguish between MALToma and an exuberant chronic gastritis. Which of the following can be helpful?
    A. Documented presence of *H pylori*
    B. Cytokeratin immunostaining
    C. Immunostaining for CD3, CD20, and CD43
    D. All of the above
    E. Both B and C

61. When MALT lymphomas transform into high-grade lesion, which of the following do they most resemble?
    A. Follicular lymphoma
    B. Diffuse large B cell
    C. Mantle cell lymphoma
    D. Burkitt lymphoma
    E. Anaplastic lymphoma

62. The most important single determinant of long-term survival in patients with MALT lymphoma is?
    A. Stage
    B. Depth of lesion
    C. Association with *H pylori* infection
    D. Distant spread of disease
    E. Delay in response to or recurrence after *H pylori* eradication

7: Gastrointestinal Tract Questions

63. Neuroendocrine tumors of the stomach are associated with all of the following, EXCEPT:
    A. Autoimmune gastritis
    B. *H pylori*-associated chronic atrophic gastritis
    C. MEN type I syndrome
    D. Zollinger-Ellison syndrome (ZES)
    E. All of the above

64. All of the following neuroendocrine tumors tend to be multiple, EXCEPT?
    A. Sporadic
    B. Autoimmune atrophic gastritis associated
    C. MEN type I associated
    D. ZES associated
    E. All demonstrate multiple lesions

65. Which of the following neuroendocrine tumors is most likely to behave malignantly?
    A. Sporadic
    B. Autoimmune atrophic gastritis associated
    C. MEN type I associated
    D. ZES associated
    E. Choices C and D

66. Treatment for sporadic neuroendocrine tumors of the stomach is?
    A. Watch and wait first
    B. Surgical resection
    C. Radiation
    D. Chemotherapy
    E. Endoscopic mucosal resection (EMR)

67. The sigmoidoscopic appearance of acute self-limited enterocolitis most resembles which of the following:
    A. Celiac disease
    B. Microscopic colitis
    C. Inflammatory bowel disease
    D. MALT lymphoma
    E. FAP

68. Which of the following findings would favor a diagnosis of inflammatory bowel disease over acute self-limited enterocolitis?
    A. Crypt abscess
    B. Inability to recover an enteric pathogen when appropriately worked-up
    C. Partial loss of intracellular mucin in cells of crypt epithelium
    D. Crypt distortion
    E. Mucosal edema most pronounced in the upper 1/3

69. Which of the following is known to yield false-negative test results for anti-tissue transglutaminase and anti-endomysial tests?
    A. Gluten-free diet
    B. Gluten-heavy diet
    C. Recent antibiotic use
    D. IgA deficiency
    E. All of the above

7: Gastrointestinal Tract Questions

70. Which of the following microscopic features is NOT associated with celiac disease?
    A. Predominantly increased eosinophils
    B. Increased intraepithelial lymphocytes
    C. Expanded lamina propria with increased plasma cells
    D. Villous blunting
    E. All of the above are associated with celiac disease

71. In patients with very early, latent, or partially treated celiac disease, what is the most sensitive histologic finding for celiac disease?
    A. Increased intraepithelial lymphocytes
    B. Expanded lamina propria with increased plasma cells
    C. Villous blunting
    D. Both B and C
    E. All of the above are seen, but more subtly

72. The increased intraepithelial lymphocytes seen in refractory (vs responsive to dietary restriction) celiac disease are usually:
    A. B cells
    B. CD8+ T cells
    C. CD8– T cells
    D. A mixture of B and T cells
    E. CD4+ T cells

73. A definitive diagnosis of celiac disease requires which of the following?
    A. Classic histologic findings
    B. Serologic tests consistent with celiac disease
    C. Clinical presentation with response to dietary modification
    D. Histologic response to dietary modification
    E. A combination of the above

74. Extraintestinal manifestations of celiac disease are seen in which of the following sites, EXCEPT:
    A. Skin
    B. Joints
    C. Uterus
    D. Liver
    E. Can be seen in all the above

75. Crohn disease is more common in which population?
    A. Western developed areas
    B. Jewish
    C. Men
    D. Both A and B
    E. All of the above

76. Which of the following is LEAST likely to be seen in Crohn disease?
    A. Skip lesions
    B. Free perforation with peritonitis
    C. Perforation with external abscess
    D. Fistulas
    E. All of the above are relatively common in Crohn disease

7: Gastrointestinal Tract Questions

77. All of the following features are associated with or is more exaggerated in Crohn disease of the small intestine vs the colon EXCEPT?
    A. More extensive submucosal fibrosis
    B. More extensive hypertrophy of the muscularis propria
    C. More extensive neuroproliferation
    D. Relatively more shallow ulcers
    E. Pyloric metaplasia

78. Which of the following features is more specific for Crohn disease than ulcerative colitis?
    A. Paneth cell hyperplasia
    B. "Creeping fat" or "fat wrapping"
    C. Non-necrotizing granulomas
    D. Necrotizing granulomas
    E. Aphthous ulcers

79. Which of the following statements is true regarding surgical treatment of Crohn disease?
    A. Surgery is curative
    B. Surgery is avoided at all costs because it exacerbates the disease
    C. Recurrences tend to occur at the site of previous surgery
    D. Both B and C
    E. None of the above

80. Which of the following associations is more common in ulcerative colitis than in Crohn disease?
    A. Perianal disease
    B. Toxic megacolon
    C. Secondary infection
    D. All of the above
    E. None of the above

81. Which of the following statement(s) is/are true regarding the development of carcinoma in patients with Crohn disease?
    A. There is no increased risk when compared to the general population
    B. Risk of developing carcinoma is related to duration of disease
    C. The incidence of carcinoma is Crohn colitis is greater than in ulcerative colitis
    D. Carcinomas that occur in Crohn disease tend to present early
    E. Both B and C

82. All of the following are features of microvillus inclusion disease, EXCEPT?
    A. Apical cytoplasmic inclusions
    B. Enterocytes lacking surface microvilli or are shortened and disorganized
    C. Diffuse villous atrophy that can be confused with celiac disease
    D. Normal neighboring Paneth and goblet cells
    E. Mononuclear inflammatory reaction

83. The inheritance pattern of microvillus inclusion disease is best described as:
    A. Autosomal recessive
    B. Autosomal dominant with variable penetrance
    C. X-linked
    D. Both A and B
    E. None of the above

7: Gastrointestinal Tract Questions

84. The etiology of Whipple disease of the small intestine is?
    A.   Infectious
    B.   Genetic
    C.   Autoimmune
    D.   Environmental toxins
    E.   Iatrogenic

85. The sine qua non of Whipple disease is?
    A.   Thickened mucosal folds
    B.   Numerous macrophages in the lamina propria with basophilic, stippled cytoplasm
    C.   Patchy coating of granular, white material
    D.   Extracellular accumulations of lipid within the lamina propria and lymphatic channels
    E.   Rounded and somewhat flattened or blunted villi

86. Which of the following is a feature of nonfunctioning duodenal neuroendocrine tumors vs those associated with Zollinger-Ellison syndrome?
    A.   Nonfunctioning tumors tend to occur at an earlier age
    B.   Nonfunctioning tumors are more likely to be infiltrative
    C.   Nonfunctioning tumors are more likely to metastasize
    D.   Tumors of the duodenal bulb are more likely to be nonfunctioning than those associated with ZES
    E.   Nonfunctioning tumors can lead to fulminant ulcer diathesis

87. Which of the following subgroups of duodenal neuroendocrine tumors is associated with von Recklinghausen disease?
    A.   Gastrin-producing (G-cell) tumor
    B.   Somatostatin-producing (D-cell) tumor
    C.   Serotonin/calcitonin-producing tumor
    D.   Poorly differentiated neuroendocrine tumor
    E.   Malignant carcinoid

88. Which of the following subgroups of duodenal neuroendocrine tumors is usually seen in the periampullary region?
    A.   Gastrin-producing (G-cell) tumor
    B.   Insulin-producing tumor
    C.   Serotonin/calcitonin-producing tumor
    D.   Poorly differentiated neuroendocrine tumor
    E.   Gangliocytic paraganglioma

89. Which of the following subgroups of duodenal neuroendocrine tumors can demonstrate pseudoacini with psammoma bodies?
    A.   Gastrin-producing (G-cell) tumor
    B.   Somatostatin-producing (D-cell) tumor
    C.   Serotonin/calcitonin-producing tumor
    D.   Poorly differentiated neuroendocrine tumor
    E.   Gangliocytic paraganglioma

90. All of the following are microscopic features of collagenous colitis, EXCEPT:
    A.   Thickened subepithelial collagen encircling superficial capillaries in the lamina propria
    B.   Thickened subepithelial collagen containing increased numbers of fibroblasts and eosinophils
    C.   Patchy increase in lymphocytes within the surface epithelium
    D.   Lack of uniform findings throughout the colon
    E.   Thickened collagen occasionally extending downward to involve the basement membrane region of the underlying crypts, in severe cases

7: Gastrointestinal Tract Questions

105. All of the following are features of untreated ulcerative colitis EXCEPT:
    A. Stricture development with chronic disease
    B. Skip areas
    C. Pseudopolyps
    D. Megacolon
    E. Ulceration with crypt abscess formation

106. Which features are seen in quiescent ulcerative colitis?
    A. Pseudopolyps
    B. Abnormal architecture
    C. Metaplastic change, including Paneth cell, pyloric gland, and squamous metaplasia
    D. Increase in mononuclear inflammatory cells and eosinophils in the lamina propria
    E. All of the above

107. Which of the following infections is both in the differential diagnosis of ulcerative colitis and a more common secondary infection?
    A. *C difficile*
    B. *Salmonella*
    C. *Shigella*
    D. *Campylobacter*
    E. *Chlamydia*

108. Extraintestinal manifestation of ulcerative colitis include all of the following, EXCEPT:
    A. Polyarthritis
    B. Dermatitis herpetiformis
    C. Uveitis
    D. Ankylosing spondylitis
    E. Sclerosing cholangitis

109. What is the incidence of carcinoma developing in patients with ulcerative colitis that extends to the hepatic flexure or more proximally?
    A. Rare
    B. 5%
    C. 15%
    D. 25%
    E. 35%

110. "Solitary rectal ulcer syndrome" refers to prolapse occurring at which of the following sites?
    A. At the margin of a colostomy
    B. At the apex of a prolapsing hemorrhoid
    C. Adjacent any polypoid lesion of the large intestine
    D. At the anterior wall of the rectum
    E. At the margin of a colonic diverticulum

111. The most important change associated with solitary rectal ulcer syndrome is which of the following?
    A. Superficial ulceration
    B. Irregularity of crypts with metaplastic-like changes in the epithelium
    C. Obliteration of lamina propria by fibrosis and smooth muscle, extending toward the lumen from a thickened muscularis mucosa
    D. Grossly well-demarcated lesion
    E. Colitis cystic profunda

7: Gastrointestinal Tract Questions

112. Which of the following best describes an "inflammatory cloacogenic polyp"?
    A. A polypoid variant of solitary rectal/mucosal prolapse syndrome
    B. Solitary rectal ulcer with extensive metaplasia
    C. Solitary rectal ulcer with dysplasia
    D. Prolapsing hemorrhoids
    E. None of the above

113. Which of the following features is seen in adenocarcinoma of the right colon vs the left colon?
    A. More common in men than women
    B. 3 times more likely to have synchronous adenomas
    C. More likely to have neuroendocrine and mucinous components
    D. Are more likely to present with signs and symptoms of obstruction
    E. None of the above (all choices more associated with left sided lesions)

114. Carcinomas related to inflammatory bowel disease generally demonstrate which of the following gross patterns?
    A. Polypoid and fungating
    B. Ulcerative and fungating
    C. Flat
    D. Exophytic/papillary, arising from a preexisting adenoma
    E. No particular gross morphology is associated

115. How much mucin does it take to be a "mucinous adenocarcinoma" of the colon?
    A. Globules of mucin present in the apical cytoplasm of the majority of cells
    B. Small pools of mucin within the epithelium
    C. 25% of the lesion mass must consist of mucin
    D. 50% of the lesion mass must consist of mucin
    E. Both A and B necessary

116. Which of the following variants of the colon/rectum has the best survival?
    A. Mucinous adenocarcinoma
    B. Signet ring carcinoma
    C. Carcinomas associated with mismatch repair deficiency (microsatellite unstable)
    D. Both A and C have a relatively good prognosis
    E. All of these variants have a very poor prognosis

117. All of the following are true statements regarding carcinomas with DNA mismatch repair deficiency (microsatellite unstable), EXCEPT:
    A. Tumor-infiltrating lymphocytes are common
    B. Tend to be polypoid or exophytic and may be multiple
    C. Present in 10%-15% of carcinomas
    D. Male predominance
    E. Most are sporadic cancers located in the right colon

118. Which of the following molecular alterations is the most commonly seen in the colon and rectum?
    A. DCC gene deletion
    B. p53 mutations
    C. Bcl-2 expression
    D. Microsatellite unstable
    E. APC/β-catenin inactivation

7: Gastrointestinal Tract Questions

119. A patient with stage III colorectal carcinoma will fare best with which of the following combinations of molecular findings?
    A. Bcl-2 expressed, p53 not overexpressed, K-ras–, DCC not expressed
    B. Bcl-2 expressed, p53 not overexpressed, K-ras+, DCC not expressed
    C. Bcl-2 not expressed, p53 overexpressed, K-ras+, DCC not expressed
    D. Bcl-2 not expressed, p53 overexpressed, K-ras+, DCC expressed
    E. Bcl-2 not expressed, p53 not overexpressed, K-ras–, DCC not expressed

120. All of the following are associated with colorectal carcinoma, EXCEPT:
    A. Juvenile polyposis syndrome
    B. Familial adenomatous polyposis
    C. Peutz-Jeghers
    D. HNPCC
    E. Lynch syndrome, type II

121. Features that would favor pseudoinvasion of an adenomatous polyp (tubular adenoma) vs true adenocarcinoma include?
    A. Abundant hemosiderin granules around the neoplastic glands
    B. Increased staining of submucosal epithelium for matrix metalloproteinase-1 (MMP-1) and p53
    C. Decreased expression of submucosal epithelium for membranous E-cadherin
    D. Irregular and/or decreased collagen deposition surrounding the submucosal glands
    E. None of the above

122. Which of the following is true regarding intestinal hamartomas (Peutz-Jeghers polyp):
    A. They occur exclusively as a component of Peutz-Jeghers syndrome
    B. They occur exclusively in the small intestine
    C. Patients with Peutz-Jeghers syndrome have an increased risk of non-GI as well as GI malignancies
    D. Both B and C are true
    E. All of the above are true

123. Which of the following statements about hyperplastic polyps is FALSE?
    A. Lesions are found predominantly in the rectum and sigmoid colon
    B. Are very often large in size, >1.5 cm
    C. Consist of a mixture of absorptive and goblet cells with well-defined brush boarders
    D. Subepithelial collagen layer along the luminal surface is often thickened
    E. Often demonstrate a characteristic splaying of the muscularis mucosae that can mimic invasion

124. Other terms used to describe inflammatory fibroid polyps include which of the following?
    A. Eosinophilic granuloma
    B. Submucosal fibroma
    C. Hemangiopericytoma
    D. Inflammatory pseudotumor
    E. All of the above have been used to describe this entity

125. All of the following histologic features distinguish sessile serrated adenoma from traditional serrated adenoma EXCEPT:
    A. Uniform dysplastic epithelium
    B. Proliferative zones located higher in the crypts, above the base
    C. Crypts that grow parallel to the muscularis mucosa, creating inverted T- or L-shaped crypts
    D. Dilated and branching crypts
    E. Serration present at the base of the crypts

7: Gastrointestinal Tract Questions

126. The classic staining pattern for sessile serrated adenomas includes which of the following:
    A. Increased staining for both hMLH1 and hMSH2
    B. Decreased staining for both hMLH1 and hMSH2
    C. Low Ki-67 labeling
    D. Both A and C
    E. Both B and C

127. All of the following features are associated with traditional serrated adenomas vs sessile serrated adenomas, EXCEPT:
    A. Uniform dysplastic epithelium
    B. Growth pattern similar to that of a hyperplastic polyp
    C. Tendency to be pedunculated
    D. Serration confined to the upper half or third of the crypts
    E. Preference for the right, rather than left colon

128. The typical behavior of giant condyloma (verrucous carcinoma) is best described as:
    A. Large lesions with high metastatic potential that are very sensitive to radiotherapy
    B. Large lesions with high metastatic potential that are insensitive to radiotherapy
    C. Locally aggressive lesions with low metastatic potential that are insensitive to radiotherapy
    D. Locally aggressive lesions with low metastatic potential that are very sensitive to radiotherapy
    E. High likelihood of progression to squamous cell carcinoma somewhere within the large lesion

129. Patients with Cowden disease are as increased risk for which of the following types of cancers?
    A. GI malignancies
    B. Breast cancer
    C. Thyroid cancers
    D. Both B and C
    E. All of the above

130. Cowden disease is associated with which mutated gene?
    A. *APC* (5q21-q22)
    B. *PTEN* (10q23)
    C. *SMAD4*
    D. *STK11*
    E. None known

131. Familial adenomatous polyposis is associated with which mutated gene?
    A. *APC* (5q21-q22)
    B. *PTEN* (10q23)
    C. *SMAD4*
    D. *STK11*
    E. None known

132. Gardner syndrome is associated with which mutated gene?
    A. *APC* (5q21-q22)
    B. *PTEN* (10q23)
    C. *SMAD4*
    D. *STK11*
    E. None known

7: Gastrointestinal Tract Questions

133. Peutz-Jegher syndrome is associated with which mutated gene?
    A.   *APC* (5q21-q22)
    B.   *PTEN* (10q23)
    C.   *SMAD4*
    D.   *STK11*
    E.   None known

134. Cronkhite-Canada syndrome is assocated with which mutated gene?
    A.   *APC* (5q21-q22)
    B.   *PTEN* (10q23)
    C.   *SMAD4*
    D.   *STK11*
    E.   None known

135. Turcot syndrome is associated with which mutated gene?
    A.   *APC* (5q21-q22)
    B.   *PTEN* (10q23)
    C.   *SMAD4*
    D.   *STK11*
    E.   None known

136. Familial juvenile polyposis is assocated with which mutated gene?
    A.   *APC* (5q21-q22)
    B.   *PTEN* (10q23)
    C.   *SMAD4*
    D.   *STK11*
    E.   None known

137. Which of the following multiple polyp syndromes is/are inherited in an autosomal-dominant fashion?
    A.   Cowden disease (multiple hamartoma syndrome)
    B.   Familial adenomatous polyposis
    C.   Hereditary nonpolyposis colorectal cancer (HNPCC)
    D.   Peutz-Jeghers syndrome
    E.   All of the above

138. Polyps of which of the following multiple polyp syndromes are NOT considered premalignant or harboring malignant potential:
    A.   Cowden disease (Multiple hamartoma syndrome)
    B.   Devon family syndrome
    C.   Intestinal ganglioneuromatosis
    D.   Familial juvenile polyposis
    E.   A, B, and C are all correct

139. Which of the following syndromes consists of GI polyposis associated with alopecia, nail atrophy, and macular hyperpigmentation of the face?
    A.   Devon family syndrome
    B.   Cronkhite-Canada syndrome
    C.   Muir-Torre syndrome
    D.   Oldfield syndrome
    E.   Ruvalcaba-Myhre-Smith syndrome

7: Gastrointestinal Tract Questions

140. Polyps of which of the following syndromes are identical to juvenile polyps?
    A. Devon family syndrome
    B. Muir-Torre syndrome
    C. Cronkhite-Canada syndrome
    D. Oldfield syndrome
    E. Turcot syndrome

141. Microsatellite instability is a feature of which of the following multiple polyp syndromes:
    A. Familial adenomatous polyposis (FAP)
    B. Gardner syndrome
    C. Familial juvenile polyposis
    D. Hereditary nonpolyposis colorectal cancer (HNPCC)
    E. Peutz-Jeghers syndrome

142. Which of the following is the most common form of familial colon cancer?
    A. Familial adenomatous polyposis
    B. Familial juvenile polyposis
    C. Hereditary nonpolyposis colorectal cancer (HNPCC)
    D. Peutz-Jeghers syndrome
    E. Turcot syndrome

143. Which of the following lesions are associated with multiple endocrine neoplasia (MEN) 2b?
    A. Sessile serrated polyps
    B. Gastrointestinal stromal tumor
    C. Hamartomatous polyps
    D. Ganglioneuroma
    E. VIP- producing pancreatic tumor

144. Which syndrome is associated with adenomatous colon polyps or colorectal cancer and either glioblastoma or medulloblastoma?
    A. Cowden
    B. Turcot
    C. Lynch
    D. Gardner
    E. Cronkhite-Canada

145. Which polyposis syndrome demonstrates the following extraintestinal manifestations: mesenteric fibromatosis, osteomas, epidermoid cyst, odontomas, and congenital hypertrophy of the retinal pigment epithelium?
    A. Cowden
    B. Turcot
    C. Lynch
    D. Gardner
    E. Cronkhite-Canada

146. Which of the colonic polyposis syndromes have been associated with cervical adenoma malignum and sex-cord tumors with annular tubules in women and Sertoli cell testicular tumors in men?
    A. Cowden
    B. MEN
    C. Lynch
    D. Peutz-Jegher
    E. Cronkhite-Canada

7: Gastrointestinal Tract Questions

147. Which other syndrome(s) can have mucocutaneous lesions similar to patients with Peutz-Jegher Syndrome?
    A. Addison disease
    B. McCune-Albright syndrome
    C. Laugier-Hunziker
    D. All the above
    E. None of the above; the lesions are pathognomonic

148. Which polyp is associated with hypokalemia?
    A. Hyperplastic
    B. Villous adenoma
    C. Tubular adenoma
    D. Hamartomatous
    E. Sessile serrated adenoma

149. The most common neoplasm of the appendix is which of the following?
    A. Adenoma
    B. Neuroendocrine tumors
    C. Hyperplastic polyp
    D. Mucinous adenocarcinoma
    E. None of the above

150. Neuroendocrine tumors of which of the following locations demonstrate Schwann-like sustentacular cells that are highlighted by immunohistochemical staining with S100?
    A. Small intestine
    B. Appendix
    C. Colon
    D. Both A and C
    E. All of the above

151. If you had to choose to have a neuroendocrine tumor of one of the following regions, which would be your first, second, and third choice?
    A. Small intestine, appendix, colon
    B. Colon, small intestine, appendix
    C. Appendix, colon, small intestine
    D. Appendix, small intestine, colon
    E. Colon, appendix, small intestine

152. Criteria for malignancy of rectal neuroendocrine tumors includes all of the following EXCEPT:
    A. Size >2 cm
    B. Invasion of muscularis propria
    C. >2 mitotic figures/hpf
    D. DNA aneuploidy
    E. All of the above

153. Which of the following immunohistochemical stains is least likely to be positive in rectal neuroendocrine tumors?
    A. Synaptophysin and chromogranin
    B. Somatostatin
    C. Serotonin
    D. Prostatic acidic phosphatase
    E. Vimentin

7: Gastrointestinal Tract Questions

154. A patient with a history of Barrett esophagus is biopsied and then 6 months later re-surveyed. The image on the left is from the first endoscopy and the one on the right is from the subsequent biopsy. Which of the following features is useful to distinguish high-grade from low-grade dysplasia?

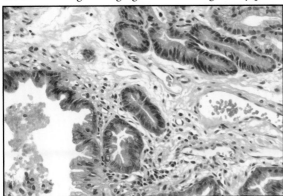 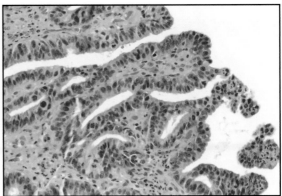

    A.   High-grade dysplasia involves the full thickness while low-grade is only present at the surface.

    B.   High-grade dysplasia demonstrates more complex architectural distortion than low-grade.

    C.   High-grade dysplasia demonstrates more cytologic atypia.

    D.   All of the above

    E.   B and C

155. Which of the following features does NOT have significant prognostic significance in the esophageal lesion shown below?

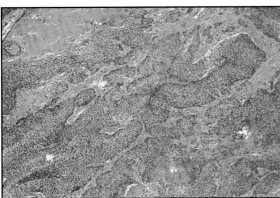

    A.   Degree of differentiation

    B.   Size of tumor

    C.   Depth of invasion

    D.   Lymph node status

    E.   All of the above have important prognostic value.

7: Gastrointestinal Tract Questions

156. The below biopsy was taken from the body of the stomach. Which of the following are potential sequelae of this gastric lesion (H&E on left, chromogranin IHC on right)?

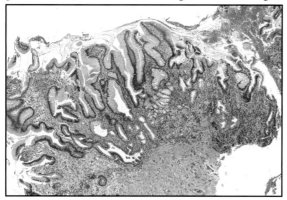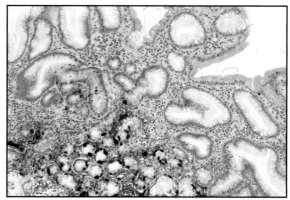

    A.   Pernicious anemia
    B.   Hypergastrinemia
    C.   Multiple small carcinoid tumors
    D.   Abnormal Schilling test
    E.   All of the above

157. The most LIKELY scenario for the findings in the following images is?

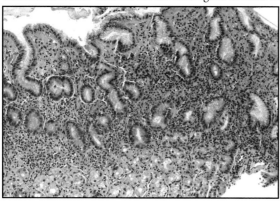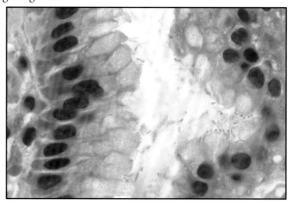

    A.   The stomach antrum of a 15-year-old from a developed area
    B.   The stomach antrum of a 45-year-old from an underdeveloped area
    C.   The stomach body of a 45-year-old from an underdeveloped area
    D.   The proximal duodenum of a 15-year-old from a developed area
    E.   The proximal duodenum of a 45-year-old from an underdeveloped area

7: Gastrointestinal Tract Questions

158. For the lesion in the gastric biopsy shown below, which one of the following choices is FALSE? The lumen surface of the gland stains for CD10.

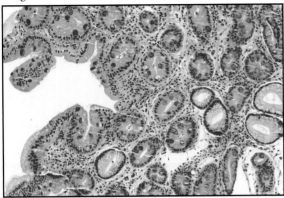

    A.   It is associated with increased risk of carcinoma.

    B.   It can be seen in cases of autoimmune gastritis.

    C.   It can result from bile reflux.

    D.   It can be seen in *H pyloric* gastritis.

    E.   All the above are true.

159. All of the following clinical features are generally associated with the gastric lesion shown below, EXCEPT:

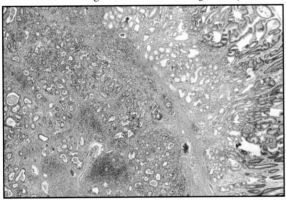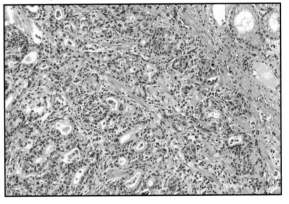

    A.   Older age

    B.   Male sex

    C.   White population in the US

    D.   Blood type A

    E.   Pernicious anemia

7: Gastrointestinal Tract Questions

164. A submucosal gastric lesion was biopsied and is shown below. Which of the following stains will MOST likely be helpful in rendering a diagnosis?

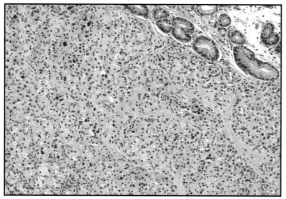

    A.   Serotonin
    B.   Chromogranin A
    C.   Synaptophysin
    D.   Epinephrine
    E.   Histamine

165. This gastric lesion pictured below is best characterized as which of the following?

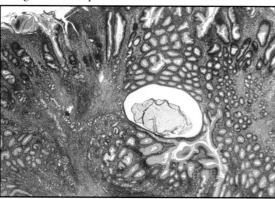

    A.   Pyloric adenoma
    B.   Intestinal metaplasia
    C.   Hyperplastic polyp
    D.   Fundic gland polyp
    E.   Intramucosal carcinoma

7: Gastrointestinal Tract Questions

166. A random esophageal biopsy was taken and is shown below. Which of the following diagnosis would be most correct?

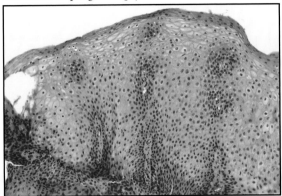

   A. No pathologic findings
   B. Gastroesophageal reflux
   C. Eosinophilic esophagitis
   D. HSV esophagitis
   E. Squamous cell dysplasia

167. Which of the following statements about the lesion shown below is FALSE?

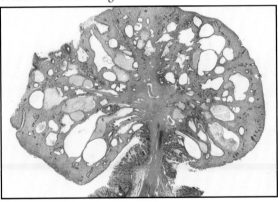
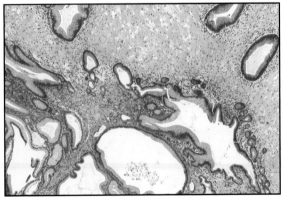

   A. It occurs mainly in the first 2 decades of life.
   B. It is usually located in the rectum.
   C. It is usually multiple and may cluster.
   D. It is associated with an increased risk of developing intestinal and gastric cancer.
   E. It consists of cystically dilated and tortuous glands in an inflamed stroma.

7: Gastrointestinal Tract Questions

168. A polypoid gastric lesion was biopsied and is depicted below. Of the following choices, which is the BEST diagnosis?

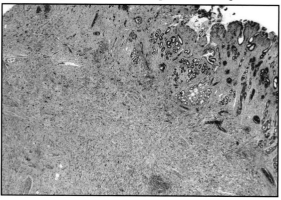 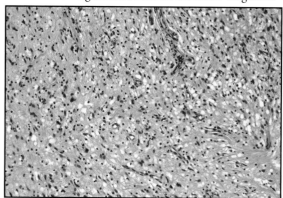

    A.   Inflammatory fibroid polyp
    B.   Fibromatosis
    C.   Gastrointestinal stromal tumor (GIST)
    D.   Eosinophilic gastritis
    E.   Pyloric adenoma

169. Given the below image, which marker is most likely to be negative in the neoplastic cells?

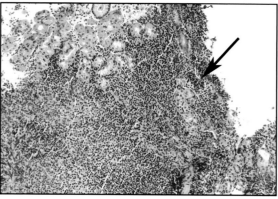

    A.   CD20
    B.   CD43
    C.   BCL-2
    D.   BCL-1/cyclin D-1
    E.   PAX5

7: Gastrointestinal Tract Questions

170. Which of the following statements regarding the esophageal lesion shown below is FALSE?

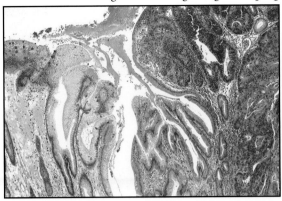

    A.   Only around 50% of these tumors have gross lesions on endoscopy.

    B.   CK20 and CK7 immunohistochemical stains distinguish between the gastric cardiac and esophageal type of this tumor.

    C.   Patients with this lesion are primarily white males.

    D.   Survival is based on tumor involvement of muscularis propria.

    E.   Proximal margin of resection should include squamous mucosa.

171. All of the following are associated with an increased risk of developing the disease displayed below in the duodenal biopsy, EXCEPT:

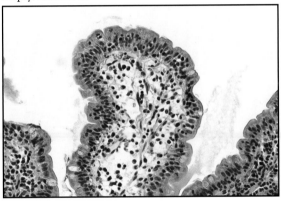 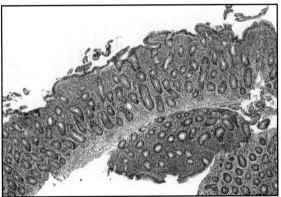

    A.   HLA antigens HLA-D2 and HLA-DQ8

    B.   Recent organ transplant

    C.   Type I diabetes

    D.   Down syndrome

    E.   Iron deficiency anemia

7: Gastrointestinal Tract Questions

172. At the time of presentation, with the disease depicted in the images, which segment of the GI tract is most likely to be involved? (Image on left luminal portion, image of right from deep/serosal side.)

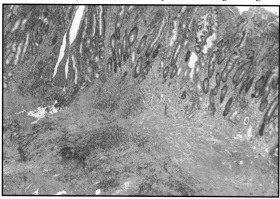 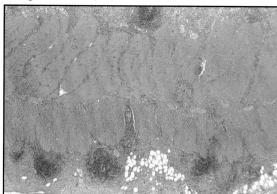

    A.   Colon alone
    B.   Both small intestine and colon
    C.   Small intestine alone
    D.   Perianal disease
    E.   Upper GI tract, including oral cavity, esophagus, stomach, and proximal duodenum

173. The below duodenal lesion stains for PAS with diastase and negative for AFB. What is the diagnosis?

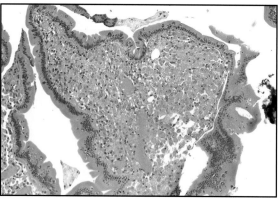 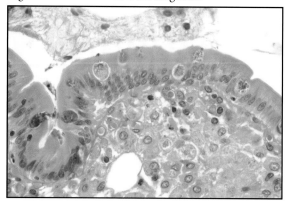

    A.   Xanthoma
    B.   *Mycobacterium avium* infection
    C.   Sarcoidosis
    D.   Microvillous inclusion disease
    E.   Whipple disease

7: Gastrointestinal Tract Questions

174. The images below demonstrate the most common duodenal neuroendocrine tumor, which is which of the following?

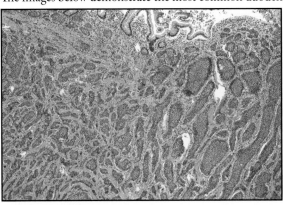 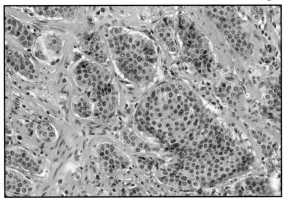

    A.   Gastrin-producing (G-cell) tumor
    B.   Somatostatin-producing (D-cell) tumor
    C.   Serotonin/calcitonin-producing tumor
    D.   Poorly differentiated neuroendocrine tumor
    E.   Gangliocytic paraganglioma

175. All of the following may be associated with disease in the images below, EXCEPT:

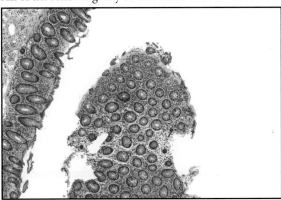 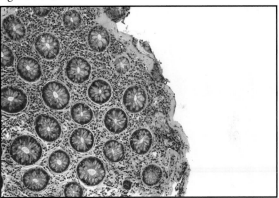

    A.   Autoimmune diseases
    B.   Celiac disease
    C.   NSAID use
    D.   A and B
    E.   All of the above

7: Gastrointestinal Tract Questions

176. The below biopsy is from a 3-day-old male infant, who has not had a bowel movement. A series of suction rectal biopsies were taken and examined under a dissecting microscopic and a representative images are shown below. Based on the image below, is the biopsy adequate for evaluation?

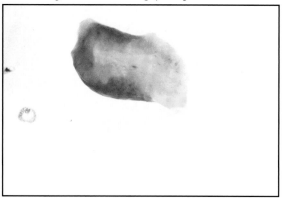 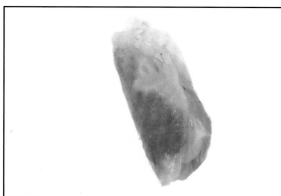

    A.   Adequate for evaluation
    B.   Inadequate for evaluation

177. A patient with a history of bone marrow transplant presents with diarrhea and abdominal pain. A colon biopsy was taken and images are shown below. What is the diagnosis?

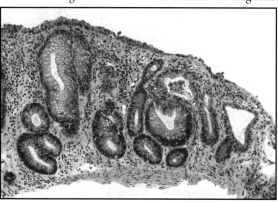 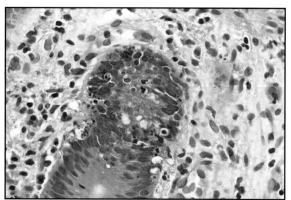

    A.   CMV colitis
    B.   T-cell enteropathic lymphoma
    C.   Graft-vs-host disease
    D.   Ischemia
    E.   Radiation effect

7: Gastrointestinal Tract Questions

178. Which of the following patients is LEAST likely to present with the disease demonstrated in the images below?

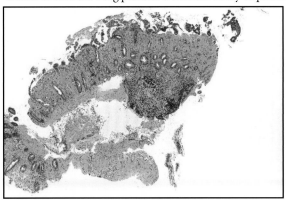 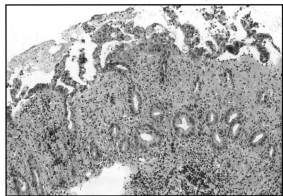

    A.   An older patient with cardiac failure
    B.   A younger patient taking psychiatric meds
    C.   An older patient with severe atherosclerotic disease
    D.   A patient with intraabdominal sepsis
    E.   A patient with digitalis toxicity

179. The colon biopsy below is most likely from which patient?

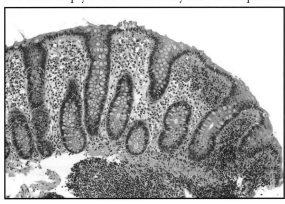 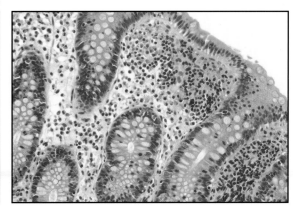

    A.   Patient with bloody diarrhea
    B.   68-year-old man
    C.   45-year-old woman
    D.   Patient with hyperkalemia
    E.   Constipated 63-year-old

7: Gastrointestinal Tract Questions

180. The images below are from the left colon of a colonic resection. What is the diagnosis?

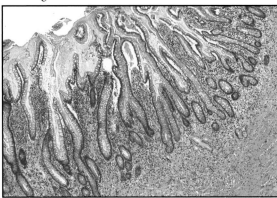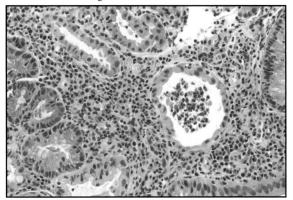

    A.   Lymphocytic colitis
    B.   Ischemic colitis
    C.   *C difficile* infection
    D.   Ulcerative colitis
    E.   *E coli* O157 infection

181. The images below are from the rectum and associated with which of the following?

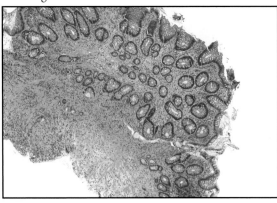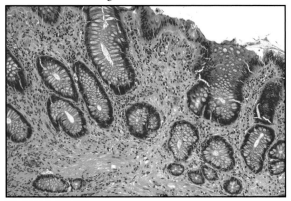

    A.   Constipation
    B.   *C difficile* infection
    C.   Crohn disease
    D.   Pelvic radiation
    E.   Diverticular disease

182. The colorectal tumor below is stained for the expression of the mismatch repair proteins. What is the most appropriate interpretation?

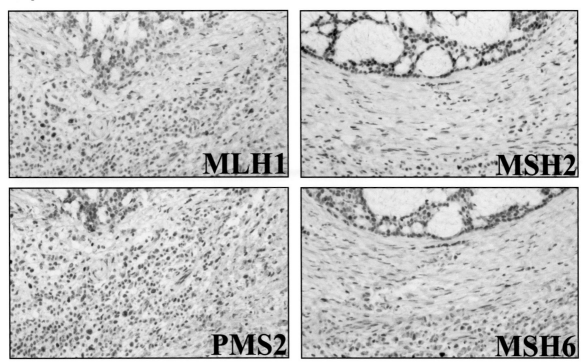

A. Mutation in the MSH2 and MSH6 gene
B. Gain of MSH2 and MSH6 expression
C. Mutation in the MLH1 and PMS gene
D. Loss of MLH1 translation
E. Loss of PMS2 translation

183. For the colonic lesion demonstrated below, what is the pT stage?

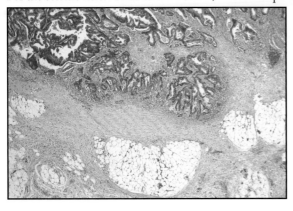 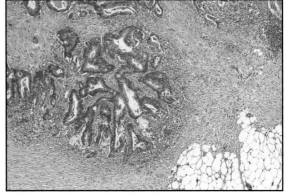

A. pT1
B. pT2
C. pT3
D. pT4
E. Cannot be determined

7: Gastrointestinal Tract Questions

184. The lesion below can occur in the small and large intestine and is associated with which of the following?

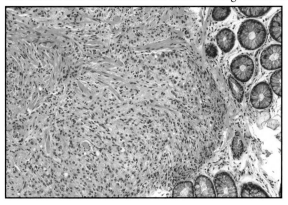 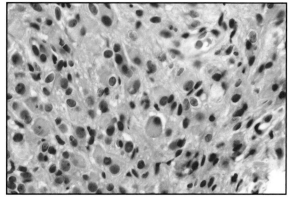

    A.   Von Recklinghausen disease
    B.   MEN IIA
    C.   MEN IIB
    D.   A and C
    E.   All of the above

185. A patient presented with acute severe abdominal pain. Below are representative sections from the segmental ileocecal resection. What clinical situation most likely represents this patient's situation?

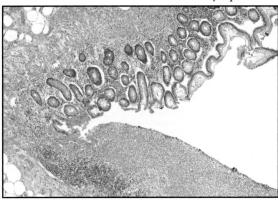 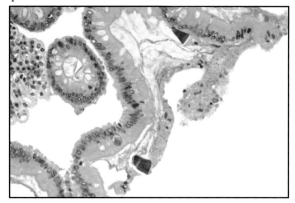

    A.   Patient on long-term antibiotics.
    B.   Patient with renal failure
    C.   Iron-deficient patient on replacement therapy
    D.   12-year-old with intussusception
    E.   Recent history of swimming in a freshwater lake

7: Gastrointestinal Tract Questions

186. The lesion shown below was biopsied from the right colon during a screening colonoscopy. Which of the following statements concerning the lesion is FALSE?

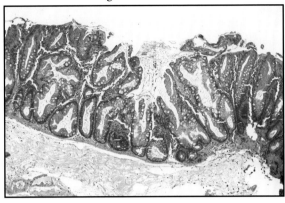 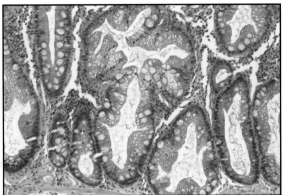

    A.   It should be treated with colectomy.
    B.   It shows decreased staining of MLH1.
    C.   It endoscopically may appear as a large mucosal fold.
    D.   It can be seen in hyperplastic polyposis syndrome.
    E.   Most have mutations in BRAF.

187. Which of the following statements about the lesion or the associated syndrome is FALSE?

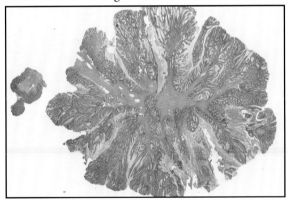 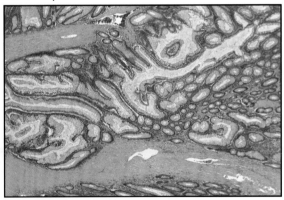

    A.   It is associated with mutation of STK11.
    B.   It most commonly occurs in the stomach.
    C.   It has increased risk of sex-cord tumor with annular tubules.
    D.   There is melanotic pigmentation in the oral cavity.
    E.   None of the above

7: Gastrointestinal Tract Questions

188. A 72-year-old man presented with rectal itching. Examination demonstrated scaly erythematous patches. A biopsy was taken and shown below. The neoplastic cells are S100 negative. Which of the following statements regarding the lesion shown in the anal biopsy below is TRUE?

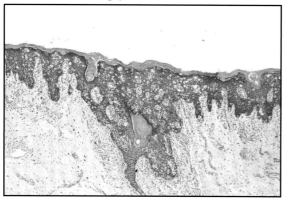 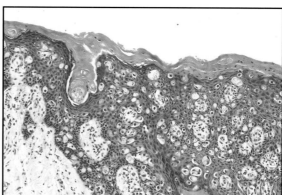

   A.   It is HPV related.
   B.   It indicates internal malignancy.
   C.   It is associated with Bowen disease.
   D.   It stains similar to apocrine tumors.
   E.   It has a poor prognosis.

189. Which of the following statements regarding the lesion demonstrated below is FALSE?

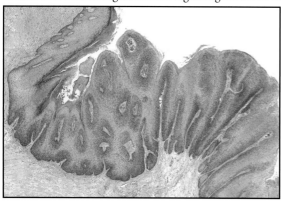 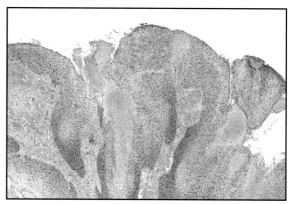

   A.   It is radiation insensitive.
   B.   It is associated with HPV type 16 and 18.
   C.   It is more common in men.
   D.   It generally does not metastasize.
   E.   It has similar morphology to giant condyloma acuminatum of Buschke-Löwenstein.

7: Gastrointestinal Tract Questions

190. The below anal lesion stains positive for c-Kit (CD117) and S100; what is the diagnosis?

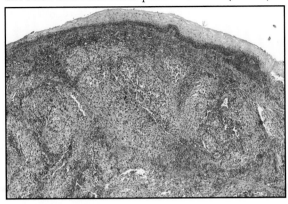 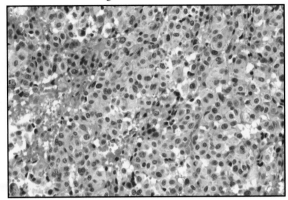

    A.   GIST
    B.   Melanoma
    C.   Leiomyoma
    D.   Schwannoma
    E.   Dendritic cell sarcoma

191. A woman presents with history of fibroid uterus and at the time of surgery, the appendix was noted to appear "abnormal" and was taken out. The image shown below is from the appendix. The neoplastic cells are positive for both alcian blue and chromogranin. All the following are TRUE about the lesion, EXCEPT?

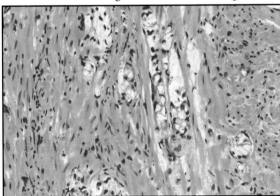

    A.   It can present as Krukenberg tumor.
    B.   Biological behavior is similar to classical carcinoid tumor.
    C.   It typically presents with acute appendicitis or asymptomatically.
    D.   It is positive for CK7.
    E.   It is positive for CK20.

7: Gastrointestinal Tract Questions

Questions 192-199

For the lesions below match the image with the appropriate diagnosis
- A.   Hyperplastic polyp
- B.   Tubular adenoma
- C.   Gangliocytic paraganglioma
- D.   Tubular villous adenoma
- E.   Inflammatory fibroid polyp
- F.   Mucinous adenocarcinoma
- G.   Signet ring adenocarcinoma
- H.   Mucocele/pseudoinvasion
- I.   Prolapse
- J.   Melanosis coli

192.

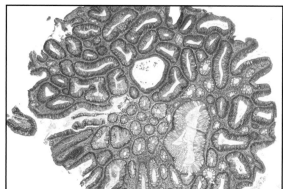 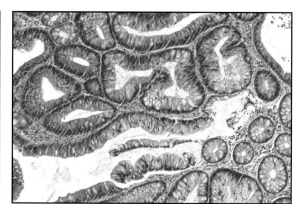

193.

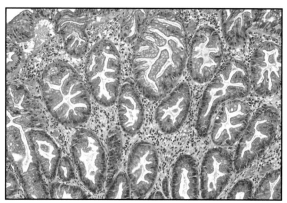

7: Gastrointestinal Tract Questions

194.

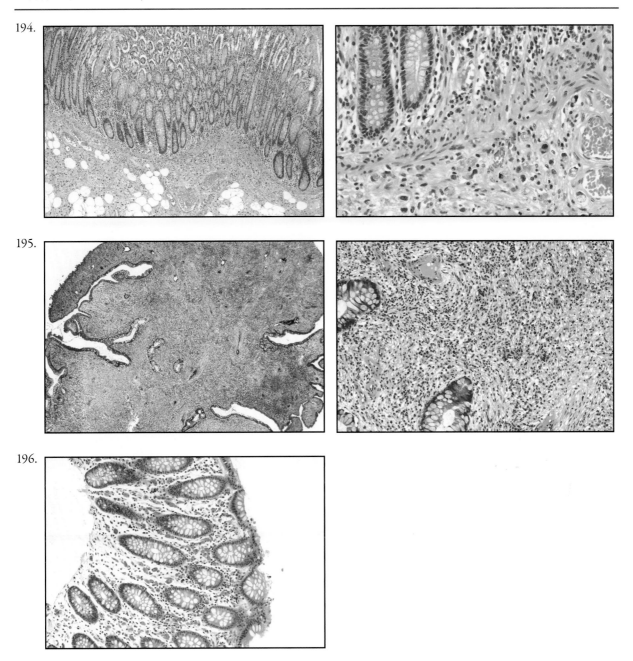

195.

196.

7: Gastrointestinal Tract Questions

197.

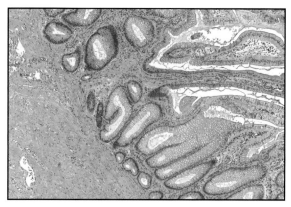

198.

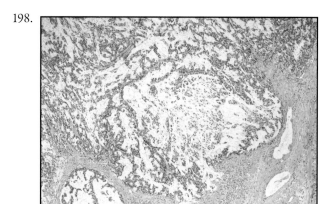

199.

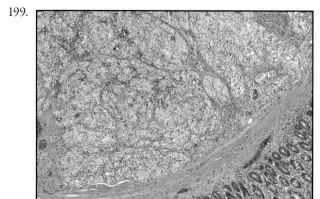
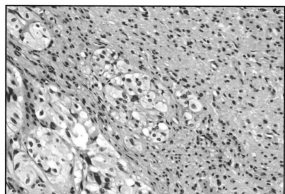

7: Gastrointestinal Tract Answers

1. D. **BOTH A AND B**
    It is often difficult to distinguish radiation atypia from dysplasia or carcinoma-in-situ. Radiation typically produces enlarged cells but both the cytoplasm and nucleus are enlarged, preserving the N:C ratio (vs dysplasia, where you would expect an increased N:C ratio). The absence of full thickness changes and a lack of mitotic figures also favor radiation atypia (thus, choice c is incorrect). Before you start agonizing over the distinction, it is prudent to confirm that the patient has, in fact, received pre-operative radiation and/or chemotherapy.
    QCSP, **Intraoperative Consultation**, p 230.

2. B. **MARGINS FOR ISCHEMIC ENTERITIS INVOLVING THE SMALL INTESTINE**
    Under normal circumstances, frozen sections should not be performed on ischemic enteritis involving the small intestine. The surgeon's macroscopic assessment of the bowel is the most significant and there is little clinical significance to mucosal ischemic changes at the surgical margin.
    QCSP, **Intraoperative Consultation**, p 230-231.

3. A. **METASTATIC LOBULAR CARCINOMA OF THE BREAST**
    Signet ring carcinoma can be very difficult to identify, especially on frozen tissue, because of its infiltrative pattern and propensity to form "skip" areas at its advancing edge. It is almost impossible on frozen section to differentiate a primary gastric signet-ring carcinoma from a metastatic lobular carcinoma. When mucinous carcinomas are seen in the ovary on frozen section, the surgeon must examine the abdominal/pelvic contents for a possible primary source. Lymphoma and endometrioid adenocarcinoma do not generally mimic signet ring carcinoma.
    QCSP, **Intraoperative Consultation**, p 230-231.

4. D. **RECTOSIGMOID COLON**
    Endometriosis has been documented to occur over a wide distribution within the pelvic and abdominal cavity. It is important to include this in the differential on "nodule(s)" picked off at the time of surgery. Microscopically you should see glands and stroma (hemosiderin-laden macrophages are a bonus). The rectosigmoid colon is the most common part of the GI tract that is involved.
    QCSP, **Intraoperative Consultation**, p 231.

5. B. **THE SURGEON WILL CREATE AN ILEAL POUCH ONLY IF THE PATIENT HAS ULCERATIVE COLITIS VS CROHN COLITIS**
    Intraoperative consultation for inflammatory bowel disease is rare, but may be warranted if the surgeon is considering an ileal pouch, which is done routinely for ulcerative colitis, but is contraindicated in Crohn colitis.
    QCSP, **Intraoperative Consultation**, p 231.

6. D. **80%**
    The majority of carcinomas occurring in the distal esophagus are adenocarcinoma. They make up 80% of all carcinomas in the lower 1/3 of the esophagus. This includes GE junction tumors, which are (currently) treated like esophageal tumors for the purpose of staging (even if some believe that GE junction tumors should be treated as a separate tumor form gastric or esophageal tumors.)
    QCSP, **Esophagus Adenocarcinoma**, p 232.

7. C. **BLACKS**
    Esophageal adenocarcinoma is associated with Barrett esophagus and has the same etiologic factors, including reflux, tobacco and alcohol use. Men are affected 3-7 times more than women and esophageal adenocarcinoma is much more common in whites than blacks, making C the correct answer to this "except" question. Squamous cell carcinoma is more common in blacks than whites.
    QCSP, **Esophagus Adenocarcinoma**, p 232.

7: Gastrointestinal Tract Answers

8. D. **50%**

Most esophageal adenocarcinomas are intestinal type. Following the similar rule of the remainder of the luminal GI tract, a tumor must be at least 50% mucinous to be considered a mucinous adenocarcinoma. Mucin may be variably seen intracellularly, within neoplastic glands, or pooling extracellularly.

QCSP, **Esophagus Adenocarcinoma**, p 232.

9. E. **ALL OF THE ABOVE**

C-myc expression is typical and the *H-ras* gene is expressed in both high-grade dysplasia and carcinoma. Approximately 60% of esophageal adenocarcinomas demonstrate TP53 mutations.

QCSP, **Esophagus Adenocarcinoma**, p 233.

10. B. **45% AND 15%-25%**

Depth of invasion, along with lymph node status and overall size, is one of the most important prognostic factors. Tumors that do not invade the muscularis propria have survival rates of 95%-100% (a lucky few). Survival drops to 45% for tumors that invade into the muscularis propria and 15%-25% for those that extend beyond it. If adjacent organs are involved, the survival rate is nil. That is why finding high grade dysplasia on a biopsy often warrants an esophagectomy (or at least a mucosal resection).

QCSP, **Esophagus Adenocarcinoma**, p 233.

11. E. **ALL OF THE ABOVE**

Esophageal adenocarcinomas typically arise from Barrett mucosa and there is often Barrett mucosa with dysplasia seen in the resection specimen (90%). When it is not seen, replacement by carcinoma is a possibility. Adenocarcinoma can also arise from foci of heterotopic gastric mucosa (inlet patch), which has an incidence of approximately 4%. When adenocarcinoma arises in submucosal glands or their ducts, it is usually adenoid cystic carcinoma and is very aggressive.

QCSP, **Esophagus Adenocarcinoma**, p 233.

12. B. **10%-20%**

Approximately 10%-20% of patients with prolonged gastroesophageal reflux disease develop Barrett esophagus. Heavy tobacco and alcohol use are associated with its development and it is usually diagnosed between 40 and 60 years of age.

QCSP, **Barrett esophagus**, p 234.

13. B. **15%-20%**

The incidence is similar to that of Barrett mucosa in all prolonged GERD sufferers, which may help you remember the figures. 10%-20% of people with prolonged GERD develop Barrett mucosa and, of these 10%-20%, 15%-20% develop dysplasia. Patients with Barrett mucosa and either low-grade dysplasia or indefinite for dysplasia typically undergo surveillance endoscopy with biopsy every 6 months for at least 2 years.

QCSP, **Barrett esophagus**, p 234.

14. C. **GOBLET CELLS**

The presence of true goblet cells, with basal nuclei and apical distention by blue mucin that stains with PAS-Alcian blue at pH 2.5, is the necessary microscopic feature for Barrett esophagus. Don't be fooled by gastric foveolar cells with neutral mucin expanding the cytoplasm or by cells that have blue mucin without the goblet shape. The metaplastic epithelium can include various cells, including colonic columnar cells, intermediate cells, Paneth cells, and endocrine cells. To diagnose "Barrett esophagus" vs "cardiac-type gastric mucosa with goblet cells" or "intestinal metaplasia," one needs both the necessary microscopic findings as well as the typical endoscopic findings of "salmon-colored mucosa."

QCSP, **Barrett Mucosa**, p 234-235.

7: Gastrointestinal Tract Answers

15. C. **ACID MUCIN STAINS BLUE, NEUTRAL MUCINS STAIN RED-PURPLE**
A PAS-Alcian blue stain performed at a low pH (2.5) can be used to help distinguish true goblet cells from gastric foveolar cells expanded by neutral mucin. The goblet cells stain blue and the gastric mucin stain red-purple. This can be useful to confirm that isolated goblet cells represent a short segment of Barrett mucosa rather than eccentric GE junction.
QCSP, **Barrett Mucosa,** p 235.

16. E. **A, B, AND C**
The transformation from normal squamous mucosa to metaplasia to dysplasia to carcinoma is multifactorial and likely involves molecular alterations such at p53 mutations (seen in 60% of Barrett dysplasia), point mutations affecting the APC suppressor gene, c-myc expression (seen in all grades of dysplasia), and H-ras expression (seen in high-grade dysplasia and carcinoma). Additional factors, such as inherited predispositions and GERD likely also contribute. Immunohistochemical staining for p53 can be utilized to highlight dysplastic epithelium. The possible role of *H pylori* in this process is currently being debated with studies supporting and not supporting an association of *H pylori* infection and Barrett mucosa.
QCSP, **Barrett Mucosa,** p 235.

17. B. **5%-10%**
After 50 years of age, 15%-20% of patients with Barrett mucosa will develop dysplasia, while 5%-10% of patients with Barrett mucosa may develop carcinoma.
QCSP, **Barrett Mucosa,** p 234-5.

18. C. **35%-50%**
The presence of high-grade dysplasia in Barrett esophagus is an indication for esophagectomy and between 35%-50% of these patients will also have an adenocarcinoma at the time of resection. However, given the trend of early diagnosis of these lesions, the more conservative approach of endoscopic mucosal resection can be utilized to remove high-grade dysplasia without esophagectomy.
QCSP, **Barrett Mucosa/Gastroesophageal Reflux,** p 237.

19. E. **ALL OF THE ABOVE ARE FEATURES OF LOW-GRADE GERD**
Choices, A through D, are all early/mild changes seen in GERD. Balloon cells may also be seen in the "midzone" of the squamous epithelium. Ballooning is caused by increased permeability of the cell membrane due to epithelial injury, which leads to accumulation of plasma proteins in the cells and subsequent swelling. Neutrophils and eosinophils may also be seen in the epithelium.
QCSP, **Gastroesophageal Reflux,** p 236.

20. B. **DYSPLASIA**
Dysplastic epithelium is not part of the spectrum of GERD, unless you are referring to Barrett esophagus with dysplasia. The epithelium and lamina propria demonstrate a marked increase in neutrophils and eosinophils. Massive edema may cause discohesive of epithelial cells. The damaged epithelium may lead to erosions, granulation tissue, inflammatory polyps, and acute or active chronic ulcers.
QCSP, **Gastroesophageal Reflux,** p 236.

21. B. **NORTHERN CHINA**
Northern China, northern Iran, along the Caspian sea, and the Transkei region of South Africa have the highest incidence of esophageal squamous cell carcinoma worldwide. Additionally, men are 3 times more affected than women.
QCSP, **Squamous Cell Carcinoma,** p 238.

7: Gastrointestinal Tract Answers

22.   C.   **GERD**

While squamous carcinoma may occur in patients with Barrett mucosa, which is related to GERD, it is not considered a risk factor and is, therefore, the correct answer to this "except" question. Dietary factors including pickled and dried vegetables, smoked meat and fish, moldy food, and diets low in β-carotene, vitamin A, B complex, C and E are all reported risk factors for esophageal squamous cell carcinoma. N-nitrosamines are also a risk factor and alcohol and tobacco use may have synergistic effects—the absorption or metabolism of tobacco-specific carcinogens may be affected by alcohol. Both radiation and thermal injury are also risk factors. Infectious agents may also play a role, like HPV, which induces papilloma formation.

Importantly, any conditions that decrease the food transit through the esophagus, results in an increased risk of squamous cell carcinoma.

QCSP, **Squamous Cell Carcinoma**, p 238.

23.   B.   **MIDDLE 1/3**

The most common location for squamous cell carcinomas of the esophagus is the middle 1/3 and least common in the upper(proximal) 1/3.

QCSP, **Squamous Cell Carcinoma**, p 238.

24.   C.   **PAPILLARY TYPE**

Early squamous cell carcinomas include the types listed in choices A-D. These may be intraepithelial (in situ, involving the full thickness of epithelium, but with intact basement membrane), intramucosal (with small groups or single cells infiltrating the basement membrane but limited to the lamina propria) or submucosal (penetrating the muscularis mucosa, but not yet reaching the muscularis propria, as in advanced cases). 50% of papillary type cancers and 35% of plaque type are submucosal. Erosive type is usually intraepithelial or intramucosal and the occult type is always intraepithelial.

QCSP, **Squamous Cell Carcinoma**, p 238-239.

25.   D.   **ALL OF THE ABOVE**

HPV-type changes, including koilocytosis, are frequently seen, while glandular differentiation can be seen focally in up to 20% cases. Additionally, small foci reminiscent of small cell undifferentiated carcinoma can also be seen in small foci of esophageal squamous cell carcinoma.

QCSP, **Squamous Cell Carcinoma**, p 238-239.

26.   C.   **SPINDLE CELL CARCINOMA/CARCINOSARCOMA**

Inflammatory cells are typically seen surrounding and intermixing with the cells of spindle cell carcinoma/carcinosarcoma. Bone, cartilage, and muscle tissue may also be present in this variant. It is important to classify/describe the sarcomatous part in case of metastasis.

QCSP, **Squamous Cell Carcinoma**, p 238-239.

27.   C.   **ELECTRON MICROSCOPY**

Electron microscopy of spindle cell carcinoma/carcinosarcoma reveals 2 groups: A true carcinosarcoma demonstrates both squamous epithelial features and mesenchymal features while sarcomatoid carcinoma demonstrates only epithelial characteristics in both the squamous and spindle cells.

QCSP, **Squamous Cell Carcinoma**, p 238-239.

28.   E.   **ALL OF THE ABOVE**

Synchronous tumors are relatively common, seen in up to 30% of cases, and are especially likely in alcoholics. Head and neck squamous cell carcinoma, gastric cancer, and primary lung cancers are also associated. In addition, Lye ingestion resulting in esophageal stricture, achalasia, Plummer-Vinson syndrome (iron deficiency anemia, stomatitis, and dysphagia), and celiac disease are associated with squamous cell carcinoma of the esophagus.

QCSP, **Squamous Cell Carcinoma**, p 238-240.

7: Gastrointestinal Tract Answers

29. A. **CORPUS-FUNDIC REGION**

The autoimmune response is primarily directed at parietal cells, which are enriched in the corpus-fundic region, which is the primary affected region. While the autoantibodies are typically directed against parietal cells, they can also be directed against the intrinsic factor (located in the parietal cell membrane) or gastrin receptor.

QCSP, **Autoimmune Gastritis,** p 240-242.

30. E. **ALL OF THE ABOVE**

Early in the disease, a mononuclear infiltrate of lymphocytes and plasma cells is seen in the gastric body or fundus, with only minimal and patchy mucosal damage. With disease progression, there is extension of this infiltrate into the deeper portion of the mucosa with progressive destruction of fundic glands in the fundus and body, while the atrium is uninvolved. Eventually, pyloric and/or intestinal metaplasia are seen. Foveolar hyperplasia and pancreatic metaplasia can also be seen. Multifocal gastric enterochromaffin cell-like (ECL) hyperplasia and multifocal carcinoid tumors can develop in the body as a side effect (specifically, developing from hyperstimulation by gastrin). Similar to carcinoid tumors, ECL hyperplasia is immunoreactive for chromogranin.

QCSP, **Autoimmune Gastritis,** p 240-242.

31. D. **IMMUNODEFICIENCY DISORDERS**

Intestinal metaplasia seen in autoimmune gastritis can undergo dysplasia and progress to adenocarcinoma. The incidence of adenocarcinoma developing is increased, at 1%-3%. Both thyroiditis and hypothyroidism are associated. Myasthenia gravis and other autoimmune disorders (which tend to run together) including Sjogren disease are also associated, as are diabetes mellitus and adrenal insufficiency. Autoimmune gastritis can also be associated with dermatitis herpetiformis, however the gastritis is NOT reversed with gluten restriction.

QCSP, **Autoimmune Gastritis,** p 240-242.

32. D. **ALL OF THE ABOVE**

While the organisms can be seen on H&E-stained sections, it is usually useful to utilize a special stain or immunohistochemical stain. While Giemsa tends to be the most utilized special stain for the identification of *H pylori,* Warthin-Starry, Dieterle, as well as a gram stain, can highlight the *H pylori* organisms. An immunohistochemical stain with antibodies to *H pylori* can also be used, however this often will distort the morphology of the organisms.

QCSP, Helicobacter pylori **Gastritis,** p 243.

33. C. **GASTROSPIRILLUM HOMINIS**

Gastrospirillum hominis, also known as *Helicobacter heilmannii* can rarely (<1%) infect adults and children and produce gastritis. These organisms have a tightly coiled "corkscrew" shape and rarely attach to the epithelium. Infections with *Gastrospirillum hominis* has been the described as the major etiological agent of infectious related gastritis is rural areas of Eastern Europe. Additionally, *Helicobacter* species that can infect humans include *Helicobacter felis, Helicobacter fennelliae,* and *Helicobacter cinaedi.*

QCSP, Helicobacter pylori **Gastritis,** p 243.

34. B. **PANETH CELLS**

Metaplasia is a response to repeated mucosal injury. Complete (mature) intestinal metaplasia looks like normal small intestine with straight crypts lined by absorptive cells with a brush border and goblet cells that secrete sialomucins. Paneth cells are sometimes seen, usually concentrated in the base of the glands. It is not a precancerous lesion. Incomplete (immature) intestinal metaplasia (type II) is architecturally distorted with irregular crypts, goblet cells and columnar cells with varying degrees of differentiation. Paneth cells are not seen and this lesion is strongly associated with subsequent development of adenocarcinoma. Incomplete (immature) intestinal metaplasia (type III) demonstrates extensive architectural distortion and is lined by undifferentiated columnar cells resembling low-grade dysplasia.

QCSP, **Atrophic Gastritis,** p 243-244.

7: Gastrointestinal Tract Answers

35. A. **PYLORIC AREA**

    Currently the literature suggest that approximately 40%-50% of gastric adenocarcinomas involve mucosa of the pyloric area, 15% arise in the cardia, 40% arise in the fundic mucosa, with 10% of those patients involving multiple areas of the stomach. Remember that adenocarcinomas involving the GE junction are staged and treated similar to esophageal tumors.
    QCSP, **Gastric Adenocarcinoma,** p 244-245.

36. B. **INTESTINAL TYPE**

    Intestinal type gastric adenocarcinoma demonstrates glands of varying degrees of differentiation and is associated with intestinal metaplasia from *Helicobacter pylori* infection.
    QCSP, **Gastric Adenocarcinoma,** p 245.

37. D. **>50% OF THE TUMOR AREA IS OCCUPIED BY MUCIN**

    Roughly 10% of gastric adenocarcinomas demonstrate excessive mucin production that can rupture cells and glands and form pools of mucin in the stroma. The term "mucinous adenocarcinoma" is appropriate if mucin occupies >50% of the area of the tumor.
    QCSP, **Gastric Adenocarcinoma,** p 246.

38. E. **UNDIFFERENTIATED CARCINOMA**

    Undifferentiated carcinoma (also classified as medullary carcinoma or lymphoepithelioma-like carcinoma) lacks structural or functional evidence of differentiation. The stroma demonstrates a prominent lymphocytic infiltrate this is rich in CD8 lymphocytes and positive for EBV-RNA.
    QCSP, **Gastric Adenocarcinoma,** p 244-7.

39. C. **E-CADHERIN/CDH1**

    Familial gastric cancer may demonstrate germline mutations in the E-cadherin/CDH1 gene with a penetrance of 70%-80%. The other molecular alterations are seen is sporadic cases. Mutated p53 tumor suppressor gene is seen and alterations to c-myc, c-erbB-2, and ras, as well as K-sam, c-met oncogenes have been identified. Loss of heterozygosity in chromosomes 7p, 17p, 1q and 5q can also be seen.
    QCSP, **Gastric Adenocarcinoma,** p 244-247.

40. C. **<50%**

    While some surgeons may seem to take the attitude that anything is possible/resectable, surgical resection for cure is generally only possible in <50% of patients with gastric carcinoma. After "resection for cure", the 5-year survival rate is around 30%. If the cancer is caught very early and no lymph node metastases are present, then the 5- and 10-year survival rates are as high as 95%. Even with early cancer, positive lymph nodes decrease survival to around 50%.
    QCSP, **Gastric Adenocarcinoma,** p 244-247.

41. E. **ALL OF THE ABOVE**

    Cancer eventually develops is approximately 40% of adenomas, while <2% of hyperplastic polyps develop carcinoma. However, an associated gastric carcinoma occurs in the stomach of approximately 6% of those with a gastric hyperplastic polyp. Chronic gastric ulceration due to *H pylori* infection is considered precancerous. Additionally, chronic atrophic gastritis is also considered premalignant.
    QCSP, **Gastric Adenocarcinoma,** p 244-247.

42. E. **ALL OF THE ABOVE**

    Gastric neoplasms are associated with Billroth II > I procedures and tend to develop 15 to 25 years out from the procedure. Immunodeficiency disorders such as common variable immunodeficiency, X-linked immunodeficiency, and infantile X-linked agammaglobulinemia are also associated, as are several hereditary tumor syndromes, including familial diffuse gastric carcinoma, HNPCC, FAP, Li-Fraumeni syndrome, Peutz-Jeghers syndrome, and hyperplastic gastric polyposis.

QCSP, **Gastric Adenocarcinoma,** p 244-247.

43.   E.   **BOTH B AND C**

Changes induced by proton pump inhibitors overlaps with features of FGPs, however changes from proton pump inhibitors typically do not demonstrate an endoscopic lesion. Conspicuous budding and tortuosity of glands is seen and microcysts of varying size are seen at different levels of the gastric glands, lined by oxyntic mucosa. Dysplasia is distinctly unusual in FGPs (<1%), unless the patient has FAP, where dysplasia may be present in 40%-45% of FGPs (consider FAP if there is dysplasia). Inflammation is usually not seen and *H pylori* infection has a very low prevalence.

QCSP, **Fundic Gland Polyp,** p 248.

44.   B.   **30%**

70% of GISTs that occur in the stomach are benign and only 30% (representing 2%-3% of malignant gastric tumors) are malignant. GISTs found in the small intestine and the colon, are more likely to be malignant. Patients with malignant GISTs are more likely to present with pain, a palpable mass and weight loss, though bleeding is the most common symptom of any GIST.

QCSP, **Gastrointestinal Stroma Tumor,** p 249.

45.   A.   **SPINDLED**

The spindle cell morphology is the most common, with epithelioid as the next most common morphologic variant. Epithelioid GISTs occur relatively more commonly in the antrum than the cardia and fundus.

QCSP, **Gastrointestinal Stroma tumor,** p 250.

46.   C.   **GENERALLY LOW MITOTIC COUNT**

Both spindled and epithelioid GISTs rarely have mitotic figures, whereas sarcomas have conspicuous mitotic figures (5/50 hpf). Cells in spindled GIST can have a single perinuclear vacuole indenting the nucleus at one end, imparting a "torch-like" appearance to the nucleus. Skeinoid fibers are extracellular globules of eosinophilic collagen most commonly seen in benign GISTs of the small intestines. Pleomorphism is most commonly seen in benign epithelioid cell tumors.

QCSP, **Gastrointestinal Stroma Tumor,** p 250-251.

47.   A.   **TUMOR SIZE AND C. MITOTIC RATE**

The location of the tumor within the GI tract, the tumor size and the mitotic rate are the most important determinants of prognosis in nonmetastatic GISTs. This is reflected in the proposed guidelines for assessing the malignant potential of gastric GISTs (separate guidelines exist for small intestinal GISTs, with lower thresholds for size and mitotic counts because GISTs of the small intestine are more likely to be malignant). Less important factors that are associated with malignancy include high cellularity and aneuploidy as well as CD34 negativity. All GISTs should be considered at least "tumors of low malignant potential".

QCSP, **Gastrointestinal Stroma Tumor,** p 252.

48.   B > A > E > (C OR D) > (D OR C).

Almost all (>90%) of GISTs in the stomach are positive for CD117 (c-Kit). 70%-80% demonstrate immunoreactivity to CD34 (usually membranous staining) and 30%-40% demonstrate reactivity to alpha-smooth muscle actin. Other smooth muscle markers may also stain. Desmin and S100 reactivity is seen rarely (<5%). As the differential diagnosis can include melanoma it is important to remember that approximately 20% of melanomas are also c-Kit positive.

QCSP, **Gastrointestinal Stroma Tumor,** p 251.

7: Gastrointestinal Tract Answers

49.   E.   **ALL OF THE ABOVE ARE ON THE DIFFERENTIAL DIAGNOSIS**

Additionally, glomus tumor and melanoma should be included on this list. These can usually be easily differentiated based on immunohistochemistry and the clinical history. For the other lesions, CD117 (c-Kit) should be negative (except in approximately 20% of melanoma). Smooth muscle markers will stain leiomyomas and their malignant counterparts. Schwannomas will be positive for S100 and negative for muscle markers. Glomus tumors are positive for smooth muscle actin and negative for keratins. Because of occasional overlapping staining patterns, you should consider ordering more than one stain in these cases because several tumors, some of which are in the differential diagnosis, can be CD117 (c-Kit) positive (small cell carcinoma, melanoma, angiosarcoma, germ cell tumor, Ewing/ PNET, angiomyolipoma, myeloid sarcoma, and fibromatosis).

QCSP, **Gastrointestinal Stroma Tumor,** p 251-252.

50.   D.   **TYROSINE KINASE INHIBITORS**

Gross total surgical resection is the treatment of choice for GISTs. However, if this cannot be achieved, then a tyrosine kinase inhibitor (Gleevec) is given as a neoadjuvant therapy in hope that the tumor will become resectable or as the only therapy. An additionally tyrosine kinase inhibitor, sunitinib (Sutent), has recently been approved as a second-line agent. There is currently no role for chemotherapy or radiation because of the success of tyrosine kinase inhibitors.

QCSP, **Gastrointestinal Stroma Tumor,** p 251.

51.   E.   **BOTH A AND C**

Gastric GISTs are linked to both NF1 and are part of Carney triad, which includes: epithelioid cell gastric sarcoma, pure cartilaginous pulmonary chondromas, and functioning extra-adrenal paragangiomas (often multifocal and causing hypertension). The epithelioid cell gastric sarcomas are usually multifocal, forming small discrete nodules and have low metastatic risk.

QCSP, **Gastrointestinal Stroma Tumor,** p 252.

52.   C.   **MODIFIED SMOOTH MUSCLE CELLS**

Glomus tumors are vascular tumors of the stomach that are typically small (>2.5 cm) and located in the muscularis propria of the antrum. Glomus cells are modified smooth muscle cells and stain for smooth muscle actin and vimentin. Individual glomus cells are surrounded by reticulin and basement membrane material, which can be demonstrated with special stains (reticulin and PAS). These lesions can cause pain, nausea and bleeding and local excision is curative.

QCSP, **Glomus Tumor,** p 252-253.

53.   B.   **DAMAGE/INFLAMMATION**

Hyperplastic polyps are the most common gastric epithelial polyp and are thought to represent excessive regeneration following mucosal damage of varying etiologies. These polyps are often seen bordering an ulcer and are often associated with *H pylori*. Additionally, they are associated with autoimmune gastritis. These polyps can be associated with dysplastic epithelium (<4%) and even adenocarcinoma (<1%). Since they are so common, approximately 20% of gastric carcinoma patients will also have a hyperplastic polyp elsewhere in the stomach.

QCSP, **Hyperplastic Polyps,** p 253-254.

54.   E.   **ALL OF THE ABOVE ARE FEATURES OF HYPERPLASTIC POLYPS**

Hyperplastic, elongated, and dilated foveolae with an edematous and inflamed stroma sums up hyperplastic polyps. The hyperplastic foveolae form infoldings, apparent branching, and cystic dilatation is almost always present in the deeper parts of the polyp. Smooth muscle fibers from the muscularis mucosa extend in bundles into the polyp. The edematous lamina propria can have plasma cells, lymphocytes—sometimes in aggregates with germinal centers, eosinophils, mast cells, and macrophages.

QCSP, **Hyperplastic Polyps,** p 253-254.

55.   E.   **ALL OF THE ABOVE**
Hyperplastic polyps are associated with a number of background gastric mucosal abnormalities that cause mucosal damage. There is a strong association with atrophic gastritis of both the autoimmune type and *H pylori* associated type. While dysplasia and adenocarcinoma within these polyps are rare, there is an increased risk (up to 6%) for synchronous or metachronous adenocarcinomas. In up to 20% of patients with gastric cancer elsewhere in the stomach, hyperplastic polyps can be seen.
QCSP, **Hyperplastic Polyps,** p 253-254.

56.   A.   **STOMACH AND TERMINAL ILEUM**
Inflammatory fibroid polyps are most typically seen in the stomach, especially the distal stomach or pyloric area, and terminal ileum. While an etiology is not known for these lesions they appear to be proliferations of perivascular cells (CD34+). They occur much less commonly in the esophagus, colon, and more proximal part of the small intestine.
QCSP, **Inflammatory Fibroid Polyp,** p 255.

57.   D.   **BOTH A AND B**
Both gastric and terminal ileal inflammatory fibroid polyps affect men slightly more commonly than women and are typically diagnosed in the 6th decade. Gastric polyps tend to be small, averaging approximately 1.5 cm in size, and sessile but may be pedunculated. They occasionally have overlying ulcers but are most commonly asymptomatic (likely related to their small size). Polyps of the terminal ileum, on the other hand, tend to be larger, are commonly extensively ulcerated, and can present with intussusception and bowel obstruction.
QCSP, **Inflammatory Fibroid Polyp,** p 255.

58.   C.   **TEND TO INVOLVE THE MUSCULARIS PROPRIA**
Inflammatory fibroid polyps of the stomach tend to fill the submucosa, with a well-defined border deeper in the submucosa and can separate glands at the base of the mucosa and spread apart the bundles of muscularis propria, but lesional cells rarely involve the muscularis propria. Their ileal counterpart, on the other hand, tends to be transmural, filling the submucosa, replacing the muscularis propria, and extending into the subserosa. Therefore, choice c does not apply to gastric lesions and is the correct choice for this "except" question. Gastric lesions are composed on plump spindle cells, while ileal lesions have cells that are more stellate than spindled and the inflammatory infiltrate is more of a mixture of plasma cells, lymphocytes, and eosinophils. The stroma of ileal lesions tends to be very edematous and the polyp can look like excessive granulation tissue, occasionally with mitotic figures and hyperchromatic nuclei near the center, which can resemble a sarcoma. Ileal inflammatory polyps lack the perivascular orientation of neoplastic cells and inflammatory cells seen in gastric lesions and their vessels tend to be more elongated than rounded. Inflammatory fibroid polyps of the esophagus tend to look like those in the terminal ileum while lesions in the colon tend to look more like those in the stomach.
QCSP, **Inflammatory Fibroid Polyp,** p 255.

59.   D.   **A SINGLE LESION**
Multifocality is a particular feature of MALToma. There may be a dominant lesion, but additional foci of smaller lesions are usually present and choice d is thus wrong, making it the correct choice for this "except" question. Lymphoepithelial lesions are pathognomonic but not always present. They consist of neoplastic lymphocytes invading and distorting the epithelium. Additionally, the epithelium demonstrates eosinophilic change as the cells are destroyed. *H pylori* gastritis is very commonly associated with the development of MALTomas, so is commonly seen in the background, as are reactive lymphoid follicles. Plasmacytoid features are seen in about 1/3 of cases.
QCSP, **MALT Lymphoma,** p 256.

60.   E.   **BOTH B AND C**
H pylori are often present in MALToma because MALToma frequently arises from chronic gastritis caused by *H pylori,* so its presence is not helpful. Cytokeratin can highlight lymphoepithelial lesions. CD3 highlights scattered

T cells among a predominance of CD20+ B cells that may aberrantly co-express CD43, which can be helpful in difficult cases.

QCSP, **MALT Lymphoma,** p 256.

61.   B.   **Diffuse large B cell**

Only a small subset of MALTomas will progress to high-grade neoplasms, which most commonly resemble (and should be diagnosed as) diffuse large B cell lymphoma, with a predominance of blasts. While both anaplastic lymphoma and Burkett lymphoma are considered high-grade lymphomas; neither is the result of a transformation event from MALT lymphoma. Both follicular lymphoma and mantle cell lymphoma are considered low-grade and while they are on the differential list for classic low-grade MALT lymphoma lesions and not a result of a transformation event from MALT lymphoma. Mantle and follicular lymphomas typically do not demonstrate lymphoepithelial lesions (some exuberant cases of follicular lymphomas can demonstrates intraepithelial infiltration.)

QCSP, **MALT Lymphoma,** p 256.

62.   A.   **Stage**

Like most neoplastic processes, stage is the single most important determinant of long-term prognosis. *H pylori* eradication with antibiotics usually causes remission, especially in the superficial lesions, though they may be slow to regress and rarely recur. Recurrences after *H pylori* eradiation often regress spontaneously. Cases that are not associated with *H pylori* and those that persist even after *H pylori* eradiation often benefit from local radiation. Distant spread of the disease is rare and when it occurs usually involves the marginal zone of the spleen.

QCSP, **MALT Lymphoma,** p 257.

63.   B.   ***H pylori* associated chronic atrophic gastritis**

There is no association with *H pylori* associated chronic gastritis and neuroendocrine tumors, therefore choice B is the correct answer to this "except" question. Autoimmune gastritis usually results from antibodies against parietal cell membranes or intrinsic factor, leading to loss of parietal cells and achlorhydria. The resulting alkaline pH causes a sustained stimulation of gastrin-secreting endocrine cells (G cells) in the antrum. Hypergastrinemia stimulates endocrine cells in the gastric body (ECL) and can result in ECL hyperplasic nodules, which can eventually lead to carcinoid tumors. High levels of serum gastrin are also seen with MEN type I and ZES, however since there are intact parietal cells, these syndromes result a hypertrophic/ hypersecretory gastropathy.

QCSP, **Neuroendocrine Tumors,** p 240, 258.

64.   A.   **Sporadic**

Neuroendocrine tumors associated with atrophic gastritis tend to be multiple, small (<1 cm) and limited to the mucosa and submucosa of the gastric fundus. Those associated with MEN type I and ZES are usually multiple and multicentric. Sporadic tumors are usually solitary and occur more commonly than those associated with MEN and ZES.

QCSP, **Neuroendocrine Tumors,** p 258.

65.   A.   **Sporadic**

Sporadic tumors are more likely to be larger and mitotically active. Tumors associated with autoimmune atrophic gastritis are small and almost always benign. Tumors associated with MEN type I and ZES can sometimes metastasize to regional lymph nodes and may cause death, usually resulting from a coexisting (usually aggressive) gastrin-producing tumor of the pancreas or duodenum.

QCSP, **Neuroendocrine Tumors,** p 240, 258.

66.   B.   **Surgical resection**

Aggressive surgical resection is the treatment of choice for solitary sporadic neuroendocrine tumors of the stomach. Since the antrum of the stomach provides the increase gastrin stimulation in autoimmune gastritis, antrectomy can

lead to regression of associated neuroendocrine lesions. In patients with MEN type I and ZES, surgical excision of a simultaneous gastrin-producing tumor can lead to regression of associated gastric neuroendocrine tumors.
QCSP, **Neuroendocrine Tumors,** p 259.

67.   C.   **INFLAMMATORY BOWEL DISEASE**
Patients with acute self-limited enterocolitis usually present with an episode of bloody diarrhea and their endoscopic examination at that time would be most similar to inflammatory bowel disease, with edema, ulceration and increased mucosal friability. However, the cases of self-limited enterocolitis usually demonstrate resolution, with normal endoscopic findings, within 2 weeks.
QCSP, **Acute Self-Limited Enterocolitis,** p 259-260.

68.   D.   **CRYPT DISTORTION**
Crypt distortion, with branching, dilation, and abnormally shaped crypts, is generally not a feature of acute-self limited enterocolitis. Crypt abscess can be seen in both conditions. Additionally, loss of mucin and mucosal edema are nonspecific features. Plasmacytosis may be seen in the upper 1/3 of the mucosa in acute self-limited enterocolitis, but basal plasmacytosis with associated lymphoid aggregates and giant cells are more often seen in inflammatory bowel disease. Enteric pathogens are only recovered 50% of the time, so the lack of recovery of an enteric pathogen is largely unhelpful. The most common causes of acute self-limited enterocolitis include *E coli* 0157:H7, *Campylobacter,* *Salmonella,* *Shigella,* and *Yersinia.* Special stains for microorganisms are usually not helpful.
QCSP, **Inflammatory Bowel Disease,** p 260.

69.   D.   **IgA DEFICIENCY**
Both the anti-tissue transglutaminase and anti-endomysial tests are IgA-based tests and false negatives are known to occur in patients with IgA deficiency.
QCSP, **Celiac Disease,** p 261.

70.   A.   **PREDOMINANTLY INCREASED EOSINOPHILS**
Eosinophils may be increased in the lamina propria and can sometimes be strikingly increased. However their increase parallels the increase in the mononuclear cells, and if there is not a comparable increase in mononuclear cells, then the diagnosis of protein/food allergies should be considered. Increases in neutrophils and histiocytes can, but are not typically seen. Increased intraepithelial lymphocytes, sometimes defined as >40 per 100 enterocytes, are seen and often demonstrates clustering in the tips of the villi. Plasma cells that are producing the IgA antibodies causing tissue damage are present in the expanded lamina propria and villous blunting occurs as the crypt zone falls behind the rate of loss of damaged surface enterocytes.
QCSP, **Celiac Disease,** p 261.

71.   A.   **INCREASED INTRAEPITHELIAL LYMPHOCYTES**
Subtle lesions that may be early, latent, or partially treated cases of celiac disease may display only intraepithelial lymphocytosis in the tips of the villi with a density similar to or more prominent than that seen in the bases. It is, however, important to note that this is not specific, and many other pathologic conditions can also cause an increase in intraepithelial lymphocytes (and flat duodenal mucosa).
QCSP, **Celiac Disease,** p 261.

72.   C.   **CD 8– T CELLS**
Biopsies from patients with refractory celiac disease (not responsive to dietary restriction) usually contain CD3+ T cells that are CD8– and CD4–. Those seen in diet sensitive forms are usually CD3+ and CD8+. It can sometimes be useful to use an immunohistochemical stain for CD3 to help identify an increase in intraepithelial lymphocytes (which are also usually CD2+).
QCSP, **Celiac Disease,** p 261.

7: Gastrointestinal Tract Answers

73.   E.   **A COMBINATION OF THE ABOVE.**
Biopsies are best signed out as "consistent with" or otherwise modified because the pathologist cannot independently diagnose celiac disease based on histologic findings. Definitive diagnosis requires a combination of clinical presentation, histology, serology and response to a gluten-free diet.
QCSP, **Celiac Disease**, p 261-262.

74.   E.   **CAN BE SEEN IN ALL THE ABOVE**
Dermatitis herpetiformis of the skin, rheumatoid arthritis affecting the joints, and dysmenorrhea and dyspareunia are all extraintestinal sites of injury seen in celiac disease. Several patterns of liver injury can be seen, with the most common (nonspecific) findings of periportal inflammation, increased number of Kupffer cells and steatosis. While there have been reports linking PBC with celiac disease, the prevalence of celiac disease in PBC patients range from 0%-11%. Additionally, various studies have reported association/occurrence of celiac disease in patient's with autoimmune hepatitis, PSC, as well as autoimmune cholangitis.
QCSP, **Crohn Disease**, p 260.

75.   D.   **BOTH A AND B**
Crohn disease is more common in Western developed countries, among Whites, and among Jewish people. 3%-11% also have a family history. Males and females are affected equally (vs a slight female predominance in ulcerative colitis). It is slightly less common than ulcerative colitis. In North America, the prevalence rate for ulcerative colitis is 201 per 100,000 and Crohn disease is 238 per 100,000. Both with prevalence rates greater in northern areas as compared to southern regions.
QCSP, **Crohn Disease**, p 262.

76.   B.   **FREE PERFORATION WITH PERITONITIS**
The inflammation of Crohn disease is transmural and ulcers commonly extend deep into the submucosa with inflammatory fissures and sinus tracts extending further. Perforation with external abscess formation and fistulas can occur, but free perforation with peritonitis is uncommon because the extensive adhesions within the viscera of the abdomen and abdominal walls due to the extensive inflammation tend to wall off the perforation and form an external abscess.
QCSP, **Crohn Disease**, p 263.

77.   D.   **RELATIVELY MORE SHALLOW ULCERS**
Disease involving the colon tends to have ulcers that are relatively shallow, limited to the mucosa and upper mucosa, when compared to small intestinal disease, thus choice D is the correct answer to this "except" question. Small intestine Crohn disease is also characterized by a reduced number of villi and hyperplasia of Paneth cells. Colonic disease has less pronounced submucosal fibrosis, muscular hypertrophy, and neuro-proliferation.
QCSP, **Crohn Disease**, p 263.

78.   C.   **NON-NECROTIZING GRANULOMAS**
Epithelioid granulomas and skip lesions along with the distribution of affected bowel are the most distinguishing features of Crohn disease vs ulcerative colitis. These are typically non-necrotizing and resemble granulomas of sarcoidosis. They can be found in about 50% of resection specimen and are suggestive if found in biopsies. Granulomas can form in response to a ruptured crypt, foreign material, or general inflammatory reaction. Ulcerative colitis cases can demonstrate Paneth cell hyperplasia (sign of chronic mucosal injury), creeping fat, and aphthous ulcers.
QCSP, **Crohn Disease**, p 264.

7: Gastrointestinal Tract Answers

79. C. **RECURRENCES TEND TO OCCUR AT THE SITE OF PREVIOUS SURGERY**

Surgery for Crohn disease can often result in extended recovery times and complications. As such, surgery should be limited in scope and reserved for intractable disease and/or complications. There is a recurrence rate of approximately 5% per year and these tend to occur at the site of prior surgery.

QCSP, **Crohn Disease,** p 264.

80. B. **TOXIC MEGACOLON**

Toxic megacolon can occur in Crohn disease and is likely related to the fibrosis associated with the disease; however, this association is more common in ulcerative colitis. Secondary infections can include *C difficile* and opportunistic infections resulting from immunosuppressive therapy.

QCSP, **Ulcerative Colitis,** p 264.

81. B. **RISK OF DEVELOPING CARCINOMA IS RELATED TO DURATION OF DISEASE**

Patients with Crohn disease have 20 times higher incidence of carcinoma in the involved area of the small intestine and the overall incidence of carcinoma developing in the colon is 3%. The development of carcinoma is directly related to disease duration and may be more common in patients with symptoms beginning prior to 30 years of age. The incidence of carcinoma in Crohn colitis is actually less than ulcerative colitis. Carcinoma tends to occur in a younger population, 10 years younger on average, and is more frequently multiple. It often presents at advanced disease.

QCSP, **Inflammatory Bowel Disease,** p 265.

82. E. **MONONUCLEAR INFLAMMATORY REACTION**

No inflammatory reaction is seen in microvillus inclusion disease, making choice D a false statement and therefore the correct answer to this "except" question. All of the other features are characteristic findings in this disease. Infants usually demonstrate was chronic intractable diarrhea, and ultimately metabolic acidosis and dehydration.

QCSP, **Microvillus Inclusion Disease,** p 265.

83. A. **AUTOSOMAL RECESSIVE**

The disease is generally inherited in an autosomal recessive pattern, though there is a late-onset form. Without life-long parenteral nutrition or a bowel transplant, patients die before 18 months of age due to complications such as sepsis, liver failure and dehydration.

QCSP, **Microvillus Inclusion Disease,** p 265-266.

84. A. **INFECTIOUS**

Whipple disease is a systemic disease (involving skin, joints, nervous system, skeletal and cardiac muscle, lung, serosal membranes, kidney, liver, spleen, and lymph nodes) caused by *Tropheryma whippelii*, a small rod-shaped bacterium. Patients with this disease may have an innate defect in cell-mediated immunity. Antibiotics (14 days of IV infusions of streptomycin and penicillin G or ceftriaxone, followed by oral TMP-SMX for 1 to 2 years) are curative.

QCSP, **Whipple Disease,** p 266.

85. B. **NUMEROUS MACROPHAGES IN THE LAMINA PROPRIA WITH BASOPHILIC, STIPPLED CYTOPLASM**

All of the answer choices listed are gross and microscopic features seen in Whipple disease, however, the most pathognomonic feature is the macrophages within the lamina propria with basophilic, stippled cytoplasm. This stippling represents granules that contain bacteria in various stages of digestion and can be highlighted by PAS with diastase (which also stains extracellular rod-shaped bacteria). The coating of white material is due to accumulation of chyle within the lymphatics of the lamina propria.

QCSP, **Whipple Disease,** p 266.

86. D. **TUMORS OF THE DUODENAL BULB ARE MORE LIKELY TO BE NONFUNCTIONING THAN THOSE ASSOCIATED WITH ZES**

Duodenal neuroendocrine tumors usually occur in the first or second portion of the duodenum. Those located in the duodenal bulb are often "nonfunctioning" and produce a milder peptic ulcer disease than that associated with ZES. All of the other choices are true for tumors occurring in association with ZES: these tumors tend to occur earlier than nonfunctioning tumors (mean age of 40 vs 65), they are more likely to be infiltrative and to metastasize. Fulminant ulcer diathesis is related to ZES.
QCSP, **Neuroendocrine Tumors,** p 267.

87. B. **SOMATOSTATIN-PRODUCING (D-CELL) TUMOR**

Approximately, 30% of somatostatin-producing (D-cell) tumors are associated with von Recklinghausen disease (also known as neurofibromatosis type I). While strong expression of somatostatin is typical of these tumors, somatostatin syndrome, with hyperglycemia, cholelithiasis, and constipation, is rare when it occurs in the duodenum/ampulla. Somatostatin syndrome occurs in the majority of somatostatin-producing NET of the pancreas. Gangliocytic paraganglioma can also express pancreatic polypeptide and somatostatin and be associated with NF I, but they have a distinct morphologic pattern.
QCSP, **Neuroendocrine Tumors,** p 267.

88. D. **POORLY DIFFERENTIATED NEUROENDOCRINE TUMOR**

Poorly differentiated neuroendocrine tumors are usually found in the periampullary region of the duodenum. The prognosis of these tumors is poor, with survival usually ranging from 6 to 18 months. Gangliocytic paraganglioma usually occur proximal to the ampulla of Vater.
QCSP, **Neuroendocrine Tumors,** p 267.

89. B. **SOMATOSTATIN-PRODUCING (D-CELL) TUMOR**

The tumor cells of duodenal neuroendocrine tumors tend to be relatively uniform with scant cytoplasm and arranged in trabeculae. Chains of micronodules extending from the main tumor can be seen. Somatostatin-producing tumors are characterized by pseudo-acini and can have psammoma bodies.
QCSP, **Neuroendocrine Tumors,** p 267.

90. E. **THICKENED COLLAGEN OCCASIONALLY EXTENDING DOWNWARD TO INVOLVE THE BASEMENT MEMBRANE REGION OF THE UNDERLYING CRYPTS, IN SEVERE CASES**

The collagen deposition seen in collagenous colitis is limited to the region just beneath the surface epithelium and it is usually irregular and while it can extend downward (demonstrate a dipping appearance) it generally does not extend downward to involve the basement membrane of the underlying crypts. Thus, this statement is false and choice E in the correct answer for this "except" question. Features of chronic colitis are also generally absent; however, Paneth cell metaplasia can be seen. All of the other choices list features commonly seen. Findings are not uniform throughout the colon, with the rectum typically being less involved. Also remember if there are no lymphocytes then it is not collagenous colitis.
QCSP, **Collagenous Colitis,** p 268.

91. C. **SMALL INTESTINE**

The small intestine is most frequently involved by and is usually the most severely affected portion of the GI tract in acute GVHD. It is rarely involved by chronic GVHD (the colon is also usually spared by chronic GVHD).
QCSP, **Graft-vs-Host Disease,** p 269.

92. B. **CHANGES PRODUCED BY SODIUM PHOSPHATE BOWEL PREPARATION**

Acute GVHD can be divided into 4 grades (I-IV), depending on the degree and extent of apoptosis/necrosis. Grade I disease has single cell necrosis with apoptotic body formation. Grade II disease is also accompanied by crypt abscesses and may be indistinguishable from changes produced by bowel preparation with a sodium phosphate solution. Grade III disease demonstrates total necrosis of individual crypts and grade IV disease has denudation of areas of bowel that can be indistinguishable from ischemic bowel disease and typhlitis. CMV colitis may coexist and can appear similar to acute GVHD, the lesions are separated by the presence of CMV inclusions (or IHC evidence).

QCSP, **Graft-vs-Host Disease,** p 269-270.

93. C. **30% OF CASES**

Approximately 30% of patients with acute GVHD will develop chronic GVHD. This is an update from the first edition of *QCSP*. Recent publications using NIH consensus criteria states that approximately 80% of patients develop acute GVHD and 35% of these patients will develop chronic GVHD. While the small intestine is most commonly and severely affected by acute disease, it is usually spared from chronic disease, as is the colon. Chronic disease is characterized by submucosal fibrosis, mucosal calcification, and focal fibrosis of the lamina propria. Remember that acute and chronic GVHD are actually different disease processes and recent treatments to reduce acute GVHD has not changed he overall chronic GVHD rates. (GI tract involved in approximately 70%-75% of cases of GVHD).

QCSP, **Graft-vs-Host Disease,** p 269-270.

94. D. **TOTAL COLONIC AGANGLIONOSIS**

80% of Hirschsprung cases occur in males, with the exception of total colonic aganglionosis in which the incidence is approximately equal in males and females. Short-segment disease is the most common variant and affects males to females at a ratio of 5:1. Overall Hirschsprung is a rare disease with an incidence of 1 in 5,000 to 30,000 live births.

QCSP, **Hirschsprung Disease,** p 270-271.

95. A. **AVOIDING PROXIMITY TO THE DENTATE LINE**

There is a normal hypoganglionotic zone in the rectum that extends proximally for 0.5 to 1.0 cm from the dentate line, therefore biopsies should be obtained proximal to this to avoid confusion. Increased numbers and dimensions of parasympathetic nerve fibers are absent in neonates and in long-segment disease, so looking for this finding is not helpful. Similarly, you will have trouble if you are looking for classic mature ganglion cells described in choice C because immature ganglion cells of the neonate appear very different. They are small, with little cytoplasm and no obvious nucleolus, and tend to cluster around small nerves like a horseshoe. Acetylcholinesterase stains can be helpful, but must be performed on frozen tissue and are technically challenging to perform. Calretinin immunohistochemical stains on formalin-fixed paraffin embedded tissue has recently gained popularity and can be helpful.

QCSP, **Hirschsprung Disease,** p 270-271.

96. C. **4%, MOTHER**

Approximately 4% of Hirschsprung cases have a familial occurrence and children with an affected mother are at greater risk than children with an affected father of having the disease, likely due to an autosomal recessive and sex-linked type inheritance. Exact genetics are poorly understood.

QCSP, **Hirschsprung Disease,** p 270-271.

97. E. **ALL OF THE ABOVE ARE ASSOCIATED**

There is a long list of associations with Hirschsprung disease (see *QCSP* p 272), including all of the above listed choices. Interestingly, molecular alterations involving the receptor tyrosine kinase gene (RET) have been found on chromosome 10q11.2, which is also involved in MEN IIa and IIb. An additional locus was mapped to the 13q22 region in a group of inbred Mennonite kindred.

QCSP, **Hirschsprung Disease,** p 271-272.

7: Gastrointestinal Tract Answers

98. C. **ACUTE INFLAMMATORY CELLS EVEN MORE PROMINENT THAN IN ACUTE SELF-LIMITED COLITIS**
While inflammatory cells, most prominently neutrophils, are often present in ischemic colitis, they are not as prominent as in acute self-limited colitis (though both processes could be present at the same time), therefore choice C is false and is the correct answer to this "except" question. Ischemic colitis is characterized by necrosis of the mucosa with sloughing of epithelium and edema of the lamina propria that can produce a polyp or mass. Capillary thrombi may be prominent. Pseudomembranes can form and tend to be diffuse, vs the patchy distribution seen in *C difficile* colitis (which is in the differential diagnosis).
QCSP, **Ischemic Colitis,** p 272-273.

99. E. **NONE OF THE ABOVE**
Clinical history and laboratory test often holds the key to diagnosis. All the above entities share overlapping histologic features. Specifically, there is often loss or paucity of mucus, surface necrosis and sloughing of epithelium. Additionally, there can by acute cryptitis and acute inflammation. While usually not present in biopsies, in resections specimens of acute ischemic colitis, thromboembolisms can be seen in the vessels. Additionally, in the resolution of many of these conditions the primarily inflammatory cell type changes from neutrophils to lymphocytes and plasma cells.
QCSP, **Ischemic Colitis,** p 273.

100. D. **DIFFUSE INCREASE IN LYMPHOCYTES AND PLASMA CELLS IN THE UPPER LAMINA PROPRIA WITH INCREASED INTRAEPITHELIAL LYMPHOCYTES**
Lymphocytic (microscopic) colitis classically presents in middle-aged or older women who present with watery diarrhea and have normal (or minimal) endoscopic findings ("microscopic" colitis). The entire colon is classically involved, with increased lymphocytes and plasma cells in the upper lamina propria and increased intraepithelial lymphocytes. The surface epithelium may be flatter than normal and has increased numbers of apoptotic bodies with conspicuous eosinophils. Crypt deformity, lymphoid nodules, thickening of the subepithelial collagen band, and gross inflammatory destruction of epithelium are not seen.
QCSP, **Lymphocytic Colitis,** p 273-274.

101. B. **WILL EVENTUALLY PROGRESS INTO COLLAGENOUS COLITIS**
While lymphocytic colitis and collagenous colitis are both considered microscopic colitides they are not thought to be the same process. Specifically, lymphocytic colitis is mostly self-limited or at least treatment-limited. There are a few cases of lymphocytic colitis that reportedly developed into collagenous colitis, but theses are rare in the literature. All of the other statements are true.
QCSP, **Lymphocytic Colitis,** p 273-274.

102. C. **SMOKERS**
There is actually a lower incidence of ulcerative colitis among smokers than the rest of the population. It is slightly more common in women than men (vs Crohn disease, which has no preference) and more common in Caucasians, Jews, and people from Western developed countries. Ulcerative colitis is the most common cause of chronic colitis in the United States.
QCSP, **Ulcerative Colitis,** p 274.

103. A. **p-ANCA**
Serum levels of antineutrophil cytoplasmic antibodies (p-ANCA) are often elevated in patients with ulcerative colitis. Anti SS-A and SS-B antibodies are related to Sjogren syndrome, anti ds-DNA is most associated with SLE, anti-RF are associated with rheumatoid arthritis and anti endomysial antibodies are seen in celiac disease.
QCSP, **Ulcerative Colitis,** p 274.

7: Gastrointestinal Tract Answers

104. C. **50%**
Approximately 90% of patients have disease limited to the rectum and sigmoid colon at presentation, and about half will have disease progression to involve more proximal portions of the bowel including the proximal transverse colon and right colon. In only 5%-10% of cases is disease limited to the rectum.
QCSP, **Ulcerative Colitis**, p 274.

105. B. **SKIP AREAS**
Skip areas of normal colon within an inflamed segment of colon are not seen in untreated ulcerative colitis but are a feature of Crohn disease, so choice b is false and therefore the correct answer to this "except" question. However relying on the presence of skip areas can be a pitfall. Specifically, you must also know the clinical and treatment history as treated ulcerative colitis can have healed areas that resemble skipped areas. Additionally, the proximal cecum and appendix may be uninvolved in ulcerative colitis and appear as a skip lesion. All of the other features can be seen in both ulcerative colitis and Crohn disease, though megacolon is more common in ulcerative colitis and the ulcerations of ulcerative colitis are more superficial.
QCSP, **Ulcerative Colitis**, p 274-275.

106. E. **ALL OF THE ABOVE**
Pseudopolyps are a good indicator of chronic disease and can persist after the acute episode has resolved. Architectural changes, including budding and branching of crypts, and metaplasia are chronic changes that persist during quiescent periods in between flares. Mononuclear inflammatory cells and eosinophils within the lamina propria and particularly between the crypts and muscularis mucosa are also a marker of quiescent disease.
QCSP, **Ulcerative Colitis**, p 275.

107. A. *C DIFFICILE*
C difficile is both a common secondary infection in people with ulcerative colitis and primary infection/overgrowth after antibiotic treatment. Among the list of conditions that could be considered within the differential diagnosis for ulcerative colitis includes, campylobacter and chlamydial infections, amebic colitis, ischemic colitis, drug reaction, vasculitis, and Crohn disease. A common secondary infection seen in Crohn disease is salmonella.
QCSP, **Ulcerative Colitis**, p 276.

108. B. **DERMATITIS HERPETIFORMIS**
Dermatitis herpetiformis is associated with celiac disease not ulcerative colitis, so choice b is the correct answer to this "except" question. Erythema nodosum and pyoderma gangrenosum are associated with ulcerative colitis, along with polyarthritis, uveitis, ankylosing spondylitis, and sclerosing cholangitis. Patients with sclerosing cholangitis have an increased risk of developing adenocarcinoma of the bile ducts.
QCSP, **Ulcerative Colitis**, p 276.

109. C. **15%**
The incidence of carcinoma in patients with ulcerative colitis reflects both the extent and duration of disease. Disease that extends to or beyond the hepatic flexure has a 15% incidence of carcinoma, whereas disease that is limited to the left side of the colon has a 5% incidence of carcinoma. After 10 years of disease, the annual incidence of carcinoma is around 1%-2%. When carcinoma does occur, it tends to occur 10 years earlier than sporadic colon cancer and dysplastic foci can usually be found elsewhere in the colon.
QCSP, **Ulcerative Colitis**, p 276.

110. D. **AT THE ANTERIOR WALL OF THE RECTUM**
Prolapsed intestinal mucosa can be found at any of the sites listed in the above choices. The best recognized site of prolapse that is referred to as "solitary rectal ulcer syndrome" (though an ulcer may not be present or there may be more than one) is the anterior or anterior lateral wall of the rectum.
QCSP, **Solitary Rectal Ulcer Syndrome**, p 277.

7: Gastrointestinal Tract Answers

123. B. **ARE VERY OFTEN LARGE IN SIZE, >1.5 CM**

The vast majority of hyperplastic polyps are small, ranging from 3 to 6 mm in size, making choice B false, and therefore the correct choice for this "false" question. Large hyperplastic polyps, >1.0 cm, are more likely to be associated with adenomatous change, seen in admixed type polyps.

QCSP, **Intestinal Polyps: Hyperplastic polyps**, p 283-284.

124. E. **ALL OF THE ABOVE HAVE BEEN USED TO DESCRIBE THIS ENTITY**

Most of these terms make some sense, if you think about the microscopic appearance of inflammatory fibroid polyps. These lesions are mesenchymal lesions limited to the submucosa (uncommonly infiltrating more deeply), and consist of fibroblasts, an inflammatory infiltrate, and a variable vascular component. The inflammatory infiltrate is mixed and has variable amount of eosinophils in addition to lymphocytes, plasma cells, macrophages, and mast cells. A vascular component may be prominent.

QCSP, **Intestinal Polyps: Inflammatory Fibroid Polyps**, p 284.

125. A. **UNIFORM DYSPLASTIC EPITHELIUM**

Uniform dysplastic epithelium and a growth pattern similar to that of a hyperplastic polyp are what characterize traditional serrated adenomas, therefore it is the correct choice to this "except" question. All of the other choices are features of sessile serrated adenomas.

QCSP, **Intestinal Polyps: Sessile Serrated Adenoma**, p 284.

126. B. **DECREASED STAINING FOR BOTH hMLH1 AND hMSH2**

This is an important point, because it addresses why we care to classify sessile serrated adenomas as a specific entity: Sessile serrated adenomas demonstrates decreased staining for hMLH1 and hMSH2 and other microsatellite instability markers, suggesting that these lesion are precursors to some colorectal adenocarcinomas, particularly those with microsatellite instability.

QCSP, **Intestinal Polyps: Sessile Serrated Adenoma**, p 284.

127. E. **PREFERENCE FOR THE RIGHT, RATHER THAN LEFT COLON**

All of the following are characteristic features of traditional serrated adenomas except for choice E, making it the correct choice for this "except" question. Sessile serrated adenomas tend to occur more commonly in the right colon, whereas traditional serrated adenoma are slightly more common in the left colon.

QCSP, **Intestinal Polyps: Traditional Serrated Adenoma**, p 285.

128. C. **LOCALLY AGGRESSIVE LESIONS WITH LOW METASTATIC POTENTIAL THAT ARE INSENSITIVE TO RADIOTHERAPY**

Giant condyloma and verrucous carcinoma are large warty lesions producing cauliflower-like growth with microscopic features typical of anal warts, though they are characterized by endophytic or downward growth of advancing tongues with intact basement membranes. Progression to dysplasia and squamous cell carcinoma has been documented but is not the typical behavior. These lesions tend to be locally aggressive, have very limited metastatic potential (nodal metastases may be seen with transformation to conventional squamous cell carcinoma), and are typically cured by excision. They are typically insensitive to radiotherapy.

QCSP, **Verrucous Carcinoma**, p 285.

129. D. **BOTH B AND C**

Manifestations of Cowden Disease include breast cancer (35%) and thyroid cancer (10%-15%), in addition to hamartomatous colonic and small intestinal polyps (35%) with no malignant potential (thus choice a is incorrect), facial trichilemmomas (85%), acral keratosis and oral mucosal papillomatosis, usually benign fibromas (8%),

lipomas (40%), hemangiomas (20%-25%), neuromas (10%), benign thyroid lesions, colloid goiter and adenoma (60%), fibrocystic changes in the breast (65%), ovarian cysts (25%), and several congenital abnormalities.
QCSP, **Multiple Polyp Syndromes**, p 285-288.

130.   B.   *PTEN* (10q23)
Cowden Disease is associated with an autosomal dominant mutation in *PTEN* (10q23).
QCSP, **Multiple Polyp Syndromes**, p 285-288.

131.   A.   *APC* (5q21-q22)
Familial adenomatous polyposis is characterized by innumerable colonic polyps (>100 polyps) along with a mutation is the *APC* gene (5q21-q22).
QCSP, **Multiple Polyp Syndromes**, p 285-288.

132.   A.   *APC* (5q21-q22)
Similar to familial adenomatous polyposis, both demonstrate innumerable colonic polyps with a mutated APC gene. In addition, there are characteristic extraintestinal manifestations in Gardner syndrome.
QCSP, **Multiple Polyp Syndromes**, p 285-288.

133.   D.   *STK11*
Peutz-Jeghers syndrome is autosomal dominant with variable penetrance and is characterized by mutation of serine threonine kinase (*STK11*) on chromosome 19q13.3.
QCSP, **Multiple Polyp Syndromes**, p 285-288.

134.   E.   **None known**
The Cronkhite-Canada syndrome is currently classified as an acquired idiopathic disease as there is no known mutated genes and no inheritance patterns.
QCSP, **Multiple Polyp Syndromes**, p 285-288.

135.   A.   *APC* (5q21-q22)
Similar to familial adenomatous polyposis, both demonstrate innumerable colonic polyposis with a mutated *APC* gene. In addition, there are characteristic extraintestinal manifestations in Turcot syndrome. Also Turcot syndrome can be seen in cases of HNPCC cases, with alteration of the expression of mis-match repair genes.
QCSP, **Multiple Polyp Syndromes**, p 285-288.

136.   C.   *SMAD4*
Familial juvenile polyposis is associated with hamartomatous polyps and mutations in *SMAD4* or *BMPR1A*.
QCSP, **Multiple Polyp Syndromes**, p 285-288.

137.   E.   **All of the above**
All of the listed multiple polyp syndromes are inherited predominantly in an autosomal dominate pattern. FAP has a very high degree of penetrance while its variant Gardner syndrome has more variable expression. Peutz-Jeghers syndrome has variable penetrance.
QCSP, **Multiple Polyp Syndromes**, p 285-288.

138.   E.   **A, B, and C are all correct**
GI polyps of Cowden disease, Devon family syndrome, and intestinal ganglioneuromatosis are not associated with the development of intestinal malignancy. Familial juvenile polyposis is associated with the development of

adenomatous polyps and adenocarcinoma of the large bowel, duodenum, stomach, or pancreas, with a 50% lifetime risk for developing colorectal cancer, usually at an early age.

QCSP, **Multiple Polyp Syndromes,** p 285-288.

139. **B.** **CRONKHITE-CANADA SYNDROME**

The syndrome described above is Cronkhite-Canada syndrome. In addition to the above, these patients often suffer from the sequelae of electrolyte disorders. Devon family syndrome is characterized by multiple inflammatory polyps in the ileum and occasionally the gastric antrum and has no extraintestinal manifestations and no association with carcinoma. Muir-Torre syndrome consists of colorectal carcinoma (often multiple) associated with genitourinary tumors, multiple sebaceous tumors, and keratoacanthomas. Oldfield syndrome is characterized by multiple adenomatous polyps throughout the GI tract, especially the colon, and multiple sebaceous cysts. Ruvalcaba-Myhre-Smith syndrome is characterize by hamartomatous intestinal polyposis (polyps are identical to juvenile polyps) and associated with macrocephaly, mental deficiency, unusual craniofacial appearance, and pigmented macules on the shaft and glans of the penis.

QCSP, **Multiple Polyp Syndromes,** p 285-288.

140. **C.** **CRONKHITE-CANADA SYNDROME**

The polyps of Cronkhite-Canada Syndrome are typically sessile and occur most frequently in the stomach, but also in the small intestine, colon, and rectum. These polyps are identical to juvenile polyps microscopically, demonstrating tortuous and cystically dilated glands filled with mucus in an edematous stroma, with increased inflammatory cells (including eosinophils), fibroblasts, and smooth muscle in the lamina propria. The major difference is seen in the intervening stroma, which, while histologically normal in juvenile polyps, also contains cystically dilated glands and an inflamed, edematous lamina propria in patients with Cronkhite-Canada syndrome. Ruvalcaba-Myhre-Smith syndrome and familial juvenile polyposis also have juvenile polyps. Ruvalcaba-Myhre-Smith syndrome may, in fact, be a variant of juvenile polyposis.

QCSP, **Multiple Polyp Syndromes,** p 285-288.

141. **D.** **HEREDITARY NONPOLYPOSIS COLORECTAL CANCER (HNPCC)**

HNPCC, also known as Lynch syndrome I and II, is an autosomal dominant disease caused by mutations in 1 of at least 4 DNA mismatch repair genes. The tumor DNA of these patients has widespread instability in short repeat sequences, termed "microsatellite instability." They still develop cancer through the adenoma-carcinoma pathway. Lynch syndrome I (hereditary site-specific colorectal cancer) is associated with an increased risk of multiple colon carcinomas that occur earlier and tend to be located in the right colon. Lynch syndrome II (cancer family syndrome) has the same risk for colon cancer and is also associated with early onset of carcinomas occurring at other sites (ovaries, endometrium, stomach, pancreas, bladder, larynx, brain).

QCSP, **Multiple Polyp Syndromes,** p 285-288.

142. **C.** **HEREDITARY NONPOLYPOSIS COLORECTAL CANCER (HNPCC)**

HNPCC (Lynch syndrome) may be the most common form of familial colon cancer, accounting for 5%-10% of all colorectal carcinomas. They tend to occur at a younger age and be right sided and patients have a high incidence of multiple cancers. As this is an autosomal dominant disorder, first-degree relatives also have a 50% risk of developing adenocarcinoma.

QCSP, **Multiple Polyp Syndromes,** p 285-288.

143. **D.** **GANGLIONEUROMA**

Similar to MEN 2a, MEN 2b patients have medullary thyroid carcinoma and pheochromocytomas and have a mutation in the RET gene. In addition, MEN 2b patients demonstrate multiple ganglioneuromas (ganglioneuromatosis) of the GI tract. They also present with neuromas of other mucosal sites and have a marfanoid body habitus. MEN 1 patients often have pancreatic neuroendocrine tumors, specifically, insulin, gastrin, or VIP producing lesions (as well as pituitary adenoma and parathyroid hyperplasia). MEN type 1 patients have a mutation in the MEN 1 gene.

QCSP, **Multiple Polyp Syndromes,** p 285-288.

144.   B.   **Turcot**

Turcot syndrome describes a polyposis syndrome associated with brain tumors. There are 2 forms of this syndrome. The first type is FAP associated with mutations in the APC gene, which most often has an associated medulloblastoma; however, astrocytomas and ependymomas have been reported. The second type is associated with lynch syndrome (HNPCC) and mutations in the MLH1 or MSH2 pathways and is associated glioblastoma multiforme.

QCSP, **Multiple Polyp Syndromes,** p 285-288.

145.   D.   **Gardner**

Gardner syndrome is a variant of familial adenomatous polyposis with autosomal dominant mutations of the APC gene. Similar to FAP, these patients have adenomatous polyposis with increased colorectal cancer risk. They also demonstrate several extraintestinal findings. Specifically, they demonstrate fibromatosis (desmoid tumors) that often involves the mesentery. Additionally, they demonstrate (and are often diagnosed by) several possible abnormalities of the jaw, including osteomas, odontomas, and impacted teeth. Additionally, they can develop epidermoid and sebaceous cysts and have an increased risk of papillary thyroid carcinoma.

QCSP, **Multiple Polyp Syndromes,** p 285-288.

146.   D.   **Peutz-Jegher**

Peutz-Jegher syndrome is associated with characteristic mucocutaneous lesions, often seen best in the oral mucosa. These patients also have increased incidence of cervical adenoma malignum (minimal deviation adenocarcinoma) and sex-cord tumors with annular tubules (SCTAT tumors) in women and Sertoli cell tumors in men. These patients are also at increased risk for developing colon, breast, stomach, small bowel and pancreatic cancers. The overall cancer risk is associated with age and reported to be 1% at age 20, 19% at age 40, 63% at age 60, and 83% at age 70.

QCSP, **Multiple Polyp Syndromes,** p 285-288.

147.   D.   **All the above**

The mucocutaneous lesions seen in Peutz-Jeghers are characteristic for the syndrome but not specific. These lesions demonstrate increased basilar melanin without in increase in the number of melanocytes, specifically, the pigment is primarily in macrophages in the dermis. Similar lesions can also be seen in other types of diseases.

QCSP, **Multiple Polyp Syndromes,** p 285-288.

148.   B.   **villous adenoma**

Villous adenomas (especially large) have been reported to cause hypokalemia secondary to secretory diarrhea. The exact etiology is unknown. While this does seem to be a random fact, similar questions have been reported to appear on the ABP board exam and past RISE.

QCSP, **Multiple Polyp Syndromes,** p 285-288.

149.   B.   **Neuroendocrine tumors**

Neuroendocrine tumors comprise nearly 75% of all benign and malignant tumors of the appendix. They are 3 times more common in women, usually small (<1 cm), located in the tip of the appendix, and rarely cause carcinoid syndrome (usually limited to cases with widespread metastasis to liver or peritoneum).

QCSP, **Multiple Polyp Syndromes,** p 285-288.

7: Gastrointestinal Tract Answers

150. **B.** **APPENDIX**

Sustentacular cells are an important component of appendiceal neuroendocrine tumors, but are generally lacking in both small intestinal and colonic neuroendocrine tumors, both of which are thought to arise from intraepithelial endocrine cells rather than from subepithelial neuroendocrine complexes (as appendiceal neuroendocrine tumors are). The exception would be the gangliocytic parapangliomas that occur in the duodenum associated with NF1. These lesions contain Schwann cell-like sustentacular cells and are S100+.

QCSP, **Neuroendocrine Tumors,** p 289-292.

151. **D.** **APPENDIX, SMALL INTESTINE, COLON**

Assuming that you are not out to collect life insurance, you would be best off having a neuroendocrine tumor of the appendix, with a 5-year survival of 95% and rate of metastases of 1.5%-10%. Second choice would be the small intestine, with a 65% 5-year survival rate and incidence of metastasis varying by size (2% if <1 cm, 50% if 1-2 cm, and 80% if >2 cm). Your colon would be, of these 3 choices, the least lucky place to have a neuroendocrine tumor, with 5-year survival rates of around only 25%.

QCSP, **Neuroendocrine Tumors,** p 289-292.

152. **E.** **ALL OF THE ABOVE**

All of the listed choices are among the criteria for malignant neuroendocrine tumors.

QCSP, **Neuroendocrine Tumors,** p 289-292.

153. **C.** **SEROTONIN**

Approximately 30% of neuroendocrine tumors of the rectum show some degree of immunoreactivity for serotonin, which is a significant portion. PAP and vimentin positivity is seen in 80%-100%, which is unique for tumors in this location. Of course, synaptophysin and chromogranin are most commonly positive, and most tumors are somatostatin positive.

QCSP, **Neuroendocrine Tumors,** p 289-292.

154. **E.** **B AND C**

The degree of dysplasia is based on the degree of architectural and/or cytologic atypia. Both lesions demonstrate Barrett esophagus, but the one on the left demonstrates low-grade dysplasia while the one on the right demonstrates high-grade dysplasia. Barrett esophagus is allowed to have some degree of architectural and cytologic atypia and even mitotic figures as long as these are restricted to deeper within the mucosa and not extending to or involving the surface. Both high- and low-grade dysplasias can involve the entire mucosal thickness and/or the surface and superficial crypt epithelium. However, high-grade dysplasia will often involve the entire gland/crypt from the base to the apical surface.

QCSP, **Barrett Mucosa and Dysplasia,** p 235.

155. **A.** **DEGREE OF DIFFERENTIATION**

The image represents a squamous cell carcinoma. Stage usually provides the most prognostic information for a cancer, which includes the tumor size, depth of invasion, lymph node status and presence/absence of metastases. The degree of differentiation does not have much prognostic significance in this tumor. Presence of esophageal strictures/obstructions greatly increases the risk of developing a squamous cell carcinoma.

QCSP, **Squamous Cell Carcinoma,** p 240.

156. **E.** **ALL OF THE ABOVE**

Loss of parietal cells in the corpus-fundus region causes achlorhydria and loss of intrinsic factor, which results in impaired absorption of vitamin B$_{12}$ in the ileum, which eventually leads to pernicious anemia. Achlorhydria simulates gastric production by G-cells (which are endocrine cells) in the stomach antrum, with ensuing hypergastrinemia. The gastrin stimulates endocrine cells in the gastric body and, given long enough; small

indolent carcinoid tumors (multiple hyperplastic nodules of G-cells) can develop. The Schilling test is abnormal in pernicious anemia, and it is corrected by the addition of intrinsic factor.
QCSP, **Autoimmune Gastritis**, p 240-242.

157. B. **The stomach antrum of a 45-year-old from an underdeveloped area**
H pylori organisms are most commonly present in the antrum of the stomach and are not commonly found in the gastric corpus-fundus or in the duodenum, and usually absent from chronic peptic ulcers. They are on the surface and within the lumina of gastric pits and do not invade the mucosa. The prevalence of *H pylori* infection increases with age and is also much more common in underdeveloped areas.
QCSP, **H pylori**, p 242.

158. A. **It is associated with increased risk of carcinoma.**
The image demonstrates a gastric biopsy with mature (complete) intestinal metaplasia, which is confirmed by staining of the brush border for CD10. This disorder can result from multiple inflammatory stimuli such as reflux of bile, autoimmune gastritis, *H pylori* gastritis. While immature (incomplete) intestinal metaplasia is considered to be precancerous, complete (mature) intestinal metaplasia is not associated with increased cancer risk.
QCSP, **Atrophic Gastritis**, p 243-4.

159. C. **White population in the US**
In the US, gastric adenocarcinomas are twice as common in the black population than the white population. Cancer usually arises in older individuals and is twice as common in men in this population. If it does strike an individual younger than 35, then the patient is 3 times more likely to be female. There is a higher incidence seen among individuals with type A blood, with patients with pernicious anemia and patients with a family history.
QCSP, **Gastric Adenocarcinoma**, p 244.

160. B. **E-cadherin/*CDH1* gene**
The gastric biopsy demonstrates an infiltration of malignant cells with signet ring features. The cells are distended by intracellular mucin, which compresses the nucleus into a crescentic (signet) shape. This type of gastric cancer is often referred to as linitis plastica carcinoma and usually does not cause a distinct mass but instead induces a fibrotic reaction as it diffusely infiltrates the stomaching, yielding the classic stiff leathery appearance. The familiar form of this lesion is associated with mutations in the E-cadherin/*CDH1* gene (similar to lobular breast cancer).
QCSP, **Gastric Adenocarcinoma**, p 244.

161. D. **They are often associated with duodenal polyposis when they arise in the duodenum.**
This statement is incorrect, as fundic gland polyps (FGPs) do not arise in the duodenum, and is therefore the correct answer to this question. There is, however, an association with increased risk for duodenal polyposis (×300) as fundic gland polyps are seen in cases of FAP. While fundic gland polyps are generally not considered precancerous, duodenal polyposis consists of either adenomas or carcinomas that tend to be periampullary. Interestingly, there is also an increased frequency of epithelial neoplasms in the colon. Middle-aged women are typically affected, with women outnumbering men 5:1, and they are found in up to 3% of routine upper GI evaluations. The body/fundus of the stomach, within the acid-secreting area, is the most common location. Histologically, they can look like PPI-related changes.
QCSP, **Fundic Gland Polyp**, p 248.

162. A. **Cardia**
Most gastric leiomyomas are confined to the stomach cardia, usually in the muscularis propria but sometimes within the muscularis mucosa, and are often multiple. They stain for the standard smooth muscle markers, including desmin, muscle-specific actin, and smooth muscle myosin, and are negative for CD34 and CD117

(c-Kit), which is helpful to distinguish them from gastrointestinal stromal tumor, which is the main differential diagnosis.

QCSP, **Gastric Leiomyoma,** p 248-249.

163. **B.** **STOMACH**

The image depicts a GI stromal tumor with the characteristic feature (artifact of formalin fixation) of perinuclear vacuoles that often appears to indent the nucleus. This diagnosis is supported by the immunostains, which rule out a leiomyoma. GISTs are also often positive for CD34 and a small percentage of tumors are S100+. The stomach is the most common location in the GI tract, with 60% of GISTs occurring here. The small intestine in the second most common location, with 20%-30% of GISTs, and <10% occur in the colon and rectum.

QCSP, **Gastrointestinal Stroma Tumor,** p 251.

164. **B.** **CHROMOGRANIN A**

The tumor in the image is a carcinoid tumor, and chromogranin A is the best choice. These tumors will also often stain for synaptophysin but less often than for chromogranin A. Additionally, these tumors are less likely to stain with any of the other choices. You could also consider Grimelius and Sevier-Munger special stain technique, in which the tumor cells would appear argyrophilic.

QCSP, **Carcinoid Tumor,** p 259.

165. **C.** **HYPERPLASTIC POLYP**

The image demonstrates a polypoid lesion within the antrum. It demonstrates hyperplastic changes with elongated foveolae with intraluminal infolding and cystic dilation. The glands are lined by mature gastric mucin cells with an edematous stroma. These lesions can demonstrate intestinal metaplasia as well as the presence of pyloric type glands. These lesions are of themselves considered nonneoplastic (regenerative polyps) in the setting of inflammatory conditions. However, these lesions can be associated with conditions that often lead to dysplasia (often p53+) and carcinoma. Hyperplastic polyps can be seen in up to 20% of patients with gastric cancer.

QCSP, **Gastric Hyperplastic Polyp,** p 253-254.

166. **B.** **GASTROESOPHAGEAL REFLUX**

The lesion demonstrates elongation of the lamina propria papillae (>2/3) of the epithelium. The biopsy also demonstrates basal layer thickening without dysplasia or atypia. There is also a mild increase in lymphocytes and eosinophils. These findings are consistent with GERD. While eosinophils are increased (maximum 2/HPF), the diagnosis falls significantly short of the criteria for eosinophilic esophagitis. Additionally, the features of HSV esophagitis, such as ulceration or viral inclusions, are not seen.

QCSP, **Gastroesophageal Reflux,** p 236-237.

167. **C.** **IT IS USUALLY MULTIPLE AND MAY CLUSTER.**

All of the above statements are true, except for choice C, making it the correct answer to this question. The image demonstrates hamartomatous overgrowth of the lamina propria with cystically dilated and tortuous glands in an inflamed stroma. Juvenile polyps are usually solitary and located in the rectum of youths, who do have an increased risk of developing intestinal and gastric cancers. These polyps are usually small, <3 cm, and up to almost 1/2 can have pink regenerative epithelial cells similar to those seen in hyperplastic polyps along with the well-formed mucus-secreting cells. The stroma has acute and chronic inflammatory cells and granulation tissue and can have a foreign-body giant cell reaction and occasionally osseous metaplasia.

QCSP, **Juvenile Polyps,** p 283.

168. **A.** **INFLAMMATORY FIBROID POLYP**

The lesion depicted demonstrates a polypoid mass with plump spindle cells. There is a prominent inflammatory infiltrate composed of eosinophils and plasma cells. As demonstrated, they can also demonstrate giant cells. These lesions demonstrate thin vessels and can be CD34 positive but are CD117 and cytokeratin negative. These lesions are usually asymptomatic but can cause outlet obstruction. When they occur in the stomach, they are often referred to as Vanek polyps.

QCSP, **Inflammatory Fibroid Polyp ,** p 255-256.

169.   D.   **BCL-1/cyclin D-1**

The picture is of low-grade extranodal marginal zone B-cell lymphoma of mucosa-associated lymphoid tissue (MALToma). Specifically, the image demonstrates a monotonous small lymphocytic infiltrate with the presence of lymphoepithelial lesions (arrow). The neoplastic cells express the B-cell markers CD19, CD20, CD79a and PAX5. Additionally, the neoplastic cells usually express bcl-2 and can demonstrate aberrant expression of CD43. The neoplastic cells in MALT lymphomas are negative for CD10, CD5, and the mantle cell lymphoma marker cyclin D-1. While the neoplastic cells will be negative for CD3 and CD5, these stains highlight the T cells in the background.

QCSP, **MALT,** p 256-258.

170.   B.   **CK20 and CK7 immunohistochemical stains distinguish between the gastric cardiac and esophageal type of this tumor.**

The lesion shown demonstrates an adenocarcinoma arising next to intestinal metaplasia. This is most consistent with the diagnosis of adenocarcinoma arising in Barrett esophagus. These patients demonstrate the same demographics as Barrett esophagus (older white males). Like most tumors, the survival is related to stage; however the penetration of the muscularis propria is of particle importance (survival is 90%-100% for tumors that do not penetrate the muscularis propria, 45% for those that penetrate, 15%-25% in those that extend beyond muscular propria, and 0% if there is invasion of other organs). As the patient already has a tendency to develop adenocarcinoma in Barrett esophagus, it is preferable to remove as much of the proximal glandular mucosa as possible. While the cytokeratin expression can be used to demonstrate primary from metastatic carcinoma and distal gastric lesions from esophageal lesions, it is fairly useless in differentiating an esophageal primary from a gastric cardiac primary lesion.

QCSP, **Adenocarcinoma of Esophagus,** p 232-233.

171.   B.   **Recent organ transplant**

Graft-vs-host disease can demonstrate flat duodenal mucosa and should be in the differential diagnosis for celiac disease given the right clinical scenario, but there is no well-established association between the 2, thus making it the correct choice in this question. Importantly, GVHD usually demonstrates a presence of apoptotic bodies in crypt base and can be associated with CMV infection. All the other choices are associated with celiac disease.

QCSP, **Celiac Disease,** p 262.

172.   C.   **Small intestine alone**

Crohn disease can affect the entire GI tract, and 45% of the time, patients initially present with disease limited to the small intestine and the terminal ileum is usually affected if the small intestine is affected. In 35% of cases, disease is in both the colon and small intestine at presentation, and in 15%-20% of cases, disease is limited to the colon. In all cases over time, 20%-25% of patients will have perianal disease, but only 5% of patients present with perianal disease. 50% of patients with Crohn disease will have proctitis. Only occasionally do patients present with lesions in the oral cavity, esophagus, stomach, and proximal duodenum.

QCSP, **Crohn Disease,** p 262-263.

173.   E.   **Whipple Disease**

The above lesion demonstrates numerous macrophages in the lamina propria with a basophilic stipple cytoplasm. A PAS-d stain would demonstrate rod-shaped bacterium. This is a case of Whipple disease, which is caused by the bacterium *Tropheryma whippelii.* The biopsy demonstrates a brush boarder that can be highlighted with a CD10 or CEA stain, and the enterocytes do not demonstrate inclusions, eliminating microvillous inclusion disease.

QCSP, **Whipple Disease,** p 266.

7: Gastrointestinal Tract Answers

174. A. **GASTRIN-PRODUCING (G-CELL) TUMOR**
Gastrin-producing, or G-cell, tumors are the most common, representing 65% of duodenal neuroendocrine tumors. 30% of these tumors have lymph node metastases at the time of diagnosis. Gangliocytic paragangliomas are very rare and considered benign.
QCSP, **Neuroendocrine Tumors,** Duodenum, p 267.

175. E. **ALL OF THE ABOVE**
Autoimmune diseases, including thyroid disease, rheumatoid joint disease, pernicious anemia, small bowel villous atrophy, iritis, and myasthenia gravis, are associated with collagenous colitis, which may also coexist with celiac disease. An etiologic association with NSAIDs may also exist. There may also be a coincidental association with colonic adenocarcinoma and Crohn disease.
QCSP, **Collagenous Colitis,** p 269.

176. A. **ADEQUATE FOR EVALUATION**
The image demonstrates a rectal biopsy. Specifically, the biopsy contains both mucosa and submucosa. Under the dissecting scope, the mucosa appears pink/tan and the submucosa is white and dense. To use a "hot dog" metaphor: the submucosa is the hot dog and the mucosa is the bun that wraps around the hot dog. In order for the biopsy to be considered adequate, the sample must contain submucosa in order to microscopically look for ganglion cells. The absence of ganglion cells would support the diagnosis of Hirschsprung disease.
QCSP, **Hirschsprung Disease,** p 270-272.

177. C. **GRAFT-VS-HOST DISEASE**
The above image from the colon demonstrates the presence of apoptotic bodies in crypt base. However, there are no viral inclusions. With the history of bone marrow biopsy, these findings are consistent with GVHD. However, the histology is not specific and an infectious etiology must be excluded. Remember that viral/infectious colitis occur along with GVHD.
QCSP, **Graft-vs-Host Disease,** P 269-270.

178. B. **A YOUNGER PATIENT TAKING PSYCHIATRIC MEDS**
While there is an association between young people taking NSAIDs and ischemic colitis, there is no well-documented link between psychiatric meds and ischemic colitis. Any cause of hypoperfusion puts patients at risk for ischemic colitis, including cardiac failure or arrhythmia, digitalis toxicity, shock, and septicemia. Arterial thrombosis can develop in the setting of atherosclerotic disease and venous thrombosis associated with intraabdominal sepsis can also lead to ischemia, as can arterial emboli. Complications of volvulus and hernias can also set the stage.
QCSP, **Ischemic Colitis,** p 273.

179. C. **45-YEAR-OLD WOMAN**
The above biopsy demonstrates a diffuse increase in lymphocytes and plasma cells in the upper lamina propria with increased intraepithelial lymphocytes. Additionally, there is no evidence of chronic mucosal change (alteration of crypt architecture) and no increase in subepithelial collagen. This is diagnostic of a lymphocytic colitis and primarily affects middle-aged women leading to watery diarrhea that can occasionally lead to hypokalemia, hypoproteinemia, and anemia.
QCSP, **Lymphocytic Colitis,** p 273-274.

180. D. **ULCERATIVE COLITIS**
The lesion demonstrates architectural changes of a chronic colitis with a Paneth-cell hyperplasia, active colitis, and a microabscess. While the features of Crohn and UC are similar on biopsy, the extent of involvement (multiple biopsies from TI through the rectum prior to treatment) can help determine and answer. *E coli* O157 is an acute

infectious colitis and would not demonstrate the findings of chronic IBD. *C difficile* infection and ischemic colitis demonstrate similar histologic findings.

QCSP, **Ulcerative Colitis,** p 274-276.

181. A. **CONSTIPATION**

The lesion demonstrates the obliteration of the lamina propria by proliferation of smooth muscle that along with fibrosis extends to the lumen from a thickened muscularis mucosa and capillary ectasia. Often the regenerative crypts will take on a diamond-shaped appearance. These lesions can be mistaken for adenocarcinoma with localized colitis cystica profunda and if the biopsy is cut tangentially, mucosal glands may be seen within a muscle and can give the false impression of an invasive carcinoma. These lesions are basically prolapse-type lesions that are caused by excess staining at defecation/constipation. The polypoid variant of the solitary rectal/mucosal prolapse syndrome is the inflammatory cloacogenic polyp.

QCSP, **Solitary Rectal Ulcer Syndrome,** p 277-278.

182. D. **LOSS OF MLH1 TRANSLATION**

In this case, there is loss of MLH1 and PMS2 protein expression. MLH1 can form homodimers with itself or heterodimers with PMS2; however PMS2 can only form heterodimers with MLH1. As such, when expression of MLH1 is lost, the expression of both proteins is lost, but PMS2 can be lost without loss of MLH1. A similar situation exist between MSH2 and MSH6, in which MSH2 can form homodimers with itself or heterodimers with MSH6, but MSH6 can only form heterodimers with MSH2. Also remember that we are looking at protein expression and you cannot directly determine the gene status of theses proteins by IHC. Specifically, the loss of MLH1 is usually by hypermethylation and not from mutations in MLH1.

QCSP, **Adenocarcinoma,** p 279-281.

183. C. **pT3**

The adenocarcinoma extends through the muscularis propria and into the subserosa tissue, which is a T3 lesion. The pathologic staging of the primary tumors is described as follows: pTis: carcinoma in situ, intraepithelial (no invasion); pTis: carcinoma in situ, invasion of lamina propria; pT1: tumor invades submucosa; pT2: tumor invades muscularis propria; pT3: tumor invades through the muscularis propria into pericolorectal tissues; pT4a: tumor penetrates the visceral peritoneum; pT4b: tumor directly invades or is adherent to other organs or structures (as listed in the CAP colon/rectum cancer protocol checklist).

QCSP, **Adenocarcinoma,** p 279-281.

184. D. **A AND C**

Ganglioneuroma of the intestine can be seen in both von Recklinghausen disease and MEN IIB, usually as multiple lesions, referred to as ganglioneuromatosis. In MEN IIB, the ganglioneuromatosis may consist of a marked accentuation of both the submucosal and myenteric nerve plexuses.

QCSP, **Ganglioneuroma,** p 282.

185. B. **PATIENT WITH RENAL FAILURE**

The images demonstrate severe ischemic-type injury with the presence of luminal necrosis and basophilic rhomboid nonpolarizing crystals. These crystals represent kayexalate. The injury is actually caused by the sorbitol component in the kayexalate prep. Kayexalate is a polystyrene polymer that is used to treat hyperkalemia in renal patients with millions of doses prescribed to patients each year. Of the other choices, long-term antibiotics treatment can lead to colonization of the colon with *C difficile*. Pills, especially iron, can induce an associated esophagitis or gastritis. In children, viral GI infections can lead to hypertrophy of Peyer patches and result in an intussusception of the terminal ileum (specifically) through the ileocecal valve. This can result in similar histologic changes (ischemia) to those pictured, but without the kayexalate crystals.

QCSP, **Ischemic Colitis,** p 273.

7: Gastrointestinal Tract Answers

186. **A.** **IT SHOULD BE TREATED WITH COLECTOMY.**

The lesion demonstrates features similar to a hyperplastic polyp; however, there is no grossly apparent polypoid lesion. Microscopically, the lesion demonstrates L-shaped or flask-shaped crypts that appear to be growing parallel to the muscularis mucosa. The lesion represents a sessile serrated adenoma and would have decreased staining for MLH1 and MSH2. While the lesion can show a high rate of DNA methylation (92%), they can also demonstrate BRAF mutations (80%), but have a low prevalence rate of KRAS or APC mutations (<5%). While these lesions are considered adenomas, the exact transformation rate into adenocarcinoma is unknown. Treatment is usually with increased surveillance similar to scheduling of patients with more classical adenomas. Colectomy usually not recommended; however, if this lesion occurs in the setting of hyperplastic polyposis syndrome, the patient might undergo colectomy.

QCSP, **Sessile Serrated Adenoma,** p 284-285.

187. **B.** **IT MOST COMMONLY OCCURS IN THE STOMACH.**

The lesion above demonstrates arborizing network of well-developed smooth muscle arising from the muscularis along with connective tissue. This would be consistent with a hamartomatous polyp (Peutz-Jeghers polyp) occurring in Peutz-Jeghers polyposis. This syndrome is autosomal dominant with a mutation of *STK11* on chromosome 19q13.3. This syndrome has multiple hamartomatous polyps and melanotic pigmentation of the mucosa of the lips, oral cavity, and genitalia as well as skin of the face, digits, palms and soles. Most patients (95%) have polyps in their small intestine (95%) while 25% of patients have polyps in the stomach, 25% in the colon, and 25% in the rectum. These patients have increased risk of adenocarcinoma of the stomach, small intestine, and colon. Additionally, there is an increased risk of malignant neoplasms occurring outside of the GI tract: including well-differentiated adenocarcinoma of the uterine cervix, pancreatic carcinoma, ovarian neoplasm (sex-cord tumor with annular tubules), ovarian mucinous tumors, breast carcinoma, as well as feminizing Sertoli tumors of the testis.

QCSP, **Peutz-Jeghers Syndrome,** p 285.

188. **D.** **IT STAINS SIMILAR TO APOCRINE TUMORS.**

The lesion shown above demonstrates malignant cells infiltrating the dermis. These cells are negative for S100, and at high power there is intracellular mucin. This morphologic picture is consistent with extramammary Paget disease. These lesions are thought to be derived from apocrine glands (although there is overlap with eccrine glands). The neoplastic cells are often positive for GCDFP (Brst-2), CK7 and/or CD20, EMA, CEA, and androgen receptor. While the mammary version of Paget disease is often associated with a breast carcinoma, in extramammary Paget disease (of the anus, vulva, and perineum), in up to 80% of these patients, their Paget disease is primary and is not associated with a current (or future) internal malignancy. There is a subset that is associated with internal malignancies; those associated with rectal carcinomas are more often CK20 and CDX2 positive and GCDFP negative. While these lesions can demonstrate squamous changes such as acanthosis, hyper/parakeratosis, and papillomatous hyperplasia, there is no associated squamous dysplasia and they are not HPV- or Bowen disease-associated. Patients are treated with wide local resections, and while there is a high local recurrence rate, the prognosis of patients with Paget disease of the anus is good (in some studies survival equals normal age-match controls).

QCSP, **Anal Paget,** p 279-281.

189. **B.** **IT IS ASSOCIATED WITH HPV TYPE 16 AND 18**

The lesion demonstrates a verrucous carcinoma. The lesion demonstrates morphologic similarities with the giant condyloma acuminatum of Buschke-Löwenstein, except this lesion demonstrates stromal invasion. The lesion is often associated with the "low-risk" HPV subtypes 6 and 11, and not with the "high-risk" HPV subtypes of 16 and 18. These lesions are best treated with wide-local excision and are often radiation insensitive. They are often locally aggressive but generally only metastasize if they progress/convert to the conventional type of squamous carcinoma.

QCSP, **Verrucous Carcinoma,** p 285.

7: Gastrointestinal Tract Answers

190. **B.** **MELANOMA**

The lesion demonstrates malignant nests of cells growing under the anal squamous mucosa. The neoplastic cells have an epithelioid appearance with eosinophilic cytoplasm and prominent nucleoli. This represents a case of primary anal melanoma. This question was designed to demonstrate a pitfall of overreliance on c-Kit staining, as over 10% of melanomas can also be positive, and not all c-Kit stromal tumors are GIST. As such, a panel of immunohistochemical staining is useful in nonepithelial tumors of the GI tract.

191. **B.** **BIOLOGICAL BEHAVIOR IS SIMILAR TO CLASSICAL CARCINOID TUMOR.**

The above lesion demonstrates cells with goblet cell/signet ring morphology in clusters. The positive chromogranin confirms the neuroendocrine differentiation of the lesion, while the positive alcian blue stain (would also be mucicarmine and PAS-D positive) confirms the mucinous differentiation. This lesion is best classified as a goblet cell carcinoid (GCC). They typically present either without specific symptoms or will acute appendicitis and present with increased stage with ~50% with metastasis at the time of diagnosis. Given the increased stage at presentation, GCC are thought to be biologically more aggressive then typical carcinoid. However, stage-to-stage comparisons of GCC to malignant carcinoid fail to demonstrate differences in prognosis. The lesion is CEA positive, demonstrates mucinous and neuroendocrine differentiation and has mixed expression of CK7 CK20, often positive for both (CK20 > CK7).
QCSP, **Appendix Carcinoid,** p 289.

192. **B.** **TUBULAR ADENOMA**

The lesion demonstrates a dysplastic (adenomatous) polyp with epithelium that demonstrates enlarged nuclei that are hyperchromatic and stratified. Additionally, the dysplastic cells have loss of mucin expression (either decreased or complete absence). Typically there is also an increase in the number apoptotic cells. These glands are not complex or cribriform in appearance (and there is no high-grade cytologic features at higher power) and this would be an example of a standard tubular adenoma with low-grade dysplastic features. In general, adenomatous polyps with >75% villous architecture are classified as villous adenomas, those with <25% as tubular adenomas and those with between 25%-75% villous architecture are classified as tubulovillous adenomas.
QCSP, **Intestinal Polyps: Adenomatous Polyp,** p 282.

193. **A.** **HYPERPLASTIC POLYP**

This lesion represents a hyperplastic polyp. Specifically, the glands have a serrated (also referred to as star-fish or saw-tooth) appearance. These changes often extend to the surface of the polyp. The cells are a mixture of absorptive and goblet cells and the nuclei are basally located and without atypia or dysplastic change.
QCSP, **Intestinal Polyps: Hyperplastic polyps,** p283-284.

194. **G.** **SIGNET RING ADENOCARCINOMA**

The lesion represents a signet ring adenocarcinoma. Specifically, the images demonstrate a colon biopsy where the submucosa and peri-colonic tissue has a cellular appearance. There are single atypical mucin producing cells seen infiltrating throughout the submucosa and peri-colonic tissue. The atypical cells have an increased amount of mucin along with an enlarged atypical nucleus, which is pushed to one side giving the cell a crescent or "signet-ring" appearance. This diffuse infiltration produces the linitis plastic (or leather bag) appearance with thickening of the colonic wall usually without a discrete mass. In general prognosis is poor.
QCSP, **Colorectal Carcinoma,** p 278-280.

195. **E.** **INFLAMMATORY FIBROID POLYP**

These images represent an inflammatory fibroid polyp. Specifically, the polyp demonstrates a primarily mesenchymal proliferation of spindle and/or stellate cells. The cells are thought to be perivascular cells and will often demonstrate a fibromyxoid appearance and CD34 positivity. Generally, these lesions are centered

7: Gastrointestinal Tract Answers

in the submucosa and demonstrate a significant vascular component. Additionally there is a prominent mixed inflammatory component, which consists of plasma cells, lymphocytes, eosinophils, and mast cells.

QCSP, **Intestinal Polyps: Inflammatory Fibroid Polyps,** p 284.

196. J. **MELANOSIS COLI**

The image demonstrates a case of melanosis coli. The epithelial portion of the mucosa appears fairly normal with collections of pigmented-laden macrophages. The pigment is usually coarsely granular, refractile, and light to dark brown. The pigment is lipofuscin and not melanin or iron. As such the pigment is positive by Fontana-Masson stain but negative by Prussian blue (iron) stain and melanin stains. It is a benign condition that most often occurs in the right colon and is related to use of herbal laxatives.

197. I. **PROLAPSE**

The image demonstrates changes of prolapse. Specifically there are long villous crypts along with thickening of the muscularis mucosa with the proliferation of muscle surrounding the glands, running perpendicular to the mucosal surface. Additionally, there are diamond (or triangle) shaped glands and glands that are displaced deeper into the muscularis mucosa. In addition to the findings seen here, one could see vascular ectasia, granulation tissue with ulceration and inflammation with possible pseudomembrane. Additionally there can be misplaced epithelium such as proctitis cystica profunda that can mimic adenocarcinoma (this can be a diagnostic dilemma in polyp stalks mimicking invasion).

QCSP, **Solitary Rectal Ulcer Syndrome,** p 277-278.

198. F. **MUCINOUS ADENOCARCINOMA**

The image is consistent with the diagnosis of a mucinous adenocarcinoma. Specifically, the lesion demonstrates pools of mucin in connective tissue with malignant cells floating in the mucin. Remember that the mucinous component must be >50% to be considered a mucinous adenocarcinoma. Around 5%-15% of colon cancers are mucinous and are usually diagnosed at a more advanced stage and as such have a worse prognosis then typical colonic adenocarcinoma.

QCSP, **Colorectal Carcinoma,** p 278-280.

199. C. **GANGLIOCYTIC PARAGANGLIOMA**

The images demonstrate a gangliocytic paraganglioma. Specifically there is a mixture of nests of eosinophilic epithelioid cells surrounded by spindle cells along with scattered Schwann cells and neuroendocrine cells (including ganglion cells). The growth pattern is similar to paraganglioma with trabecular growth pattern.

The higher-power image (on the right) demonstrated neurofibrillary cells with large cells with gangliocytic differentiation. These lesions typically occur in the middle age and can be associated with NF-1.

QCSP, **Neuroendocrine Tumors,** p 267.

Chapter 8

Liver, Gallbladder, and Extrahepatic Bile Ducts

1. Microscopic findings in alcohol-related fatty liver disease include all the following EXCEPT:
   - A. Ballooning degeneration
   - B. Mallory hyaline (Mallory-Denk bodies)
   - C. Neutrophil infiltrate
   - D. Periportal necrosis/interface hepatitis
   - E. Steatosis

2. Mallory hyaline (Mallory-Denk bodies) consists of:
   - A. Enlarged mitochondria
   - B. Dying hepatocytes
   - C. Cytoskeleton intermediate filaments
   - D. Viral particles
   - E. A1-AT (α-1-antitrypsin)

3. Which of the following statements concerning α-1-antitrypsin (A1-AT) deficiency is FALSE?
   - A. There is an increased risk of hepatocellular carcinoma.
   - B. Approximately 10% will die from liver failure.
   - C. Misfolded A1-AT proteins are retained in the Golgi bodies.
   - D. Patients who have the homozygous null phenotype develop pulmonary disease but not liver disease.
   - E. The only treatment for associated liver disease is transplant.

4. Which autoantibody is NOT associated with autoimmune hepatitis?
   - A. Antimitochondrial antibodies
   - B. Antinuclear antibodies (ANA)
   - C. Anti-smooth muscle antibodies (SMA)
   - D. Liver-kidney microsome type 1 antibodies (anti-LKM)
   - E. Antisoluble liver antigen/liver pancreas (anti-SLA/LP)

5. Which statement best describes the typical microscopic features of autoimmune hepatitis?
   - A. Hepatocytes contain intracytoplasmic eosinophilic granules
   - B. Fine chickenwire fibrosis
   - C. Periportal inflammation with germinal center formation
   - D. Dense periportal lymphocytic infiltrate with plasma cells
   - E. Zone 3 necrosis

6. Autoimmune hepatitis is associated with all the following autoimmune diseases EXCEPT:
   - A. Rheumatoid arthritis
   - B. Sjögren syndrome
   - C. Ulcerative colitis
   - D. Crohn disease
   - E. Thyroiditis

7. All of the following statements concerning cirrhosis are TRUE, EXCEPT:
   - A. Ito cells become activated and acquire contractile properties similar to myofibroblasts.
   - B. The fibrous bands of cirrhosis represent type I and type III collagen.
   - C. Cirrhosis from any etiology has the same outcome/prognosis.
   - D. Biopsies from cirrhotic livers are often fragmented.
   - E. Cirrhosis differs histologically from congenital hepatic fibrosis because of the intact acinar architecture.

8: Liver, Gallbladder, and Extrahepatic Bile Ducts Questions

8. Which of the following is the MOST characteristic finding in a liver biopsy of graft-vs-host disease (in the correct clinical setting)?
   A. Dense lymphocytic infiltrate
   B. Fibrosis
   C. Nuclear vacuolization
   D. Loss of bile ducts
   E. Central lobular necrosis

9. Characteristic findings of congenital hepatic fibrosis include all the following EXCEPT:
   A. It presents between 1 and 2 years of age with an enlarged, firm liver.
   B. It is frequently associated with abnormalities in the kidneys and pancreas (usually cystic changes).
   C. Patients have normal liver function tests.
   D. Patients usually die from hepatic failure.
   E. Fibrosis has normal vascular relationships.

10. Which is the most common microscopic finding in the liver of cystic fibrosis patients?
    A. Steatosis
    B. Chronic portal inflammation
    C. Bile duct necrosis
    D. Bile duct proliferation
    E. Ballooning hepatic necrosis

11. Etiologies for macrovesicular steatosis include all the following EXCEPT:
    A. Obesity
    B. HCV
    C. Malnutrition
    D. Total parenteral nutrition
    E. Corticosteroids

12. Which of the following features are more typically seen in alcohol-related fatty liver disease than in non-alcohol-related fatty liver disease?
    A. Mallory-Denk bodies
    B. Cirrhosis
    C. Perivenular fibrosis
    D. Mononuclear lymphocytic infiltrate
    E. Zone 3 fatty change

13. Etiologies for microvesicular steatosis include all the following EXCEPT:
    A. Pregnancy
    B. Wilson disease
    C. Reye syndrome
    D. Valproate toxicity
    E. HIV drug toxicity

14. Mallory-Denk bodies may be seen in association with all the following, EXCEPT:
    A. Copper toxicity
    B. Amiodarone toxicity
    C. Alcohol-related liver disease
    D. Primary biliary cirrhosis
    E. Angiomyolipoma

8: Liver, Gallbladder, and Extrahepatic Bile Ducts Questions

15. When comparing alcohol-related steatohepatitis with non-alcohol-related steatohepatitis, all of the following is TRUE, EXCEPT:
    A. In alcohol-related steatohepatitis, the AST>ALT while in non-alcohol-related steatohepatitis the ALT>AST
    B. Fatty change is more pronounced in non-alcohol-related steatohepatitis.
    C. Mallory-Denk bodies are more plentiful in alcohol-related steatohepatitis.
    D. Satellitosis is more common in non-alcohol-related steatohepatitis.
    E. Sclerosing hyaline necrosis is seen in alcohol-related steatohepatitis but not in non-alcohol-related steatohepatitis.

16. Megamitochondria are seen in all the following EXCEPT:
    A. α-1-antitrypsin deficiency
    B. Wilson disease
    C. Alcohol-related liver disease/steatohepatitis
    D. Pregnancy
    E. Fatty liver of pregnancy

17. Which is the most reliable method for the diagnosis of hemochromatosis?
    A. Molecular testing for the HFE gene
    B. Quantitative hepatic iron content
    C. Iron staining of the liver biopsy
    D. Skin pigmentation
    E. Serum iron concentration

18. All the following are established etiologies of neonatal hepatitis EXCEPT:
    A. TORCH infections
    B. Inborn errors of metabolism
    C. α-1-antitrypsin deficiency
    D. Niemann-Pick type A and C disease
    E. Wilson disease

19. Which of the following microscopic features would be more consistent with biliary atresia than neonatal hepatitis?
    A. Extensive bile ductular proliferation
    B. Prominent canalicular cholestasis
    C. Fatty change and prominent cholestatic rosettes
    D. Giant multinucleated hepatocytes
    E. Nuclear viral inclusions

20. Primary biliary cirrhosis is associated with all the following, EXCEPT:
    A. CREST syndrome
    B. Osteoporosis
    C. Celiac disease
    D. Ulcerative colitis
    E. Sjögren syndrome

21. Which autoantibody is most closely associated with primary biliary cirrhosis?
    A. Anti-smooth muscle antibodies (SMA)
    B. Liver-kidney microsome type 1 antibodies (anti-LKM)
    C. Antimitochondrial antibodies
    D. Antinuclear antibodies (ANA)
    E. Antisoluble liver antigen/liver pancreas antibodies (anti-SLA/LP)

22.   Which of the following stains can demonstrate a chronic cholestatic condition?
    A.   Rhodamine
    B.   Prussian blue
    C.   Trichrome
    D.   Reticulin
    E.   PAS

23.   Which of the following is/are NOT common microscopic findings seen in liver biopsies of patients with primary biliary cirrhosis?
    A.   Irregular and hyperplastic bile duct epithelium
    B.   Ductular proliferation
    C.   Bile duct loss
    D.   Dense periportal inflammation
    E.   All these findings are associated with PBC

24.   Which of the following statements concerning primary sclerosing cholangitis is FALSE?
    A.   Men are affected more frequently.
    B.   The disease may affect any part of the biliary tree including the gallbladder.
    C.   The diagnosis is typically made on liver biopsy.
    D.   There is an increased risk for development of cholangiocarcinoma.
    E.   The median survival is 10-12 years.

25.   Which of the following abnormalities in immunoglobulins or autoantibodies is specific for primary sclerosing cholangitis?
    A.   ANA
    B.   AMA
    C.   Elevated IgG
    D.   Elevated IgM
    E.   None of the above

26.   Which of the following is/are NOT associated with veno-occlusive disease?
    A.   Hypervitaminosis A
    B.   Bone marrow transplant s/p alkylating agents
    C.   Pyrrolizidine alkaloid ingestion
    D.   Chemotherapeutic agents
    E.   All of the above are associated.

27.   Which of the following viral infections has the greatest incidence of fulminant hepatitis following acute infection?
    A.   HAV
    B.   HBV
    C.   HCV
    D.   HDV
    E.   HEV

28.   Which of the following findings is more consistent with chronic than acute viral hepatitis?
    A.   Hepatocellular injury in zone 3
    B.   Perivenular cholestasis
    C.   Interface hepatitis
    D.   Confluent necrosis
    E.   Fulminant hepatitis

8: Liver, Gallbladder, and Extrahepatic Bile Ducts Questions

29. Which of the following statements concerning Wilson disease (hepatolenticular degeneration) is FALSE?
    A. The defective gene is located on chromosome 13q-14.3.
    B. The condition is transmitted as an autosomal dominant trait.
    C. It can occasionally present at fulminant hepatic failure.
    D. The earliest histologic changes include hepatocellular ballooning and glycogenated nuclei.
    E. End-stage disease is characterized by hepatic necrosis and collapse.

30. Which of the following findings is LEAST specific for the diagnosis of Wilson disease?
    A. Low serum ceruloplasmin levels
    B. Serum copper levels
    C. Increased urinary copper excretion
    D. Kayser-Fleischer rings
    E. Increased quantitative copper in a liver biopsy

31. Which of the following immunohistochemical or special stains would be the MOST usefully in rendering the diagnosis of Angiomyolipoma?
    A. PAS
    B. Melan-A
    C. Smooth muscle actin
    D. CD34
    E. Sudan black

32. Which of the following microscopic feature(s) is/are seen in the majority of the cases of angiomyolipoma?
    A. Adipose tissue and thick-walled blood vessels
    B. Smooth muscle cells arranged in a solid or trabecular pattern
    C. Extramedullary hematopoiesis
    D. A and B
    E. A, B, and C

33. All of the following are associated etiologic agents/conditions for hepatic angiosarcoma, EXCEPT:
    A. Androgenic steroids
    B. Vinyl chloride
    C. Arsenic
    D. Infantile hemangioendothelioma
    E. Epithelioid hemangioendothelioma

34. Which of the following markers is NOT expressed by hepatic angiosarcoma?
    A. Fli-1
    B. CD34
    C. Keratin
    D. HerPar-1
    E. Factor VIII

35. Which immunohistochemical stain is the LEAST helpful in differentiating bile duct hamartoma/adenoma from metastatic adenocarcinoma?
    A. MOC-31
    B. Dpc4 (smad4)
    C. B72.3
    D. Mesothelin
    E. Monoclonal CEA

8: Liver, Gallbladder, and Extrahepatic Bile Ducts Questions

50. Which of the following immunohistochemical stains is LEAST helpful in differentiating epithelioid hemangioendothelioma from metastatic adenocarcinoma?
    A. CD34
    B. MOC-31
    C. Pankeratin
    D. Factor VIII
    E. CD31

51. Which of the following microscopic descriptions is LEAST compatible with a diagnosis of epithelioid hemangioendothelioma?
    A. Papillary tufts in vascular spaces
    B. Myxoid background
    C. Mucin staining of neoplastic cells
    D. Biphenotypic appearance of neoplastic cells, spindle-shaped and epitheloid cells
    E. Obliteration of central venules

52. Which of the following elements is NOT seen in hepatoblastoma?
    A. Keratinized squamous cells
    B. Extramedullary hematopoiesis
    C. Trabecular pattern
    D. Pale bodies
    E. Osteoid

53. Multinucleated giant cells seen in hepatoblastoma will often stain for which of the following?
    A. hCG
    B. α-fetoprotein
    C. CD68
    D. Erythropoietin
    E. Chromogranin

54. Which of the following histological type/pattern of hepatoblastoma has the best prognosis?
    A. Fetal pattern
    B. Embryonal pattern
    C. Macrotrabecular pattern
    D. Small cell undifferentiated pattern
    E. Mixed pattern with osteoid

55. Which of the following neoplasms do NOT typically demonstrate mucoid/myxoid stroma?
    A. Epithelioid hemangioendothelioma
    B. Fibrolamellar hepatocellular carcinoma
    C. Hepatoblastoma
    D. Mesenchymal hamartoma
    E. Embryonal sarcoma

56. Which of the following neoplasms CANNOT be seen at birth?
    A. Neuroblastoma
    B. Hepatoblastoma
    C. Hemangioma
    D. Nasopharyngeal teratoma
    E. All of the above can be present at birth.

8: Liver, Gallbladder, and Extrahepatic Bile Ducts Questions

57. Which of the following tumors is LEAST likely to demonstrate increased serum α-fetoprotein levels?
    A. Fibrolamellar hepatocellular carcinoma
    B. Endodermal sinus tumor
    C. Hepatoblastoma
    D. Undifferentiated embryonal sarcoma, hepatic
    E. Conventional hepatocellular carcinoma

58. Which of the following features could differentiate hepatic adenoma from focal nodular hyperplasia?
    A. Lack of bile ducts
    B. Steatosis
    C. Mallory-Denk bodies
    D. Scar and fibrosis
    E. Lack of bile ductules

59. Which of the following stain(s) can be expressed in both hepatocellular adenoma and hepatocellular carcinoma?
    A. Glypican-3
    B. CD34
    C. α-fetoprotein
    D. Pankeratin
    E. B and D

60. Hepatocellular adenomas have been associated with all the following, EXCEPT:
    A. Oral contraceptive steroids
    B. Anabolic steroids
    C. Sex hormone-producing ovarian tumor
    D. Vascular insult
    E. Type Ia or III glycogen storage disease

61. Which of the following findings would MOST strongly argue against the diagnosis of hepatocellular adenoma?
    A. Multiple lesions
    B. Cirrhosis
    C. Male gender
    D. Rupture and hemorrhage
    E. Intact reticulin framework

62. Which lesion can have a microscopic appearance reminiscent of fibroadenoma of the breast?
    A. Bile duct adenoma
    B. Bile duct hamartoma
    C. Mesenchymal hamartoma
    D. Embryonal sarcoma
    E. Von Meyenburg complex

63. Which lesion is MOST likely to be seen in association with hepatic hemangioma?
    A. Nodular regenerative hyperplasia
    B. Focal nodular hyperplasia
    C. Hepatic adenoma
    D. Hepatocellular carcinoma
    E. Epithelioid hemangioendothelioma

8: Liver, Gallbladder, and Extrahepatic Bile Ducts Questions

64. Which of the following stains is usually NEGATIVE in focal nodular hyperplasia?
    A. CD34
    B. PAS
    C. Rhodamine
    D. CK7
    E. α-1-antitrypsin

65. Which of the following lesions is/are associated with use of chemotherapy drugs?
    A. Nodular regenerative hyperplasia
    B. Venous-occlusive disease
    C. Steatohepatitis
    D. B and C
    E. A, B, and C

66. Which finding would NOT support a finding of nodular regenerative hyperplasia?
    A. Similar appearance of lesional and surrounding normal hepatocytes
    B. Collapse of the reticulin network
    C. Atrophic hepatocytes
    D. Fibrosis
    E. Portal hypertension

67. What is/are the accepted type(s) of gallbladder metaplasia?
    A. Squamous metaplasia
    B. Gastric metaplasia
    C. Intestinal metaplasia
    D. B and C
    E. A, B, and C

68. Which of the following statements concerning extrahepatic bile duct carcinoma is FALSE?
    A. Up to 95% of the lesions are well to moderately differentiated.
    B. Usually, the only evidence of malignancy is the presence of perineural invasion or occasional desmoplastic response.
    C. The majority of the lesions are Klatskin tumors.
    D. Papillary lesions have a worse prognosis.
    E. There is an increased risk for the development of extrahepatic bile duct carcinoma in patients with primary biliary cirrhosis.

69. Which of the following statements concerning biliary (hepatobiliary) cystadenocarcinoma is TRUE?
    A. It has the same sex and age distribution as biliary cystadenoma.
    B. The presence of ovarian stroma indicates a worse prognosis.
    C. It oftentimes is identified in an extrahepatic location.
    D. The stroma stains positive for ER and PR.
    E. Lesional ovarian-type stroma is present in both men and women.

70. Histologically, biliary (hepatobiliary) cystadenomas most closely resemble which of the following neoplasms?
    A. Choledochal cyst
    B. Pancreatic mucinous cystic neoplasm
    C. Retention cyst
    D. Pancreatic serous cystadenoma
    E. Biliary adenomyoma

8: Liver, Gallbladder, and Extrahepatic Bile Ducts Questions

71. What is the most common location for biliary (hepatobiliary) cystadenoma?
    A. Intrahepatic
    B. Common bile duct
    C. Cystic duct
    D. Hepatic duct
    E. Gallbladder

72. Which of the following is NOT associated with an increased risk of gallbladder carcinoma?
    A. Porcelain gallbladder
    B. Abnormal choledochopancreatic junction
    C. Hispanic ethnic group
    D. Biliary atresia
    E. Familial adenomatosis polyposis

73. The biopsy is from a 52-year-old male that presents with GI bleeding and elevated LFTs. Which of the following diagnoses is most consistent with the biopsy?

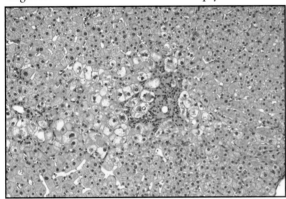 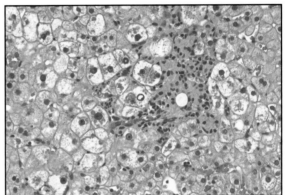

    A. Autoimmune hepatitis
    B. α-1-antitrypsin
    C. HCV infection
    D. Alcoholic liver disease
    E. Chronic venous congestion

74.   The patient's liver biopsy is shown below. What additional lesion/condition is the patient most likely to have?

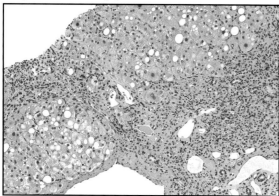 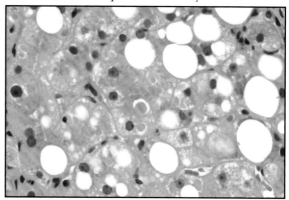

    A.   Extrahepatic cholangiocarcinoma
    B.   Hepatocellular carcinoma
    C.   Emphysema
    D.   Hepatocellular adenoma
    E.   Hepatocellular siderosis

75.   A 27-year-old female presents to the doctor with fatigue, itching, joint stiffness and amenorrhea. A metabolic panel demonstrates elevated liver function test (ALT: 306, AST: 286, ALK Pho: 65). Her viral hepatitis serologies are negative. A liver biopsy is performed and shown below. Which is the most likely diagnosis?

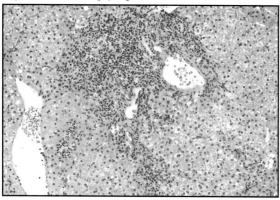 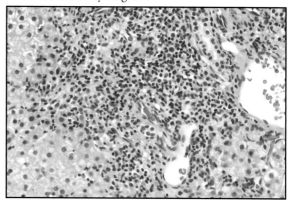

    A.   Primary sclerosing cholangitis
    B.   Autoimmune hepatitis
    C.   Alcohol liver disease
    D.   Sarcoidosis
    E.   Hepatitis B infection

8: Liver, Gallbladder, and Extrahepatic Bile Ducts Questions

76. The biopsy and radiograph are from a 36-year-old male. Which of the following conditions is most likely to be associated with this diagnosis?

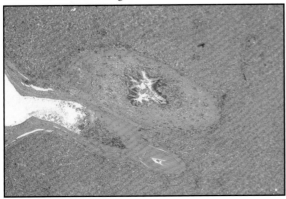 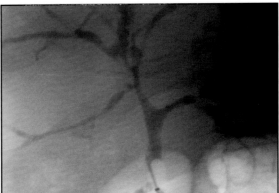

    A.   Crohn disease
    B.   Ulcerative colitis
    C.   Celiac disease
    D.   Sjögren syndrome
    E.   Rheumatoid arthritis

77. A 45-year-old woman presented with a hepatic mass that was biopsied and shown below. What is the diagnosis?

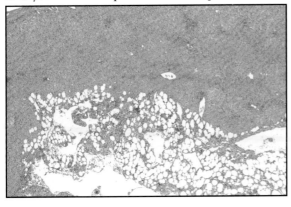 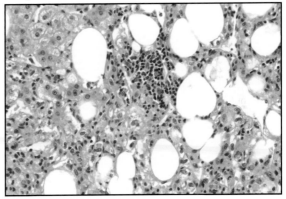

    A.   Leiomyosarcoma
    B.   Malignant fibrous histiocytoma
    C.   Hepatocellular carcinoma
    D.   Angiomyolipoma
    E.   Embryonal sarcoma

8: Liver, Gallbladder, and Extrahepatic Bile Ducts Questions

82. A 26-year old male with acute leukemia underwent myeloablative therapy, which was complicated by an admission for pneumonia. After 4 months, the patient developed a rise in his transaminases. A liver biopsy was performed. What is the most likely diagnosis?

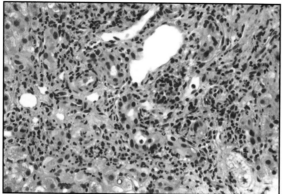

   A.   CMV hepatitis
   B.   Graft-vs-host disease
   C.   PTLD
   D.   Autoimmune hepatitis
   E.   Drug-induced hepatitis

83. Which of the following conditions is MOST often associated with the following biopsy? (H&E stain on the left and trichrome on the right)

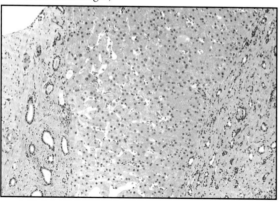 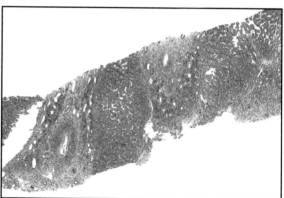

   A.   Caroli syndrome
   B.   Hepatocellular carcinoma
   C.   Iron overload
   D.   CREST syndrome
   E.   Retroperitoneal fibrosis

Questions 84 and 85:

On physical exam, an 8-year-old boy was found to have an enlarged liver. Subsequent blood test demonstrated elevated LFTs. A biopsy was performed and shown below:

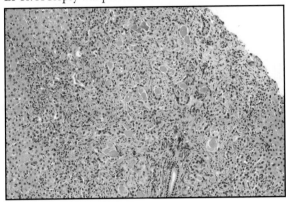 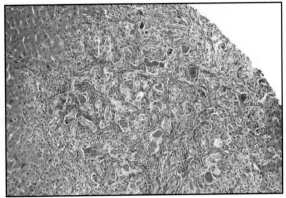

84. What is the correct diagnosis?
   A. Hereditary hemochromatosis
   B. Biliary atresia
   C. Amyloidosis
   D. Cystic fibrosis
   E. Mesenchymal hamartoma

85. The genetic abnormality MOST likely associated with the above biopsy occurs on which chromosome?
   A. Chromosome 7
   B. Chromosome 21
   C. Chromosome 13
   D. Chromosome 12
   E. Chromosome 18

86. Which of the following is the LEAST likely to result in the changes demonstrated in the following biopsy?

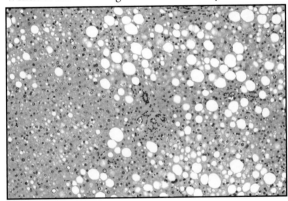 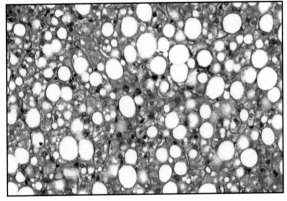

   A. Obesity
   B. Total parenteral nutrition
   C. Malnutrition
   D. Diabetes mellitus
   E. Corticosteroids

8: Liver, Gallbladder, and Extrahepatic Bile Ducts Questions

87. The following biopsy is from a 41-year-old man. Which of the following statements concerning the diagnosis of the biopsy is FALSE? (H&E on the left and Prussian blue stain on the right)

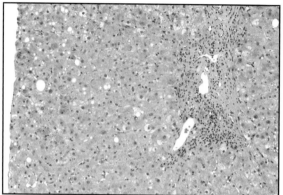 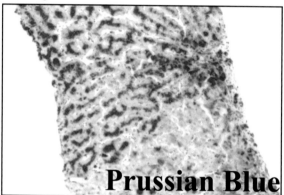

    A.   Acquired hemochromatosis is associated with a prominent lymphocytic response.

    B.   There is increased risk of HCC.

    C.   It affects females at a younger age.

    D.   Hepatic iron index of greater or equal to 2.0 is diagnostic of hemochromatosis.

    E.   It demonstrates initial iron accumulation in the periportal hepatocytes.

88. Which of the following is LEAST likely to be an etiology for the following lesion? (H&E stain on the left and trichrome strain on the right)

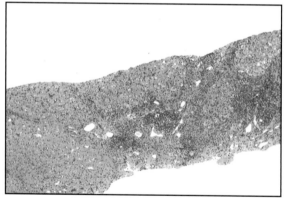 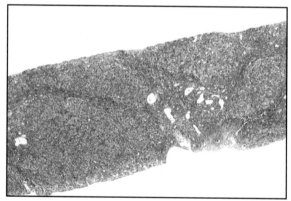

    A.   Alcohol use

    B.   HCV infection

    C.   Acute acetaminophen overdose

    D.   Autoimmune hepatitis

    E.   Wilson disease

8: Liver, Gallbladder, and Extrahepatic Bile Ducts Questions

Questions 89 and 90:

A 65-year-old woman presents with chronic right upper quadrant pain. A routine laparoscopic cholecystostomy was performed, and representative sections are shown below.

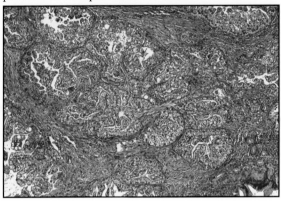 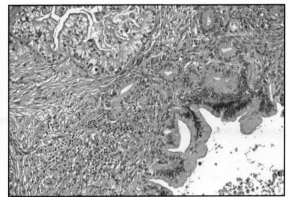

89. The above lesion is LEAST likely to be positive for which marker by immunohistochemistry?
    A. Cytokeratin 7
    B. Cytokeratin 20
    C. Cytokeratin 19
    D. CA19-9
    E. CEA-M

90. Which of the following statements regarding the above lesion is FALSE?
    A. 50% of cases are inoperable at time of diagnosis.
    B. Extension into liver is present in 20% of cases.
    C. Presence in 10% of gallbladders removed in patients over age 65.
    D. It is associated with K-ras codon 12 mutation.
    E. Chemotherapy and radiation therapy are of little value.

91.   A 54-year-old woman presents with itching and a clinical work-up demonstrated elevated alkaline phosphatase and positive AMA. A biopsy was performed and shown below. Which of the following statements regarding the diagnosis is FALSE?

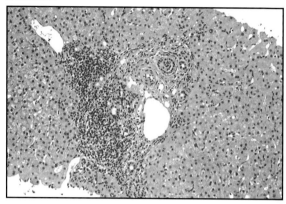 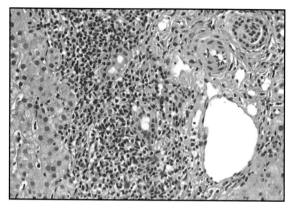

    A.   It is usually anti-M2 positive.
    B.   Without treatment the natural course of disease results in cirrhosis and liver failure.
    C.   Histologic evaluation is required for the diagnosis.
    D.   It predominately affects women.
    E.   All the above are true.

92.   The below biopsy was taken from someone with elevated transaminases and alkaline phosphatase. Which of the follow choices would be the LEAST likely etiology for the findings?

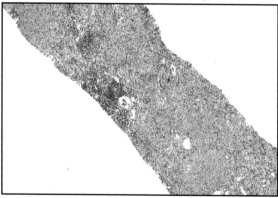 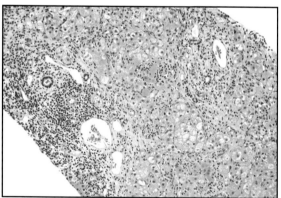

    A.   Hepatitis B virus
    B.   Hepatitis C virus
    C.   Isoniazid
    D.   Tamoxifen
    E.   Autoimmune hepatitis

8: Liver, Gallbladder, and Extrahepatic Bile Ducts Questions

93. A 17-year-old was brought to the ER by his parents with symptoms of frank psychosis. His drugs of abuse screen was negative and his metabolic panel was normal expect for mildly elevated transaminases. A liver biopsy was performed and is shown below. Which of the following is the BEST diagnosis?

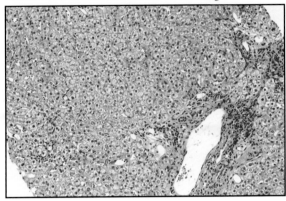
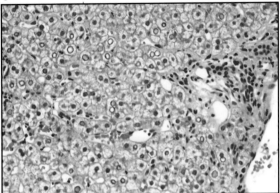

- A. Acute hepatitis A
- B. Wilson disease
- C. Vitamin A overdose
- D. Diabetic glycogenosis
- E. Tricyclic antidepressant

94. A 55-year-old man presents with isolated thrombocytopenia. Otherwise his peripheral blood counts are normal and he has a normal bone marrow biopsy. Imaging demonstrates an enlarged liver with multiple hypo- and hyper-dense areas. A biopsy was performed, and 2 low-magnification images and 1 high-magnification image are shown below. What is the diagnosis?

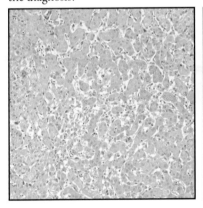
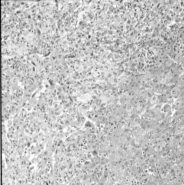
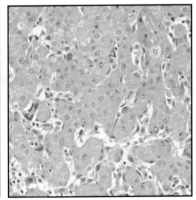

- A. Hepatocellular carcinoma
- B. Metastatic colon cancer
- C. Hemangioma
- D. Angiosarcoma
- E. Cholangiocarcinoma

8: Liver, Gallbladder, and Extrahepatic Bile Ducts Questions

95. A 68-year-old male was undergoing a Whipple resection of pancreatic adenocarcinoma. During the abdominal survey, the surgeon found a grey-white lesion of the liver that measured 0.5 × 0.4 cm. The biopsy of this lesion is shown below. What is the diagnosis?

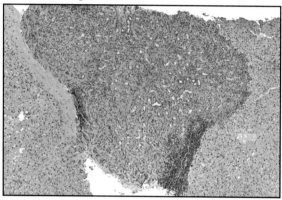 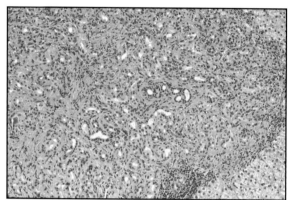

   A.   Metastatic pancreatic adenocarcinoma
   B.   Bile duct adenoma
   C.   Bile duct hamartoma
   D.   Mesenchymal hamartoma
   E.   Intrahepatic cholangiocarcinoma

96. A 60-year-old Japanese woman presents with upper abdominal pain and weight loss. Imaging demonstrates a large solitary mass. Images from the resection specimen are shown below. Which of the following statements concerning the diagnosis is FALSE?

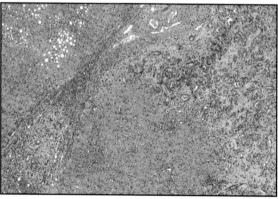 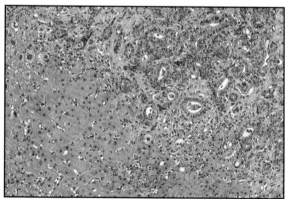

   A.   The neoplastic cells are negative for Hall stain.
   B.   The neoplastic cells are often PAS-D positive.
   C.   There is elevated serum AFP and CEA.
   D.   80% of patients present with unresectable tumors.
   E.   All the above are true.

8: Liver, Gallbladder, and Extrahepatic Bile Ducts Questions

97.   A 53-year-old man was involved in an automobile accident. CT scan of the abdomen demonstrated multiple nodules within the liver, ranging in size from 1-4 cm. After stabilization and treatment of his injuries, one of his liver masses was biopsied. The lesion is shown below. What is the diagnosis?

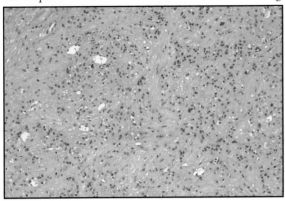 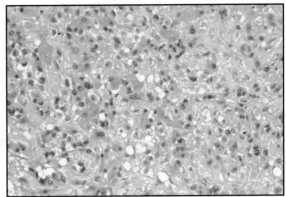

    A.   Epithelioid hemangioendothelioma
    B.   Mesenchymal hamartoma
    C.   Sclerosing hemangioma
    D.   Chondrosarcoma
    E.   Angiosarcoma

98.   The below lesion was resected from a 32-year-old female. What is the diagnosis?

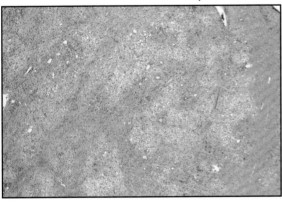 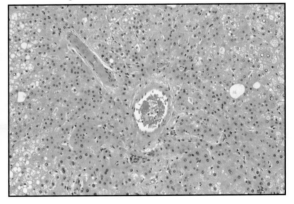

    A.   Nodular regenerative hyperplasia
    B.   Hepatocellular carcinoma
    C.   Focal nodular hyperplasia
    D.   Hepatic adenoma
    E.   Steatohepatitis

99. A 48-year-old female presents with right upper quadrant pain and an ultrasound was found to have a 15-cm multilocular cystic mass. The lesion was resected and representative sections shown below. Which of the following statements concerning the diagnosis is FALSE?

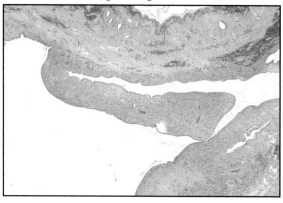 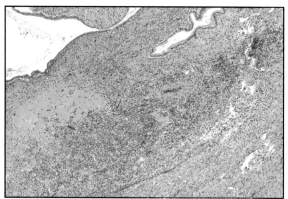

    A. It occurs predominately in women.
    B. Stroma stains for ER and PR.
    C. It is a precursor lesion for cystadenocarcinoma.
    D. Extrahepatic lesions almost always develop into a carcinoma.
    E. There are increased intracystic and serum levels of CA19-9.

100. A 38-year-old woman presented with epigastric pain, and a HIDA scan was consistent with cholecystitis. The patient was scheduled for a laparoscopic cholecystectomy and upon adnominal survey; the liver demonstrated multiple subcentimeter white-grey nodules on the capsule of the liver. One of the lesions was biopsied and representative images are shown below. What is the diagnosis?

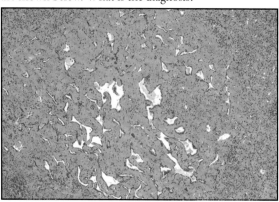 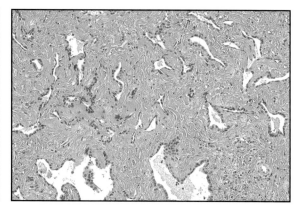

    A. Metastatic gallbladder carcinoma
    B. Bile duct hamartoma
    C. Peribiliary gland hamartoma
    D. Cholangiocarcinoma
    E. Biliary cystadenoma

101. A 28-year-old woman presents with right lower quadrant pain. A CT scan demonstrates an inflamed appendix. Additionally, the CT scan demonstrates a solitary liver lesion involving the right lobe. What of the following statements concerning the below lesion is FALSE?

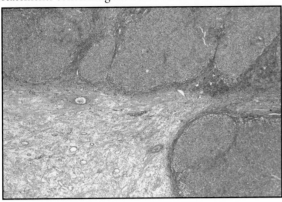 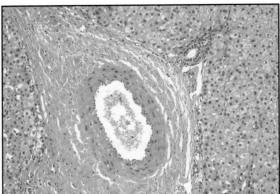

    A. It is caused by oral contraceptive use.

    B. It can be associated with meningiomas.

    C. There is increased risk of berry aneurysm.

    D. It is hypervascular on angiography.

    E. All the above are true.

102. Which of the following statements regarding the lesion demonstrated below is TRUE?

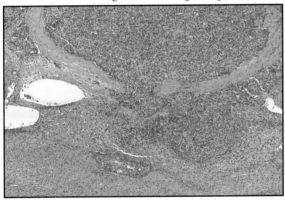 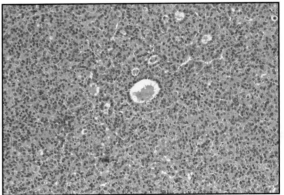

    A. It always occurs in a background of cirrhosis.

    B. Elevated serum AFP levels >10× the upper limit are diagnostic of the above lesion.

    C. Chronic HCV is a greater risk factor than chronic HBV.

    D. It typically develops from hepatic adenoma.

    E. CD34 highlights the lesion.

103. A 48-year-old presents with thrombocytopenia, ascites, and bleeding esophageal varices. He ultimately went to transplant, and representative sections are shown below. What is the diagnosis?

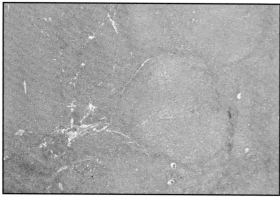

 A. Hepatic adenoma
 B. Hepatocellular carcinoma
 C. Focal nodular hyperplasia
 D. Nodular regenerative hyperplasia
 E. Congenital fibrosis

104. A 31-year old woman had a cholecystectomy, and upon gross inspection, multiple stones were identified along with a thickened gall bladder wall. Representative sections are taken and shown below. What is the diagnosis?

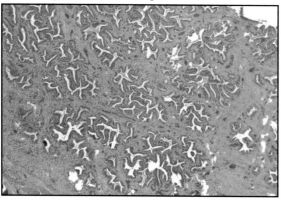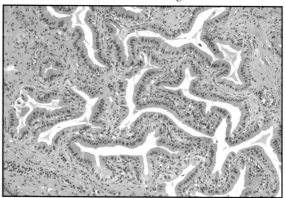

 A. Chronic cholecystis
 B. Gallbladder adenocarcinoma
 C. Pancreatic adenocarcinoma
 D. Adenomyoma/adenomyomatosis
 E. Extrahepatic bile duct carcinoma

8: Liver, Gallbladder, and Extrahepatic Bile Ducts Questions

105. A 64-year-old woman presented with early satiety and upon imaging was found to have a multiloculated intrahepatic cyst. A resection was performed, and representative images are shown below. What is the diagnosis?

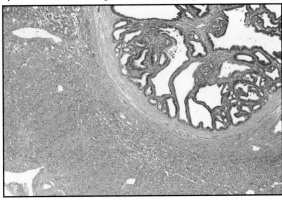 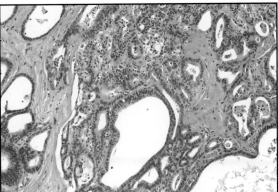

    A.   Biliary cystadenoma
    B.   Biliary papillomatosis
    C.   Polycystic liver disease
    D.   Biliary cystadenocarcinoma
    E.   Acinar hepatocellular carcinoma

106. A 3-month-old infant presents with jaundice. Laboratory findings of cholestasis were present; however, no abnormality was found on ultrasound or physical exam. The liver was biopsied and shown below. What is best the diagnosis?

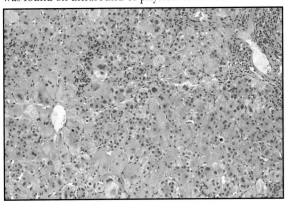 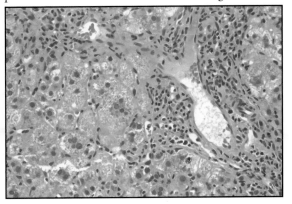

    A.   Extramedullary hematopoiesis
    B.   Neonatal hepatitis
    C.   Alagille syndrome
    D.   Biliary atresia
    E.   Hemophagocytic syndrome

8: Liver, Gallbladder, and Extrahepatic Bile Ducts Answers

1.   D.   **PERIPORTAL NECROSIS/INTERFACE HEPATITIS**

The injury pattern seen in alcohol-related fatty liver disease is primarily found in zone 3 (perivenular). Microscopically, alcohol-related fatty liver disease demonstrates steatosis and an inflammatory infiltrate (lobular in the early phase, portal in the later phases of the disease). A diagnosis of steatohepatitis can be made if the following additional histologic features are present: ballooning degeneration of hepatocytes and/or perisinusoidal/perivenular fibrosis (chicken wire pattern). Mallory-Denk bodies are a microscopic finding supporting the clinical impression of an alcohol-related fatty liver disease.

QCSP, **Alcohol-Related Fatty Liver Disease,** p 296.

2.   C.   **CYTOSKELETON INTERMEDIATE FILAMENTS**

Mallory hyaline consists of clumps, strands, or perinuclear rings of intermediate filaments. Mallory hyaline is chemotactic for neutrophils. Mallory hyaline stains positive for ubiquitin and p62 and occasionally cytokeratins such as CK20. Of note, Councilman bodies are apoptotic hepatocytes.

QCSP, **Alcohol-Related Fatty Liver Disease,** p 296.

3.   C.   **MISFOLDED A1-AT PROTEINS ARE RETAINED IN THE GOLGI BODIES.**

A mutated A1-AT gene leads to misfolding of the A1-AT protein and inhibition of trafficking of the protein from the ER to the Golgi body. Misfolded A1-AT proteins are therefore retained in the endoplasmic reticulum. Patients with A1-AT deficiency have an increased risk of hepatocellular carcinoma and cholangiocarcinoma. The most common phenotype, PIMM (wild type), is associated with normal A1-AT serum levels. Patients who are homozygous, PIZZ, demonstrate A1-AT serum levels that are 10% of normal. Patients with the null phenotype fail to make A1-AT and will develop pulmonary disease without liver disease. It is the build-up of A1-AT that causes liver damage. While the pulmonary symptoms can be treated with aerosol delivered replacement A1-AT, liver transplant is the only treatment for the liver disease. Approximately 72% of patients will die from complications from pulmonary emphysema and another 10% from cirrhotic related disease.

QCSP, **A1-AT Deficiency,** p 297-298.

4.   A.   **ANTIMITOCHONDRIAL ANTIBODIES**

Antimitochondrial antibodies are associated with primary biliary cirrhosis, especially anti-M2. Autoimmune hepatitis is divided into 3 types. Type I is associated with ANA and SMA; type II is associated with anti-LKM (ANA and SMA negative); type III is associated with anti-SLA/LP (ANA and LKM negative).

QCSP, **Autoimmune Hepatitis,** p 298-300.

5.   D.   **DENSE PERIPORTAL LYMPHOCYTIC INFILTRATE WITH PLASMA CELLS**

The typical microscopic features of autoimmune hepatitis include a dense uniform periportal infiltrate of lymphocytes and plasma cells (especially at the interface as well as throughout the lobule; eosinophiles can also be part of the infiltrate), pyknotic necrosis, interface hepatitis, hepatocellular ballooning, and architectural disruption and cell drop-out in centrilobular areas. Additionally, autoimmune hepatitis can demonstrate bridging necrosis, rosette formation, and multinucleated giant hepatocytes.

QCSP, **Autoimmune Hepatitis,** p 298-300.

6.   D.   **CROHN DISEASE**

Autoimmune hepatitis has been associated with other autoimmune disorders including rheumatoid arthritis, thyroiditis, Sjögren syndrome, and ulcerative colitis; as well as autoimmune hemolytic anemia, idiopathic thrombocytopenic purpura, and proliferative glomerulonephritis. Crohn disease has been associated with primary sclerosing cholangitis and not autoimmune hepatitis.

QCSP, **Autoimmune Hepatitis,** p 298-300.

7.   C.   **CIRRHOSIS FROM ANY ETIOLOGY HAS THE SAME OUTCOME/PROGNOSIS.**
All forms of cirrhosis, regardless of etiology, have an improved survival if the underlying etiology is treated. The 5-year survival for cryptogenic cirrhosis is the worst with 25%. The 5-year survival for alcohol-related cirrhosis and active hepatitis (viral)-related cirrhosis is approximately 50%, while the survival for hemochromatosis-related cirrhosis is 70%.
QCSP, **Cirrhosis,** p 300-302.

8.   D.   **LOSS OF BILE DUCTS**
Bile duct damage, while often quite variable, is a characteristic finding in graft-vs-host disease. Specifically, in a patient with a bone marrow transplant, damage to >50% of the bile ducts is presumptive evidence of GVHD. The bile duct damage is characterized by vacuolated or acidophilic cytoplasm, individual cell loss, and pleomorphic nuclei. The lymphocyte infiltrate is typically sparse and within the portal tracts, especially within the epithelial layer of the bile ducts. The hepatocyte damage seen in GVHD is typically single cell ballooning degeneration and scattered focal necrosis.
QCSP, **Graft-vs-Host Disease,** p 302-303.

9.   D.   **PATIENTS USUALLY DIE FROM HEPATIC FAILURE.**
Aside from the increased risk of portal hypertension, which may require a shunting procedure, there is no evidence that this condition limits life expectancy. Microscopically, the liver demonstrates fibrosis without hepatic necrosis or inflammation. While there can be evidence of cholangitis or cholestasis (often seen when associated with Caroli disease), there should be no neocholangigensis.
QCSP, **Congenital Hepatic Fibrosis,** p 303.

10.   A.   **STEATOSIS**
Steatosis is the most common hepatic lesion in a patient with cystic fibrosis. However, the most reliable diagnostic feature is stellate scarring with dilated bile ducts with inspissated eosinophilic (PAS-positive) material. Additionally, liver biopsies can demonstrate a portal inflammatory infiltrate, bile duct proliferation, and bile duct cellular degeneration and necrosis.
QCSP, **Cystic Fibrosis,** p 303-304.

11.   D.   **TOTAL PARENTERAL NUTRITION**
The etiologies for macrovesicular steatosis include alcohol, obesity, diabetes mellitus, corticosteroids, malnutrition, and HCV. Total parenteral nutrition results in microvesicular steatosis.
QCSP, **Fatty Liver,** p 304-306.

12.   A.   **MALLORY-DENK BODIES**
The true best discriminator between alcohol-related and non-alcohol-related fatty liver disease is an accurate (truthful) clinical history. The histological overlap is often too great to distinguish both entities on morphology alone. Mallory hyaline is more specific for alcohol-related fatty liver disease; however, it may also be present in non-alcohol-related fatty liver disease. When Mallory hyaline is present in non-alcohol-related fatty liver disease, it tends to be sparser. Additionally, both types of fatty liver disease demonstrate infiltration by a mixed population of immune cells including neutrophils and mononuclear lymphocytes. Although alcohol-related liver disease tends to demonstrate a more intense neutrophil infiltrate. The pattern of fibrosis and distribution of fatty change are similar in both entities as well.
QCSP, **Fatty Liver,** p 304-306.

13.   B.   **WILSON DISEASE**
Wilson disease demonstrates glycogenated nuclei but typically does not demonstrate fatty change. The etiologies for microvesicular steatosis include fatty liver of pregnancy, Reye syndrome, total parenteral nutrition, and certain

drugs. While alcohol usually leads to a macrovesicular steatosis, there is a variant of alcohol-induced liver injury known as alcoholic foamy degeneration, which presents with microvesicular steatosis.
QCSP, **Fatty Liver,** p 304-306.

14.   E.   **ANGIOMYOLIPOMA**
Mallory-Denk bodies can been seen in a variety of disorders, including fatty liver disease, Wilson disease, cholestatic diseases, hepatocellular carcinoma, hepatocellular adenoma, and amiodarone toxicity. Mallory-Denk bodies can be highlighted by a trichrome stain or immunohistochemical stains for p62, ubiquitin, and cytokeratins CK8/CK18.
QCSP, **Fatty Liver,** p 304-306.

15.   D.   **SATELLITOSIS IS MORE COMMON IN NON-ALCOHOL-RELATED STEATOHEPATITIS.**
Satellitosis is the ringing of neutrophils around Mallory-Denk body containing hepatocytes and is more often seen in alcohol-related liver disease. Sclerosing hyaline necrosis is characterized by extensive hepatocyte necrosis in a perivenular pattern with associated fibrous deposition. This can occlude the terminal hepatic venules leading to portal hypertension (in the absence of cirrhosis). Mallory-Denk bodies are typically more plentiful in alcohol-related steatohepatitis and remain even after disappearance of fatty changes.
QCSP, **Fatty Liver,** p 304-306.

16.   A.   **α-1-ANTITRYPSIN DEFICIENCY**
Megamitochondria are primarily seen in alcohol-related liver disease, but can also be seen in Wilson disease, normal pregnancy as well as fatty liver of pregnancy. Patients with α-1-antitrypsin liver disease do not have megamitochondria but do have globules of misfolded α-1-antitrypsin. Both megamitochondria and α-1-antitrypsin globules have a similar eosinophilic appearance histologically. However, megamitochondria are PAS negative and primarily in zone 3 hepatocytes, while α-1-antitrypsin globules are PAS positive and primarily in the periportal region.
QCSP, **Fatty Liver,** p 304-306.

17.   B.   **QUANTITATIVE HEPATIC IRON CONTENT**
The most reliable method for hemochromatosis diagnosis is the quantitation of iron in dry/unfixed liver tissue. "Bronzing" of the skin can be seen in 75%-80% of patients. Molecular testing for the HFE gene (chromosome 6) can identify patients who are heterozygous or homozygous. But not all cases of hemochromatosis have a genetic cause and not all patients with HFE mutations develop symptomatic hemochromatosis. Iron staining of the biopsy can demonstrate the presence of stainable iron stores; however, this can be nonspecific, as several conditions can lead to increased stainable iron in the liver without dramatic increase in quantitative iron. Serum iron concentration, serum ferritin, transferrin saturation, and total iron-binding capacity are often elevated in hemochromatosis but are not as specific as the quantitative determination of the iron content in liver tissue.
QCSP, **Hemochromatosis,** p 306-307.

18.   E.   **WILSON DISEASE**
Neonatal hepatitis accounts for around 35% of all cases of neonatal cholestasis. While the etiology is usually unknown, the established etiologies include infectious agents (such as CMV, rubella, herpes simplex, *Toxoplasma gondii,* varicella, coxsackievirus, HIV, treponema), disorders of amino acid metabolism (tyrosinemia), disorders of carbohydrate metabolism (glycogen storage disease, galactosemia, fructosemia), inborn errors of bile synthesis, and α-1-antitrypsin disease.
QCSP, **Neonatal Hepatitis,** p 307-309.

8: Liver, Gallbladder, and Extrahepatic Bile Ducts Answers

19.   A.   **EXTENSIVE BILE DUCTULAR PROLIFERATION**
Neonatal hepatitis can demonstrate a mild inflammatory infiltrate in the portal tracts with occasional bile ductular proliferation. An extensive amount of ductular proliferation in the majority of the portal tracts should make one consider neonatal hepatitis. Both can demonstrate giant multinucleated hepatocytes and cholestasis, while cholestatic rosettes are more common in neonatal hepatitis. Additionally, viral inclusions are seen in neonatal hepatitis (CMV and HSV) but not biliary atresia.
QCSP, **Neonatal Hepatitis,** p 307-309.

20.   D.   **ULCERATIVE COLITIS**
Ulcerative colitis is more closely associated with primary sclerosing cholangitis. Several autoimmune/degenerative diseases are associated with primary biliary cirrhosis including Sjögren syndrome, CREST syndrome, osteoporosis, autoimmune thyroiditis, rheumatoid arthritis, renal tubular acidosis, celiac disease, and HLA-DR8.
QCSP, **Primary Biliary Cirrhosis,** p 309-310.

21.   C.   **ANTIMITOCHONDRIAL ANTIBODIES**
Primary biliary cirrhosis patients have elevated alkaline phosphatase levels. Approximately 90% of patients have detectable antimitochondrial antibodies (often referred to as M2) against the E2 subunit of pyruvate dehydrogenase complex. This protein is found in mitochondria and in the epithelial cells lining the intralobular bile ducts. These patients also have elevated immunoglobulins, specifically IgM.
QCSP, **Primary Biliary Cirrhosis,** p 309-310.

22.   A.   **RHODAMINE**
Rhodamine can be used to stain copper. Excess copper is typically excreted in the bile; however if bile epithelium is damaged, there is decreased copper excretion and increased intrahepatic copper. Prussian blue is used to stain iron, trichrome stain highlights collagen and fibrosis, and a reticulin stain highlights the reticular fibers and the lobular architecture. In the liver, PAS highlights α-1-antitrypisin globules but can also highlight the residual basement membrane in injured or destroyed bile ducts.
QCSP, **Primary Biliary Cirrhosis,** p 309-310.

23.   E.   **ALL THESE FINDINGS ARE ASSOCIATED WITH PBC.**
The progression of the disease is divided into 4 stages. Stage I (florid duct lesion) is characterized by the destruction of septal and intralobular bile ducts with granulomatous inflammation and the presence of irregular and hyperplastic bile duct epithelium. Stage II (ductular proliferation) shows a decrease in the active bile duct damage with proliferation of bile ductules as well as periportal interface hepatitis. Stage III (bridging and septal fibrosis) demonstrates progressive loss of bile ducts with increased septal fibrosis. The pattern of inflammation and fibrosis produces a halo effect at low power. Stage IV (cirrhosis) is end-stage cirrhosis.
QCSP, **Primary Biliary Cirrhosis,** p 309-310.

24.   C.   **THE DIAGNOSIS IS TYPICALLY MADE ON LIVER BIOPSY.**
As compared to other autoimmune liver diseases, primary sclerosing cholangitis occurs more often in men than women. The histologic findings may be heterogeneous and are not always diagnostic. On ERCP, there is a characteristic beaded appearance of the intrahepatic biliary ducts with irregular strictures and secondary dilations. There is an increased risk of cholangiocarcinoma and gallbladder carcinoma in patients with primary sclerosing cholangitis. The survival of patients is approximately 10-12 years.
QCSP, **Primary Sclerosing Cholangitis,** p 311-312.

25.   E.   **NONE OF THE ABOVE**
While patients with primary sclerosing cholangitis can have elevated ANA (80% of patients) or hypergammaglobulinemia (30% of patients), these are not specific for the disease. PBC patients demonstrate

313

8: Liver, Gallbladder, and Extrahepatic Bile Ducts Answers

AMA and elevated IgM. Elevated ANA can also be seen in autoimmune hepatitis and PBC-autoimmune overlap syndrome.

QCSP, **Primary Sclerosing Cholangitis,** p 311-312.

26.   E.   ALL OF THE ABOVE ARE ASSOCIATED.

Veno-occlusive disease (VOD) is thought to occur secondary to damage to the endothelium of the central vein or centrilobular sinusoids initiating a fibrotic cascade leading to fibrous occlusion. All the mentioned agents are associated with the development of VOD. Other agents associated with VOD are azathioprine in renal transplant, hepatic irradiation, arsenic poisoning, thorotrast exposure, etc.

QCSP, **Veno-Occlusive Disease,** p 312-313.

27.   D.   HDV

HBV patients with coinfection or superinfection of hepatitis D have the greatest incidence of fulminant hepatitis, approximately 1%-10% and 5%-20%, respectively. The other infections listed have an incidence of fulminant hepatitis at around 0.2%. Survival rate for fulminant hepatitis is 5%-20%.

QCSP, **Viral Hepatitis,** p 313-317.

28.   C.   INTERFACE HEPATITIS

Chronic viral hepatitis demonstrates accentuation of the inflammatory response in the portal and periportal regions often demonstrating interface hepatitis (piecemeal necrosis). In acute hepatitis the inflammatory infiltrate is often located in zone 3. While portal inflammation can be seen in acute hepatitis, the inflammation in acute hepatitis is typically composed of a mixed infiltrate and restricted to portal fibrous tissue. However, a severe acute viral hepatitis can cause spillover of the inflammation into the periportal parenchyma, resembling interface hepatitis.

QCSP, **Viral Hepatitis,** p 313-317.

29.   B.   THE CONDITION IS TRANSMITTED AS AN AUTOSOMAL DOMINANT TRAIT.

Wilson disease is an autosomal recessive disease with the defective gene located on 13q-14.3 encoding a P-type ATPase that transports copper. The remaining answers are true.

QCSP, **Wilson Disease,** p 317-318.

30.   B.   SERUM COPPER LEVELS

The key finding is the accumulation of copper in the liver and other organs (brain, cornea, kidney, striated muscle, bones and joints). This manifests as Kayser-Fleischer rings, increased quantitative copper in the liver biopsy, as well as low serum ceruloplasmin and increased urinary copper excretion. Serum copper levels have little value in the work-up for Wilson disease.

QCSP, **Wilson Disease,** p 317-318.

31.   B.   MELAN-A

Angiomyolipoma belongs to a group of tumors known as PEComas (perivascular epithelioid cell tumors, which include cardiac rhabdomyoma, lymphangiomyomatosis, and clear cell "sugar" tumor of the lung). This group of tumors is positive for Melan-A and HMB-45, and focally positive for S100, since these tumors are an admixture of adipose tissue and thick-walled blood vessels. In angiomyolipomas, the endothelial cells are positive for CD34. A Sudan black highlights the lipomatous part of the tumor.

QCSP, **Angiomyolipoma,** p 318-319.

8: Liver, Gallbladder, and Extrahepatic Bile Ducts Answers

32. **D. A AND B**

The microscopic features of angiomyolipoma include a mixture of adipose tissue along with thick-walled blood vessels. The stromal cells demonstrated smooth muscle differentiation. These tumors can also demonstrate extramedullary hematopoiesis; however, this feature is only present in a minority of cases.

QCSP, **Angiomyolipoma,** p 318-319.

33. **E. EPITHELIOID HEMANGIOENDOTHELIOMA**

Hepatic angiosarcoma can be associated with an etiologic agent in 25%-45% of cases. These include thorotrast (radiographic contrast), vinyl chloride, arsenic, androgenic steroids, cooper sulfate, estrogenic steroids, radiotherapy, etc. Additionally, angiosarcomas can occur in children in the setting of infantile hemangioendothelioma. There is no known risk of developing angiosarcoma in the setting of epithelioid hemangioendothelioma.

QCSP, **Angiosarcoma,** p 319-320.

34. **D. HERPAR-1**

Angiosarcoma typically expresses endothelial markers such as CD31, CD34, ulex lectin, factor VIII, and Fli-1. Factor VIII is typically thought to be the most sensitive and specific marker for hepatic angiosarcoma. The malignant cells can also express keratin, which can be a pitfall. Entrapped hepatocytes will express HerPar-1, but the neoplastic cells of angiosarcoma are negative for this marker.

QCSP, **Angiosarcoma,** p 319-320.

35. **A. MOC-31**

Both bile duct hamartoma and metastatic adenocarcinoma can express MOC-31. Bile duct adenoma/hamartoma is usually positive for Dpc4 but negative for mesothelin, B72.3, and monoclonal CEA. Metastatic pancreatic adenocarcinoma can lose expression of Dpc4, but express B72.3, mesothelin, and monoclonal CEA.

QCSP, **Bile Duct Adenoma,** p 320; Odze, p 1310.

36. **A. IT IS USUALLY A SOLITARY LESION.**

Bile duct hamartomas are usually multiple small lesions (<0.5 cm). They consist of irregularly cystically dilated biliary ducts with bile (or eosinophilic material) embedded in a densely fibrous/hyalinized stroma without a significant inflammatory infiltrate. These lesions have been associated with polycystic kidney disease, Caroli disease, portal hypertension and congenital hepatic fibrosis. No cellular atypia is seen in this lesion.

QCSP, **Bile Duct Adenoma/Bile Duct Microhamartoma,** p 320-321.

37. **D. BILE IS PRESENT WITHIN BILE LUMENS.**

Bile duct adenomas are composed of, usually solitary, small well-formed ducts that contain intracytoplasmic mucin (positive for mucicarmine or alcian blue stain). These ducts are not dilated and do not contain bile. The stroma can be sclerotic or edematous and fibrous. The stroma can contain inflammatory cells including lymphoid follicles and granulomas.

QCSP, **Bile Duct Adenoma/Bile Duct Microhamartoma,** p 320-321.

38. **B. CD5**

Cholangiocarcinoma can be challenging to differentiate from pancreatic ductal adenocarcinoma; however, there are a few stains that assist in arriving at the correct diagnosis. Specifically, a greater proportion of cholangiocarcinomas will stain for CD5 and MUC2 than pancreatic ductal adenocarcinoma. Both types of tumors stain positive for p-CEA, MOC-31, CK 7/CK19, and Ber-EP4.

QCSP, **Cholangiocarcinoma,** p 322.

8: Liver, Gallbladder, and Extrahepatic Bile Ducts Answers

39.   E.   **IT IS ASSOCIATED WITH CIRRHOSIS.**

Bile duct carcinoma (intrahepatic cholangiocarcinoma) often presents as a multicentric disease resembling metastatic disease. The lesions typically occur in noncirrhotic livers. Intrahepatic cholangiocarcinoma is a mucin-secreting tumor highlighted by alcian blue or mucicarmine stains. The same neoplastic glands may demonstrate heterogeneity of the cells from a cuboidal or columnar appearance to a papillary pattern. It is often difficult to determine the presence of carcinoma at time of frozen section. Often times, perineural invasion may be the only definite sign of malignancy. Additionally, when a stromal reaction is evident, it appears as concentric layering of the cellular stroma around the neoplastic glands.

QCSP, **Cholangiocarcinoma,** p 322.

40.   A.   **ECHINOCOCCUS GRANULOSUS**

The *Echinococcus* species is a cyclophyllidae parasite that causes hydatid disease. Humans are an accidental host and are also considered the end host. The majority of cases of echinococcal (hydatid) cyst are the result of *Echinococcus granulosus* infection. All the above listed species of *Echinococcus* have been identified as causative agents in human disease, except *Echinococcus shiquicus. Echinococcus multilocularis* has the worst prognosis, leading to progressive disease resulting in death unless radical hepatic resection eliminates all disease.

QCSP, **Echinococcal Cyst,** p 323-324.

41.   B.   **DIAGNOSIS IS USUALLY MADE BY FNA.**

Echinococcal cysts are usually asymptomatic until they are >10 cm in size. The walls of the cyst typically calcify aiding the diagnosis by CT scan. Additionally, serologic testing can detect infection. Skin tests as well as peripheral blood analysis to detect eosinophilia, however, are only worthwhile if the cyst/parasites are viable. While it is common for the cyst to calcify, calcification of the germinal layer (layer that gives rise to the brood capsules) indicates that the cyst is dead. The mass effect of the cyst on the surrounding liver tissue can result in hepatic atrophy. The surrounding liver tissue can also demonstrate associated portal inflammation with eosinophiles. While infection with *E granulosus* often results in a single large cyst, infection with *E multilocularis* is a more insidious infection, which can clinically mimic a hepatic malignancy or a "metastasis." While surgery is the preferred method of treatment, inoperable patients can be treated with aspiration, instilment of a scolicidal agent and reaspiration. Problems with FNA of the cyst include rupture, possible dissemination of the disease and anaphylaxis.

QCSP, **Echinococcal Cyst,** p 323-324.

42.   A.   **THE INTRACELLULAR AND EXTRACELLULAR EOSINOPHILIC GLOBULES STAIN FOR α-FETOPROTEIN.**

Microscopically, embryonal sarcoma demonstrates variably sized intracellular and extracellular eosinophilic globules, which contain α-1-chymotrypsin, albumin, and α-1-antitrypsin but NOT α-fetoprotein. Embryonal sarcoma is an aggressive malignancy with a poor prognosis; often patients are dead within 1 year of diagnosis. It can extend into the vena cava and into the heart. Several reports suggest that embryonal sarcoma may arise from mesenchymal hamartomas because both demonstrate 19q chromosomal abnormalities. Extramedullary hematopoiesis can be seen in approximately 50% of cases.

QCSP, **Embryonal Sarcoma,** p 324-325.

43.   B.   **ANABOLIC STEROIDS**

High-risk factors for the development of hepatocellular carcinoma include infections by HBV and HCV (greatest risk for HBV infection), hemochromatosis, tyrosinemia, porphyria cutanea tarda, and hypercitrullinemia. Lower-risk factors include PBC, PSC, congenital hepatic fibrosis, biliary atresia, Wilson disease, oral contraceptives, and anabolic steroids.

QCSP, **Hepatocellular Carcinoma,** p 325-328.

8: Liver, Gallbladder, and Extrahepatic Bile Ducts Answers

44.   C.   β-CATENIN

β-catenin is not a reliable differentiating marker between HCC and adenocarcinoma, NOS. There is a subpopulation of HCC that has β-catenin mutations that lead to nuclear accumulation and subsequent positive nuclear staining. These tumors are typically lower grade and have a better prognosis than tumors with overexpression of β-catenin in the cytoplasm. MOC-31 is a specific and sensitive marker for adenocarcinoma and usually negative in HCC (except the mixed HCC and cholangiocarcinoma). HCC is usually positive for HepPar-1 (except for the poorly differentiated HCC). CEA-polyclonal demonstrates a canalicular pattern in HCC, while adenocarcinomas show a cytoplasmic or membranous pattern. CEA-monoclonal IHC is typically negative in HCC but is often positive in other adenocarcinomas, such as pancreatic and colorectal adenocarcinoma.

QCSP, **Hepatocellular Carcinoma**, p 325-332; Odze, p 1304-1305.

45.   B.   RETICULIN

One of the major features separating well-differentiated HCC from benign proliferation/neoplasms is the size of the cell plate. If the plate is 3 cells or more in thickness, the lesion is consistent with HCC. A reticulin stain highlights the thickened plates as well as the loss of the reticulin framework seen in early HCC. While the other stains are useful in the work up of various hepatic processes, they are usually useless in differentiating a benign hepatic lesion from HCC. In addition to reticulin, glypican-3 has shown promise in differentiating HCC from other liver lesions.

QCSP, **Hepatocellular Carcinoma**, p 325-328.

46.   A.   BILE PRODUCTION BY NEOPLASTIC CELLS

The pathognomonic feature of HCC is the production of bile by the tumor cells or the presence of bile canaliculi (usually seen by EM). While elevated serum AFP is present in the majority of HCC cases, it is not specific for HCC, as germ-cell tumors can secrete high levels of AFP. While cirrhosis is a typical finding in livers with HCC, it is neither sensitive nor specific for the diagnosis of HCC. Elevated serum CEA is seen in a variety of neoplastic processes, such as medullary thyroid, breast, colorectal, liver, lung, ovarian, pancreatic, and prostatic carcinomas. LOH in 8p is a common finding in HCC as well as colorectal, renal, prostatic, and breast carcinoma.

QCSP, **Hepatocellular Carcinoma**, p 325-328.

47.   A.   THE MAJORITY OF PATIENTS HAVE ELEVATED α-FETOPROTEIN LEVELS.

Unlike conventional HCC, the fibrolamellar variant does not typically demonstrate elevated α-fetoprotein levels. Additionally, in comparison to conventional HCC, the fibrolamellar variant occurs in younger patients and often (90%) occurs in noncirrhotic livers. The increased number/volume of mitochondria gives the tumor its oncocytic appearance. Focal nodular hyperplasia (FNH) can be seen at the edge of fibrolamellar HCC. This is believed to be due vascular abnormalities cause by the tumor. FNH is NOT considered a precursor lesion to fibrolamellar HCC.

QCSP, **Fibrolamellar Hepatocellular Carcinoma**, p 328-329.

48.   D.   THE PATIENT IS 2 YEARS OLD.

Infantile hemangioendothelioma is almost always present in patients under the age of 6 months. Kasabach-Merritt syndrome is a consumptive thrombocytopenia and coagulopathy seen in patients with vascular tumors. This can lead to disseminated intravascular coagulation. Electron microscopy of the tumor demonstrates Weibel-Palade bodies, which are storage granules containing von Willebrand factor and P-selectin in endothelial-derived cells. The center of the lesion is particularly at risk for developing cavernous changes with intravascular thrombosis as well as dystrophic calcifications.

QCSP, **Infantile Hemangioendothelioma**, p 329-330.

8: Liver, Gallbladder, and Extrahepatic Bile Ducts Answers

49. **B. CUTANEOUS HEMANGIOMAS**

Patients with infantile hemangioendothelioma commonly demonstrate cutaneous hemangiomas as well as hemangiomas of other organs. Additionally, there are reports of angiosarcoma development even after regression of infantile hemangioendothelioma. There is no association between infantile hemangioendothelioma and epithelioid hemangioendothelioma, undifferentiated sarcoma, or intrauterine exposure to oral contraceptive.
QCSP, **Infantile Hemangioendothelioma,** p 329-330.

50. **C. PANKERATIN**

Epithelioid hemangioendothelioma is typically positive for CD31, CD34, and factor VIII. MOC-31 is a fairly sensitive marker for adenocarcinoma. Epithelioid hemangioendothelioma can be positive for keratin stains, especially low-molecular-weight keratins, such as CK7. Additionally, entrapped normal liver parenchyma will stain positive for a pankeratin stain.
QCSP, **Epithelioid Hemangioendothelioma,** p 330-331.

51. **C. MUCIN STAINING OF NEOPLASTIC CELLS**

The intracytoplasmic vacuoles in the neoplastic cells can mimic signet-ring cells. High-power examination of the vacuolated cells ("blister cells") in epithelioid hemangioendothelioma can demonstrate RBCs within these incipient vascular lumina. Since these vacuoles represent vascular lumina, they do not stain for mucin, unlike signet-ring carcinoma.
QCSP, **Epithelioid Hemangioendothelioma,** p 330-331.

52. **D. PALE BODIES**

It is believed that hepatoblastoma arises from multipotential blastema, due to the various observed tissue types such as osteoid, neural tissue, cartilage, striated muscle, keratinized squamous cell, etc. Extramedullary hematopoiesis is often associated with the "fetal component" (epithelial type). Hepatoblastoma demonstrates multiple growth patterns including the trabecular pattern. Pale bodies are "ground glass" intracytoplasmic inclusions seen in fibrolamellar hepatocellular carcinoma and stain positive for fibrinogen.
QCSP, **Hepatoblastoma,** p 331-333.

53. **A. hCG**

In cases where the patient presents with precocious puberty or virilization, the hepatoblastoma will demonstrate multinucleated giant cells that morphologically mimic syncytiotrophoblasts. These cells stain positive for human chorionic gonadotropin, but not α-fetoprotein.
QCSP, **Hepatoblastoma,** p 331-333.

54. **A. FETAL PATTERN**

The fetal pattern typically has the best prognosis, while the small cell undifferentiated and the macrotrabecular patterns have a worse prognosis. Interestingly, tumors with osteoid can be associated with a better prognosis. Osteoid is often seen in treated tumor sections.
QCSP, **Hepatoblastoma,** p 331-333.

55. **B. FIBROLAMELLAR HEPATOCELLULAR CARCINOMA**

Epithelioid hemangioendothelioma demonstrates a myxohyaline matrix. The small cell undifferentiated pattern of hepatoblastoma can demonstrate mucoid stroma, while the mixed epithelial/mesenchymal type can demonstrate myxoid change. Embryonal sarcoma demonstrates a mucopolysaccharide myxoid stroma, while mesenchymal hamartoma often exhibits edematous myxoid stroma.
QCSP, **Epithelioid Hemangioendothelioma,** p 330-331.

8: Liver, Gallbladder, and Extrahepatic Bile Ducts Answers

56. E. **ALL OF THE ABOVE CAN BE PRESENT AT BIRTH.**

    Neuroblastoma, hemangioma, and teratomas can all be present at birth and can be detected by prenatal ultrasound. Approximately 5% of hepatoblastoma patients will have signs of disease at birth.

    QCSP, **Hepatoblastoma,** p 331-333.

57. D. **UNDIFFERENTIATED EMBRYONAL SARCOMA, HEPATIC**

    Elevated α-fetoprotein levels can be seen in all these hepatic lesions except for undifferentiated embryonal sarcoma. This is in stark contrast to the embryonal components of hepatoblastoma and testicular germ-cell tumor, which express high levels of α-fetoprotein. Yolk sac tumors (endodermal sinus tumor) are known to express high levels of AFP. In patients with conventional HCC, only 30%-40% of patients have elevated AFP levels, while <10% of fibrolamellar hepatocellular carcinoma patients demonstrate elevated serum AFP.

    QCSP, **Embryonal Sarcoma,** p 324-325.

58. E. **LACK OF BILE DUCTULES**

    The differential between hepatic adenoma and focal nodular hyperplasia can be challenging on biopsy. Both hepatic adenoma and focal nodular hyperplasia lack true bile ducts; however, bile ductules are present in focal nodular hyperplasia, often within the fibrous tissue. Bile ductules are absent in liver cell adenomas. While focal nodular hyperplasia demonstrates central (or eccentric) scar tissue, larger hepatic adenomas that have infracted will also have scar tissue. Steatosis and Mallory-Denk bodies/hyaline are nonspecific findings that can be seen in either lesion.

    QCSP, **Hepatocellular (Liver Cell) Adenoma,** p 334-335.

59. E. **B AND D**

    Hepatocellular carcinoma expresses α-fetoprotein (30%-40% of cases), while hepatocellular adenomas are negative. Additionally, glypican-3 is proposed as a new specific marker to differentiate benign from malignant lesions (some well-differentiated HCCs are negative). Both hepatocellular adenoma and carcinoma can stain positive for pankeratin (especially, low-molecular-weight cytokeratins, such as CK8 and CK18). While capillarization of sinusoids (expression of CD34 by cells in the hepatic sinusoids) is typical of hepatocellular carcinoma, it can also be seen in cases of hepatocellular adenoma.

    QCSP, **Hepatocellular (Liver Cell) Adenoma,** p 334-335.

60. D. **VASCULAR INSULT**

    The etiologies associated with hepatocellular adenoma are the exposure to sex hormones (which include oral contraceptives), anabolic steroids, estrogens, and sex hormone-producing ovarian tumor. Additionally, hepatocellular adenoma can be seen in patients with types Ia, III, or IV glycogen storage disease. Vascular insults are thought to be the cause of focal nodular hyperplasia.

    QCSP, **Hepatocellular (Liver Cell) Adenoma,** p 334-335.

61. B. **CIRRHOSIS**

    By definition, hepatocellular adenoma CANNOT occur in a background of cirrhosis (such lesions would probably be best classified as macroregenerative nodules vs dysplastic nodule vs well-differentiated HCC). While most adenomas occur in women of reproductive age, approximately 5% occur in males. Most adenomas (70%) consist of a solitary lesion, but multiple lesions can occur, especially in patients taking anabolic steroids. Large hepatocellular adenomas can rupture and lead to hemoperitoneum. The amount of reticulin is usually retained in hepatocellular adenoma, but can be slightly reduced.

    QCSP, **Hepatocellular (Liver Cell) Adenoma,** p 334-335.

8: Liver, Gallbladder, and Extrahepatic Bile Ducts Answers

62.   C.   **MESENCHYMAL HAMARTOMA**

Mesenchymal hamartoma demonstrates branched (often cystically dilated) bile ducts in a myxoid (often edematous) stroma, which can resemble a fibroadenoma of the breast. Additionally, the stroma demonstrates numerous thick-walled veins and foci of extramedullary hematopoiesis.

QCSP, **Mesenchymal Hamartoma,** p 335-336.

63.   B.   **FOCAL NODULAR HYPERPLASIA**

Focal nodular hyperplasia is associated with vascular abnormalities such as hepatic hemangioma. Additionally, some of these patients may demonstrate telangiectasias of the brain, berry aneurysms, dysplastic systemic arteries, and portal vein atresia. Focal nodular hyperplasia is thought arise as a result of a vascular injury/insult.

QCSP, **Focal Nodular Hyperplasia,** p 336-337.

64.   A.   **CD34**

Unlike HCC (and occasionally hepatic adenoma), focal nodular hyperplasia does not demonstrate capillarization of the sinusoids and as such does not demonstrate sinusoidal staining by CD34. The bile ductular proliferation seen primarily in the septa would be highlighted by CK7 or CK19 stains. PAS staining can highlight Mallory hyaline seen in hepatocytes adjacent to the fibrous septa. Additionally, α-1-antitrypsin and copper (rhodamine) staining can be seen in hepatocytes adjacent to the fibrous septa. Generally features of cholestasis are seen in the hepatocytes near the fibrous septa.

QCSP, **Focal Nodular Hyperplasia,** p 336-337.

65.   E.   **A, B, AND C**

All of the above lesions can be associated with exposure to chemotherapeutic agents. Additionally, hypersensitivity, toxic hepatitis, and chronic hepatitis (methotrexate) can be seen with chemotherapeutic agent exposure.

QCSP, **Nodular Regenerative Hyperplasia,** p 337-338.

66.   D.   **FIBROSIS**

Fibrosis is not seen in nodular regenerative hyperplasia. Nodular regenerative hyperplasia contains hepatocytes similar to the surrounding normal parenchyma (lipid/glycogen content). These lesions usually arise from a periportal position. The regenerative nodule lacks the normal reticulin network, which is usually collapsed around the periphery of the nodule along with atrophic hepatocytes. These lesions can cause narrowing/obliteration of the portal veins, resulting in portal hypertension.

QCSP, **Nodular Regenerative Hyperplasia,** p 337-338.

67.   E.   **A, B, AND C**

There are 3 types of metaplasia recognized in the gallbladder. The least common is squamous metaplasia. Of note, the presence of squamous metaplasia should prompt the pathologist to search for the often-associated dysplasia and/or carcinoma. The most common type of metaplasia is gastric metaplasia, which can be seen in up to 1/2 of patients with cholelithiasis. Another type is intestinal metaplasia demonstrating goblet cells with acid mucin (alcian blue-positive mucin). Intestinal metaplasia is associated with an increased risk for the development of gallbladder carcinoma.

QCSP, **Adenomyoma and Adenomyomatosis,** p 338-339.

68.   E.   **THERE IS AN INCREASED RISK FOR THE DEVELOPMENT OF EXTRAHEPATIC BILE DUCT CARCINOMA IN PATIENTS WITH PRIMARY BILIARY CIRRHOSIS.**

Bile duct carcinoma is usually well differentiated, often to the degree that it is difficult to separate benign from reactive glands. Oftentimes, the diagnosis requires the presence of perineural invasion or the presence of a desmoplastic response. The perihilar-located tumors (Klatskin tumors) have a worse prognosis than the more distally located tumors. Papillary tumors have a better prognosis (probably secondary to mass effect and early symptoms) and are only superficially invasive.

QCSP, **Bile Duct Carcinoma - Extrahepatic,** p 339-340.

69.　D.　**THE STROMA STAINS POSITIVE FOR ER AND PR.**

The stroma is typically cellular resembling ovarian-type stroma. Similar to ovarian mucinous neoplasms and pancreatic mucinous cystic neoplasms, the stroma stains positive for the estrogen and progesterone receptor. The presence of ovarian-type stroma is associated with a more favorable prognosis. However, the stroma is only present in women and NOT men. These tumors are found in an intrahepatic location, representing 1% of primary malignant liver neoplasms. Biliary cystadenomas occur primarily in women (95%); however, biliary cystadenocarcinomas affect both older men and women equally.

QCSP, **Biliary Cystadenocarcinoma,** p 340-341.

70.　B.　**PANCREATIC MUCINOUS CYSTIC NEOPLASM**

Both hepatobiliary cystadenomas and pancreatic mucinous cystic neoplasms demonstrate dense cellular subepithelial spindle cell stroma, resembling ovarian stroma. Biliary cystadenomas are mostly mucinous with intestinal-type epithelium with goblet cells. Interestingly, a focal hyalinized collagenous zone is frequently present between the epithelium and dense stroma, resembling collagenous colitis. Choledochal cysts can demonstrate surface columnar epithelium with dense fibrous tissue and smooth muscle in the cyst wall.

QCSP, **Biliary Cystadenoma,** p 341-342.

71.　A.　**INTRAHEPATIC**

Approximately 85% of biliary cystadenomas occur in an intrahepatic location. The intrahepatic lesion can give rise to biliary cystadenocarcinoma; however, extrahepatic lesions have not been shown to undergo malignant transformation.

QCSP, **Biliary Cystadenoma,** p 341-342.

72.　D.　**BILIARY ATRESIA**

Gallbladder carcinoma is associated with an abnormal choledochopancreatic junction, in which the bile duct and the pancreatic duct combine prior to the sphincter of Oddi (which allows reflux of the pancreatic secretions into the biliary system). Additionally, an increased risk for the development of gallbladder carcinoma is seen with porcelain gallbladder, familial adenomatosis polyposis, as well as gallstones. There is an unusually high incident of gallbladder carcinoma in the Native American and Hispanic populations. There is no described link between biliary atresia and gallbladder cancer. This may be secondary to the removal of the gallbladder in the Kasai procedure or subsequent liver transplant.

QCSP, **Gallbladder Carcinoma,** p 342-344.

73.　D.　**ALCOHOLIC LIVER DISEASE**

The above biopsy demonstrates large ballooning hepatocytes with Mallory hyaline. The cells are surrounded by neutrophils and perihepatocyte fibrosis. Additionally, megamitochondria are present in the biopsy. While steatosis is not readily evident in this biopsy, it is often present, but not necessary for the diagnosis. Autoimmune hepatitis and chronic HCV typically demonstrates a periportal infiltrate (which is predominantly lymphocytes). Chronic venous congestion would lead to zone 3-hepatocyte atrophy, without inflammation.

QCSP, **Alcoholic Liver Disease,** p 295-297.

74.　C.　**EMPHYSEMA**

The biopsy demonstrates a chronic active hepatitis with portal and periportal inflammation and portal fibrous expansion. There is also a bile ductal reaction and periportal steatosis. Importantly, the high power field view

demonstrates solid intrahepatic eosinophilic globules. These finding are most consistent with α-1-antitrypin deficiency. As such, the patient most likely has emphysema or emphysematous changes within the lung.
QCSP, **A1-AT Deficiency,** p 297-8.

75. B. **Autoimmune hepatitis**

Both the biopsy and clinical history are most consistent with autoimmune hepatitis. Specifically, the patient is a young female with AST/ALT levels >1.5 times her ALK Phos level. Her viral hepatitis panels are negative, suggesting against hepatitis B. The biopsy demonstrates a dense periportal infiltrated with interface hepatitis and lobular activity.
QCSP, **Autoimmune Hepatitis,** p 298-300.

76. B. **Ulcerative colitis**

The above biopsy demonstrates concentric periductal fibrosis and a mild to moderate lymphocytic infiltrate. This is most consistent with a diagnosis of primary sclerosing cholangitis. From the choices, ulcerative colitis is most often associated with PSC, up to 75% of patients with PSC also having a history of ulcerative colitis. Only 10% of patients with PSC also have Crohn. Celiac disease can be associated with primary biliary cirrhosis, while Sjögren syndrome and rheumatoid arthritis can be associated with either PBC or autoimmune hepatitis.
QCSP, **Primary Sclerosing Cholangitis,** p 311-312.

77. D. **Angiomyolipoma**

The above biopsy demonstrates an admixture of adipose tissue, thick-walled blood vessels, and smooth muscle along with extramedullary hematopoiesis. This is most consistent with the diagnosis of angiomyolipoma.
QCSP, **Angiomyolipoma,** p 318-319.

78. C. *E granulosus* **infection**

The specimen demonstrates features consist with an *Echinococcus granulosus* infection. The specimen demonstrates a cyst with 3 layers: the adventitial layer (outermost) with dense fibrovascular tissue and inflammatory cell; laminated membrane (middle layer, chitinous layer), which consists of avascular material that is eosinophilic and refractile with no nuclei; and the germinal layer (innermost), which contains nuclei that give rise to the brood capsule (heads of adult tapeworms). The cyst of *E multilocularis* is typically multicystic with a very thin laminated wall and lacks a germinal layer.
QCSP, **Echinococcal Cyst,** p 323-324.

79. B. **Embryonal sarcoma**

The biopsy demonstrates malignant stellate and spindle-shaped cells in a loose mucopolysaccharide myxoid stroma. The biopsy is from the edge of the lesion and demonstrates entrapped hepatocytes. This is most consistent with embryonal sarcoma. (Not shown here, about 50% of embryonal sarcoma demonstrates hematopoietic activity.) Mesenchymal hamartoma demonstrates immature mesenchymal tissue with bland stellate or spindle cells dispersed in edematous myxoid stroma that contains various amounts of collagen, bile ducts, blood vessels, and hepatocytes. Infantile hemangioendothelioma usually occurs in infants under 6 months and is a "benign" vascular proliferation. Hepatoblastoma causes elevated α-fetoprotein in 90% of patients.
QCSP, **Embryonal Sarcoma,** p 324-325.

80. D. **Fibrolamellar hepatocellular carcinoma**

The biopsy demonstrates atypical hepatocytes with deeply eosinophilic cytoplasm and enlarged nuclei with prominent nucleoli. Additionally, there are hyaline globules with the neoplastic cells as well as a (rare) pale body. These findings are most consistent with a fibrolamellar variant of hepatocellular carcinoma. The lesion also demonstrates bile ducts arguing against a hepatocellular adenoma. There is no central scar as seen in focal nodular hyperplasia, and the lesion is hepatocyte in nature, ruling out a primary cholangiocarcinoma.

QCSP, **Fibrolamellar Hepatocellular Carcinoma,** p 328-329.

81. D. **HEPATOBLASTOMA**

The excision consists of a hepatocellular neoplasm that resembles fetal hepatocytes. The mass shows a mixture of hepatocytes growing in cords and nests separated by collagen. There is little to no intact architecture, with lack of portal architecture and bile ducts. There is a variation in dark and light zones secondary to fat and glycogen distribution.

QCSP, **Hepatoblastoma,** p 331-333.

82. B. **GRAFT-VS-HOST DISEASE**

The above biopsy demonstrates a portal tract with multiple injured bile ducts/ductules. The duct epithelium demonstrates a "dysplastic appearance" with nuclear pleomorphism and loss of polarity of the duct cells. Given the appropriate clinical history, the above histology is most consistent with chronic graft-vs-host disease (GVHD). Additionally, a typical finding would be the variability in the bile duct damage; however, if >50% of bile ducts are damaged (in a patient with the correct clinical history), the presumptive diagnosis would be GVHD. These inflammatory reactions can lead to loss of bile ducts. It is important to differentiate GVHD from a viral hepatitis, as this might delay the start of appropriate therapy. CMV hepatitis is more often seen in the immunocompromised and the characteristic findings include neutrophilic "microabscesses" and presence of typical CMV viral inclusions.

QCSP, **Graft-vs-Host Disease,** p 331-333.

83. A. **CAROLI SYNDROME**

The biopsy demonstrates fibrosis with a lack of an inflammatory response. This is consistent with congenital hepatic fibrosis, which is associated with Caroli syndrome (dilation of intra- or extrahepatic bile ducts], renal medullary tubular ectasia, and polycystic kidney disease. In addition, there is conflicting data on whether congenital fibrosis imposes an increased risk of developing cholangiocarcinoma or hepatocellular carcinoma.

QCSP, **Congenital Hepatic Fibrosis,** p 303.

84. D. **CYSTIC FIBROSIS**

The biopsy demonstrates dilated bile ductules filled with (pathognomonic) pink concretions and amorphous material. This material would be PAS-d resistant but negative for mucin stains. Additionally, other typical findings, such as bile ductular proliferation, chemical (sclerosing) cholangitis, chronic inflammation, and biliary fibrosis, are present. EM would demonstrate filamentous material in the bile ducts. These changes may develop into secondary biliary cirrhosis.

QCSP, **Cystic Fibrosis,** p 303-304.

85. A. **CHROMOSOME 7**

The biopsy demonstrates an area of stellate scarring with proliferating, dilated bile ducts/ductules filled as an inspissated eosinophilic material. These findings are consistent with cystic fibrosis. The mutated gene is located on chromosome 7 and involves the CFTR gene. The best-known mutation is the deletion of the 3 nucleotides coding for phenylalanine at position 508. Wilson disease has been associated with the *ATP7B* gene on chromosome 13 (13q-14.3). The *ATP7B* gene encodes a transmembrane copper-transporting ATPase, which is located on the canalicular aspect of hepatocytes. The *PEX1* gene associated with Zellweger syndrome is located on chromosome 12.

QCSP, **Cystic Fibrosis,** p 303-304.

8: Liver, Gallbladder, and Extrahepatic Bile Ducts Answers

86.   B.   **TOTAL PARENTERAL NUTRITION**
The biopsy demonstrates macrovesicular steatosis with minimal pericellular fibrosis. With the exception of total parenteral nutrition (choice B), all of the choices are associated with macrovesicular steatosis. Additionally, the biopsy demonstrates fatty change primarily involving zones 2-3, which is the typical pattern. However, accumulation of fat in the periportal region is seen in patients receiving total parenteral nutrition, with kwashiorkor, and HIV-infected patients.
QCSP, **Fatty Liver,** p 304-306.

87.   C.   **IT AFFECTS FEMALES AT A YOUNGER AGE.**
The treatment of iron overload/hemochromatosis is through period phlebotomies. The disease is often delayed in females who are premenopausal secondary to menses. Iron accumulation and subsequent cirrhosis leads to a 20%-25% increase in the incidents of hepatocellular carcinoma. The hepatic iron index (HII) is a calculation of the quantitative iron in hepatic tissue (micromoles of iron/dry weight of liver tissue) divided by the patient's age. Patients that are normal have a HII of <1; those that are heterozygous for the mutation can have a HII that varies between <1 and up to 1.9. The patients who are homozygous for the mutation have a HII of >2.0. Brown pigment that starts to accumulate in the perivenular hepatocytes is often lipofuscin, as iron begins to accumulate in the periportal hepatocytes.
QCSP, **Hemochromatosis,** p 306-307.

88.   C.   **ACUTE ACETAMINOPHEN OVERDOSE**
The H&E stain and the trichrome stain demonstrate the formation of regenerative hepatocyte nodules and complete fibrosis meeting the criteria of cirrhosis. There is also decrease separation of the portal tracts and terminal venules as well as an increase in the ratio of venules to portal tracts. Acute acetaminophen overdose generally results in an acute fulminant hepatitis with centrilobular collapse. The use of trichrome stains can be misinterpreted under such circumstances in which the acinar collapse may be confused with fibrosis. A reticulin stain is useful to help differentiate fibrosis from acinar collapse and loss of lobular architecture.
QCSP, **Cirrhosis,** p 300-302.

89.   B.   **CYTOKERATIN 20**
The above image demonstrates a gallbladder carcinoma. These lesions are typically positive for cytokeratins 7 and 19 as well as CA19-9 and p53. The lesion is typically CEA-M positive but CEA-P negative. Cytokeratin 20 can be positive in up to 25% of these lesions (more often positive in gallbladder carcinoma than in other bile duct lesions). These lesions can also be CDX-2 positive, but the staining pattern is often weak and patching.
QCSP, **Gallbladder Carcinoma,** p 342-343.

90.   B.   **EXTENSION INTO LIVER IS PRESENT IN 20% OF CASES.**
The above lesion demonstrates a gallbladder carcinoma. These lesions are inoperable in approximately 50% of cases at the time of diagnosis. Additionally, approximately 80% of these lesions demonstrate extension into the liver, and 50%-80% demonstrate lymph node metastasis. The K-ras codon 12 mutation as well as mutations in the APC gene, amplification of the c-erb-2 gene, and increased expression of the p53 protein have all been described.
QCSP, **Gallbladder Carcinoma,** p 342-343.

91.   C.   **HISTOLOGIC EVALUATION IS REQUIRED FOR THE DIAGNOSIS**
The biopsy along with the patient's clinical values is consistent with the diagnosis of primary biliary cirrhosis. The diagnosis of PBC can be made by the presence of biochemical evidence of cholestatic injury (ie, elevated alkaline phosphatase from >6 months) and the presence of an antimitochondrial antibody (specifically anti-M2). A liver biopsy is not required for the diagnosis, but can assist in making the diagnosis in patients that are AMA negative or with other nontypical findings. This autoimmune liver disease is usually asymptomatic, with pruritus being the initial presenting symptom only to be followed much later by jaundice. Without treatment, the natural course

of the disease is to liver failure and cirrhosis with a 5-year survival, from time of diagnosis, of 65%. There is a dramatic increase in the female-to-male ratio of approximately 9-10:1.

QCSP, **Primary Biliary Cirrhosis,** p 309-310.

92.   D.   **TAMOXIFEN**
The biopsy was taken from a patient with chronic active hepatitis C. The biopsy demonstrates findings typical of chronic viral hepatitis including portal inflammation that is composed primarily of lymphocytes. This case also demonstrates interface hepatitis (piecemeal necrosis) as well as scattered apoptotic hepatocytes. While these findings are typical, they are not specific for viral hepatitis. Specifically, these findings can be seen in autoimmune hepatitis and some forms of drug-induced liver disease. There is a long list of drugs and different morphologic findings associated with drug-induced liver disease. Specifically, isoniazide, halothane, methotrexate, valproic acid, amiodarone, and herbal medications have been reported to induce a chronic hepatitis pattern similar to chronic viral hepatitis. However, tamoxifen, corticosteroids, and certain anti-HIV drugs tend to induce a steatohepatitis-like injury.

QCSP, **Viral Hepatitis,** p 313-317.

93.   B.   **WILSON DISEASE**
The patient's history and biopsy results are consistent with Wilson disease. Specifically, the biopsy demonstrates a mild periportal inflammatory infiltrate along with glycogenation of periportal hepatocytes. Often patients will present with neuropsychiatric symptoms ranging from depression to frank psychosis and often with Parkinson-like movement disorders. Many of the biopsy findings are nonspecific and in addition to the findings above can demonstrate macro or microvesicular steatosis and the presence of Mallory hyaline. While rare, the first presentation can be fulminant hepatic failure. A vitamin A overdose would result in hypertrophy of hepatic stellate cells and resulting sinusoidal dilation and peliosis. Generally when tricyclic antidepressants cause hepatic damage, they demonstrate a pattern of cholestatic hepatitis but can also demonstrate spotty, submassive, or massive necrosis.

QCSP, **Wilson Disease (Hepatolenticular Degeneration),** p 317-318.

94.   D.   **ANGIOSARCOMA**
The biopsy shown above demonstrates a trabecular pattern with colonization of the sinusoids by large atypical cells. These cells demonstrate poorly defined cell borders with large prominent nucleoli. In the image on the upper left, the neoplastic cells are spindled, forming nodules reminiscent of fibrosarcoma. These cells express endothelial markers CD34, CD31, factor VIII, and FLI-1; however, they lack expression of HHV8. Thrombocytopenia is seen in approximately 50% of cases, with 30% demonstrating hemoperitoneum.

QCSP, **Angiosarcoma,** p 319-320.

95.   B.   **BILE DUCT ADENOMA**
This is a common differential (especially for intraoperative frozen consultation) in which a benign lesion can grossly be concerning for a malignant deposit. The pictured lesion is a bile duct adenoma with small (not dilated or cystic) acini and ducts embedded in a mature fibrous stroma. Bile duct hamartomas demonstrate dilated bile duct structures and usually occur as multiple lesions. While well-differentiated pancreatic carcinomas can have a low-powered bland appearance, carcinomas always demonstrate some cytologic atypia, including variable size from cell to cell and increased nuclear-to-cytoplasmic ratio, all of which are absent in the pictured biopsy. Also, the pictured lesion lacks a desmoplastic response, typically of metastatic lesions.

QCSP, **Bile Duct Adenoma (Peribiliary Gland Hamartoma),** p 320-321.

96.   C.   **THERE IS ELEVATED SERUM AFP AND CEA.**
The presentation as well as the histology is consistent with an intrahepatic cholangiocarcinoma. The lesion demonstrates malignant glands within a dense sclerotic/fibrotic background with concentric layering of stroma

around the neoplastic glands. While the images demonstrate bile plugs, the neoplastic cells would not stain for bile (Hall stain). Remember that bile production is pathognomonic for hepatocellular tumors. However, unlike hepatocellular tumors, cholangiocarcinomas demonstrate intracellular mucin that would stain by PAS-D. Unfortunately, approximately 80% of the patients that present with intrahepatic cholangiocarcinoma have unresectable disease, and since there is no (yet) proven role for chemotherapy and radiation, the prognosis is poor. This lesion is derived from biliary epithelium, and as such serum levels for CEA and CA19-9 would be increased, but AFP should be normal (except in mixed HCC and cholangiocarcinomas, in which all 3 can be elevated). Remember that CEA and CA19-9 can also be elevated in benign biliary lesions.

QCSP, **Bile Duct Carcinoma—Intrahepatic (Cholangiocarcinoma),** p 322.

97.   A.   **EPITHELIOID HEMANGIOENDOTHELIOMA**
The lesion demonstrates a mixture of spindle cells and epithelioid cells in a myxoid and slightly sclerotic background. On high magnification, blister cells can be seen. These are cells with prominent intracytoplasmic vacuoles that can contain RBCs. While the neoplastic cells are too atypical to be a hemangioma, they do not demonstrate the atypia or mitotic activity seen in angiosarcoma. Epithelioid hemangioendotheliomas are typically asymptomatic and slow growing, and on imaging can be calcified and by contrast imaging often appear avascular. The neoplastic cells are positive for endothelial markers (ie, CD31, CD34, and factor VIII) and sometimes can express low-molecular-weight keratins (ie, CK7 and CK18), but are CEA negative.

QCSP, **Epithelioid Hemangioendothelioma,** p 330-331.

98.   D.   **HEPATIC ADENOMA**
This lesion represents a hepatic adenoma. The lesion demonstrates loss of acinar structures with loss of portal tracts and bile ducts. However, the lesion but does not demonstrate cytologic atypia or increased N/C ratio. While the lesion demonstrates thickened plates, they are <3 cells thick, and can be highlighted by reticulin staining. Lipid accumulation in adenomas is common.

QCSP, **Hepatocellular (Liver Cell) Adenoma,** p 334.

99.   D.   **EXTRAHEPATIC LESIONS ALMOST ALWAYS DEVELOP INTO A CARCINOMA.**
The images and history are consistent with the diagnosis of biliary cystadenoma. The sections demonstrate an epithelial lining that resembles biliary or gastric foveolar cells. There is a cellular stroma that is ovarian-like in appearance and would be positive by ER and PR immunostains. Additionally, the stroma can stain for SMA, vimentin, and inhibin, while the epithelial cells are usually positive for CK7/19, EMA, CEA, and CA19-9. Patients usually have increased serum and intracystic levels of CA19-9. The lesion predominantly occurs in women and, when it does occur in men, lacks the ovarian-like stroma. Cystadenocarcinoma can arise from a preexisting cystadenoma; however, this is limited to intrahepatic lesions. Specifically, even if extrahepatic biliary cystadenomas demonstrate dysplasia, there is not good evidence to support their malignant transformation into an extrahepatic biliary cyst adenocarcinoma.

QCSP, **Biliary Cystadenoma,** p 341-342.

100.   B.   **BILE DUCT HAMARTOMA**
The pictured lesion is a classic example of a bile duct hamartoma (von Meyenburg complex). This lesion, similar to bile duct adenoma (peribiliary gland hamartoma), is often sampled at the time of surgery because of the similar gross appearance to metastatic disease. The bile duct hamartoma demonstrates dilated ducts that are often branched or angulated. While grossly the lesion is concerning for a metastatic lesion, there is typically no cytologic atypia in this lesion.

QCSP, **Bile Duct Microhamartoma (von Meyenburg Complex),** p 321.

8: Liver, Gallbladder, and Extrahepatic Bile Ducts Answers

101.　A.　**IT IS CAUSED BY ORAL CONTRACEPTIVE USE.**

The images demonstrate a focal nodular hyperplasia (FNH) with a central scar area and fibrous septa dividing the lesion in lobules resembling focal cirrhosis. Bile ducts are seen within the lesion. While oral contraceptive use can be associated with growth of the lesion, it is not an apparent etiologic factor. These lesions are thought to be caused by a vascular malformation and, when FNHs are multiple, are associated with other vascular anomalies such as berry aneurysm, portal vein atresia, hepatic hemangioma, and telangiectasias of the brain. Additionally, FNHs are associated with meningiomas and astrocytomas.

QCSP, **Focal Nodular Hyperplasia,** p 336-337.

102.　E.　**CD34 HIGHLIGHTS THE LESION.**

The lesion demonstrates atypical hepatocytes forming pseudoglandular structures along with thickened cell plates (>3 cells thick). The hepatocytes also demonstrate large nuclei with distinct nucleoli, along with rare giant cell formation and mitotic figures. These findings are consistent with the conventional type of hepatocellular carcinoma. Serum AFP levels in normal adults are around 0-9 ng/mL and often elevated in people with chronic liver disease or other hepatic injury (usually not elevated after resection or biopsy). However, values >500 ng/mL are indicative of hepatocellular carcinoma, germ cell tumors (nonseminomatous), or metastatic tumors to the liver. Other processes that can cause elevated AFP include pregnancy, ataxia telangiectasia, and GI malignancies. The major identified risk factors for the development of HCC include processes that cause chronic hepatic damage and cirrhosis. However, hepatocellular carcinoma can occur in the setting of a noncirrhotic liver, but hepatic adenomas are not a precursor lesion for hepatocellular carcinoma. Infection with HBV appears to be more carcinogenic than infection with HCV. A finding that vascular endothelium cells (that are CD34 positive) replace the "liver sinusoidal endothelial cells" (CD31positive and CD34 negative) is consistent with hepatocellular carcinoma. This replacement results in the typical FNA appearance of HCC in which there are round-shaped collections of malignant hepatocytes surrounded by an endothelial wrap/rim.

QCSP, **Hepatocellular Carcinoma,** p 325-328.

103.　D.　**NODULAR REGENERATIVE HYPERPLASIA**

The lesion demonstrates a diffuse nodularity with hyperplastic hepatocytes in the center of the nodule with atrophic hepatocytes along the edge (this is highlighted by a reticulin stain). The hepatocytes demonstrate variable orientation to one another. There is a history of portal hypertension, which always raises the possibility of cirrhosis. However, there is no fibrosis in the biopsy, as demonstrated by trichrome stain, ruling out cirrhosis and congenital fibrosis. The lesion can be associated with immunologic disorders, neoplastic disorders, drugs and toxins (especially platinum-based chemotherapeutic agents and azathioprine/imuran), vascular disorders, and transplantation (probably drug related).

QCSP, **Nodular Regenerative Hyperplasia,** p 337-338.

104.　D.　**ADENOMYOMA/ADENOMYOMATOSIS**

The lesion demonstrates a thickened gallbladder with benign appearing glands of columnar epithelium embedded in bundles of smooth muscle characteristic of adenomyoma/adenomyomatosis. The term "adenomyoma" is used for a focal lesion and "adenomyomatosis" for diffuse disease. The lesion is thought to be a form of diverticular disease of the gallbladder in which the Rokitansky-Aschoff sinuses extend deep into the muscle layer and are surrounded by hypertrophic smooth muscle. While not seen in this case, these lesions can demonstrate areas of high-grade dysplasia and even carcinoma.

QCSP, **Adenomyoma and Adenomyomatosis,** p 338-339.

105.　D.　**BILIARY CYSTADENOCARCINOMA**

The images and history are consistent with the diagnosis of biliary cystadenocarcinoma. The sections demonstrate dilated cystic areas with a benign flattened cuboidal epithelial lining. In close association are glands that demonstrate complex tubulopapillary growth pattern. These glands demonstrate solid areas with cytologic atypia, mitosis, and stroma evasion. The diagnosis of biliary cystadenocarcinoma can be rendered in the absence of

8: Liver, Gallbladder, and Extrahepatic Bile Ducts Answers

stromal invasion, when in the presence of high-grade dysplasia. Cystadenocarcinoma often arise from a preexisting cystadenoma. This lesion lacks ovarian stroma, which predicts a worse prognosis. Given the rarity of this primary lesion, metastatic disease from pancreas, ovary, or appendix must be considered.

QCSP, **Biliary Cystadenocarcinoma,** p 340-341.

106. **B.** **NEONATAL HEPATITIS**

The images demonstrate the presence of lobular disarray with multiple giant multinucleated hepatocytes and a pseudoacinar change. There is a mild portal infiltrate with intact biliary structures without edema, fibrosis or ductular reaction. Additionally, there is hepatocyte cholestasis and multiple canalicular bile plugs. There are diffuse patches of extramedullary hematopoiesis, which is a common finding in neonatal hepatitis; however extramedullary hematopoiesis is not the best diagnosis for this case. While biliary atresia can resemble neonatal hepatitis, it is usually associated with less giant cell formation and inflammation and generally demonstrates a ductular proliferation with edema and fibrosis. Alagille syndrome is characterized with a paucity of interlobular bile ducts (along with abnormal facies, vertebral anomalies, cardiac anomalies, renal anomalies and various other abnormalities). There is no evidence of hemophagocytosis in this specimen.

QCSP, **Neonatal Hepatitis,** p 307-309.

Chapter 9

Pancreas

1. The presence of metastatic disease during intraoperative consultation (frozen section) usually obviates resection.
   A. True
   B. False

2. Extensive sampling of mucinous pancreatic neoplasms is required in order to identify an invasive component.
   A. True
   B. False

3. Ductal adenocarcinomas of the pancreas:
   A. Represent 85% of all pancreatic tumors
   B. Typically occur in men under 40 years of age
   C. Are commonly located in the tail of the pancreas
   D. Rarely metastasize
   E. Demonstrate 95% survival at 5 years

4. Which following features distinguish ductal adenocarcinoma of the pancreas from chronic pancreatitis?
   A. Loss of lobular architecture
   B. Irregular, complex, or incomplete glands
   C. Preserved islets of Langerhans
   D. A and B
   E. A and C

5. Pancreatitis, hypoglycemia, hypercalcemia, endocarditis, and migratory thrombophlebitis (Trousseau sign) are all associated with which of the following?
   A. Acinar cell carcinoma
   B. Pancreatoblastoma
   C. Pancreatic (ductal) adenocarcinoma
   D. Pancreatic neuroendocrine neoplasm
   E. Solid-pseudopapillary neoplasm

6. All of the following are TRUE about pancreatic (ductal) adenocarcinoma EXCEPT:
   A. The cut surface is typically ill-defined, yellow-white, and hard.
   B. Perineural invasion is rarely seen.
   C. Changes of pancreatitis may accompany the tumor.
   D. Obstructive tumors involving the head of the pancreas often result in dilation of the common bile and pancreatic ducts.
   E. 70% of patients experience concomitant symptoms of diabetes mellitus.

7. Microscopic variants of pancreatic (ductal) adenocarcinoma include which of the following?
   A. Adenosquamous carcinoma
   B. Clear cell carcinoma
   C. Signet ring cell carcinoma
   D. Mucinous noncystic carcinoma
   E. All of the above

9: Pancreas Questions

8. Molecular alterations in pancreatic (ductal) adenocarcinoma involve which of the following?
    A. EGFR
    B. p16
    C. K-ras
    D. A and C
    E. B and C

9. All of the following are TRUE about serous cystic neoplasms EXCEPT:
    A. Serous cystadenocarcinomas are common.
    B. Serous cystic neoplasms occur in the elderly with a slight female predominance.
    C. Serous microcystic adenomas are composed of innumerable small cysts lined by a single layer of small, cuboidal epithelial cells with clear cytoplasm and a round central nucleus with an inconspicuous nucleolus.
    D. Serous oligocystic adenomas contain few irregularly arranged cysts filled with clear watery fluid and are separated by broad fibrous septa.
    E. PAS without diastase staining highlights the cells lining the cysts, confirming the presence of intracytoplasmic glycogen.

10. The cytoplasm of the cells in serous cystic neoplasms is rich in which of the following?
    A. Mitochondria
    B. Lysosomes
    C. Golgi
    D. Glycogen
    E. Neurosecretory granules

11. Serous microcystic adenomas are associated with which of the following?
    A. von Hippel-Lindau disease
    B. Evan syndrome
    C. Gallstones
    D. All of the above
    E. A and B only

12. Mucinous cystic neoplasms of the pancreas occur almost exclusively in young to middle-aged men.
    A. True
    B. False

13. A 35-year-old woman presents with vague abdominal pain and a palpable abdominal mass. Imaging shows a large pancreatic mass in the tail of the pancreas, which does not communicate with the main duct system. Surgical excision yields a mucin-producing tumor mass. The clinical history and gross impression are most likely consistent with a diagnosis of:
    A. Pseudocyst
    B. Intraductal papillary mucinous neoplasm (IPMN)
    C. Mucinous cystic neoplasm
    D. Solid-pseudopapillary tumor
    E. Lymphoepithelial cyst

9: Pancreas Questions

14. Features that distinguish mucinous cystic neoplasms from intraductal papillary neoplasms include which of the following?
    A. Localization to the body or tail of pancreas
    B. Cysts which do not communicate with the main duct system
    C. Subepithelial stroma reminiscent of ovarian-type stroma
    D. All of the above
    E. None of the above

15. Failure to completely resect a mucinous cystadenoma of the pancreas may result in recurrence or death of the patient from invasive mucinous cystadenocarcinoma.
    A. True
    B. False

16. All of the following are TRUE about intraductal papillary mucinous tumors EXCEPT:
    A. The majority of cases occur in the head of the pancreas.
    B. The pancreatic parenchyma surrounding the dilated ducts is atrophic and fibrotic and exhibits changes of chronic pancreatitis.
    C. The subepithelial stroma is reminiscent of ovarian stroma.
    D. The tumor directly communicates with the duct system, predominantly involving the major ducts.
    E. Prognosis is generally good.

17. Intraductal papillary mucinous neoplasms (IPMNs):
    A. Commonly occur in elderly men
    B. Present with obstruction of the main pancreatic duct due to viscous mucin production
    C. Typically occur in the head of the pancreas
    D. Are classified based on the degree of dysplasia and presence of invasion
    E. All of the above

18. Parenchymal invasion is seen in what percentage of IPMN cases?
    A. 80%-90%
    B. 50%-60%
    C. 10%-20%
    D. <5%
    E. Never

19. Periodic-acid-Schiff (PAS) with diastase stains the apical cytoplasm of tumor cells in acinar cell carcinoma. Which of the following imparts this reactivity and the finely granular cytoplasmic appearance?
    A. Mitochondria
    B. Golgi
    C. Zymogen granules
    D. Lysosomes
    E. None of the above

20. All of the following are TRUE about acinar cell carcinoma EXCEPT:
    A. The mean age of presentation is 55-60 years, although there have been case reports in children.
    B. Survival at 3 years is 95%.
    C. Tumor cells are typically arranged in large lobules separated by fibrous strands; within nodules, acinar areas alternate with solid areas.
    D. Tumor cells in the acinar areas form small lumina, are uniform in size with abundant finely granular eosinophilic cytoplasm and uniform round basal nuclei with prominent nucleoli.
    E. Mitotic activity in the acinar areas is usually <1 mitosis/10 hpf.

9: Pancreas Questions

21. All of the following are TRUE regarding solid-pseudopapillary tumors EXCEPT:
    A. They predominantly occur in adolescent girls and young women.
    B. The cut surface is typically lobulated, light brown, and soft with foci of cystic change, hemorrhage, and necrosis, and may resemble a pseudocyst.
    C. Large numbers of variably sized intracellular and extracellular eosinophilic globules may be present.
    D. Mitotic figures are typically abundant.
    E. The majority of tumors are benign and cured by surgical excision.

22. The tumor cells of solid-pseudopapillary tumor have which of the following immunophenotypes?
    A. NSE+, vimentin+, focal cytokeratin+, mucicarmine and PAS−
    B. NSE−, vimentin+, focal cytokeratin+, synaptophysin and chromogranin−
    C. NSE+, vimentin+, focal cytokeratin+, synaptophysin and chromogranin+
    D. NSE−, vimentin+, cytokeratin−, mucicarmine and PAS+
    E. None of the above

23. Which key histologic feature distinguishes pancreatoblastoma from acinar cell carcinoma?
    A. Tumor cells that have abundant finely granular eosinophilic cytoplasm
    B. Tumor cells arranged in acinar and solid patterns
    C. Fibrous bands traversing the tumor
    D. Squamoid cell nests (squamoid corpuscles)
    E. None of the above

24. Pancreatoblastoma in children is associated with which of the following?
    A. Familial adenomatous polyposis
    B. Beckwith-Wiedemann syndrome
    C. Zollinger-Ellison syndrome
    D. Carney triad
    E. Carney syndrome

25. Absolute criteria for malignancy in pancreatic endocrine tumors include the following EXCEPT:
    A. Gross invasion of adjacent organs
    B. Metastasis to regional lymph nodes, liver, or other distant sites
    C. Angioinvasion
    D. Tumor size, mitotic rate, Ki-67 labeling index
    E. All of the above are unequivocal evidence of malignancy

9: Pancreas Questions

Questions 26-30:

Correctly match the following functioning pancreatic endocrine neoplasms with their respective syndrome/disease association:
A. Insulinoma
B. Gastrinoma
C. VIPoma
D. Enterochromaffin cell tumor
E. Glucagonoma

26. Zollinger-Ellison syndrome

27. Whipple triad

28. WDHA syndrome

29. Carcinoid syndrome

30. Glucagonoma syndrome

31. Which of the following functioning endocrine tumors of the pancreas are associated with MEN I (Wermer syndrome)?
A. Insulinoma
B. Glucagonoma
C. Somatostatinoma
D. A and B
E. A, B, and C

32. The most common functioning endocrine neoplasm of the pancreas is:
A. Somatostatinoma
B. Gastrinoma
C. Insulinoma
D. Enterochromaffin cell tumor
E. Glucagonoma

33. A 65-year-old man presents with weight loss and jaundice. Imaging shows a large pancreatic mass invading adjacent organs and widespread metastatic disease. Tumor cells are arranged in nests and sheets and are characterized by markedly hyperchromatic round to oval nuclei, inconspicuous nucleoli, and poorly defined cell borders with frequent mitoses and foci of necrosis. The tumor cells are immunoreactive for NSE, synaptophysin, and cytokeratin with a high Ki-67 (Mib-1) labeling index. The tumor cells are negative for CD45 and CD99 (MIC2). The clinical presentation and histologic features in conjunction with the immunophenotype are most consistent with a diagnosis of:
A. Poorly differentiated/high-grade endocrine neoplasm (small cell carcinoma)
B. Well-differentiated neuroendocrine neoplasms
C. Lymphoma
D. PNET/Ewing
E. Pancreatoblastoma

9: Pancreas Questions

34. The gross image shown represents a resection specimen from an 80-year-old man with a pancreatic head mass. The most likely diagnosis is:

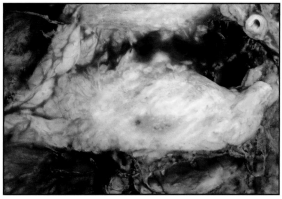

    A.   Pancreatic (ductal) adenocarcinoma
    B.   Pancreatoblastoma
    C.   Pancreatic neuroendocrine neoplasm
    D.   Intraductal papillary mucinous neoplasm (IPMN)
    E.   Solid-pseudopapillary tumor

35. The lesion seen in this image is immunoreactive with all of the following markers EXCEPT:

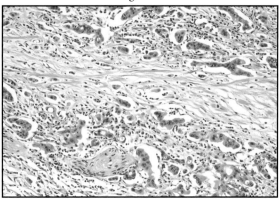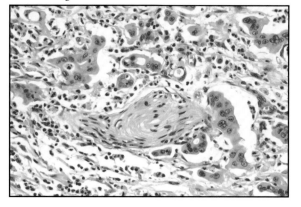

    A.   MUC-1
    B.   MUC-2
    C.   MUC-3
    D.   CEA
    E.   Cytokeratin

9: Pancreas Questions

36. A 60-year-old woman has an incidental finding on imaging, which shows a mass in the body of the pancreas characterized by honeycombing and a central stellate scar. The resection specimen is shown in the image. These findings are typical of the following diagnosis:

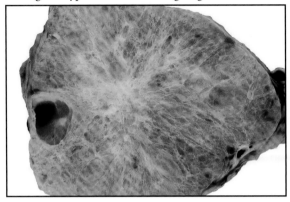

A. Pseudocyst
B. Lymphoepithelial cyst
C. Mucinous cystic neoplasm
D. Serous cystic neoplasm
E. None of the above

37. The pancreatic neoplasm shown in the image represents which of the following?

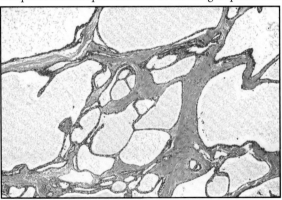 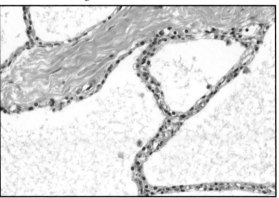

A. Serous microcystic adenoma
B. Serous oligocystic adenoma
C. Serous cystadenocarcinoma
D. A or B
E. None of the above

9: Pancreas Questions

38. The image represents a large pancreatic tail mass in a 40-year-old woman. The subepithelial stroma is immunoreactive to which of the following?

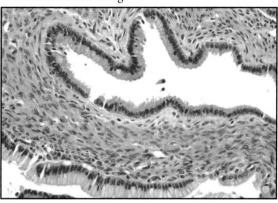 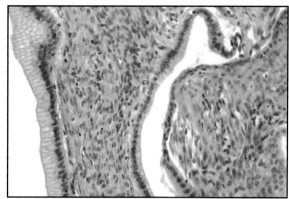

    A.   Vimentin
    B.   SMA
    C.   Inhibin
    D.   Estrogen and progesterone receptor
    E.   All of the above

39. A 65-year-old men presents with acute pancreatitis and is found to have a pancreatic head mass. Imaging shows that the mass communicates with the main pancreatic duct, which is dilated. A Whipple procedure is performed to excise the mass. The microscopic image is most consistent with a diagnosis of:

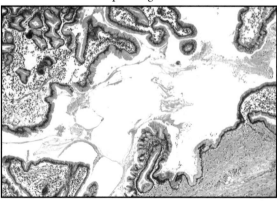 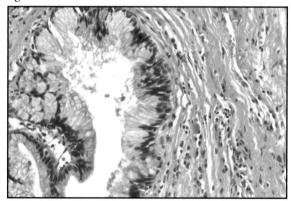

    A.   Mucinous cystic neoplasm
    B.   Intraductal papillary mucinous neoplasm
    C.   Chronic pancreatitis
    D.   Ductal adenocarcinoma
    E.   None of the above

9: Pancreas Questions

40. A 60-year-old man presents with polyarthralgia, eosinophilia, extrapancreatic disseminated fat necrosis, and nonbacterial thrombotic endocarditis. He is found to have a well-circumscribed, nodular, soft mass in the head of the pancreas (see microscopic image). The clinical, gross, and microscopic features are most consistent with a diagnosis of:

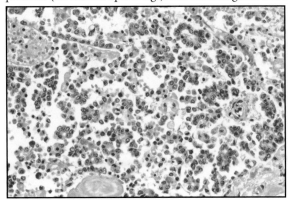 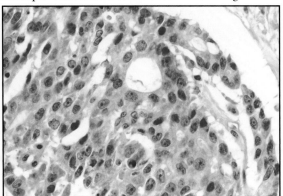

    A.   Acinar cell carcinoma

    B.   Pancreatic endocrine neoplasm

    C.   Ductal adenocarcinoma

    D.   Solid-pseudopapillary tumor

    E.   Pancreatoblastoma

41. A 15-year-old girl presents with vague abdominal discomfort and is found to have a distal pancreatic mass on CT scan. The microscopic image shown is most consistent with a diagnosis of:

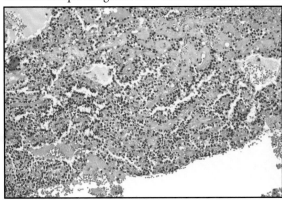 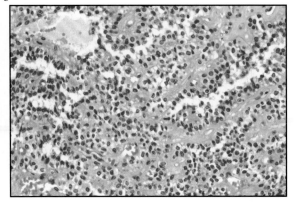

    A.   Papillary mucinous carcinoma

    B.   Solid-pseudopapillary tumor (Gruber-Frantz tumor)

    C.   Pancreatoblastoma

    D.   Acinar cell carcinoma

    E.   Pancreatic endocrine tumor

9: Pancreas Questions

42. The entity shown in this image most likely presented in which of the following patients?

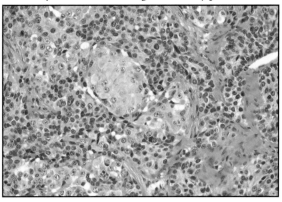 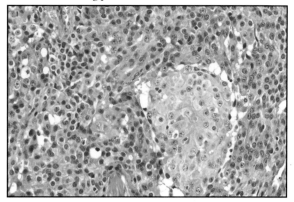

    A.   65-year-old woman with jaundice
    B.   25-year-old woman with vague abdominal pain
    C.   4-year-old asymptomatic boy with an abdominal mass
    D.   60-year-old man with anorexia, weight loss, and abdominal pain
    E.   A and D

43. A patient presents with unexplained hypoglycemia and is found to have a pancreatic mass. Histologic examination establishes the diagnosis of an insulinoma (see image). The most distinguishing microscopic feature of this entity is:

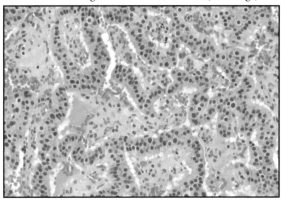

    A.   Fibrous capsule
    B.   Ribbon-like or trabecular architecture
    C.   Uniformly round to oval nuclei with finely dispersed and stippled chromatin
    D.   Presence of amyloid in fibrovascular stroma adjacent to tumor cells
    E.   Lack of nucleoli

9: Pancreas Questions

44. The tumor shown in the image was an incidentally discovered mass in the tail of the pancreas. Tumor cells showed strong and diffuse immunoreactivity with chromogranin, synaptophysin, and neuron-specific enolase. The diagnosis is:

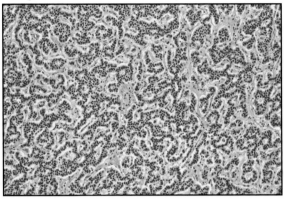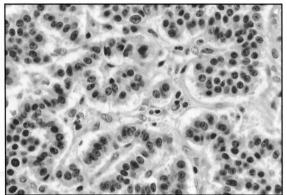

    A.   High-grade/poorly differentiated neuroendocrine tumor (small cell carcinoma)

    B.   Low-grade/well-differentiated neuroendocrine tumor (nonfunctioning)

    C.   Acinar cell carcinoma

    D.   Solid pseudopapillary tumor

    E.   Ductal adenocarcinoma

9: Pancreas Answers

1.   A.   **TRUE**

Surgery is usually intended as a curative measure in the setting of pancreatic cancer. Since there may be significant morbidity associated with this type of intervention compromising the patient's subsequent quality of life, the presence of metastatic disease typically aborts the procedure. Approximately 20% of patients with clinically resectable disease on initial presentation demonstrate evidence of metastasis intraoperatively.

QCSP, **Intraoperative Consultation,** p 346.

2.   A.   **TRUE**

An invasive component may be quite focal and only found on extensive sampling of the lesion. Since the prognosis may be significantly impacted, identification of such a focus, however minute, is critical.

QCSP, **Intraoperative Consultation,** p 347.

3.   A.   **REPRESENT 85% OF ALL PANCREATIC TUMORS**

Ductal adenocarcinomas represent 85% of all pancreatic tumors. They typically occur in the elderly (60-80 years) and exhibit a slight male predominance. 2/3 of cases are located in the head of the pancreas, while only 1/3 of cases are located in the body or tail. Ductal adenocarcinomas grow rapidly and are often unresectable on clinical presentation due to widespread extrapancreatic growth. The prognosis is poor with <5 percent of patients experiencing survival beyond 5 years.

QCSP, **Ductal Adenocarcinoma,** p 347-349.

4.   D.   **A AND B**

Ductal adenocarcinoma can be grossly and microscopically difficult to distinguish from chronic pancreatitis, particularly on frozen preparations. A diagnosis of adenocarcinoma is favored by the presence of irregular, often incomplete glandular structures lined by atypical cells in the setting of lobular disarray. Perineural invasion, necrosis, prominent mitotic activity, and mucin production also are helpful features. It is important to keep in mind that ductal carcinoma and chronic pancreatitis of the adjacent nonneoplastic parenchyma often coexist.

QCSP, **Ductal Adenocarcinoma,** p 347.

5.   C.   **PANCREATIC (DUCTAL) ADENOCARCINOMA**

Ductal carcinoma can be associated with pancreatitis, hypoglycemia, hypercalcemia, endocarditis, and migratory thrombophlebitis (Trousseau sign). Acinar cell carcinomas can be associated with peripheral eosinophilia and lipase hypersecretion syndrome (polyarthralgia, extrapancreatic disseminated fat necrosis, nonbacterial thrombotic endocarditis). Pancreatoblastoma can be associated with Beckwith-Wiedemann syndrome. The pancreatic neuroendocrine neoplasms are associated with the effects of the overexpressed hormone.

QCSP, **Ductal Adenocarcinoma,** p 347.

6.   B.   **PERINEURAL INVASION IS RARELY SEEN.**

Perineural invasion is present in up to 90% of cases.

QCSP, **Ductal Adenocarcinoma,** p 347.

7.   E.   **ALL OF THE ABOVE**

All of the answers listed represent variants of pancreatic (ductal) adenocarcinoma. Additional variants include mixed ductal-endocrine carcinoma, undifferentiated (anaplastic) carcinoma, and undifferentiated carcinoma with osteoclast-like giant cells. While it is useful to be familiar with the broad histologic spectrum of pancreatic ductal carcinoma, the prognosis of all variants listed is poor with the anaplastic variant imparting a particularly dismal chance of survival.

QCSP, **Ductal adenocarcinoma,** p 348.

8.   E.   **B AND C**
Up to 95% and 90% of patients with pancreatic (ductal) adenocarcinoma exhibit molecular alterations involving the p16 and K-ras genes, respectively.
QCSP, **Ductal Adenocarcinoma,** p 349.

9.   A.   **SEROUS CYSTADENOCARCINOMAS ARE COMMON.**
Serous cystadenocarcinomas are rare tumors. These lesions are most common in the elderly and exhibit a slight female predominance. Serous microcystic and oligocystic adenomas are predominantly distinguished from each other by their gross appearance. The cells lining the cyst walls in both entities are filled with intracytoplasmic glycogen, which is best seen on PAS without diastase staining.
QCSP, **Serous Cystadenocarcinomas,** p 349.

10.   D.   **GLYCOGEN**
A PAS stain without diastase highlights the glycogen-rich cytoplasm in tumor cells of serous cystic neoplasms.
QCSP, **Serous Microcystic Adenoma,** p 350.

11.   D.   **ALL OF THE ABOVE**
Serous microcystic adenomas are associated with von Hippel-Lindau disease (retinal angiomatosis, cerebellar hemangioblastoma, renal cell carcinoma, pheochromocytoma, and renal, liver, lung, pancreas, and spleen cysts) and Evan syndrome (autoimmune hemolytic anemia, idiopathic thrombocytopenic purpura). Coincidental associations include gallstones, diabetes mellitus, and extrapancreatic malignancies.
QCSP, **Serous Microcystic Adenoma,** p 351.

12.   B.   **FALSE**
Mucinous cystic neoplasms of the pancreas occur almost exclusively in young to middle-aged women.
QCSP, **Mucinous Cystic Neoplasms,** p 352.

13.   C.   **MUCINOUS CYSTIC NEOPLASM**
Mucinous cystic neoplasms occur in young to middle-aged women, most commonly in the body or tail of the pancreas. Clinical presentation includes vague abdominal pain and a palpable abdominal mass. The external surface of the specimen is lobulated and glistening. The cut surface reveals a single cyst or multiple cysts filled with thick gelatinous material. The cyst lining can be smooth or contain papillary excrescences. In contrast to IPMNs, the cysts do not communicate with the duct system.
QCSP, **Mucinous Cystic Neoplasms,** p 352.

14.   D.   **ALL OF THE ABOVE**
Mucinous cystic neoplasms commonly occur in young women and involve the tail of the pancreas. They do not communicate with the main duct system and are histologically characterized by subepithelial stroma reminiscent of ovarian-type stroma. In contrast, IPMNs are seen in elderly men and involve the head of the pancreas. The lesion is typically in continuity with the main duct system.
QCSP, **Mucinous Cystic Neoplasms,** p 352.

15.   A.   **TRUE**
The treatment of mucinous cystic neoplasms is complete resection. Either internal or external drainage of a mucinous cystic tumor or incomplete excision may result in recurrence as an invasive cystadenocarcinoma. If unresectable, mucinous cystadenocarcinoma has the same prognosis as invasive ductal carcinoma.
QCSP, **Mucinous Cystic Neoplasms,** p 353.

9: Pancreas Answers

16. C. **THE SUBEPITHELIAL STROMA IS REMINISCENT OF OVARIAN STROMA.**
    The main differential diagnosis for IPMN is a mucinous cystic neoplasm. The radiologic and gross impression is important, because IPMNs are connected to the main duct system and its branches, while mucinous cystic neoplasms are not. In addition, a very helpful histologic feature is the ovarian-type stroma, which is prominent in mucinous cystic neoplasms but not seen in IPMNs. Other helpful features include location and patient demographic, with IPMNs occurring more commonly in the head of the pancreas of older men, while mucinous cystic neoplasms typically arise in the tail of the pancreas of younger women.
    QCSP, **IPMN,** p 353-354.

17. E. **ALL OF THE ABOVE**
    Unlike mucinous cystic neoplasms, which are common in young women and occur in the tail of the pancreas, IPMNs typically present in elderly men and preferentially involve the head of the pancreas. Due to their connection to the duct system, IPMNs may present with obstruction of the main pancreatic duct secondary to viscous mucus plugging. This latter feature can be appreciated on endoscopic examination and may clinch the diagnosis prior to resection. IPMNs can be prognostically stratified by taking into account the degree of ductal dysplasia and the presence of invasion.
    QCSP, **IPMN,** p 353-354.

18. C. **10%-20%**
    10%-20% of IPMNs invade either focally or diffusely into the adjacent pancreatic parenchyma. These lesions are better classified as papillary mucinous carcinomas.
    QCSP, **Papillary Mucinous Carcinoma,** p 355.

19. C. **ZYMOGEN GRANULES**
    The apical portion of the tumor cells contains dense zymogen granules of various sizes. These granules show reactivity with PAS-D staining and impart a fine granular appearance to the cytoplasm.
    QCSP, **Acinar Cell Carcinoma,** p 355.

20. B. **SURVIVAL AT 3 YEARS IS 95%.**
    Survival in acinar carcinoma is poor, with only 25% of patients living at 3 years despite surgical resection and adjuvant therapy. Of note, well-differentiated acinar cell carcinomas are sometimes difficult to distinguish from normal acinar pancreatic tissue or other well-differentiated tumors with acinar architecture. The most helpful histologic feature is the presence of prominent nucleoli, which supports the diagnosis of acinar cell carcinoma.
    QCSP, **Acinar Cell Carcinoma,** p 356.

21. D. **MITOTIC FIGURES ARE TYPICALLY ABUNDANT.**
    Mitotic figures are rare in solid-pseudopapillary tumors. Marked mitotic activity, perineural invasion, angioinvasion, marked nuclear atypia, and necrosis are suggestive of malignant potential.
    QCSP, **Solid-Pseudopapillary Tumors,** p 356-357.

22. A. **NSE+, VIMENTIN+, FOCAL CYTOKERATIN+, MUCICARMINE AND PAS–**
    The tumor cells are immunoreactive with NSE and vimentin. Focal positivity is seen with cytokeratin. Tumor cells also stain for CD10 and β-catenin (nuclear labeling). Mucicarmine is negative. PAS is negative in the tumor cells but highlights the eosinophilic globules. In contrast to neuroendocrine tumors, the tumor cells in solid-pseudopapillary neoplasm are negative or only weakly and focally positive for chromogranin and synaptophysin.
    QCSP, **Solid-Pseudopapillary Tumors,** p 357.

9: Pancreas Answers

23. D. **SQUAMOID CELL NESTS (SQUAMOID CORPUSCLES)**
     Answers A-C are histologic features found in both acinar cell carcinoma and pancreatoblastoma. Squamoid corpuscles, however, are a key feature of pancreatoblastoma. The squamoid nests consist of whorled polygonal epithelial cells with eosinophilic cytoplasm. Central keratinization as well as foci of necrosis can also be seen.
     QCSP, **Pancreatoblastoma,** p 358-359.

24. B. **BECKWITH-WIEDEMANN SYNDROME**
     Pancreatoblastoma in children is associated with Beckwith-Wiedemann syndrome (11p15), which is characterized by exophthalmos, macroglossia, giantism, hemihypertrophy, pancreatic islet cell hyperplasia, pancreatoblastoma, enlarged adrenal glands with cortical cytomegaly, adrenal cortical carcinoma, neuroblastoma, renal medullary cysts, and a predisposition to develop Wilms tumor. Pancreatoblastoma in adults is associated with FAP (>100 GI tract polyps, autosomal dominant, involving APC gene). Zollinger-Ellison syndrome includes gastrinomas, massive gastric acid hypersecretion with elevated basal serum gastrin levels, and peptic ulceration (multiple and occur in unusual sites). Carney triad consists of gastric leiomyosarcoma, pulmonary chondroma, and extra-adrenal paraganglioma. Carney syndrome includes myxomas, lentiginous and blue nevi, and endocrine tumors.
     QCSP, **Pancreatoblastoma,** p 359.

25. D. **TUMOR SIZE, MITOTIC RATE, KI-67 LABELING INDEX.**
     The biologic behavior of pancreatic endocrine tumors (especially well-differentiated subtypes) is quite difficult to predict. Proposed criteria for malignancy include the presence of invasion of adjacent organs, unequivocal metastases, and large vessel invasion. Tumor size >2 cm, mitotic rate (>2 mitosis per 10 Hpf), and an elevated Ki-67 labeling index confer a poor prognosis but are insufficient for a diagnosis of malignancy.
     QCSP, **Endocrine Tumors,** p 360.

26. B. **GASTRINOMA**
     Gastrinoma: Zollinger-Ellison syndrome (gastrinomas, massive gastric acid hypersecretion with elevated basal serum gastrin levels, peptic ulceration [multiple and in unusual sites])
     QCSP, **Well-Differentiated Endocrine Tumors,** p 360-361.

27. A. **INSULINOMA**
     Insulinoma: Whipple triad (symptomatic hypoglycemia, low fasting glucose, improvement of symptoms when glucose is raised to normal levels)
     QCSP, **Well-Differentiated Endocrine Tumors,** p 360-361.

28. B. **VIPOMA**
     VIPoma: WDHA syndrome (watery diarrhea, hypokalemia, achlorhydria)
     QCSP, **Well-Differentiated Endocrine Tumors,** p 360-361.

29. D. **ENTEROCHROMAFFIN CELL TUMOR**
     Enterochromaffin cell tumor: carcinoid syndrome (diarrhea, cutaneous flushing, hypotension, bronchospasm, right heart endocardial fibrosis, mesenteric and retroperitoneal fibrosis)
     QCSP, **Well-Differentiated Endocrine Tumors,** p 360-361.

30. E. **GLUCAGONOMA**
     Glucagonoma: glucagonoma syndrome (this syndrome consists of necrolytic migratory erythema, stomatitis, diabetes mellitus, weight loss, anemia, depression, and deep venous thrombosis)
     QCSP, **Well-Differentiated Endocrine Tumors,** p 360-361.

9: Pancreas Answers

44. B. **LOW-GRADE/WELL-DIFFERENTIATED NEUROENDOCRINE TUMOR (NONFUNCTIONING)**
The image demonstrates a well-differentiated neuroendocrine tumor. The majority of these lesions are nonfunctioning. They consist of islet A and pancreatic polypeptide cells. As they do not demonstrate signs of hormone hyperfunction, they most often present with expanding mass, pain, jaundice, and/or ascites.
QCSP, **Nonfunctioning Tumors,** p 362.

Chapter 10

Upper Aerodigestive Tract

1. The fossa of Rosenmüller is located in which of the following anatomic regions of the upper aerodigestive tract?
   A. Oropharynx
   B. Nasal cavity and paranasal sinuses
   C. Nasopharynx
   D. Hypopharynx
   E. Larynx

2. The juxtaoral organ of Chievitz can be mistaken for invasive squamous cell carcinoma.
   A. True
   B. False

3. A 32-year-old man is seen by his PCP for a white patch located on the mucosal aspect of the lower lip. The patient has been using chewing tobacco daily for 10 years. The PCP suspects leukoplakia and performs a biopsy. Which of the following regarding leukoplakia is TRUE?
   A. It has a high risk of malignant transformation.
   B. It is easily scraped off.
   C. The speckled variant is less likely to transform into invasive squamous cell carcinoma than typical leukoplakia.
   D. Histologic findings include epithelial thickening, hyperkeratosis, and acanthosis.
   E. The white patch will most likely persist even if the patient ceases his tobacco use.

4. The same patient returns to the PCP 16 years later, at the age of 48. He now presents with an irregular red patch involving the floor of his mouth. The patient has continued using chewing tobacco during this interval. The PCP is concerned for erythroplakia and performs a biopsy. Which of the following regarding erythroplakia is FALSE?
   A. It most commonly involves the lips.
   B. Compared to leukoplakia and erythroleukoplakia, it poses a higher risk of subsequent squamous cell carcinoma.
   C. Histologic findings include atrophic epithelium, subepithelial vascular telangiectasia, and inflammation.
   D. Most cases contain foci of high-grade dysplasia or carcinoma in situ.

5. Pure verrucous carcinoma is incapable of metastasis.
   A. True
   B. False

6. Which of the following statements regarding olfactory neuroblastoma is FALSE?
   A. The tumor cells generally stain for neuron-specific enolase, synaptophysin, and neurofilament protein.
   B. Chromogranin is not a reliable marker for diagnosis.
   C. The sustentacular cells at the border of tumor cell nests stain for S100.
   D. Approximately 30% of cases will stain for cytokeratin.
   E. Olfactory neuroblastoma is rapidly progressive; recurrences beyond 10 years are exceedingly rare.

7. Melanotic neuroectodermal tumor of infancy is incapable of metastasis.
   A. True
   B. False

8. Inverted papillomas are sometimes associated with squamous cell carcinoma and may demonstrate HPV positivity.
   A. True
   B. False

10: Upper Aerodigestive Tract Questions

9. A 59-year-old man presents with epistaxis and dull, constant facial pain. An exophytic mass of the left ethmoid sinus is biopsied, and the pathologist renders a diagnosis of sinonasal squamous cell carcinoma. Which of the following statements regarding sinonasal squamous cell carcinoma is FALSE?
    A. Carcinomas occurring in the nasal cavity have a better prognosis compared to their counterparts in the sinuses.
    B. Sinonasal squamous cell carcinomas of the nasal cavity are associated with smoking and industrial exposure to nickel ore, chromium, radium, and isopropyl alcohol.
    C. Squamous cell carcinoma of the maxilla is associated with chronic sinusitis and Thorotrast administration.
    D. Squamous cell carcinoma of the maxillary antrum has a 5% chance of bilateral involvement.
    E. Recurrence of sinonasal squamous cell carcinoma generally occurs >10 years after initial diagnosis.

10. Which of the following statements is TRUE regarding keratinizing squamous cell carcinoma of the nasopharynx?
    A. It is more likely than undifferentiated carcinomas to have locally advanced growth and invasion.
    B. It is less likely than undifferentiated carcinomas to metastasize to lymph nodes.
    C. It is less likely than undifferentiated carcinomas to be immunoreactive for EBV.
    D. All of the above
    E. None of the above

11. Which of the following statements regarding nasopharyngeal carcinomas is FALSE?
    A. Keratinizing squamous cell carcinoma is the least radiosensitive type.
    B. Radiation-induced nasopharyngeal carcinoma is not associated with EBV.
    C. Stage I undifferentiated carcinoma (confined to the nasopharynx) has a >90% survival rate.
    D. The incidence of nasopharyngeal carcinoma is lower in patients with blood group B.
    E. These tumors most commonly arise near the eustachian tube opening in the fossa of Rosenmüller.

12. Radiation therapy has been shown to be effective for nasopharyngeal angiofibromas.
    A. True
    B. False

13. Which of the following statements regarding adenosquamous carcinoma of the head and neck is FALSE?
    A. Approximately 40% of patients are alive 15 years after diagnosis.
    B. Distant metastases develop in 80% of patients with primary tumors >1.0 cm in size.
    C. Metastases usually contain all 3 histologic components.
    D. All of the above
    E. None of the above

14. Radiation therapy has been shown to be highly effective for treating spindle cell carcinoma.
    A. True
    B. False

15. A 62-year-old man with a 50-pack/year smoking history is referred to an otolaryngologist for persistent hoarseness and new onset hemoptysis. Laryngoscopy reveals an ulcerated supraglottic mass, and a biopsy is performed. A diagnosis of lymphoepithelial carcinoma is rendered. Which of the following statements regarding lymphoepithelial carcinoma of the hypopharynx, larynx, and trachea is FALSE?
    A. Ethanol abuse and smoking history are significant risk factors.
    B. EBV infection is not commonly associated with lymphoepithelial carcinoma in these anatomic sites.
    C. Men are more likely to be affected by lymphoepithelial carcinoma in these anatomic sites.
    D. Metastatic lymphoepithelial carcinoma with a Regaud histologic pattern can be mistaken for sinus histiocytosis.
    E. Regardless of stage, survival rates are <50%.

10: Upper Aerodigestive Tract Questions

16. A 49-year-old man is seen by his PCP for a raised, partially ulcerated mass on the floor of his mouth. A biopsy is performed, and a photomicrograph of the lesion is shown below. Which of the following statements regarding this lesion of the oral cavity and oropharynx is FALSE?

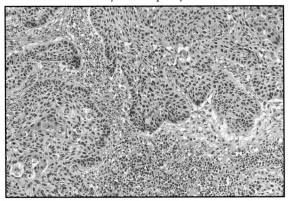

    A.   It is more common in men.

    B.   It represents >90% of all intraoral malignancies.

    C.   Significant tobacco and ethanol use act synergistically to increase the risk of developing this lesion.

    D.   25% of cases arise in the floor of mouth, the lateral-ventral tongue, and the soft palate-retromolar trigone-anterior tonsillar pillar region.

    E.   It is most frequently diagnosed between the 5th and 8th decades of life.

17. A photomicrograph of verrucous carcinoma is shown below. Which of the following statements regarding verrucous carcinoma is FALSE?

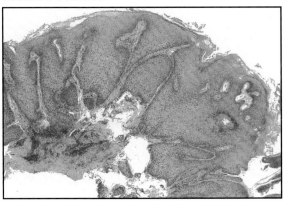

    A.   It most commonly arises in the buccal mucosa.

    B.   It is exquisitely well-differentiated and exhibits orderly maturation of both superficial and deep epithelium.

    C.   It is strongly associated with tobacco use (particularly the chewing-type).

    D.   It is strongly associated with ethanol use.

    E.   Approximately 30% of cases are associated with HPV infection (types 6, 11, and 16).

10: Upper Aerodigestive Tract Questions

18.   A 15-year-old male is referred to an otolaryngologist for a polypoid mass arising in the roof of the nasal fossa. The biopsy is shown below. A karyotype demonstrates trisomy 8q. The most likely diagnosis is:

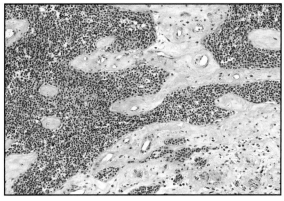

  A.   Ewing sarcoma
  B.   Olfactory neuroblastoma
  C.   Oncocytic papilloma
  D.   Pituitary adenoma
  E.   Melanoma

19.   A photomicrograph of Ewing sarcoma is shown below. Which of the following statements is TRUE regarding Ewing sarcoma?

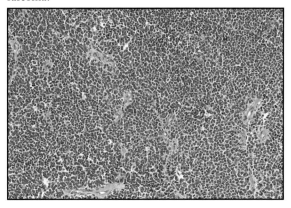

  A.   Homer Wright rosettes are found only rarely.
  B.   The tumor cells are negative for CD99 and vimentin.
  C.   Ewing sarcoma of the head and neck has a worse prognosis overall than Ewing sarcoma occurring at other anatomic sites.
  D.   5-year survival is only around 10%-20%.
  E.   Approximately 80% of cases of Ewing sarcoma occur in the head and neck.

10: Upper Aerodigestive Tract Questions

20. A photomicrograph of a nasal lesion is shown below. Which of the following statements regarding this lesion is FALSE?

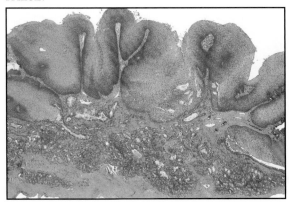

    A. It is the most common type of Schneiderian papilloma.

    B. It is composed of thin fibrovascular stalks covered by 5-30 layers of epithelium (squamous, ciliated columnar, and intermediate cells).

    C. It is strongly associated with squamous cell carcinoma.

    D. Among the 3 types of Schneiderian papillomas, fungiform papillomas have the lowest rate of recurrence following excision.

    E. It only rarely occurs bilaterally.

21. A photomicrograph of an oncocytic papilloma is shown below. Which of the following statements regarding oncocytic papilloma is FALSE?

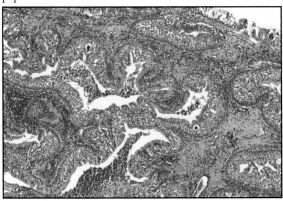

    A. It is the rarest type of Schneiderian papilloma.

    B. It frequently demonstrates HPV positivity.

    C. Immunohistochemical stains for cytokeratin are frequently positive.

    D. It is associated with squamous cell carcinoma.

    E. It frequently exhibits both inverted and exophytic patterns of growth.

22. A 55-year-old man undergoes biopsy of a fungating pink mass located in the ethmoid sinus. A photomicrograph of the lesion is shown below. Which of the following is TRUE regarding this tumor?

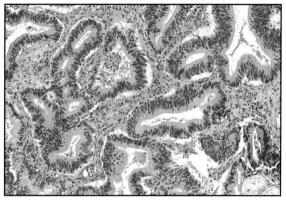

    A.   It is associated with chronic exposure to leather dust and fine hardwood dust.

    B.   Sporadic cases without carcinogen primarily involve the maxillary antrum and occur in women.

    C.   It can resemble signet ring carcinoma.

    D.   All of the above

    E.   None of the above

23. A 56-year-old woman presents with proptosis and periorbital swelling. A large fungating mass in the nasal cavity is detected, and a biopsy is performed, which is interpreted as sinonasal undifferentiated carcinoma (SNUC). A photomicrograph of the lesion is shown below. Which of the following statements is FALSE regarding SNUC?

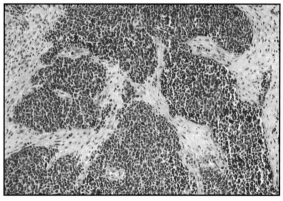

    A.   It is somewhat more common in females.

    B.   The median survival after diagnosis is 4 years.

    C.   Olfactory neuroblastoma is an important consideration in the differential diagnosis.

    D.   All of the above

    E.   None of the above

10: Upper Aerodigestive Tract Questions

24. A 48-year-old man presents with hearing loss and headache. A mass is found in the nasopharynx. A photomicrograph of the lesion is shown below. Which of the following is FALSE regarding this tumor?

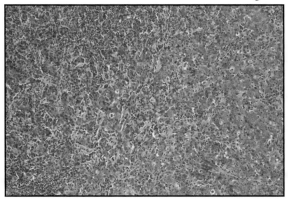

   A. It has a bimodal age distribution with peaks in the 2nd and 6th decades.
   B. EBV infection is present in 20% of cases.
   C. Primary radiation therapy is the treatment of choice.
   D. Metastases can resemble either Hodgkin lymphoma or sinus histiocytosis.
   E. Between 50%-80% of patients present with cervical lymphadenopathy.

25. A 63-year-old man with dysphonia and hemoptysis is noted to have a large, exophytic laryngeal mass on laryngoscopy. A biopsy is performed, and a photomicrograph of the lesion is shown below. An alcian blue stain is positive. The most likely diagnosis is:

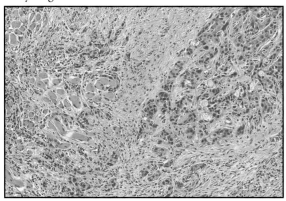

   A. Basaloid squamous cell carcinoma
   B. Lymphoepithelial carcinoma
   C. Necrotizing sialometaplasia
   D. Adenosquamous carcinoma
   E. Acinic cell carcinoma

26.   A 48-year-old man is referred to an otolaryngologist for an exophytic mass arising from the vermillion border of the lower lip. He has a 30-year history of chewing tobacco use and poor dentition. A biopsy is performed, and the pathologist renders a diagnosis of spindle cell carcinoma. A photomicrograph of the lesion is shown below. Which of the following statements regarding spindle cell carcinoma is FALSE?

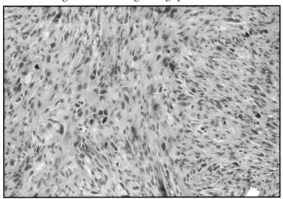

A.   The most common sites include the tongue, vermillion border of the lower lip, alveolar ridge, and gingiva.
B.   The diagnosis depends on the presence of malignant spindle cells and squamous cell carcinoma.
C.   The spindle cell component can assume numerous histologic patterns.
D.   Metastatic lesions can be composed entirely of the spindle cell component.
E.   Approximately 80% of patients will have multiple synchronous or metachronous primary carcinomas of the upper respiratory or digestive tracts.

27.   A 68-year-old man is diagnosed with papillary squamous cell carcinoma of the supraglottis. A photomicrograph of the lesion is shown below. Which of the following is FALSE regarding papillary squamous cell carcinoma?

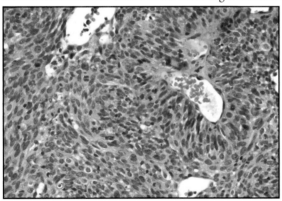

A.   The role of HPV is currently unknown.
B.   Smoking and ethanol use are strongly associated with this carcinoma.
C.   It has a better prognosis than typical squamous cell carcinoma.
D.   It is most commonly found in the subglottis.
E.   Men are more likely to develop this lesion.

28.   A 62-year-old man is referred to an otolaryngologist for an ulcerated mass arising from the left palatine tonsil. A biopsy is performed, and the pathologist renders a diagnosis. A photomicrograph of the lesion is shown below. The most likely diagnosis is:

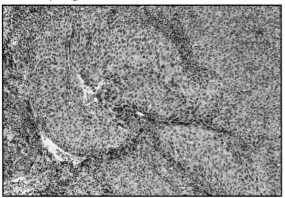

    A.   Spindle cell carcinoma
    B.   Papillary squamous cell carcinoma
    C.   Lymphoepithelial carcinoma
    D.   Adenosquamous carcinoma
    E.   Basaloid squamous cell carcinoma

10: Upper Aerodigestive Tract Answers

1. C. **NASOPHARYNX**

   The fossa of Rosenmüller is a recess located behind the eustachian tubes in the nasopharynx. It is an important anatomic landmark, because it is the most common site for nasopharyngeal carcinomas. This is a picky question, I know, but it does represent useful Boards fodder.

   QCSP, **Intraoperative Consultation,** p 364.

2. A. **TRUE**

   The juxtaoral organ of Chievitz is a structure located in the retromolar trigone, which consists of basaloid or squamoid epithelial cells arranged in nests that may be in close proximity to nerve fibers. Histologically, this can be misinterpreted as invasive squamous cell carcinoma with perineural involvement. This is another esoteric question, but can come in handy to avoid a treacherous diagnostic pitfall with potentially devastating consequences.

   QCSP, **Intraoperative Consultation,** p 365.

3. D. **HISTOLOGIC FINDINGS IN LEUKOPLAKIA INCLUDE EPITHELIAL THICKENING, HYPERKERATOSIS, AND ACANTHOSIS.**

   Leukoplakia is a benign lesion of the oral mucosa that usually develops on the lips, buccal mucosa, alveolar ridges and sulci, and palate. Physical examination reveals a discrete white patch, which cannot be scraped from the mucosal surface. Leukoplakia represents the initial mucosal response following injury due to carcinogens. It has a low risk of malignant transformation. Removal of the irritant will result in spontaneous resolution of the lesion. In contrast, erythroleukoplakia (mixed white and red patches, or "speckled leukoplakia") has a high risk of progression to squamous cell carcinoma. Histologically, leukoplakia is characterized by epithelial thickening, hyperkeratosis, and acanthosis. Dysplasia is not typically present.

   QCSP, **Squamous Cell Carcinoma,** p 365-366.

4. A. **IT MOST COMMONLY INVOLVES THE LIPS.**

   Erythroplakia is a red patch of the oral mucosa which most frequently involves the floor of the mouth, retromolar trigone, mandibular gingiva and sulcus, tongue, or palate. Compared to leukoplakia and erythroleukoplakia, this lesion has a much higher risk of progression to squamous cell carcinoma. Histologic findings include thin, atrophic epithelium, subepithelial vascular telangiectasia, and inflammation. Most cases will demonstrate foci of high-grade dysplasia or carcinoma in situ.

   QCSP, **Squamous Cell Carcinoma,** p 366.

5. A. **TRUE**

   A pure verrucous carcinoma, while locally invasive, is incapable of metastasis. However, if invasive foci of lesser differentiated squamous cell carcinoma are present at the deep margin (20% of cases), the lesion should be classified as a verrucous carcinoma with coexisting foci of squamous cell carcinoma, alerting the clinician to its potential for metastasis. Verrucous carcinomas are typically resected, although advanced disease can also be treated with radiation. Chemotherapy has not proven beneficial. Approximately 85% of patients treated with complete surgical excision achieve tumor control. Lesions that are treated solely with radiation can undergo anaplastic transformation within months of therapy.

   QCSP, **Verrucous Carcinoma,** p 369-370.

6. E. **OLFACTORY NEUROBLASTOMA IS RAPIDLY PROGRESSIVE; RECURRENCES BEYOND 10 YEARS ARE EXCEEDINGLY RARE.**

   Olfactory neuroblastoma is generally a slowly progressive tumor, and recurrences do occur >10 years after diagnosis. The greatest chance for cure is achieved by total surgical excision with chemoradiation (75% chance of cure). In up to 20% of cases, nodal and bone metastases can occur.

   QCSP, **Olfactory Neuroblastoma,** p 370-371.

10: Upper Aerodigestive Tract Answers

7.   B.   **FALSE**

Approximately 7% of these tumors metastasize. Common locations include the lymph nodes, adrenal glands, liver, bone, and soft tissue. For a more extensive description of this tumor, please see chapter 17 (Mandible and Maxilla).

QCSP, **Melanotic Neuroectodermal Tumor of Infancy,** p 372.

8.   A.   **TRUE**

Inverted papillomas represent approximately 45% of all Schneiderian papillomas and usually occur between the ages of 30 and 50. Grossly, these lesions are firm and polypoid and almost always arise from the lateral nasal wall or paranasal sinuses. The overlying mucosa is intact. Histologically, these papillomas are characterized by deeply invaginated nests or cords of squamous epithelium that extend into the underlying stroma. The papillomas are lined by 5-30 layers of squamous, ciliated columnar, or intermediate cells with intermixed mucus-secreting cells. Rarely, the inverted papilloma can have an exophytic surface component. These lesions have a recurrence rate of approximately 45%, with a rate as high as 70% following simple local excision. Unlike fungiform papillomas, inverted papillomas have an association with squamous cell carcinoma, which may be present in or adjacent to the papilloma. A metachronous carcinoma can occur after excision of the papilloma in 3% of patients. Although HPV infection has the strongest association with fungiform papillomas, occasional cases of inverted papilloma have also demonstrated HPV positivity, particularly types 6, 11, 16, and 18.

QCSP, **Schneiderian Papilloma,** p 373-374.

9.   E.   **RECURRENCE OF SINONASAL SQUAMOUS CELL CARCINOMA GENERALLY OCCURS >10 YEARS AFTER INITIAL DIAGNOSIS.**

Sinonasal squamous cell carcinomas of the nasal cavity and the sinuses differ in their demographics and pathophysiology. While tumors occurring in the nasal cavity are commonly associated with smoking and industrial exposure, tumors occurring in the sinuses are usually accompanied by chronic sinusitis or a history of Thorotrast administration. The prognosis of nasal cavity lesions is typically better than that of sinus lesions. The latter also exhibits an increased incidence of bilaterality. Both lesions can and do recur, usually within 2 years of diagnosis.

QCSP, **Sinonasal Carcinoma,** p 375-377.

10.   D.   **ALL OF THE ABOVE**

Compared to undifferentiated nasopharyngeal carcinomas, keratinizing squamous cell carcinoma is more likely to exhibit local invasion and advanced growth and less likely to be immunoreactive for EBV and metastasize to lymph nodes.

QCSP, **Nasopharyngeal Carcinoma,** p 377-378.

11.   D.   **THE INCIDENCE OF NASOPHARYNGEAL CARCINOMA IS LOWER IN PATIENTS WITH BLOOD GROUP B.**

Compared to differentiated carcinoma and undifferentiated carcinoma, keratinizing squamous cell carcinoma is the least radiosensitive. The cases of radiation-induced nasopharyngeal carcinoma are not associated with EBV. Stage I undifferentiated carcinoma (limited to the nasopharynx) has a 98% survival rate. Nasopharyngeal carcinomas classically arise in the fossa of Rosenmüller. Interestingly, patients with blood group A have a lower incidence of nasopharyngeal carcinomas.

QCSP, **Nasopharyngeal Carcinoma,** p 377-378.

10: Upper Aerodigestive Tract Answers

12. A.   **TRUE**

Nasopharyngeal angiofibromas most frequently occur in adolescent males. These lesions usually present as bilateral nasal obstruction (95%) and are frequently accompanied by epistaxis (70%). Grossly, these benign lesions appear as red polypoid masses that arise in the lateral nasopharynx or posterior nasal cavity. The mass can sometimes extend into the anterior nasal cavity, orbit, or pterygomaxillary fossa. Histologically, these lesions are composed of dense collagenized fibrous tissue containing numerous vascular channels that are usually thin-walled and lacking an elastic membrane. The fibrous component can vary in both cellularity and quantity of collagen present. The endothelial cells are positive for CD34, CD31, and factor VIII-related antigen, while the stromal cells are positive for vimentin and testosterone. Radiotherapy has been shown to produce dramatic tumor regression, and can produce permanent symptom control in 80% of patients. However, most cases are treated with complete surgical excision followed by oral estrogen therapy. Chemotherapy has a role in the treatment of aggressive, unresectable lesions. Between 35%-60% of these lesions recur, depending on the completeness of excision.

QCSP, **Nasopharyngeal Angiofibroma,** p 379.

13. A.   **APPROXIMATELY 40% OF PATIENTS ARE ALIVE 15 YEARS AFTER DIAGNOSIS.**

Adenosquamous carcinoma is highly aggressive, with only 25% of patients surviving 10 years after diagnosis. There are no survivors 15 years after diagnosis. Distant metastases develop in approximately 80% of patients with primary tumors >1.0 cm in size and usually contain all 3 histologic components (see previous question).

QCSP, **Adenosquamous Carcinoma,** p 383-384.

14. B.   **FALSE**

The overall mortality rate for spindle cell carcinoma is 60%-65%, with a mean survival of <2 years. The most important prognostic factor is the presence of cervical node metastases. Tumor size and depth of invasion appear to have no effect on prognosis. Primary radiation therapy is ineffective for spindle cell carcinoma, with a failure rate of 80%.

QCSP, **Spindle Cell Carcinoma,** p 386.

15. E.   **REGARDLESS OF STAGE, SURVIVAL RATES ARE <50%.**

Although lymphoepithelial carcinoma of the hypopharynx, larynx, and trachea histologically resembles undifferentiated nasopharyngeal carcinoma, there is no association with EBV infection. The inflammatory infiltrate characteristic of these lesions consists of lymphocytes and plasma cells, which dissect between tumor foci and obscure the neoplastic epithelial component. There are 2 major patterns: Regaud and Schmincke. The Regaud pattern is characterized by neoplastic cells in obvious bundles and trabeculae that are surrounded and separated by lymphocytes and plasma cells. Nodal metastases of such lesions can be mistaken for sinus histiocytosis. The Schmincke pattern, on the other hand, is characterized by individual neoplastic epithelial cells that are surrounded and obscured by the prominent lymphoid background. Metastatic lesions of this type can be mistaken for Hodgkin or non-Hodgkin lymphoma. Approximately half of lymphoepithelial carcinomas will have a variable squamous cell component with overlying carcinoma in situ. These carcinomas are far more common in men (4:1) with an average age of 60 years at the time of diagnosis. Ethanol abuse and smoking are strong risk factors, while EBV infection does not appear to be associated with this neoplasm in the hypopharynx, larynx, and trachea. These carcinomas are actually quite rare in these anatomic sites, and when present are most commonly supraglottic. The majority of patients present with hoarseness, cough, sore throat, dysphagia, neck mass, and/or hemoptysis. These lesions are treated primarily with radiation therapy. Survival rates are excellent, and range from 98% survival in stage I lesions to 75% in stage IV-B lesions.

QCSP, **Lymphoepithelial Carcinoma,** p 387.

10: Upper Aerodigestive Tract Answers

16. **D.** **25% OF CASES ARISE IN THE FLOOR OF MOUTH, THE LATERAL-VENTRAL TONGUE, AND THE SOFT PALATE-RETROMOLAR TRIGONE-ANTERIOR TONSILLAR PILLAR REGION.**

The image demonstrates a squamous cell carcinoma. Squamous cell carcinoma of the oral cavity and oropharynx more commonly develops in men and most cases occur between the 5th and 8th decades of life. While tobacco use appears to be the most significant risk factor, combined tobacco and ethanol abuse synergistically increase the risk of carcinoma. Squamous cell carcinoma represents >90% of all intraoral malignancies, and approximately 75% of these carcinomas arise in the semicircular region of the mouth (floor of mouth, lateral-ventral tongue, and soft palate-retromolar trigone-anterior tonsillar pillar region). Histologically, squamous cell carcinomas can be well differentiated (with nests of large squamous cells and prominent keratinization), moderately differentiated (with small nests of mitotically active squamous cells and less prominent keratinization), or poorly differentiated (with minute nests or individual cells, diffuse infiltration, and brisk mitotic activity). The presence of either single cell keratinization or keratin pearl formation below the overlying epithelium is diagnostic of invasion.

QCSP, **Squamous Cell Carcinoma,** p 365.

17. **D.** **IT IS STRONGLY ASSOCIATED WITH ETHANOL USE.**

Verrucous carcinoma is a rare variant of squamous cell carcinoma, representing only 1% of all squamous cell neoplasms of the head and neck. Most of these carcinomas arise in the buccal mucosa, with the gingiva, tongue, palate, and tonsillar pillar being affected less frequently. Most cases are diagnosed in the 7th decade of life, and men are more commonly affected. Grossly, these lesions are circumscribed, nodular masses that have a cobblestone or smooth red to white surface with a tan-gray cut surface and a distinct margin of invasion. Histologically, these carcinomas are extremely well differentiated with hyperplastic growth and orderly maturation in both the superficial and deep portions of the tumor. The surface is composed of prominent papillae ("church spires") that are covered by parakeratotic and orthokeratotic squamous cells, with keratin that fills the surface crevices. Growth at the tumor base is characterized by well-demarcated, broad, bulbous ridges and nests of well-differentiated squamous cells with surrounding lymphoplasmacytic inflammatory cell infiltrate. Invasion is characterized by small irregular nests of cells. Vascular or perineural invasion is never present. While tobacco (especially chewing tobacco) is a major etiologic agent, ethanol use does not appear to be associated with verrucous carcinoma. Approximately 30% of these carcinomas are associated with HPV (types 6, 11, and 16).

QCSP, **Verrucous Carcinoma,** p 369-370.

18. **B.** **OLFACTORY NEUROBLASTOMA**

Olfactory neuroblastoma typically arises within the roof of the nasal fossa, involves the cribriform plate, and presents as a polypoid mass producing epistaxis or nasal obstruction. The mass is typically soft, red-gray, and highly vascular. These tumors have a bimodal age distribution, with peak incidences in adolescence (15 years) and adulthood (55 years). Histologically, these tumors are composed of nests of small cells with minimal cytoplasm and round nucleoli with speckled chromatin. Minimal nuclear pleomorphism is present, and the nests of cells are separated by stroma. Mitotic activity is variable from tumor to tumor. Well-formed rosettes are rare (Flexner-Wintersteiner rosettes rarer than Homer Wright rosettes). Ewing sarcomas can have a similar presentation and histologic picture, but the characteristic cytogenetic finding is t(11;22). Trisomy 8q, on the other hand, is associated with some cases of olfactory neuroblastoma.

QCSP, **Olfactory Neuroblastoma,** p 370-371.

10: Upper Aerodigestive Tract Answers

19. **A.** **HOMER WRIGHT ROSETTES ARE FOUND ONLY RARELY.**

Ewing sarcoma/primitive neuroectodermal tumor is a rare malignancy that usually arises in children and young adults. Approximately 20% of these tumors occur in the head and neck, particularly in the maxillary sinus. These lesions have a better prognosis compared to those occurring at other anatomic sites. Grossly, these tumors are gray-white with foci of hemorrhage. Histologically, they are composed of dense, uniform small to medium-sized round cells with fine chromatin and minimal cytoplasm. Mitotic activity is usually quite brisk. While helpful in making the diagnosis, true Homer Wright rosettes are not commonly present. The tumor cells are positive for both vimentin and CD99, with variable positivity for S100, neurofilament protein, neuron-specific enolase, CD57, synaptophysin, and chromogranin. The overall 5-year survival is 60%-70%.

QCSP, **Ewing Sarcoma (EWS)/Primitive Neuroectodermal Tumor (PNET),** p 371-372.

20. **C.** **IT IS STRONGLY ASSOCIATED WITH SQUAMOUS CELL CARCINOMA.**

Fungiform papillomas are the most common type of Schneiderian papilloma, representing 50% of all Schneiderian papillomas. They generally arise in individuals between the ages of 20 and 40. Grossly, these lesions are tan-gray, exophytic, and firm, and generally arise from the nasal septum. These lesions rarely occur bilaterally and are not associated with an increased risk of squamous cell carcinoma. Histologically, fungiform papillomas have an exophytic architecture with branching fibrovascular stalks covered by 5-30 layers of epithelium composed of squamous, ciliated columnar, and intermediate cells. Following surgical excision, fungiform papillomas have a 20% recurrence rate, which is the lowest rate of recurrence among the different types of Schneiderian papillomas.

QCSP, **Schneiderian Papilloma,** p 373-374.

21. **B.** **IT FREQUENTLY DEMONSTRATES HPV POSITIVITY.**

Oncocytic papillomas are the rarest type of Schneiderian papilloma (5%). Grossly, they are single or multifocal polypoid lesions that involve the lateral nasal wall or paranasal sinuses. Histologically, most of these lesions have both inverted and exophytic patterns of growth. The exophytic component consists of fibrovascular cores covered by 3-8 layers of epithelium. The inverted component is characterized by nests and cords of epithelial cells. The epithelial cells are polygonal to columnar cells with copious eosinophilic and granular cytoplasm with round, uniform nuclei and inconspicuous nucleoli. Ciliated cells may cover the epithelium, and mucous-filled microcysts are sometimes present. The epithelial cells are immunoreactive with cytokeratin. These papillomas have a recurrence risk of 45% following surgical excision. Unlike the fungiform and inverted papillomas, oncocytic papillomas have no known association with HPV. However, like the inverted papillomas, oncocytic papillomas are associated with squamous cell carcinoma.

QCSP, **Schneiderian Papilloma,** p 373-374.

22. **D.** **ALL OF THE ABOVE**

Sinonasal intestinal-type adenocarcinoma most commonly occurs in men (80%), and usually arises in the ethmoid sinuses. There is a strong association between this tumor and chronic exposure to leather dust and fine hardwood dust. However, sporadic tumors of this type without obvious carcinogen exposure primarily occur in women and involve the maxillary antrum. Histologically, these tumors are composed of cells that mimic normal or neoplastic intestinal mucosa. Occasionally, these neoplasms can resemble signet ring carcinomas.

QCSP, **Sinonasal Carcinoma,** p 375-377.

23. **B.** **THE MEDIAN SURVIVAL AFTER DIAGNOSIS IS 4 YEARS.**

SNUCs are highly aggressive neoplasms with a median survival of only 4 months after diagnosis. Unlike most sinonasal tumors, SNUCs are somewhat more common in females (average age at diagnosis is 55). Olfactory neuroblastoma is an important consideration in the differential diagnosis. SNUCs are not associated with EBV. The lesion is typically immunoreactive with cytokeratin and EMA. About 1/2 of cases express neuron-specific enolase.

QCSP, **Sinonasal Carcinoma,** p 375-377.

10: Upper Aerodigestive Tract Answers

24.   B.   **EBV INFECTION IS PRESENT IN 20% OF CASES.**

Undifferentiated nasopharyngeal carcinomas (lymphoepitheliomas) have a bimodal age distribution (2nd and 6th decades), and are associated with EBV in virtually all cases. They are best treated with primary radiation therapy and are only rarely resected. Between 50%-80% of patients present with cervical lymphadenopathy due to metastases from occult primary lesions. Histologically, these undifferentiated carcinomas are composed of large tumor cells with eosinophilic or amphophilic cytoplasm, indistinct cell borders, round to oval vesicular nuclei and large central nucleoli. A prominent inflammatory infiltrate consisting of lymphocytes, plasma cells, and occasional eosinophils is present and typically manifests itself in 2 patterns: Regaud and Schmincke. The Regaud pattern showcases neoplastic cells arranged in cohesive nests and trabeculae separated by inflammatory cells. Metastatic carcinomas exhibiting this type of inflammatory distribution can resemble sinus histiocytosis. The Schmincke pattern is characterized by an admixture of neoplastic cells and inflammatory cells resulting in individual carcinoma cells scattered amongst a prominent lymphoid background. Metastatic carcinomas with the Schmincke pattern can resemble Hodgkin or non-Hodgkin lymphoma.

QCSP, **Nasopharyngeal Carcinoma,** p 377-378.

25.   D.   **ADENOSQUAMOUS CARCINOMA**

Adenosquamous carcinoma is an aggressive neoplasm that arises from the surface epithelium or minor salivary glands of the tongue, larynx, nasal cavity, and floor of mouth. The tumor is more common in men, with an average age of 60 years at the time of diagnosis. Grossly, it presents as small, erythroplakic ulcers or as swollen submucosal nodules. Laryngeal tumors are usually bulky, exophytic, and ulcerated. Histologically, adenosquamous carcinoma consists of 3 components, ie, squamous cell carcinoma, adenocarcinoma, and admixture of glandular mucous cells and cells with squamoid differentiation. Mucicarmine, PAS with diastase, and alcian blue stains highlight the presence of intracellular mucin. The glandular component expresses low molecular weight cytokeratin and CEA, while both squamous and glandular components express high molecular weight keratin.

QCSP, **Adenosquamous Carcinoma,** p 383.

26.   E.   **APPROXIMATELY 80% OF PATIENTS WILL HAVE MULTIPLE SYNCHRONOUS OR METACHRONOUS PRIMARY CARCINOMAS OF EITHER THE UPPER RESPIRATORY OR DIGESTIVE TRACTS.**

Spindle cell carcinoma is a variant of squamous cell carcinoma composed of a biphasic population of cells: typical squamous cell carcinoma and malignant spindle cells. The spindle cell component can assume a variety of histologic patterns. These include occasional cells that resemble rhabdomyoblasts, dense cell proliferations that resemble fibrosarcoma, edematous myxoid stroma with atypical bipolar spindled cells, and osteoclast-like giant cells. Metastatic lesions can be composed entirely of the squamous cell component, entirely of the spindle cell component, or a combination of the 2. These tumors most commonly arise in the larynx, lower lip, tongue, alveolar ridge, and gingiva and are more common in men (especially in the 6th decade). Major etiologic factors include tobacco and ethanol use, poor dental hygiene, and prior radiation. Approximately 20% of patients will have multiple synchronous carcinomas of the upper respiratory and digestive tracts, consistent with a field effect secondary to a carcinogen. Approximately 1/2 of these tumors will demonstrate cytokeratin staining in the spindle cell component.

QCSP, **Spindle Cell Carcinoma,** p 385-386.

10: Upper Aerodigestive Tract Answers

27.   D.   **IT IS MOST COMMONLY FOUND IN THE SUBGLOTTIS.**

Papillary squamous cell carcinoma is a variant of squamous cell carcinoma composed of thin fibrovascular cores covered by neoplastic squamous cells. These tumors are most commonly found in the larynx (especially the supraglottis) and hypopharynx, with only rare involvement of the subglottis. Men are more likely to develop this variant, particularly in the 6th and 7th decades of life. As with other squamous cell carcinomas, this tumor is strongly associated with ethanol use and smoking. Keratosis is frequently present, as are foci of hemorrhage and necrosis. Invasion is characterized by single neoplastic cells or nests of cells surrounded by prominent lymphoplasmacytic inflammation at the tumor/stromal interface. The role of HPV in these carcinomas has not been determined. Compared to typical squamous cell carcinoma, the papillary variant has a better prognosis. It is treated with surgical excision and occasional radiation therapy.

QCSP, **Papillary Squamous Cell Carcinoma,** p 386-387.

28.   E.   **BASALOID SQUAMOUS CELL CARCINOMA**

The basaloid variant of squamous cell carcinoma occurs predominantly in the oral cavity (base of tongue, palatine tonsil, and pyriform sinus), larynx, and nasopharynx. Smoking, heavy ethanol use, and HPV infection have all been associated with this variant. The average age at diagnosis is 60 years with a male predominance. Histologically, this tumor is composed of nests and cords of crowded basaloid cells occasionally exhibiting single cell and comedo-type necrosis. Nuclear palisading at the periphery of the basaloid component is often seen. Cytologic features include moderate pleomorphism, hyperchromatic nuclei, and plentiful mitotic figures. Immunohistochemical staining is generally weakly positive for cytokeratin and occasionally positive for S100 and neuron-specific enolase. P16 immunoreactivity suggests HPV infection. Basaloid squamous cell carcinoma is treated with radical surgical excision followed by adjuvant radiation and chemotherapy.

QCSP, **Basaloid Squamous Cell Carcinoma,** p 384-385.

Chapter 11

Lung

1. The cyst wall of a bronchogenic cyst consists of which of the following?
   A. Ciliated cuboidal or columnar respiratory epithelium surrounded by a fibromuscular wall with islands of cartilage and nests of bronchial glands
   B. Gastric-type epithelium
   C. Squamous and muscular lining
   D. Mesothelial lining
   E. None of the above

2. Pulmonary sequestration most commonly affects which portion of the lung?
   A. Right lower lobe
   B. Left lower lobe
   C. Right upper lobe
   D. Left upper lobe
   E. No predilection for site

3. Which alveolar hemorrhage syndrome is characterized by antibodies to the glomerular basement membrane (type IV collagen), which cross-react with the pulmonary basement membrane causing sudden onset of hemoptysis, anemia, azotemia, and diffuse pulmonary infiltrates?
   A. Goodpasture syndrome
   B. Idiopathic pulmonary hemosiderosis
   C. Wegener granulomatosis
   D. Acute lupus pneumonitis
   E. Henoch-Schönlein purpura

4. Wegener granulomatosis can affect which of the following site(s)?
   A. Lung
   B. Kidney
   C. Peripheral nerves and central nervous system
   D. Skin and breast
   E. All of the above

5. Which laboratory test(s) is/are most commonly abnormal in Wegener granulomatosis?
   A. Platelet count
   B. c-ANCA
   C. p-ANCA
   D. ANC (absolute neutrophil count)
   E. A and B

6. Diffuse alveolar damage is the pathologic manifestation of which clinical entity?
   A. Acute respiratory distress syndrome (ARDS)
   B. Pneumonia
   C. Pulmonary hemorrhage
   D. Pulmonary edema
   E. Pulmonary emboli

11: Lung Questions

7. Usual interstitial pneumonia:
   A. Occurs in young women
   B. Affects predominantly the upper lung lobes
   C. Is clinically called idiopathic pulmonary fibrosis
   D. Has characteristic hyaline membranes
   E. Has an excellent prognosis when treated early

8. Respiratory bronchiolitis-associated interstitial lung disease most closely histologically resembles which of the following?
   A. Usual interstitial pneumonia
   B. Desquamative interstitial pneumonia
   C. Nonspecific interstitial pneumonia
   D. Acute interstitial pneumonia
   E. Bronchiolitis-obliterans organizing pneumonia

9. An otherwise healthy woman develops a sudden onset of respiratory distress and progresses to respiratory failure after a flu-like illness. CT scan shows extensive and symmetric bilateral airspace consolidation ("white-out"). The clinical team has excluded potential causes such as trauma, sepsis, shock, aspiration, infectious agents, and drug toxicity. A biopsy shows diffuse alveolar damage in various stages. The clinical diagnosis is most likely:
   A. Acute respiratory distress syndrome
   B. Nonspecific interstitial pneumonia
   C. Acute interstitial pneumonia
   D. Idiopathic pulmonary fibrosis
   E. Cryptogenic organizing pneumonia

10. Giant cell interstitial pneumonia is a result of which of the following?
    A. Viral illness
    B. Duplication of chromosome 22
    C. Bacterial infection
    D. Aspiration
    E. Inhalation of hard metal

11. The lymphoid infiltrate in lymphoid interstitial pneumonia is clonal.
    A. True
    B. False

12. Sarcoidosis is:
    A. Limited to the perihilar lymph nodes and the lung parenchyma
    B. A diagnosis of exclusion
    C. Characterized by necrotizing granulomas
    D. More commonly seen in Caucasians than African-Americans
    E. Characterized by asteroid and Schaumann bodies, which are exclusively seen in sarcoidosis

13. Loeffler syndrome is a mild, self-limited asymptomatic disease characterized by transient pulmonary infiltrates and peripheral eosinophilia that spontaneously resolve.
    A. True
    B. False

11: Lung Questions

14. All of the following are characteristic features of small cell carcinoma of the lung EXCEPT:
    A. Nuclear molding
    B. Scant cytoplasm
    C. Prominent nucleoli
    D. Brisk mitotic activity
    E. Extensive necrosis and apoptosis

15. The Azzopardi effect is seen in which lung neoplasm?
    A. Squamous cell carcinoma
    B. Adenocarcinoma
    C. Small cell carcinoma
    D. Bronchioloalveolar carcinoma
    E. Inflammatory myofibroblastic tumor

16. Large cell carcinoma of the lung is a diagnosis of exclusion.
    A. True
    B. False

17. Adenosquamous carcinoma is a carcinoma that contains both squamous carcinomatous and adenocarcinomatous components. What minimum percentage of each component is required to make the diagnosis of adenosquamous carcinoma?
    A. 5%
    B. 15%
    C. 25%
    D. 50%
    E. There is no defined percentage.

18. All of the following are TRUE about sarcomatoid carcinomas of the lung EXCEPT:
    A. Most patients have a history of smoking.
    B. They are large peripheral tumors.
    C. Histologically, these are poorly-differentiated tumors with a sarcoma-like differentiation.
    D. The tumor cells are positive for cytokeratin, vimentin, and smooth muscle actin.
    E. They carry a better prognosis than other non-small cell carcinomas of the lung.

19. Criteria for separating typical from atypical carcinoid tumors of the lung include which of the following?
    A. Cellular pleomorphism
    B. Mitotic activity
    C. Necrosis
    D. B and C
    E. All of the above

20. The most common salivary gland tumor in an endobronchial location is:
    A. Acinic cell carcinoma
    B. Adenoid cystic carcinoma
    C. Low-grade mucoepidermoid carcinoma
    D. Pleomorphic adenoma (benign mixed tumor)
    E. Epithelial-myoepithelial carcinoma

11: Lung Questions

21. A 25-year-old man presents with cough and hemoptysis and is found to have an endobronchial polypoid mass. Histologically, the lesion consists of an admixture of glandular mucin-secreting cells, intermediate cells, and squamous cells. Mitotic activity and nuclear pleomorphism are sparse. There is no evidence of necrosis. The diagnosis is:
    A. Adenocarcinoma
    B. Mucous gland adenoma
    C. Adenoid cystic carcinoma
    D. Low-grade mucoepidermoid carcinoma
    E. Adenosquamous carcinoma

22. All of the following are TRUE about Langerhans cell histiocytosis (LCH) EXCEPT:
    A. It is not associated with a history of smoking.
    B. It is composed of discrete stellate peribronchial nodules.
    C. Langerhans cells are large with folded nuclei, inconspicuous nucleoli and indistinct cytoplasm.
    D. Langerhans cells are positive for S100 and CD1a.
    E. Electron microscopy shows characteristic Birbeck granules.

23. Pleuropulmonary blastoma is:
    A. Composed of a primitive appearing mesenchyme
    B. Usually found peripherally as a large solitary mass
    C. Commonly found in children <12 years of age
    D. A rare entity
    E. All of the above

24. The proliferating smooth muscle population in lymphangioleiomyomatosis is immunopositive for which of the following?
    A. Desmin
    B. HMB-45
    C. CD1a
    D. A and B
    E. None of the above

25. The differential diagnosis for small, well-circumscribed lesions of the lung in asymptomatic patients includes which of the following?
    A. Clear cell tumor (sugar tumor)
    B. Carcinoid tumor
    C. Hamartoma
    D. Granular cell tumor
    E. All of the above

11: Lung Questions

26. The lung lesion shown in the image is from a newborn infant with respiratory distress. Which of the following is TRUE about this entity?

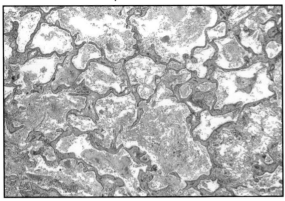

- A. It is a highly aggressive neoplasm.
- B. Several types of these lesions exist, all curable by surgical resection.
- C. The lesion involutes over time and has no clinical significance.
- D. Only female infants are affected.
- E. The entity may be complicated by the development of carcinoma (usually mucinous bronchioloalveolar carcinoma).

27. The image shows the exudative phase of diffuse alveolar damage. What is the histologic hallmark of this phase?

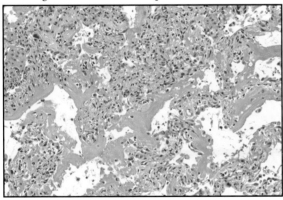

- A. Fibroblasts in the alveolar spaces
- B. Type II pneumocyte proliferation
- C. Fibrin thrombi
- D. Squamous metaplasia of the bronchial epithelium
- E. Edema accompanied by inflammatory cells as well as hyaline membranes lining the alveolar spaces

11: Lung Questions

28. A 50-year-old man presents with dyspnea. Chest X-ray shows a reticular pattern involving the periphery of the lung and the lung bases. A CT scan demonstrates peripheral honeycombing. The image shown is characterized by temporal heterogeneity. The diagnosis is:

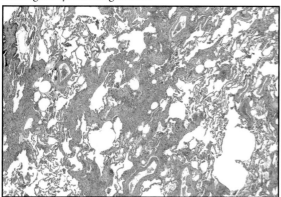 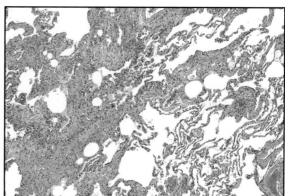

    A.   Desquamative interstitial pneumonia (DIP)
    B.   Respiratory bronchiolitis-associated interstitial lung disease (RBILD)
    C.   Usual interstitial pneumonia (UIP)
    D.   Nonspecific interstitial pneumonia (NSIP)
    E.   Diffuse alveolar damage, exudative phase (DAD)

29. The alveolar spaces in desquamative interstitial pneumonia (see image) are filled with:

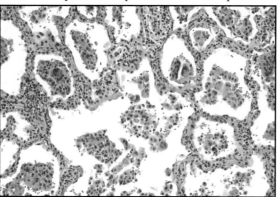

    A.   Desquamated alveolar epithelial lining cells
    B.   Macrophages
    C.   Plasma cells
    D.   Neutrophils
    E.   Lymphocytes

11: Lung Questions

30. The interstitial lung process shown in the image is:

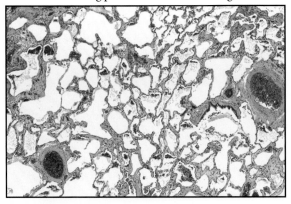

    A.   Temporally heterogeneous
    B.   Temporally homogeneous
    C.   Linked to a poor outcome
    D.   A and C
    E.   B and C

31. Polypoid fibromyxoid lesions (Masson bodies), as shown in the image below, are characteristic for which lung process?

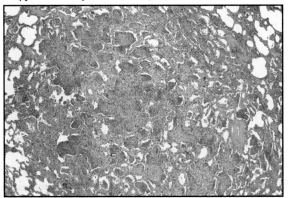 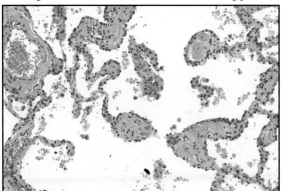

    A.   Usual interstitial pneumonia
    B.   Nonspecific interstitial pneumonia
    C.   Lymphoid interstitial pneumonia
    D.   Desquamative interstitial pneumonia
    E.   Bronchiolitis obliterans-organizing pneumonia

11: Lung Questions

32. The lung process shown in the image below is negative on polarized light. Which of the following would be the most likely diagnosis?

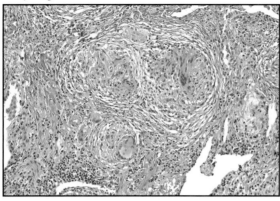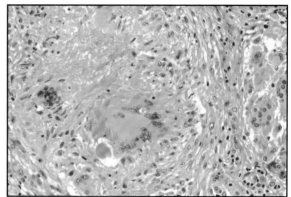

    A. Mycobacterial infection
    B. Fungal infection
    C. Sarcoidosis
    D. Langerhans cell histiocytosis
    E. Talc granulomatosis

33. A farmer presents with shortness of breath. A lung biopsy is remarkable for patchy interstitial pneumonia, non-necrotizing granulomas with scattered giant cells, and chronic bronchiolitis. The cause of this patient's clinical symptoms is most likely which of the following?

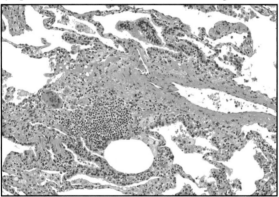

    A. *Actinomyces*
    B. Idiopathic
    C. Parasites
    D. *Mycobacterium*
    E. Blastomycosis

11: Lung Questions

34. The type of pneumonia depicted in the image below can be seen in association with which of the following?

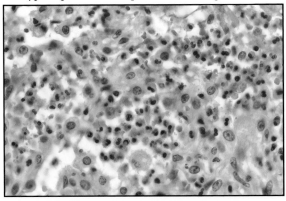

    A. Parasites
    B. Asthma
    C. Drug toxicity
    D. Hypersensitivity to *Aspergillus*
    E. All of the above

35. The image shown is from a lung wedge resection from an AIDS patient with shortness of breath and a dry cough. All of the following are TRUE about this entity EXCEPT:

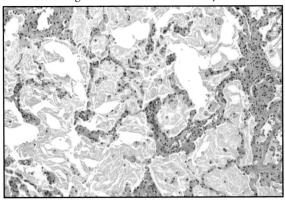

    A. Etiologic factors include exposure to mineral dust.
    B. It can be seen in patients with hematologic malignancies or AIDS.
    C. The intraalveolar material is strongly PAS positive.
    D. The intraalveolar accumulation of the brightly eosinophilic material is due to a genetic defect in the surfactant-secreting ability of type I pneumocytes.
    E. The intraalveolar accumulation of the brightly eosinophilic material is due to an acquired defect in the clearance of surfactant by macrophages.

11: Lung Questions

36. The lung tumor shown:

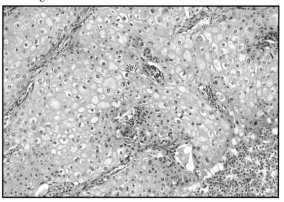

    A.   Occurs predominantly peripherally

    B.   Is linked to smoking

    C.   Most commonly affects women

    D.   Is associated 90% of the time with human papillomavirus

    E.   Is cytokeratin negative

37. The intercellular bridges of the lung tumor shown in the image correspond to which structure on electron microscopy?

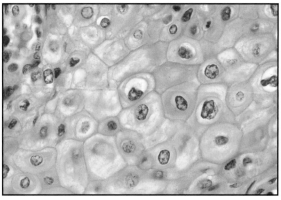

    A.   Gap junctions

    B.   Desmosomes

    C.   Microvilli

    D.   Secretory granules

    E.   None of the above

11: Lung Questions

38. The lung tumor shown is associated with which of the following?

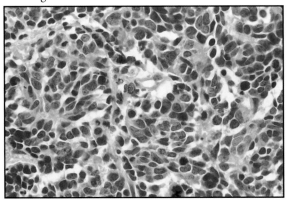

    A.   Syndrome of inappropriate ADH secretion
    B.   Ectopic Cushing syndrome
    C.   Eaton-Lambert syndrome
    D.   A and C only
    E.   A, B, and C

39. Which of the following immunohistochemical profiles is consistent with the lung tumor shown in this image:

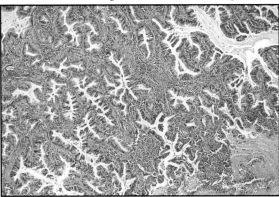

    A.   Cytokeratin 7+, cytokeratin 20−, EMA+, TTF1+
    B.   Cytokeratin 7−, cytokeratin 20+, EMA+, TTF1+
    C.   Cytokeratin 7−, cytokeratin 20−, EMA−, TTF1+
    D.   Cytokeratin 7+, cytokeratin 20−, EMA−, TTF1−
    E.   Cytokeratin 7+, cytokeratin 20+, EMA+, TTF1−

11: Lung Questions

44. A 40-year-old woman with a history of tuberous sclerosis presents with dyspnea. Chest X-ray reveals an interstitial infiltrate. CT scan shows marked cystic change throughout the lung parenchyma. A photomicrograph of the lesion is shown below. The diagnosis is:

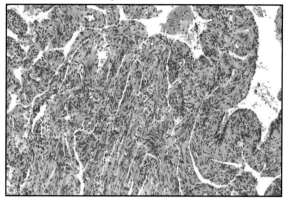

   A. Inflammatory myofibroblastic tumor
   B. Lymphangioleiomyomatosis (LAM)
   C. Benign metastasizing leiomyoma
   D. Meningothelial-like nodule (chemodectoma)
   E. Spindle cell sarcoma

45. The lung lesion shown in the picture consists of spindled fibroblasts and myofibroblasts admixed with plasma cells and lymphocytes. 65% of these lesions involve a chromosomal aberration of which gene?

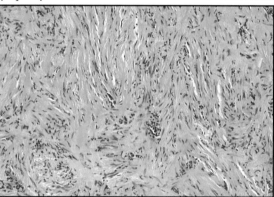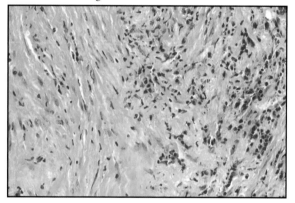

   A. ALK
   B. TSC-1
   C. TSC-2
   D. B and C
   E. None of the above

11: Lung Questions

46. Which of the following is TRUE regarding the lung lesion shown in the image?

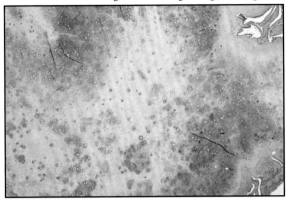

A. It is characterized by rapid expansile growth with central necrosis.
B. It is part of Carney triad.
C. It represents <1% of coin lesions.
D. It is composed of cartilage, adipose tissue, and lung epithelium.
E. Surgery followed by chemotherapy and radiation can potentially cure this aggressive neoplasm.

47. The neoplastic cells shown in the image are immunopositive for which of the following?

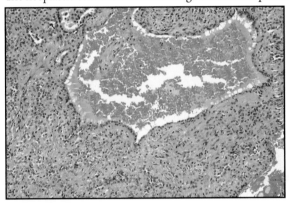

A. CD31
B. Factor VIII
C. CD34
D. TTF-1
E. All of the above

11: Lung Questions

48. This 1.0-cm well-circumscribed lung lesion was discovered incidentally in an asymptomatic patient. Which of the following is TRUE about this lesion?

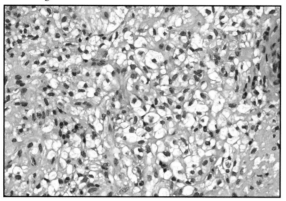

   A.   It is a neoplasm of adolescents.

   B.   Mitoses are usually prominent but necrosis is characteristically absent.

   C.   Nuclei show the classic neuroendocrine (salt-and-pepper) chromatin.

   D.   The optically clear cytoplasm is an artifact related to formalin fixation.

   E.   Tumor cells are uniformly positive for HMB-45.

49. The tumor shown in the image is:

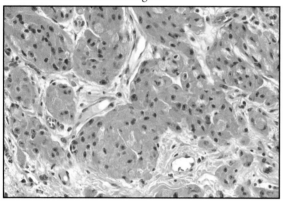 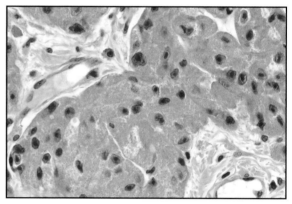

   A.   Immunonegative for S100

   B.   Most commonly located within a bronchus, usually near a bifurcation

   C.   Rich in mitochondria, which give the cytoplasm its eosinophilic granular appearance

   D.   Usually metastatic to the lung rather than a lung primary

   E.   A low-grade neuroendocrine tumor

11: Lung Questions

50.   This small lesion was incidentally seen on histologic examination of a lung at autopsy. Which of the following is/are TRUE about this entity?

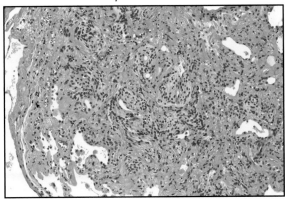

A.   It is 5-6 times more common in women than men.

B.   It is seen in association with thromboembolic disease in 50% of cases.

C.   The immunophenotype and ultrastructure are similar to meningioma.

D.   The lesion has no clinical significance but may be mistaken for carcinoid tumorlets or lymphangioleiomyomatosis histologically.

E.   All of the above

11: Lung Answers

1. A. **CILIATED CUBOIDAL OR COLUMNAR RESPIRATORY EPITHELIUM SURROUNDED BY A FIBROMUSCULAR WALL WITH ISLANDS OF CARTILAGE AND NESTS OF BRONCHIAL GLANDS**
    Enteric cysts are located in the posterior mediastinum and are lined by gastric epithelium. Esophageal cysts have a squamous lining and a muscular wall reminiscent of the esophagus. Pericardial cysts are located in the right or left cardiophrenic angles and have a mesothelial lining.
    QCSP, **Bronchogenic Cyst**, p 391.

2. B. **LEFT LOWER LOBE**
    Both extra- and intralobar sequestration more often involves the left lung, 65 and 55% respectively. Additionally, 65% of extralobar sequestrations occur between the lower lung and diaphragm, and 15% occur within or below the diaphragm. Intralobular sequestrations are most commonly found in the medial aspect of the lower lobe.
    QCSP, **Pulmonary Sequestration**, p 393.

3. A. **GOODPASTURE SYNDROME**
    Goodpasture syndrome is characterized by anti-GBM (glomerular basement membrane) antibodies. These antibodies cross-react with the lung/alveolar basement membrane inducing the sudden onset of hemoptysis, anemia, azotemia and diffuse pulmonary infiltrates. Idiopathic pulmonary hemosiderosis (IPH) presents similarly to Goodpasture syndrome but with increased serum IgA and without anti-GBM. Lupus presents with the histologic pattern identical to Goodpasture (alveolar space filled with blood and hemosiderin-laden macrophages), but demonstrates antibodies to double-stranded DNA, Sm, cardiolipin and ANA. Henoch-Schönlein purpura is a small-vessel vasculitis that presents with IgA and C3 complexes.
    QCSP, **Alveolar Hemorrhage Syndromes**, p 394.

4. E. **ALL OF THE ABOVE**
    Wegener granulomatosis can involve multiple organ systems. While sometimes it just involves the respiratory tract, it often involves the kidneys, peripheral nerves, orbit, CNS, joints, skin, breast, etc.
    QCSP, **Wegener Granulomatosis**, p 397.

5. B. **c-ANCA**
    In Wegner granulomatosis, up to 90% of patients are positive for c-ANCA, also referred to as anti-PR3 (antibodies directed against neutrophil serine proteinase 3). p-ANCA, also referred to as anti-MPO (antibodies directed against myeloperoxidase) stains the cytoplasm of neutrophils and monocytes. p-ANCA is present in only a few cases of Wegener granulomatosis. c-ANCA and p-ANCA are often positive in inflammatory bowel disease, pulmonary embolus, collagen vascular disease, microscopic polyarteritis, and crescentic glomerulonephritis.
    QCSP, **Wegener Granulomatosis**, p 397.

6. A. **ACUTE RESPIRATORY DISTRESS SYNDROME (ARDS)**
    Diffuse alveolar damage (DAD) is the pathologic finding for the clinical diagnosis of ARDS. There is a lengthy list of possible causes for ARDS that includes infection, sepsis, drugs, systemic shock, radiation, collagen vascular disease, burns, trauma, cardiopulmonary bypass, etc.
    QCSP, **Diffuse Alveolar Damage**, p 398.

7. C. **IS CLINICALLY CALLED IDIOPATHIC PULMONARY FIBROSIS**
    Usual interstitial pneumonia is a disease of patients between 40-70 years of age with an average age of onset at age 60. Patients complain of an insidious onset of dyspnea. The disease process affects predominantly the periphery of the lung and the lower lobes. However, as the disease progresses, the process moves centrally, terminating in end-stage honeycombing. Clinically, UIP is referred to as idiopathic pulmonary fibrosis. Hyaline membranes are not a histologic hallmark of UIP. They are seen in DAD in the exudative phase. DAD can be superimposed on UIP,

especially during an acute exacerbation of UIP. UIP has a poor prognosis, with death typically occurring within 3-6 years of diagnosis.

QCSP, **Usual Interstitial Pneumonia,** p 399.

8. B. **DESQUAMATIVE INTERSTITIAL PNEUMONIA**
Respiratory bronchiolitis-associated interstitial lung disease is thought to be a more localized form (localized to the peribronchial parenchyma) of desquamative interstitial pneumonia.

QCSP, **Respiratory Bronchiolitis-Associated Interstitial Lung Disease,** p 401.

9. C. **ACUTE INTERSTITIAL PNEUMONIA**
Acute interstitial pneumonia is rare. It occurs in healthy immunocompetent individuals, who rapidly progress to respiratory failure without any known cause. The clinical findings resemble ARDS, but the usual causes of ARDS, such as trauma, sepsis, shock, aspiration, infection, and drug toxicity, are ruled out. The histology is identical to diffuse alveolar damage (hence the clinical name acute interstitial pneumonia or, histologically, idiopathic diffuse alveolar damage). The entity usually has a rapidly fatal course.

QCSP, **Acute Interstitial Pneumonia,** p 401.

10. E. **INHALATION OF HARD METAL**
Giant cell interstitial pneumonia (GIP) is a pneumoconiosis that results from the inhalation of hard metal (a mixture of tungsten carbide and cobalt with or without other metals such as titanium, chromium, tantalum, and nickel).

QCSP, **Giant Cell Interstitial Pneumonia,** p 402.

11. B. **FALSE**
Lymphoid interstitial pneumonia (LIP) is characterized by a polymorphous interstitial infiltrate composed of lymphoid cells (mixture of B and T cells), plasma cells, and large mononuclear cells. LIP may rarely evolve into a low-grade lymphoma.

QCSP, **Lymphoid Interstitial Pneumonia,** p 403.

12. B. **A DIAGNOSIS OF EXCLUSION**
Sarcoidosis can be a systemic disease process. It most commonly affects the perihilar lymph nodes and the lung parenchyma but can involve other sites as well. The classic presentation is bilateral and symmetric hilar lymphadenopathy with or without lung parenchyma involvement in an African-American patient. Histologically, sarcoidosis is characterized by nonnecrotizing granulomas. Punctate foci of necrosis can rarely be seen. It is prudent to rule out an infectious etiology (microbiology and special stains) before rendering the diagnosis of sarcoidosis. Inclusions such as asteroid and Schaumann bodies are helpful features but can be seen in other granulomatous diseases.

QCSP, **Sarcoidosis,** p 404.

13. A. **TRUE**
Loeffler syndrome is a mild, self-limited disease. It is a simple eosinophilic pneumonia which is usually asymptomatic, with peripheral eosinophilia and pulmonary infiltrates.

QCSP, **Eosinophilic Pneumonia,** p 406.

14. C. **PROMINENT NUCLEOLI**
Small cell carcinoma has nuclei with *absent or inconspicuous* nucleoli.

QCSP, **Small Cell Carcinoma,** p 410.

11: Lung Answers

15.　C.　**SMALL CELL CARCINOMA**

The Azzopardi effect refers to the purple-staining DNA material seen impregnating the blood vessels in small cell carcinoma of the lung.

QCSP, **Small Cell Carcinoma,** p 410.

16.　A.　**TRUE**

Large cell carcinoma of the lung is characterized by sheets of large epithelial cells without evidence of differentiation on routine stains. It is a diagnosis of exclusion after ruling out squamous, glandular, or neuroendocrine tumors. The tumors are usually large and peripherally located. Of note, large cell carcinoma is not synonymous with large cell neuroendocrine carcinoma. The latter has neuroendocrine differentiation (chromogranin, synaptophysin, NSE positivity) and has a worse prognosis (similar to small cell carcinoma).

QCSP, **Large Cell Carcinoma,** p 416.

17.　A.　**5%**

A minimum of 5% of adenocarcinomatous differentiation in a predominantly squamous lesion or 5% of squamous carcinomatous differentiation in a predominantly adenocarcinoma lesion is required for the diagnosis of an adenosquamous carcinoma.

QCSP, **Adenosquamous Carcinoma,** p 417.

18.　E.　**THEY CARRY A BETTER PROGNOSIS THAN OTHER NON-SMALL CELL CARCINOMAS OF THE LUNG**

All the above statements regarding sarcomatoid carcinoma are true except the comment on the prognosis. Typically patients with a sarcomatoid carcinoma have a poor prognosis with a 5 year survival for stage I lesions of only 20%.

QCSP, **Sarcomatoid Carcinoma,** p 418.

19.　D.　**B AND C**

Criteria for separating typical from atypical carcinoid tumors include necrosis and increased mitotic activity (>2 mit/10 HPFs). Cellular pleomorphism is no longer a differentiating feature. Cellular pleomorphism may be observed in typical carcinoids in the absence of necrosis and increased mitotic activity. The presence or absence of metastasis is also *not* a differentiating feature. Even typical carcinoid tumors have the potential to metastasize.

QCSP, **Carcinoid Tumor,** p 420.

20.　B.　**ADENOID CYSTIC CARCINOMA**

Adenoid cystic carcinoma is the most common salivary gland tumor in the lung but still only represents <0.2% of all primary lung tumors. In general they arise in large cartilage-bearing bronchi and usually extends into the bronchial lumen resulting in symptoms of chronic bronchial obstruction/irritation.

QCSP, **Adenoid Cystic Carcinoma,** p 422.

21.　D.　**LOW-GRADE MUCOEPIDERMOID CARCINOMA**

The microscopic description is consistent with a mucoepidermoid carcinoma, which generally consists of an admixture of squamous cells, intermediate cells, and mucin-secreting/glandular cells. Intermediate cells or transition cells are oval to polygonal with eosinophilic cytoplasm and are typically intermixed with the glandular cells.

QCSP, **Mucoepidermoid Carcinoma,** p 424.

22.　A.　**IT IS NOT ASSOCIATED WITH A HISTORY OF SMOKING.**

Langerhans cell histiocytosis is a smoking-related lung disease.

QCSP, **Langerhans Cell Histiocytosis,** p 426.

23.   E.   **ALL OF THE ABOVE**

Pleuropulmonary blastoma is a rare entity that typically affect children younger than 12. These lesions are classified into 3 types from multicystic, cystic with thickened areas (nodular), and solid masses. Microscopically the lesion demonstrates embryonic-appearing mesenchyme, which can demonstrate features of malignant sarcomas including rhabdomyosarcoma, liposarcoma, chondrosarcoma and undifferentiated sarcoma. The lesions often have entrapped epithelial structures, however the lesions do not have a malignant epithelial component

QCSP, **Pleuropulmonary Blastoma**, p 428.

24.   D.   **A AND B**

The smooth muscle proliferation of lymphangioleiomyomatosis will stain for the muscle markers desmin and smooth muscle actin. Additionally the smooth muscle proliferation in this lesion is positive for HMB-45 (which is negative in normal smooth muscle).

QCSP, **Lymphangioleiomyomatosis**, p 428.

25.   E.   **ALL OF THE ABOVE**

Several lesions can present as small, well-circumscribed lesions of the lung. These are often asymptomatic and are incidentally found. Such lesions include clear cell tumor (sugar tumor), carcinoid tumor, hamartoma and granular cell tumor.

QCSP, **Clear Cell Tumor**, p 433.

26.   E.   **THE ENTITY MAY BE COMPLICATED BY THE DEVELOPMENT OF CARCINOMA (USUALLY MUCINOUS BRONCHIOLOALVEOLAR CARCINOMA).**

The image shows CPAM (congenital pulmonary airway malformation). It is usually seen in stillborn or newborn infants with respiratory distress. It is slightly more common in boys than girls. Several types of CPAM exist; type 0 is incompatible with life, and only type 1 and 4 CPAM can be cured by surgery alone.

QCSP, **Congenital Pulmonary Airway Malformation**, p 392.

27.   E.   **EDEMA ACCOMPANIED BY INFLAMMATORY CELLS AS WELL AS HYALINE MEMBRANES LINING THE ALVEOLAR SPACES**

Choices A-D are all histologic hallmarks of DAD in the proliferative (fibroblastic) phase.

QCSP, **Diffuse Alveolar Damage**, p 399.

28.   C.   **USUAL INTERSTITIAL PNEUMONIA (UIP)**

DIP is a disease of smokers and radiologically shows ground-glass opacities. Histologically, the alveolar spaces are filled with macrophages. RBILD is thought to be the same process as DIP, but the disease is patchy rather than diffuse, affecting mainly the peribronchiolar areas. NSIP can look radiologically similar to UIP, involving the periphery of the lung and the lung bases; however, the interstitial process is histologically uniform and lacks the temporal heterogeneity of UIP. DAD is most commonly the histologic correlate to ARDS. Radiologically, both lung fields are opacified ("complete white-out") in DAD, and hyaline membranes are classically observed in the exudative phase.

QCSP, **Usual Interstitial Pneumonia**, p 399.

29.   B.   **MACROPHAGES**

The most prominent histologic finding in DIP is the filling of the alveolar space with macrophages. Typically these macrophages are pigmented and stain positive with an iron stain.

QCSP, **Desquamative Interstitial Pneumonia**, p 400.

11: Lung Answers

30.   B.   **TEMPORALLY HOMOGENEOUS**

The image shows nonspecific interstitial pneumonia (NSIP), a patchy homogeneous process. This disease entity is important to distinguish from UIP. The majority of NSIP patients recover with corticosteroids. In contrast, UIP is often rapidly fatal. Choices A and C describe UIP.

QCSP, **Nonspecific Interstitial Pneumonia,** p 402.

31.   E.   **BRONCHIOLITIS OBLITERANS-ORGANIZING PNEUMONIA**

Masson bodies are polypoid fibromyxoid lesions seen in a patchy distribution within the alveoli, alveolar ducts, and respiratory bronchioles in bronchiolitis obliterans-organizing pneumonia (BOOP).

QCSP, **Bronchiolitis Obliterans-Organizing Pneumonia (BOOP),** p 403-404.

32.   C.   **SARCOIDOSIS**

The process represents sarcoidosis of the lung. The lesion demonstrates well-circumscribed, non-necrotizing granulomas. While mycobacterial and fungal infections result in granuloma formation, they are usually associated with necrosis. Additionally, the lack of polarizable particles in the lung lesion would argue against the presence of talc.

QCSP, **Sarcoidosis,** p 404.

33.   A.   *ACTINOMYCES*

Farmer's lung is the most well-known entity in the rubric of hypersensitivity pneumonitis. It is caused by repeated exposure to *Actinomyces* in moldy hay, leading to fever, malaise, cough, and breathlessness. With continued exposure, patients can enter the chronic stage and pulmonary fibrosis can occur. Hypersensitivity pneumonitis is characterized histologically by a triad of chronic interstitial infiltrate composed of lymphocytes and plasma cells in association with poorly-formed nonnecrotizing granulomas with scattered giant cells and bronchiolitis.

QCSP, **Hypersensitivity Pneumonitis,** p 405.

34.   E.   **ALL OF THE ABOVE**

The image shows eosinophilic pneumonia, which can be seen in association with all of the listed choices.

QCSP, **Eosinophilic Pneumonia,** p 406.

35.   D.   **THE INTRAALVEOLAR ACCUMULATION OF THE BRIGHTLY EOSINOPHILIC MATERIAL IS DUE TO A GENETIC DEFECT IN THE SURFACTANT-SECRETING ABILITY OF TYPE I PNEUMOCYTES.**

The image shows pulmonary alveolar proteinosis, which can occur due to occupational exposure (mineral dust) or in patients with hematologic malignancies or AIDS. The granular eosinophilic material within the alveolar spaces is caused by an acquired defect of surfactant removal by macrophages.

QCSP, **Pulmonary Alveolar Proteinosis,** p 406.

36.   B.   **IS LINKED TO SMOKING**

Lung cancer has a strong association with smoking. Squamous cell carcinoma occurs predominantly centrally, although 35% occur peripherally. It more commonly affects men. Squamous cell carcinomas are associated with HPV 20% of the time. The tumor is uniformly cytokeratin positive.

QCSP, **Squamous Cell Carcinoma,** p 408.

37.   B.   **DESMOSOMES**

The key features of squamous differentiation include intercellular bridges (desmosomes) and keratinization.

QCSP, **Squamous Cell Carcinoma,** p 408.

11: Lung Answers

38.   E.   **A, B, AND C**

The image demonstrates a small cell carcinoma. The cells have a scant cytoplasm and an increased N:C ratio with finely granulated nuclear chromatin, nuclear molding, and absent nucleoli. Small cell carcinoma can present with paraneoplastic manifestations such as SIADH, ectopic Cushing syndrome, and Eaton-Lambert syndrome. These syndromes are the result of production of ectopic hormones such as ADH and ACTH. Eaton-Lambert syndrome is a myasthenia-like paraneoplastic syndrome that demonstrates muscle weakness of the arms and legs.
QCSP, **Small Cell Carcinoma,** p 410.

39.   A.   **CYTOKERATIN 7+, CYTOKERATIN 20–, EMA+, TTF1+**

The image demonstrates a primary lung adenocarcinoma. These tumors are typically positive for pan-keratin and EMA, CK7, TTF1, Napsin A, CEA, LeuM1, Ber-Ep4, B72.3 (and others). Lung adenocarcinomas are typically negative for CK20. Additionally, cases with neuroendocrine differentiation can expression NSE and CD57 as well as chromogranin and/or synaptophysin.
QCSP, **Adenocarcinoma,** p 411.

40.   A.   **TRUE**

This lesion is a mucinous bronchioloalveolar carcinoma with mucin filled (goblet-like) cells growing in a lepidic growth pattern along the alveolar walls. In general the mucinous type have a worse prognosis. The best prognosis is seen in those with a peripherally located solitary non-mucinous bronchioloalveolar carcinoma.
QCSP, **Bronchioloalveolar Carcinoma,** p 414.

41.   E.   **IS IMMUNOREACTIVE FOR TTF-1 AND CK7**

Bronchioloalveolar carcinoma, nonmucinous type, is shown in the image. This entity presents as a peripheral consolidation and has a better prognosis than its mucinous counterpart.
QCSP, **Bronchioloalveolar Carcinoma,** p 415.

42.   A.   **CAN PRESENT IN AN ENDOBRONCHIAL LOCATION AS A LARGE, POLYPOID, FLESHY MASS**

The image shows a typical carcinoid tumor (well-differentiated neuroendocrine carcinoma). These tumors can present in an endobronchial location or in a peripheral location. The latter is associated with spindle cell morphology. Nuclei have the characteristic salt-and-pepper chromatin, which is finely speckled with inconspicuous nucleoli. Typical carcinoids are indolent, low-grade neuroendocrine neoplasms with an excellent 5-year survival. Carcinoid tumors are the most common lung tumors of childhood.
QCSP, **Carcinoid Tumor,** p 420.

43.   D.   **WEIBEL-PALADE BODIES**

This lesion represents a pulmonary epithelioid hemangioendothelioma (also known as an intravascular bronchoalveolar tumor). This lesion is a vascular tumor and would demonstrate Weibel-Palade bodies by EM.
QCSP, **Epithelioid Hemangioendothelioma,** p 427.

44.   B.   **LYMPHANGIOLEIOMYOMATOSIS (LAM)**

LAM is exclusively seen in women, usually of reproductive age. It commonly presents as a diffusely infiltrative and microcystic lesion. The image shows a nodular smooth muscle proliferation. The lesion can arise from blood vessels, lymphatics, and distal airways. HMB-45 positivity is characteristic, distinguishing it from the other entities listed.
QCSP, **Lymphangioleiomyomatosis,** p 428.

11: Lung Answers

45.   A.   **ALK**

These images demonstrate an inflammatory myofibroblastic tumor. This lesion often has expression of ALK by IHC and rearrangement of the ALK gene by FISH/molecular studies. TSC-1 and TSC-2 are the germ-line mutations associated with lymphangioleiomyomatosis.

QCSP, **Inflammatory Myofibroblastic Tumor,** p 430.

46.   B.   **IT IS PART OF CARNEY TRIAD.**

The image shows a pulmonary hamartoma. It is the most common incidental lung lesion (coin lesion). It is characterized by very slow growth and treated by simple enucleation. Hamartomas are lung masses composed of cartilage, adipose tissue, connective tissue and smooth muscle. The glandular epithelium is entrapped bland lung parenchyma (technically not a true component of the lesion). Pulmonary chondromatous hamartomas are part of Carney triad (the other 2 components are gastric epithelioid leiomyosarcoma and extraadrenal paraganglioma).

QCSP, **Hamartoma,** p 431.

47.   D.   **TTF-1**

Sclerosing hemangioma is the most common peripheral *benign* glandular tumor of the lung. It is an epithelial tumor, not a vascular lesion. It has prominent vascular patterns with blood lakes; however, the blood-filled spaces are not lined by endothelial cells. Rather, they are lined by epithelial cells that are positive for TTF-1 (also positive for cytokeratin, vimentin, and EMA). The tumor cells are negative for CD31, CD34, and factor VIII.

QCSP, **Sclerosing Hemangioma,** p 432.

48.   E.   **TUMOR CELLS ARE UNIFORMLY POSITIVE FOR HMB-45.**

Clear cell tumors (sugar tumors) are neoplasms of adults, with a median age of 50 at the time of discovery. The tumor is generally discovered incidentally in an asymptomatic patient and is usually small (2.0 cm or less). Mitoses and necrosis are absent. Nuclei may be small with dense chromatin or large with vesicular chromatin. The clear cytoplasm is related to the high glycogen content of the cells. The tumor cells are uniformly positive for HMB-45. Recent studies show that clear cell tumors of the lung may belong to the PEComa (perivascular epithelioid cell tumors) family due to HMB-45 positivity.

QCSP, **Clear Cell Tumor,** p 433.

49.   B.   **MOST COMMONLY LOCATED WITHIN A BRONCHUS, USUALLY NEAR A BIFURCATION**

Granular cell tumors can occur in the lung periphery but are most commonly located within a bronchus near a bifurcation. The cytoplasm is eosinophilic and granular due to the abundance of secondary lysosomes. Tumor cells are immunopositive for S100. There are no reports to date of a malignant granular cell tumor arising as a primary neoplasm in the lung.

QCSP, **Granular Cell Tumor,** p 434.

50.   E.   **ALL OF THE ABOVE**

The image represents a meningothelial-like nodule with its characteristic "zellballen" appearance and discrete swirled nests of pink spindle cells surrounding a small network of delicate capillaries. The lesion resembles the "zellballen" pattern of paragangliomas. However, immunophenotype and ultrastructure mimic a meningioma with EMA and vimentin positivity, and keratin, S100, and neuroendocrine marker negativity. It is important not to mistake these lesions for carcinoid tumorlets or LAM.

QCSP, **Meningothelial-Like Nodules,** p 435.

Chapter 12

Pleura and Peritoneum

1. Which of the following is the most common presentation for malignant mesothelioma?
   - A. A 5-year-old girl whose mother worked in a shipyard while pregnant with her
   - B. The 5-year-old girl's 25-year-old mother, who has lived near or worked in that shipyard since she was 5 years old
   - C. A 65-year-old man who has worked in the same shipyard since he was 30
   - D. A 95-year-old woman who spent much of her life traveling in India
   - E. A and C are both common presentations, representing 2 peaks in age groups affected.

2. Which of the following is the most common site for the development of malignant mesothelioma?
   - A. Pleura
   - B. Peritoneum
   - C. Pericardium
   - D. Tunica vaginalis of testis
   - E. Mediastinum

3. Malignant mesothelioma tends to begin initially as small foci of tumor that develop into plaque-like lesions and spread outward. Which of the following is NOT characteristic of the way malignant mesothelioma tends to spread?
   - A. Pleural malignant mesothelioma likes to spread into the soft tissues of the chest wall as the disease advances.
   - B. Peritoneal malignant mesothelioma likes to spread into the abdominal wall as the disease advances.
   - C. 50% of patients with peritoneal malignant mesothelioma will have metastatic disease at the time of diagnosis.
   - D. Sarcomatous mesothelial lesions in the pleura are especially likely to spread via blood-borne metastases.
   - E. Malignant mesothelioma of the pericardium may focally invade myocardium but does not involve the endocardium or enter the heart chamber.

4. The desmoplastic form of sarcomatoid malignant mesothelioma can be difficult to distinguish from reactive pleural fibrosis. All of the following features are helpful EXCEPT:
   - A. Foci of obvious malignant features
   - B. Invasion of the chest wall
   - C. Necrosis
   - D. Invasion of the lungs characterized by invasion of the alveolar septa
   - E. None of the above is helpful.

5. Which immunohistochemical stain(s) can be used to help distinguish mesotheliomas from benign mesothelial proliferations?
   - A. Calretenin
   - B. Ki-67
   - C. p53
   - D. None of the above
   - E. All of the above

6. Which of the following is the most common location of solitary fibrous tumor?
   - A. Visceral pleura
   - B. Parietal pleura
   - C. Diaphragmatic pleura
   - D. Mediastinal pleura
   - E. Both A and B are about equally likely.

12: Pleura and Peritoneum Questions

7. Which of the following histologic features should make you concerned for malignant solitary fibrous tumor?
    A. Variable arrangement of spindled cells within the lesion ("patternless pattern")
    B. Prominent areas of hyalinization
    C. Vascularity with narrow clefts rather than wide-open branching channels
    D. >4 mitotic figures/hpf
    E. Focal areas of myxoid or cystic change

8. Hypoglycemia can been seen in association with which of the following tumors?
    A. Mesothelioma
    B. Solitary fibrous tumor
    C. Fibrosarcoma
    D. Pancreatic epithelial neoplasms
    E. All of the above

9. Which of the following order reflects the most common to least common major histotype of malignant mesothelioma seen in pleural tumors? (Hint: the most common variant is pictured here.)

    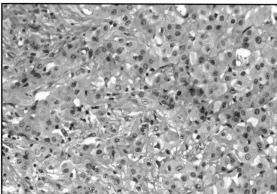

    A. Biphasic > sarcomatous > epithelial > poorly differentiated
    B. Epithelial > sarcomatous > mixed > poorly differentiated
    C. Epithelial > biphasic > sarcomatous > poorly differentiated
    D. Sarcomatous > epithelioid > biphasic > poorly differentiated
    E. Sarcomatous > poorly differentiated > epithelioid > biphasic

12: Pleura and Peritoneum Questions

10. Which histologic subtype of malignant mesothelioma (pictured here) is rare in the peritoneum?

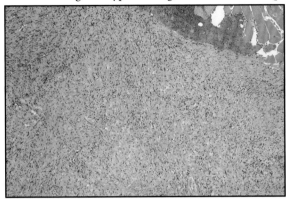 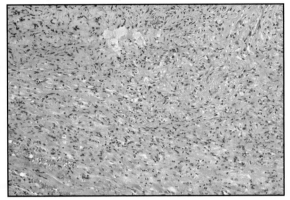

    A. Epithelial
    B. Sarcomatous
    C. Biphasic
    D. Poorly differentiated
    E. Well-differentiated papillary

11. Which variant of malignant mesothelioma (pictured here) is more common in women in their 3rd and 4th decades?

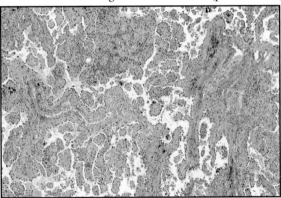

    A. Poorly differentiated
    B. Well-differentiated papillary mesothelioma
    C. Malignant mesothelioma of the tunica vaginalis
    D. Localized malignant mesothelioma
    E. Lymphohistiocytoid mesothelioma

12: Pleura and Peritoneum Questions

12. Which of the following immunohistochemical stain(s) is/are useful to help distinguish tubulopapillary form of epitheloid mesothelioma (depicted here) from adenocarcinoma?

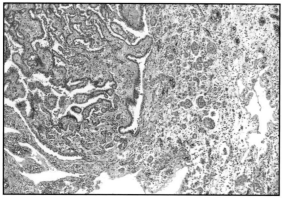

    A.   CEA
    B.   Leu-M1 (CD15)
    C.   Ber-EP4
    D.   Calretinin
    E.   All of the above

13. Which 2 of the following immunostains are most commonly positive in the lesion depicted below (select 2 choices)?

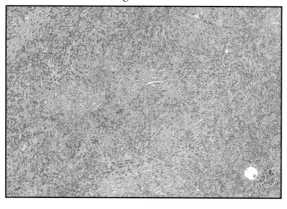 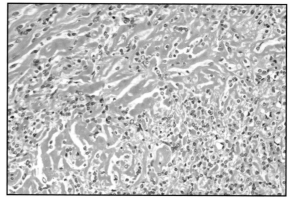

    A.   S100
    B.   SMA
    C.   CD34
    D.   CD99
    E.   EMA

12: Pleura and Peritoneum Answers

1.   C.   **A 65-YEAR-OLD MAN WHO HAS WORKED IN THE SAME SHIPYARD SINCE HE WAS 30**
   75% of people affected by malignant mesothelioma are men and most are in the 6th to 8th decade of life. There is an epidemiologic link between asbestos exposure and the development of this neoplasm, and a shipyard is an example of a common site of exposure. The average interval from first exposure to asbestos and the development of malignant mesothelioma is about 35 years. The man in choice C fits all of these characteristics.
   QCSP, **Malignant Mesothelioma,** p 438.

2.   A.   **PLEURA**
   Approximately 65%-75% of mesothelioma involves the pleura. The peritoneum is the next most commonly involved location, with 25% of cases. The pericardium is a relatively rare site, with only 2% of mesotheliomas arising there, and the tunica vaginalis of the testis is even less common. Advanced disease in any of the first 3 sites can lead to spread of the neoplasm into the mediastinum as well as into other serosal cavities.
   QCSP, **Malignant Mesothelioma,** p 438.

3.   B.   **PERITONEAL MALIGNANT MESOTHELIOMA LIKES TO SPREAD INTO THE ABDOMINAL WALL AS THE DISEASE ADVANCES.**
   Peritoneal malignant mesothelioma will progress to encase the abdominal visceral pleura with obliteration of the peritoneal cavity; however, it rarely involves the abdominal wall except at the site of surgical scars. All of the other statements are true.
   QCSP, **Malignant Mesothelioma,** p 438.

4.   D.   **INVASION OF THE LUNGS CHARACTERIZED BY INVASION OF THE ALVEOLAR SEPTA**
   Choice D is unhelpful and therefore the right answer to this question. Invasion of the lungs by sarcomatoid malignant mesothelioma is characterized by filling of alveolar spaces without invasion of the septa. The first 3 choices are also features that help distinguish this malignant neoplasm from a reactive process.
   QCSP, **Malignant Mesothelioma,** p 439.

5.   C.   **P53**
   Mesotheliomas often express the infamous tumor suppressor gene p53. Calretinin will stain both, and ki-67 can be elevated in reactive processes.
   QCSP, **Malignant Mesothelioma,** p 440.

6.   A.   **VISCERAL PLEURA**
   Most solitary fibrous tumors of the pleura and peritoneum are located in the thoracic cavity and are asymptomatic. Approximately 65% of solitary fibrous tumors are attached to the visceral pleura, sometimes by a broad-based pedicle. Less commonly, they arise from the parietal diaphragmatic, or mediastinal pleura. They have also been reported in sites unrelated to serosal surfaces, including the lung, liver, thyroid, nasal passages, meninges, skin, soft tissue, and breast.
   QCSP, **Solitary Fibrous Tumor,** p 441.

7.   D.   **>4 MITOTIC FIGURES PER HPF**
   Solitary fibrous tumors are characterized by bland spindle-shaped cells randomly arranged throughout the tumor and often described as demonstrating a "patternless pattern." Areas of hyalinization are often prominent and usually present, with dense collagen and "cracks" between the cells and this collagen or parallel "wires" of collagen. Vascularity may vary between narrow clefts and wide-open branching channels that are reminiscent of hemangiopericytoma. Focal areas of myxoid or cystic change can be seen, as can necrosis; however, tumors with areas of hemorrhage and/or necrosis should raise your level of suspicion. Finding >4 mitotic figures per hpf is

characteristic of malignant lesions. These tumors also tend to be more pleomorphic, cellular, and often have a prominent fascicular pattern.

QCSP, **Solitary Fibrous Tumor,** p 441.

8. E. **ALL OF THE ABOVE**
    Hypoglycemia occurs in approximately 5% of solitary fibrous tumors and is more common in women. It may also be seen in mesothelioma, fibrosarcoma, hemangiopericytoma, and other nonpancreatic mesenchymal and epithelial neoplasms.

    QCSP, **Solitary Fibrous Tumors,** p 442.

9. C. **EPITHELIAL > BIPHASIC > SARCOMATOUS > POORLY DIFFERENTIATED**
    Among pleural tumors, 50% are epithelial, 25% biphasic, 15%, sarcomatous, and 10% poorly differentiated.

    QCSP, **Malignant Mesothelioma,** p 438.

10. B. **SARCOMATOUS**
    Among peritoneal tumors, 75% are epithelial. The sarcomatous type is rare. Well-differentiated papillary mesothelioma variant is usually seen in the peritoneum.

    QCSP, **Malignant Mesothelioma,** p 439.

11. B. **WELL-DIFFERENTIATED PAPILLARY MESOTHELIOMA**
    Well-differentiated papillary mesothelioma is a special variant. It is considered to be more of an intermediate malignancy, with well-developed papillary or tubule-papillary architecture and cuboidal or flat cells with bland nuclear features in a single layer. Psammoma bodies can be seen. It is more common in women in the 3rd and 4th decades.

    QCSP, **Malignant Mesothelioma,** p 439-440.

12. E. **ALL OF THE ABOVE**
    All of these stains and more can help to distinguish adenocarcinoma from tubulopapillary mesothelioma. Mesotheliomas and not adenocarcinomas will usually stain with calretinin. Adenocarcinomas much more commonly express CEA, Leu-M1 (CD15), and Ber-EP4, as well as B72.3. Both mesothelioma and adenocarcinoma can stain for cytokeratins; the mesotheliomas generally express high molecular weight cytokeratins. A special stain for mucicarmine can also be helpful, as it is usually positive in adenocarcinoma and negative in mesothelioma. None of these stains is seen 100% of the time in one and never in the other neoplasm, so you should always order a panel.

    QCSP, **Malignant Mesothelioma,** p 440.

13. 5. **C AND D**
    The lesion demonstrates a patternless pattern with varying cellular and hypocellular areas with a collagenized background typical of solitary fibrous tumors. Approximately 90%-95% of solitary fibrous tumors will express CD34 and bcl-2, and up to 70%-90% will express CD99. 20%-30% will express SMA and/or EMA. Cytokeratin, desmin, and S100 stains are typically negative.

    QCSP, **Solitary Fibrous Tumor,** p 441.

Chapter 13

Mediastinum

1. Which mediastinal compartment is the most common site for germ cell tumors?
    A. Anterior
    B. Posterior
    C. Superior
    D. Inferior
    E. Middle

2. Klinefelter syndrome is associated with which of the following extragonadal germ cell tumor(s)?
    A. Choriocarcinoma
    B. Embryonal carcinoma
    C. Yolk sac tumor
    D. Germinoma (seminoma)
    E. All of the above

3. A mediastinal germ cell tumor can be accompanied by this synchronous hematologic malignancy:
    A. Nodular sclerosing Hodgkin lymphoma
    B. Diffuse large B-cell lymphoma
    C. Chronic lymphocytic leukemia
    D. Anaplastic large cell lymphoma
    E. Mantle cell lymphoma

4. Choriocarcinomas of the mediastinum are most commonly encountered in pure rather than in mixed form.
    A. True
    B. False

5. Patients with choriocarcinoma present with highly elevated β-hCG levels. Which of the following statements explains the β-hCG immunoreactivity in *embryonal carcinomas* and *germinomas (seminomas)*?
    A. The tumor cells aberrantly express β-hCG.
    B. It is nonspecific staining and should be ignored.
    C. Embryonal carcinomas and germinomas (seminomas) can have small numbers of syncytiotrophoblasts, which express β-hCG.
    D. Embryonal carcinomas and germinomas can have small numbers of cytotrophoblasts, which express β-hCG.
    E. C and D

6. All of the following are TRUE regarding germinoma (seminoma) EXCEPT:
    A. It typically occurs in men between the 2nd and 4th decades.
    B. It is characterized microscopically by sheets of large polygonal cells with distinct cell membranes, clear cytoplasm, and round nuclei with prominent nucleoli.
    C. It exhibits fibrous septations and a stroma infiltrated by lymphocytes
    D. It tends to be widely invasive at time of diagnosis and has a poor prognosis.
    E. It is associated with Klinefelter syndrome (47,XXY karyotype).

7. The most common germ cell neoplasm of the mediastinum is which of the following?
    A. Choriocarcinoma
    B. Embryonal carcinoma
    C. Germinoma
    D. Yolk sac tumor
    E. Mature teratoma

13: Mediastinum Questions

8. The most common germ cell neoplasm of the mediastinum seen in women is which of the following?
    A. Germinoma (dysgerminoma)
    B. Mature cystic teratoma
    C. Choriocarcinoma
    D. Yolk sac tumor
    E. Malignant mixed germ cell tumor

9. Malignant teratomas:
    A. Occur exclusively in women
    B. Typically occur as carcinomas rather than sarcomas
    C. Are associated with Turner syndrome (45X)
    D. Can present as rhabdomyosarcoma, myxoid liposarcoma, and glioblastoma multiforme
    E. All of the above

10. Schiller-Duval bodies and eosinophilic hyaline droplets are key microscopic features in the diagnosis of:
    A. Choriocarcinoma
    B. Embryonal carcinoma
    C. Yolk sac tumor
    D. Seminoma
    E. None of the above

11. Embryonal carcinoma, yolk sac, and choriocarcinoma are more commonly seen as a component of a malignant mixed germ cell neoplasm than in pure form.
    A. True
    B. False

12. Which germ cell tumor component(s) is/are least likely to be positive for cytokeratin?
    A. Germinoma (seminoma)
    B. Choriocarcinoma
    C. Embryonal carcinoma
    D. Yolk sac tumor
    E. A and C

13. Which mediastinal compartment is the most common site of neurogenic tumors?
    A. Anterior
    B. Posterior
    C. Superior
    D. Inferior
    E. Middle

14. Which marker is universally positive in neurogenic tumors?
    A. S100
    B. Cytokeratin
    C. EMA
    D. Chromogranin
    E. Synaptophysin

15. Malignant peripheral nerve sheath tumors arising in the setting of neurofibromatosis have a worse prognosis compared to sporadic cases.
    A. True
    B. False

13: Mediastinum Questions

16. Neuroblastomas are associated with amplification of which of the following oncogenes?
    - A. EGFR
    - B. Ras
    - C. Ret
    - D. N-myc
    - E. K-ras

17. Which rosettes are typically seen in neuroblastoma?
    - A. True rosettes
    - B. Flexner-Wintersteiner rosettes
    - C. Perivascular pseudorosettes
    - D. Homer Wright rosettes
    - E. A and D

18. Neurofibromas:
    - A. Are the most common neurogenic tumor of the mediastinum
    - B. Are usually encapsulated lesions
    - C. Grow within a nerve, imparting a fusiform appearance
    - D. Are characterized by pleomorphic cells with multinucleated giant cells, hemorrhage, and brisk mitotic activity
    - E. Are negative for S100, unlike other neural lesions in the mediastinum

19. Patients with neurofibromatosis type 1 can have neurofibromas of the mediastinum. Which other lesions are associated with NF type 1?
    - A. Café-au-lait spots
    - B. Axillary freckling
    - C. Optic gliomas
    - D. Lisch nodules
    - E. All of the above

20. The NF1 tumor suppressor gene is located on which chromosome?
    - A. 11
    - B. 14
    - C. 17
    - D. 22
    - E. X

21. The sustentacular cells surrounding the zellballen nests in paragangliomas are immunoreactive for which of the following markers?
    - A. Chromogranin
    - B. Synaptophysin
    - C. S100
    - D. Neuron-specific enolase
    - E. A and B

22. Which panel of immunohistochemical stains would confirm the diagnosis of peripheral neuroectodermal tumor?
    - A. CD99+, chromogranin−, CD56−, keratin−, vimentin+
    - B. CD99−, chromogranin+, CD56+, keratin−, vimentin+
    - C. CD99−, chromogranin+, CD56+, keratin+, vimentin+
    - D. CD99+, chromogranin+, CD56+, keratin+, vimentin−
    - E. None of the above

13: Mediastinum Questions

23. The most common neurogenic tumor of the mediastinum is:
    A. Paraganglioma
    B. Schwannoma
    C. Primitive neuroectodermal tumor
    D. Neuroblastoma
    E. Ganglioneuroma

24. A dumbbell-shaped mass extending from the posterior mediastinum into the spinal canal of a patient with the Carney complex is characteristic of which subtype of schwannoma?
    A. Ancient schwannoma
    B. Cellular schwannoma
    C. Glandular schwannoma
    D. Melanocytic schwannoma
    E. Neuroblastoma-like schwannoma

25. The most common neoplasm of the mediastinum in adults is:
    A. Schwannoma
    B. Germinoma (seminoma)
    C. Thymoma
    D. Lymphoma
    E. Mature teratoma

26. Thymomas occur most commonly in which compartment of the mediastinum?
    A. Anterior
    B. Posterior
    C. Superior
    D. Inferior
    E. Middle

27. Thymomas are composed of:
    A. Nonneoplastic epithelial cells only
    B. Nonneoplastic epithelial cells and neoplastic lymphoid cells
    C. Neoplastic epithelial cells and nonneoplastic lymphoid cells
    D. Neoplastic lymphoid cells only
    E. A or D but never both

28. Thymomas are associated with all of the following EXCEPT:
    A. Myasthenia gravis
    B. Epstein-Barr virus
    C. Pure red cell aplasia
    D. Collagen vascular diseases
    E. Hypogammaglobulinemia

29. Thymic carcinoids are most frequently associated with which of the following?
    A. Cushing syndrome
    B. Hypertrophic osteoarthropathy
    C. Lambert-Eaton syndrome
    D. Myasthenia gravis
    E. Aplastic anemia

13: Mediastinum Questions

30. The tumor cells in thymic carcinoids are typically positive for which of the following?
    A. Neuron-specific enolase
    B. Chromogranin
    C. Synaptophysin
    D. Cytokeratin
    E. All of the above

31. All of the following statements are true regarding thymic carcinomas EXCEPT:
    A. Most cases occur in middle-aged adults.
    B. They are associated with paraneoplastic syndromes and pure red cell aplasia.
    C. They are characterized by marked cytologic atypia and numerous mitotic figures
    D. Histologic subtypes include squamous cell carcinoma, basaloid carcinoma, mucoepidermoid carcinoma, and adenocarcinoma.
    E. Factors associated with poor prognosis include poor differentiation, infiltrative margins, and brisk mitotic activity.

32. Which of the following statements regarding CASTLE is/are TRUE:
    A. The term is an acronym for "carcinoma showing thymus-like elements."
    B. It typically involves the lower pole of the thyroid.
    C. It resembles thyroid carcinoma of the squamous or the lymphoepitheliomatous type.
    D. Primary undifferentiated or squamous cell carcinoma of the thyroid and metastatic carcinoma of unknown origin are important differential considerations.
    E. All of the above

33. The most common location of ectopic cervical thymomas is which of the following?
    A. Anterior/lateral neck
    B. Deep to the sternocleidomastoid muscle
    C. A and B

34. All of the following statements are TRUE regarding ectopic hamartomatous thymomas EXCEPT:
    A. They are not found within the thymus.
    B. They arise from the thymic anlage associated with branchial pouches.
    C. They are composed of several haphazardly arranged elements including spindled, adipose, squamous, and/or glandular cells.
    D. Recurrence rates are high, and metastatic disease has been reported.
    E. The differential diagnoses include mixed tumor of salivary or sweat gland, peripheral nerve sheath tumor, spindle cell carcinoma, and synovial sarcoma.

35. A 15-year-old boy presents with worsening dyspnea and a nodule near the lower pole of the thyroid compressing the trachea. A biopsy demonstrates a densely cellular lesion traversed by irregular sclerotic bands. The tumor cells are bland and arranged in a spindled and glandular pattern. No mitotic figures or inflammatory infiltrates are present. Which of the following lesions could be consistent with the patient's clinical presentation and tumor morphology?
    A. Immature teratoma
    B. Synovial sarcoma
    C. Spindle epithelial tumor with thymus-like elements (SETTLE)
    D. A and B
    E. A, B, and C

13: Mediastinum Questions

36. The most common microorganism detected in sclerosing mediastinitis is:
    A. *Aspergillus*
    B. *Cryptococcus*
    C. *Histoplasma*
    D. *Mucor*
    E. *Nocardia*

Questions 37 and 38 are based on these images:

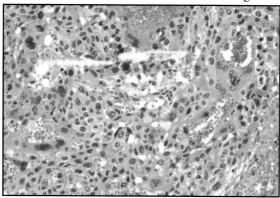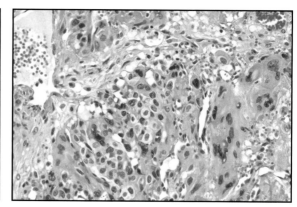

37. A 35-year-old man presents with gynecomastia, decreased libido, and testicular atrophy. Imaging demonstrates a mediastinal mass, the biopsy of which is shown in the image below. The most likely immunohistochemical profile of the neoplastic population is:
    A. Cytokeratin +, β-hCG+, PLAP+, EMA+
    B. Cytokeratin +, CD30+, PLAP+, EMA–
    C. Cytokeratin –, CD117+, PLAP+, EMA–
    D. Cytokeratin +, α-1-antitrypsin +, PLAP+, CEA+
    E. None of the above

38. Which serologic marker is most likely elevated in this patient due to the tumor?
    A. α-fetoprotein
    B. Cortisol
    C. β-hCG
    D. Testosterone
    E. Estrogen

13: Mediastinum Questions

39. The anterior mediastinal tumor depicted in this image extensively invaded the adjacent tissue at the time of diagnosis. Immunohistochemical stains for cytokeratin, PLAP, and CD30 were positive, while EMA and α-fetoprotein were negative. The diagnosis is:

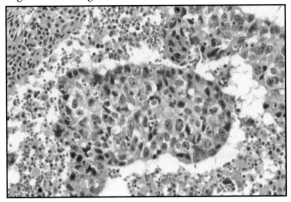

   A. Choriocarcinoma
   B. Thymic carcinoma
   C. Metastasis
   D. Embryonal carcinoma
   E. Germinoma (seminoma)

40. The mediastinal mass depicted in this image has the following immunohistochemical profile:

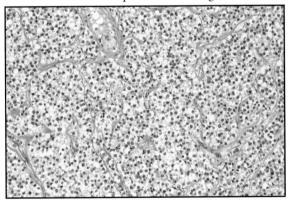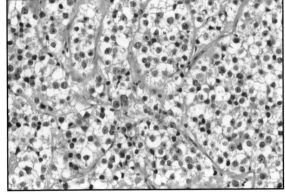

   A. Cytokeratin +, EMA+, PLAP+, CD117+
   B. Cytokeratin +, EMA−, PLAP+, CD117+
   C. Cytokeratin −, EMA−, PLAP+, CD117+
   D. Cytokeratin +, EMA+, PLAP−, CD117+
   E. Cytokeratin +, EMA+, PLAP−, CD117−

13: Mediastinum Questions

41. A 40-year-old woman presents with a well-circumscribed, cystic mediastinal mass, which is shown in this image. Which of the following statements is/are TRUE regarding this lesion?

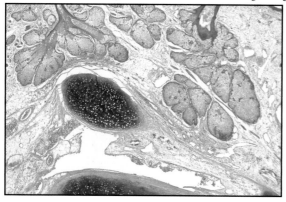 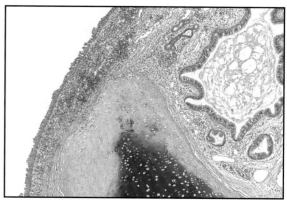

    A.   It is composed of an abnormal mixture of tissues derived from 2 or 3 embryonic layers.

    B.   The most frequently encountered tissue is skin and its appendages.

    C.   Many cases contain large areas of immature neural tissue.

    D.   A and B

    E.   A and C

42. All of the following are true regarding the mediastinal tumor shown in this image EXCEPT:

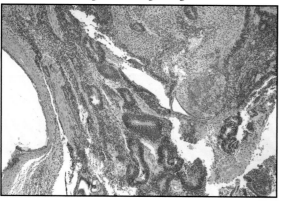 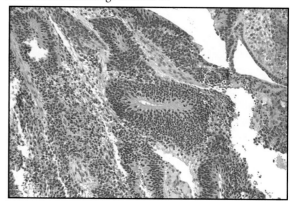

    A.   It is most frequently encountered in children and adolescents.

    B.   It usually invades surrounding structures.

    C.   Immature elements may be seen which include ectodermal, mesodermal, and endodermal tissue.

    D.   Large areas of immature neural tissue are commonly present.

    E.   It is usually pure and devoid of malignant germ cell tumor components.

13: Mediastinum Questions

Questions 43 and 44 are based on these images:

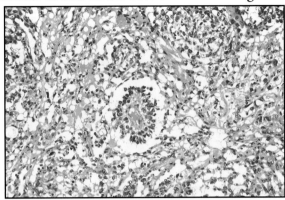 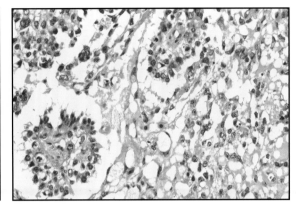

43. A 25-year-old man presents with a large, widely invasive mediastinal mass and elevated α-fetoprotein levels. The clinical history and the microscopic image confer a diagnosis of:
    A. Choriocarcinoma
    B. Immature teratoma
    C. Yolk sac tumor
    D. Embryonal carcinoma
    E. Thymic carcinoma

44. The following immunophenotype would confirm the diagnosis in the previous case:
    A. Cytokeratin +, β-hCG+, PLAP+, EMA+
    B. Cytokeratin +, CD30+, PLAP+, EMA−, α-fetoprotein +
    C. Cytokeratin −, CD117+, PLAP+, EMA−
    D. Cytokeratin +, α-1-antitrypsin +, PLAP+, CEA+, α-fetoprotein +
    E. None of the above

45. The tumor shown in this image:

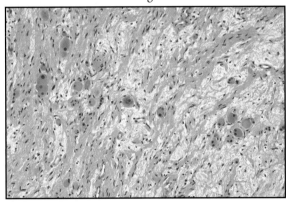 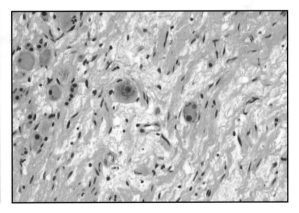

    A. Is the most common neurogenic tumor of the mediastinum
    B. Occurs in the anterior mediastinum and retroperitoneum of children and young adults
    C. Is a result of maturation within a neuroblastoma
    D. Is characterized by immature ganglion cells, Schwann cells, and nerve fibers
    E. Is treated by surgical resection followed by radiation and chemotherapy

13: Mediastinum Questions

46. Polygonal tumor cells with granular cytoplasm arranged in Zellballen nests bordered by capillaries are characteristic of this neurogenic tumor:

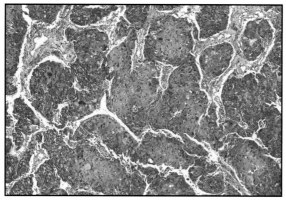 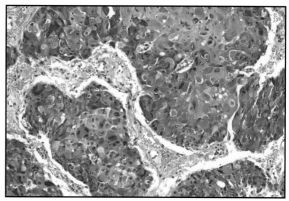

    A. Paraganglioma
    B. Schwannoma
    C. Primitive neuroectodermal tumor
    D. Neuroblastoma
    E. Ganglioneuroma

47. The main differential diagnoses for the mediastinal tumor shown are:

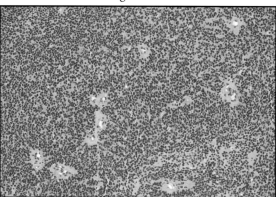

    A. Neuroblastoma
    B. Small cell carcinoma
    C. Peripheral neuroectodermal tumor
    D. A and B
    E. A, B, and C

13: Mediastinum Questions

48. The gross and microscopic images shown represent a solitary lesion in the posterior mediastinum, which was discovered incidentally on a routine chest X-ray. The diagnosis is:

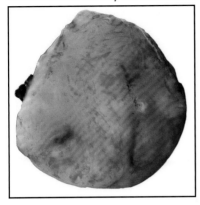 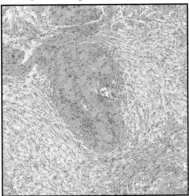 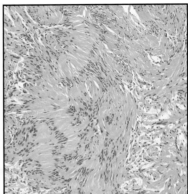

    A. Paraganglioma
    B. Schwannoma
    C. Ganglioneuroma
    D. Ganglioneuroblastoma
    E. Neurofibroma

49. Which important microscopic feature(s) shown in the image is/are helpful in separating lymphocytic thymomas from lymphomas?

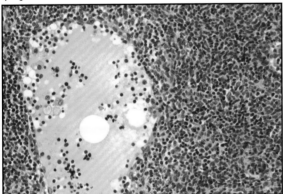

    A. Fibrous septation
    B. Tingible body macrophages
    C. Perivascular spaces/serum lakes
    D. Microcystic change
    E. All of the above

13: Mediastinum Questions

50.   All of the following statements are true regarding thymomas EXCEPT:

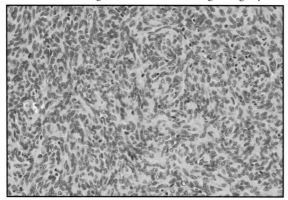

A.   Thymomas are composed of a mixture of neoplastic epithelial cells and nonneoplastic lymphocytes of varying proportions.
B.   Histologic subtypes of thymoma include lymphocyte-predominant thymomas, mixed epithelial and lymphocytic thymomas, and epithelial thymomas.
C.   Clear cell thymomas can resemble renal cell carcinoma.
D.   Spindle cell thymomas have a worse prognosis than epithelial thymomas with polygonal epithelial cells
E.   Epstein-Barr virus is not associated with thymomas.

51.   The thymic epithelial tumor shown in the image was grossly hemorrhagic and focally necrotic. The diagnosis is:

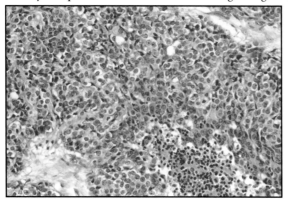

A.   Thymoma, mixed epithelial and lymphocyte type
B.   Thymoma, lymphocytic predominant type
C.   Thymoma, epithelial predominant type
D.   Thymic carcinoid
E.   Thymic carcinoma

13: Mediastinum Questions

52. A 45-year-old man presents with superior vena cava syndrome. Imaging demonstrates asymmetric widening of the mediastinum with a projection of a mass into the upper lung field. The differential diagnosis for the microscopic image shown includes:

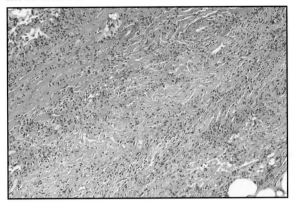

    A.   Solitary fibrous tumor
    B.   Nodular sclerosing Hodgkin lymphoma
    C.   Sclerosing mediastinitis
    D.   Malignant desmoplastic mesothelioma
    E.   All of the above

13: Mediastinum Answers

1.   A.   **ANTERIOR**
The anterior compartment is the most common site for mediastinal germ cell tumors and lymphoproliferative disorders, while the posterior compartment more commonly gives rise to neurogenic tumors such as schwannoma and ganglioneuromas.
QCSP, **Germ Cell Tumors**, p 447.

2.   E.   **ALL OF THE ABOVE**
Patients with Klinefelter syndrome (47,XXY) are at substantial risk for developing *any* kind of extragonadal germ cell tumor. The incidence of Klinefelter syndrome in patients with a mediastinal germ cell tumor is 30-40 times greater than the incidence of Klinefelter syndrome in the general population.
QCSP, **Germ Cell Tumors**, p 445-450.

3.   D.   **ANAPLASTIC LARGE CELL LYMPHOMA**
Germ cell tumors are occasionally accompanied by synchronous hematologic malignancies, typically in the form of anaplastic large cell lymphoma, but also malignant histiocytosis, and acute myelomonocytic leukemia.
QCSP, **Germ Cell Tumors**, p 445-450.

4.   B.   **FALSE**
Choriocarcinoma is most commonly seen as a component of a mixed germ cell tumor. Pure choriocarcinoma of the mediastinum is extremely rare.
QCSP, **Choriocarcinomas**, p 445.

5.   C.   **EMBRYONAL CARCINOMAS AND GERMINOMAS (SEMINOMAS) CAN HAVE SMALL NUMBERS OF SYNCYTIOTROPHOBLASTS, WHICH EXPRESS β-hCG.**
Elevations in serum AFP are often accompanied by mild increases in serum β-hCG levels in patients with embryonal carcinomas and germinomas due to the presence of scattered syncytiotrophoblasts. The presence of cytotrophoblasts warrants a diagnosis of choriocarcinoma.
QCSP, **Embryonal Carcinoma**, p 446.

6.   D.   **IT TENDS TO BE WIDELY INVASIVE AT TIME OF DIAGNOSIS AND HAS A POOR PROGNOSIS.**
Germinomas are exquisitely radiosensitive. Surgical cure is achieved in most patients following primary radiation therapy. Long-term survival is approximately 80%.
QCSP, **Germinoma**, p 446-447.

7.   E.   **MATURE TERATOMA**
The most common germ cell neoplasm of the mediastinum is the mature teratoma, representing about 10%-20% of all tumors in this location.
QCSP, **Benign Teratoma**, p 447.

8.   B.   **MATURE CYSTIC TERATOMA**
Germinoma, yolk sac tumor, and malignant mixed germ cell tumor all exhibit a marked male predominance. The vast majority of mediastinal germ cell neoplasms occurring in women are mature cystic teratomas.
QCSP, **Benign Teratoma**, p 447.

9.   D.   **CAN PRESENT AS RHABDOMYOSARCOMA, MYXOID LIPOSARCOMA, AND GLIOBLASTOMA MULTIFORME**
Malignant teratomas and other germ cell tumors are almost exclusively seen in males and present with cough, dyspnea, chest pain, fatigue, and weight loss. These tumors are typically sarcomas rather than carcinomas and can present as rhabdomyosarcoma, myxoid liposarcoma, angiosarcoma, chondrosarcoma, leiomyosarcoma,

glioblastoma multiforme, and many more. Germ cell neoplasms of the mediastinum are associated with Klinefelter syndrome (47,XXY).

QCSP, **Malignant Teratoma**, p 448-449.

10. C. **YOLK SAC TUMOR**

Schiller-Duval bodies are papillae composed of a central vessel covered by columnar tumor cells. Eosinophilic hyaline droplets are often present in and between the tumor cells. A PAS stain will highlight these droplets. They are resistant to digestion with diastase.

QCSP, **Yolk Sac Tumor**, p 449-450.

11. A. **TRUE**

Germinoma occurs most commonly in pure form. The tumors listed are more frequently encountered in combination with each other or in combination with an immature teratoma.

QCSP, **Mixed Germ Cell Tumors**, p 450.

12. A. **GERMINOMA (SEMINOMA)**

Nonseminomatous germ cell tumors are generally positive for cytokeratin.

QCSP, **Mixed Germ Cell Tumors**, p 450.

13. B. **POSTERIOR**

Mediastinal germ cell tumors and lymphoproliferative disorders typically occur in the anterior compartment, while neurogenic tumors occur in the posterior compartment.

QCSP, **Neurogenic Tumors**, p 451.

14. A. **S100**

S100 staining is observed in all neurogenic tumors, although the degree of staining between tumors can vary.

QCSP, **Neurogenic Tumors**, p 451.

15. A. **TRUE**

Approximately 5% of patients with neurofibromatosis (NF) type 1 develop malignant peripheral nerve sheath tumor (MPNST), typically arising out of a preexisting neurofibroma. On the other hand, 1/2 of all cases of MPNST occur in patients with NF type 1. These tumors are associated with alterations involving chromosome 17 at a site away from the NF type 1 gene locus, which may provide a pathogenesis for the worse prognosis associated with these cases.

QCSP, **Malignant Peripheral Nerve Sheath Tumor**, p 451.

16. D. **N-MYC**

Many cases of neuroblastoma are associated with N-myc amplification, which is considered a negative prognostic indicator.

QCSP, **Neuroblastoma**, p 452.

17. D. **HOMER WRIGHT ROSETTES**

The rosettes seen in neuroblastoma are Homer Wright rosettes, which are characterized by a central collection of neuropil surrounded by a mantle of neuroblasts. True rosettes and perivascular pseudorosettes are seen in ependymomas, which rarely occur in the mediastinum. Perivascular pseudorosettes have a central blood vessel surrounded by cytoplasmic processes of neoplastic ependymal cells. True rosettes, in contrast, have an empty lumen. Flexner-Wintersteiner rosettes are true rosettes seen in retinoblastoma.

QCSP, **Neuroblastoma**, p 452.

13: Mediastinum Answers

34.   D.   **RECURRENCE RATES ARE HIGH, AND METASTATIC DISEASE HAS BEEN REPORTED.**
Ectopic hamartomatous thymomas most commonly occur in middle-aged men. They typically arise from the thymic anlage associated with branchial pouches, although they do not occur within normal mediastinal thymus (hence "ectopic"). Like other hamartomas, they are composed of haphazardly arranged tissue elements such as adipose, squamous, and glandular cells. Hamartomas are benign malformations and do not recur or metastasize.
QCSP, **Ectopic Hamartomatous Thymoma,** p 464.

35.   E.   **A, B, AND C**
While this question was targeted at SETTLE, a comprehensive differential diagnosis for this clinical presentation and morphologic appearance would also include synovial sarcoma and immature teratoma.
QCSP, **SETTLE,** p 465.

36.   C.   *HISTOPLASMA*
Histoplasma capsulatum is the most common organism identified in sclerosing mediastinitis. A silver stain is helpful in highlighting the organisms in tissue. Overall, approximately 50% of cases of sclerosing mediastinitis result from fungal infections; the remaining 50% have no obvious etiology. Less common organisms associated with this entity include *Aspergillus, Cryptococcus,* and *Mucor.* Other cases may be associated with sarcoidosis, syphilis, chest trauma, *Nocardia, Actinomyces,* and methysergide (antimigraine agent).
QCSP, **Mediastinal Fibrosis,** p 466.

37.   A.   **CYTOKERATIN +, β-hCG+, PLAP+, EMA+**
The image represents choriocarcinoma of the mediastinum. It consists of an admixture of mononuclear cytotrophoblasts and giant multinucleated syncytiotrophoblasts. Answers B, C, and D represent the immunohistochemical profiles of embryonal carcinoma, germinoma (seminoma), and yolk sac tumor, respectively.
QCSP, **Choriocarcinoma,** p 445.

38.   C.   **β-hCG**
While we always think of choriocarcinoma as the classic tumor associated with an elevated β-hCG level, it is important to remember that scattered syncytiotrophoblasts can also be present in germinomas and embryonal carcinomas. As a result, patients with these tumors may also present with mild β-hCG elevations. In contrast to syncytiotrophoblasts, cytotrophoblasts are only seen in choriocarcinoma and are required for the diagnosis. Moreover, β-hCG levels are usually extremely high in choriocarcinomas.
QCSP, **Choriocarcinoma,** p 445.

39.   D.   **EMBRYONAL CARCINOMA**
Embryonal carcinomas are usually extensively invasive at the time of diagnosis. The cut surface of the tumor is hemorrhagic and necrotic. Microscopic features include sheets, tubules, and papillary structures of large polygonal cells containing round to oval nuclei with prominent nucleoli, pale cytoplasm, and indistinct cell borders. Mitotic figures are easily identified. The tumor cells are immunoreactive for cytokeratin, PLAP, and CD30, but negative for EMA. α-fetoprotein is only positive in 30%-35% of cases. The main differential diagnoses include primary thymic carcinoma and metastatic carcinoma from other sites. The immunoprofile for embryonal carcinoma is critical in distinguishing this entity from thymic carcinoma or metastatic disease. CD30 is particularly helpful in differentiating germinoma (seminoma) from embryonal carcinoma. Choriocarcinoma is EMA positive and has strong β-hCG reactivity, in contrast to embryonal carcinoma.
QCSP, **Embryonal carcinoma,** p 446-447.

40.   C.   **CYTOKERATIN −, EMA−, PLAP+, CD117+**
The image is that of a germinoma (seminoma). The tumor exhibits sheets of large polygonal cells with distinct cell borders, clear cytoplasm, and a large nucleus containing a single prominent nucleolus. There is a loose

lymphocytic infiltrate. The classic germinoma is negative for cytokeratin and EMA and positive for PLAP and CD117.

QCSP, **Germinoma,** p 447.

41.   D.   **A AND B**
The macroscopic description in conjunction with the microscopic image represents a mature cystic teratoma. Immature neural elements would be consistent with an immature teratoma, but are not seen in this image.

QCSP, **Benign Teratoma,** p 448.

42.   E.   **IT IS USUALLY PURE AND DEVOID OF MALIGNANT GERM CELL TUMOR COMPONENTS.**
The microscopic image depicts frequent immature neural elements, consistent with an immature teratoma. Immature teratomas frequently undergo malignant transformation, and should be sampled carefully, since malignant germ cell tumor foci may be minute.

QCSP, **Benign Teratoma,** p 448.

43.   C.   **YOLK SAC TUMOR**
Yolk sac tumors usually occur in men in their 20s and are large and invasive at the time of diagnosis. They may be seen in the pure form or in combination with immature teratoma or other malignant germ cell tumors (especially embryonal carcinoma). Microscopically, the tumor can vary widely in microscopic appearance. Classically, the neoplasm exhibits a reticular pattern with various sized spaces lined by flattened cells and Schiller-Duval bodies (papillae composed of a central vessel covered by columnar tumor cells). Eosinophilic hyaline droplets in and between tumor cells are also a helpful feature.

QCSP, **Yolk Sac Tumor,** p 449-450.

44.   D.   **CYTOKERATIN +, α-1-ANTITRYPSIN +, PLAP+, CEA+, α-FETOPROTEIN +**
Answers A, B, C, are the immunoprofiles for choriocarcinoma, embryonal carcinoma, and germinoma (seminoma), respectively. Embryonal carcinoma can also cause an elevation of serum α-fetoprotein. However, only one third of cases of embryonal carcinomas are positive for α-fetoprotein by immunohistochemistry. In contrast, yolk sac tumors strongly express α-fetoprotein.

QCSP, **Yolk Sac Tumor,** p 450.

45.   C.   **IS A RESULT OF MATURATION WITHIN A NEUROBLASTOMA**
The image represents a ganglioneuroma, which is histologically characterized by mature ganglion cells, Schwann cells and nerve fibers. They are a result of maturation within a neuroblastoma and occur in the posterior mediastinum. The most common neurogenic tumor of the mediastinum is the schwannoma. Local resection is adequate treatment.

QCSP, **Ganglioneuroma,** p 451.

46.   A.   **PARAGANGLIOMA**
Paraganglioma in the mediastinum typically arises from the aortopulmonary region (ie, superior or middle compartment) or the sympathetic paraganglia in the posterior compartment. The tumor is characterized by zellballen nests of polygonal tumor cells with granular cytoplasm which are lined by capillaries. None of the other tumors listed exhibits a nested growth pattern.

QCSP, **Paraganglioma,** p 454.

47.   E.   **A, B, AND C**
The image shows a small round blue cell tumor. The most likely diagnoses to consider are neuroblastoma (especially in small children), PNET, and small cell carcinoma (metastasis from lung primary).

QCSP, **Primitive Neuroectodermal Tumor,** p 454-455.

13: Mediastinum Answers

48.   B.   **SCHWANNOMA**

Schwannomas are typically discovered incidentally. The tumor arises from a peripheral nerve and is almost always solitary. Compact cellular growth called "Antoni A" areas alternate with myxoid paucicellular foci referred to as "Antoni B" areas. Palisading tumor cell nuclei, also known as Verocay bodies, are occasionally associated with Antoni A areas. Thick-walled, hyalinized vessels are very characteristic of this tumor and can aid in the diagnosis. *QCSP,* **Schwannoma,** p 455.

49.   C.   **PERIVASCULAR SPACES/SERUM LAKES**

Perivascular spaces/serum lakes are shown in this image of a lymphocyte-predominant thymoma. These spaces are seen around the capillary or venule-sized intratumoral vessels. The area between the vessel and the basement membrane of the epithelial cells is filled with proteinaceous eosinophilic transudate. Lymphocytes, erythrocytes, and foamy macrophages may be suspended in the contents of the serum lakes. Fibrous septations are seen in thymomas. The septations divide the tumor into well-defined lobules and characteristically form acute angles at points of intersection. Tingible body macrophages can be seen in thymomas or lymphomas. Thymomas can have a low power "starry sky" pattern like Burkitt lymphoma. However, the lymphocytes in thymomas are small and mature and never neoplastic. Microcystic change is also a helpful feature in thymomas, but is not present in this image. *QCSP,* **Thymoma,** p 456.

50.   D.   **SPINDLE CELL THYMOMAS HAVE A WORSE PROGNOSIS THAN EPITHELIAL THYMOMAS WITH POLYGONAL EPITHELIAL CELLS.**

Spindle cell thymomas are a subtype of epithelial thymomas and are associated with a favorable prognosis. *QCSP,* **Thymoma,** p 458.

51.   E.   **THYMIC CARCINOMA**

This image is an example of thymic carcinoma. The neoplastic population consists of large, atypical epithelioid tumor cells with irregular chromatin and conspicuous nucleoli. While mitotic activity and necrosis are not prominent in this image, the degree of cellular atypia is more than would be expected in a typical thymoma and clinches the diagnosis. *QCSP,* **Thymic Carcinoma,** p 460.

52.   E.   **ALL OF THE ABOVE**

The clinical history and radiographic appearance is classic for sclerosing mediastinitis; however, all of the choices mentioned should be considered because they represent diagnostic pitfalls. While there are no immunohistochemical stains diagnostic of sclerosing mediastinitis, a panel of stains may be required to rule out these mimickers. *QCSP,* **Mediastinal Fibrosis,** p 466.

Chapter 14

Lymph Node

1. Follicular dendritic cell sarcoma tends to be an indolent disease except for what site(s)?
    A. Lung
    B. Intraabdominal
    C. Any extranodal site
    D. Nodes other than cervical
    E. Supraclavicular lymph nodes

2. Which of the following immunoprofiles is most consistent with follicular dendritic cell sarcoma?
    A. CD21+/CD35+/CD79a–
    B. CD21+/CD35+/CD79a+
    C. CD3–/CD20+/CD30+
    D. CD21–/CD30+/CD35–
    E. CD10+/CD20+/bcl-2+

3. Various bacterial infections can be distinguished from histiocytic necrotizing lymphadenitis primarily based on which of the following feature(s)?
    A. Follicular hyperplasia
    B. Histiocytes
    C. Granulocytes
    D. Reactive immunoblasts
    E. A and C

4. All of the following organisms have been associated with suppurative lymphadenitis EXCEPT:
    A. *Bartonella henselae*
    B. *Tropheryma whippelii*
    C. *Chlamydia trachomatis*
    D. *Staphylococcus* species
    E. *Yersinia enterocolitica*

5. Which of the following statements regarding Kikuchi-Fujimoto disease is FALSE?
    A. Patient typically presents with elevated WBC count
    B. Seen in young patients of Asian descent
    C. Contain large discrete areas of eosinophilic necrosis
    D. Usually lacks granulocytes
    E. Can be seen following diffuse large B-cell lymphoma

6. Calcium oxalate crystals, sometimes forming large, concentric calcifications, are associated with which inflammatory/hyperplastic disease of the lymph nodes?
    A. Lymphogranuloma venereum
    B. Cat-scratch disease
    C. Sarcoidosis
    D. Dermatopathic lymphadenitis
    E. Toxoplasmosis

7. The characteristic triad of findings in toxoplasmosis includes all EXCEPT:
    A. Marked follicular hyperplasia
    B. Effacement of nodal architecture
    C. Epithelioid histiocytes
    D. Reactive monocytoid B-cell proliferation distending sinuses
    E. None of the above

8. What is the causative agent of cat-scratch fever?
    A. *Tularemia*
    B. *Bordetella*
    C. *Parainfluenza*
    D. *Bartonella*
    E. *Mycoplasma*

9. Which special stain can be useful in identifying the causative agent of cat-scratch fever?
    A. PAS light green
    B. Warthin-Starry
    C. Brown-Hopps
    D. GMS
    E. PAS without diastasis

10. Which of the following organisms is the causative agent of lymphogranuloma venereum?
    A. *Haemophilus ducreyi*
    B. *Calymmatobacterium granulomatis*
    C. *Chlamydia trachomatis*
    D. *Chlamydia pneumoniae*
    E. EBV

11. In patients with HIV, the most typical histological finding within the lymph node is?
    A. Florid reactive hyperplasia
    B. Hodgkin lymphoma
    C. Lymphocyte depletion
    D. Vascular proliferation
    E. Necrosis

12. A positive Fascin stain confirms that the AIDS virus infects which cell type?
    A. Follicular dendritic cell
    B. Germinal center B-cell
    C. Interfollicular T-cell
    D. Endothelial cell
    E. Histiocytes

13. All of the following are features of AIDS-related lymphadenopathy EXCEPT:
    A. Florid follicular hyperplasia
    B. Dumbbell- or serpentine-shaped follicles
    C. Absent mantle zone
    D. Intrafollicular plasma cells and tingible-body macrophages
    E. Suppurative lymphadenitis

14: Lymph Node Questions

14. Which of the following entities is least associated with a HIV infection?
    A. Primary effusion lymphoma
    B. Plasmablastic lymphoma
    C. Kaposi sarcoma
    D. Extranodal marginal zone B-cell lymphoma
    E. Mycobacterial spindle cell tumor

15. The atypical lymphocytes seen in the peripheral blood smear of patients with infectious mononucleosis are?
    A. CD19+ B cells
    B. CD4+ T-helper cells
    C. CD8+ cytotoxic T cells
    D. CD4+ CD8+ T cells
    E. CD3+ CD8– CD4– T cells

16. Which of the following features are more specific for infectious mononucleosis than lymphoma?
    A. Necrosis
    B. EBV+ lymphocytes
    C. CD15+ lymphocytes
    D. CD30+ lymphocytes
    E. Paracortical distribution of the large lymphoid cells

17. All of the following are features of hyaline-vascular Castleman disease EXCEPT:
    A. Onion skinning of small lymphocytes around germinal centers
    B. Interfollicular vascularity with small blood vessels radially penetrating follicles
    C. Multiple germinal centers per follicle
    D. Enlarged follicles
    E. Single mass, often mediastinal

18. Multicentric Castleman disease is associated with which infection?
    A. HHV-8
    B. EBV
    C. CMV
    D. HIV
    E. HHV6

19. Multicentric Castleman disease is associated with which syndrome?
    A. POEMS
    B. WAGR
    C. Coffin-Siris
    D. Carney syndrome
    E. Carney triad

20. Which of the following is NOT associated with Castleman disease?
    A. Non-Hodgkin lymphoma
    B. Follicular dendritic cell tumor
    C. Kaposi sarcoma
    D. All of the above are associated with Castleman disease
    E. None of the above

21. Which cytokine is associated with the systemic manifestations of Castleman disease?
    A. IL-1
    B. IL-2
    C. IL-5
    D. IL-6
    E. IL-10

22. Which of the following statements concerning dermatopathic lymphadenitis is FALSE?
    A. Demonstrates presence of pale nodules with numerous histiocytes
    B. Can demonstrates melanotic pigment
    C. Caused by skin antigens presented by S100+ cells
    D. Mixed lymphocytic infiltrate
    E. A precursor lesion for mycosis fungoides

23. Which of the following is/are more commonly seen and/or seen to a greater degree in sinus histiocytosis with massive lymphadenopathy (Rosai-Dorfman disease) vs Langerhans cell histiocytosis?
    A. CD1a expression
    B. Emperipolesis
    C. Presence of eosinophils
    D. Massively dilated sinuses
    E. Choices B and D

24. Which of the following is NOT a feature of sinus histiocytosis with massive lymphadenopathy (Rosai-Dorfman disease)?
    A. Plasma cells
    B. Histiocytes
    C. Emperipolesis
    D. Birbeck granules by electron microscopy
    E. Polyclonal hypergammaglobulinemia, anemia, and leukocytosis

25. Which of the following statements best describes sinus histiocytosis with massive lymphadenopathy (Rosai-Dorfman disease)?
    A. Histiocytes comprising the lesion express S100 protein, CD68 and CD1a.
    B. Women are more often affected than men.
    C. 10% of patients present with soft tissue involvement.
    D. The condition is frequently preceded by a viral illness.
    E. Patients typically present with bilateral painful lymphadenopathy.

26. Which statement best describes progressive transformation of germinal centers?
    A. A malignant process that has a rapid and fulminant clinical course
    B. A precursor lesion for classical Hodgkin lymphoma
    C. An incidental finding characterized by atypical follicular hyperplasia and mantle zone expansion with migration of small lymphocytes into germinal centers
    D. Localized lymphadenopathy characterized by abnormal follicles containing radially penetrating hyalinized capillaries
    E. A low-grade lymphoma associated with EBV infection

14: Lymph Node Questions

27. With which lymphoma is progressive transformation of germinal centers most often associated?
    A. Classical Hodgkin lymphoma
    B. Nodular lymphocyte-predominant Hodgkin lymphoma
    C. Follicular lymphoma
    D. Diffuse large B-cell lymphoma
    E. T-cell/histiocyte-rich B-cell lymphoma.

28. Which of the following organisms has been associated with bacillary angiomatosis?
    A. HHV-8
    B. *Bartonella henselae*
    C. *Brucella abortus*
    D. CMV
    E. *Mycoplasma pneumoniae*

29. Which of the following statements regarding Kaposi sarcoma is FALSE?
    A. Extracellular and cytoplasmic hyaline globules are present in a minority of these tumors.
    B. No single chromosomal abnormality is associated with this tumor.
    C. Immunohistochemical stains for FLI-1 are usually positive.
    D. The spindle cells demonstrate strong immunoreactivity for CD31 and CD34.
    E. Hyaline globules are accentuated by the use of a PAS stain.

30. Classic Reed-Sternberg cells are most frequently seen in what 2 subtypes of Hodgkin lymphoma?
    A. Nodular lymphocyte-predominant Hodgkin lymphoma
    B. Lymphocyte-rich Hodgkin lymphoma
    C. Nodular sclerosis Hodgkin lymphoma
    D. Mixed cellularity Hodgkin lymphoma
    E. Lymphocyte-depleted Hodgkin lymphoma

31. The obliterative "syncytial variant" is a variant of which type of classical Hodgkin lymphoma?
    A. Mixed cellularity Hodgkin lymphoma
    B. Lymphocyte-depleted Hodgkin lymphoma
    C. Lymphocyte-rich Hodgkin lymphoma
    D. Nodular sclerosing Hodgkin lymphoma
    E. Lymphocyte-predominant nodular Hodgkin lymphoma

32. Pleomorphic/sarcomatoid Reed-Sternberg cells are a key feature of which variant of classical Hodgkin lymphoma?
    A. Nodular sclerosing Hodgkin lymphoma
    B. Mixed cellularity Hodgkin lymphoma
    C. Lymphocyte-depleted Hodgkin lymphoma
    D. Lymphocyte-rich Hodgkin lymphoma
    E. None of the above

33. Adverse prognostic factors in Hodgkin lymphoma include all of the following EXCEPT?
    A. Stage III or IV disease
    B. Absence of B symptoms
    C. Old age
    D. Splenic involvement
    E. Extranodal involvement

34. EBV is most closely associated with which subtype of Hodgkin lymphoma?
    A. Nodular lymphocyte-predominant Hodgkin lymphoma
    B. Lymphocyte-rich Hodgkin lymphoma
    C. Nodular sclerosis Hodgkin lymphoma
    D. Mixed cellularity Hodgkin lymphoma
    E. Lymphocyte-depleted Hodgkin lymphoma

35. Which of the following markers is NOT expressed by L&H cells?
    A. CD45
    B. CD20
    C. PAX5
    D. EMA
    E. CD15

36. Which of the following variants of Hodgkin lymphoma is associated with or related to T-cell/histiocyte-rich B-cell lymphoma?
    A. Nodular sclerosing Hodgkin lymphoma
    B. Lymphocyte-rich Hodgkin lymphoma
    C. Mixed cellularity Hodgkin lymphoma
    D. Nodular lymphocyte-predominant Hodgkin lymphoma
    E. Lymphocyte-depleted Hodgkin lymphoma

37. What is the most common genetic alteration seen in precursor B-cell lymphoblastic leukemia/lymphoma?
    A. t(9;22)(q34;q11.2) *BCR/ABL*
    B. t(12;21)(p13;q22) *TEL1/AML1*
    C. t(4;11)(q21;q23) *AF4/MLL*
    D. Hypodiploidy
    E. Polysomy

38. Factors associated with a worse prognosis for precursor B-cell lymphoblastic leukemia include all of the following EXCEPT:
    A. Hyperdiploidy (>50)
    B. Age <1
    C. High white blood cell count
    D. t(9;22)(q34;q11.2) *BCR/ABL*
    E. t(4;11)(q21;q23) *AF4/MLL*

39. Which of the following factors is consistent with a favorable prognosis in precursor B-cell lymphoblastic leukemia/lymphoma?
    A. Hypoploidy
    B. t(9;22)(q34;q11.2)
    C. t(4;11)(q21;q23)
    D. Age less than 2 years
    E. t(12;21)(p13;q22)

40. The blast in B-cell lymphoblastic leukemia can express all the following except?
    A. TdT
    B. CD24
    C. CD22
    D. Surface immunoglobulin light chain
    E. CD10

41. Which of the following phenotypes is associated with B-cell acute lymphoblastic leukemia with an 11q23 (MLL) translocation?
    A. CD19+ CD22+ TdT+ CD9–
    B. CD19+ CD79a+ CD10+ CD25+
    C. CD19+ TdT+ CD10+ CD45–
    D. CD19+ TdT+ CD20+, CD34–
    E. CD19+ TdT+ CD9+ CD10– CD15+

42. Which of the following is true of precursor T-cell lymphoblastic leukemia/lymphoma?
    A. The great majority of children treated with aggressive chemotherapy will achieve complete remission.
    B. All other factors being equal, a 6-month-old diagnosed with this lymphoma would have a better prognosis than a 5-year-old.
    C. A deletion of 12p is seen in approximately 30% of patients.
    D. All other factors being equal, a 15-year-old diagnosed with this lymphoma would have a better prognosis than a 5-year-old.
    E. Almost all cases have translocations involving the T-cell receptor genes.

43. Which of the following markers on T-ALL is associated with a worse prognosis and a specific genetic alteration?
    A. CD33
    B. CD117
    C. CD79a
    D. CD1a
    E. CD7

44. Which of the following statements concerning lineage designation is FALSE?
    A. Myeloperoxidase expression is specific for myeloid lineage.
    B. Clonal TCR-γ chain PCR is specific for T-cell lineage.
    C. Strong CD19 expression plus 1 other B-cell marker is required for B-cell lineage.
    D. TdT is not specific for a cell lineage.
    E. All the above are true.

45. Which of the following flow cytometry results is most consistent with a diagnosis of CLL/SLL:
    A. CD19+, CD5+, CD23+, CD10+, FMC7+
    B. CD19+, CD5–, CD23–, CD10+, FMC7–
    C. CD19+, CD5+, CD23+, CD10–, FMC7–
    D. CD19+, CD5–, CD23–, CD10+, FMC7+
    E. CD19+, CD5+, CD23–, CD10–, FMC7+

46. Which of the following cytogenetic alterations is typically seen in CLL/SLL?
    A. Trisomy 12
    B. Deletion of 13q14
    C. Deletion of 11q22-23
    D. Deletion of 17p13
    E. All can be seen in CLL/SLL

47. Which of the following does NOT indicate a poor prognosis in CLL/SLL?
    A. Expression of Zap70
    B. Expression of CD38
    C. IGHV unmutated
    D. Richter syndrome
    E. All the above indicate a poor prognosis.

14: Lymph Node Questions

48. A 60-year-old man presents with complaints of visual impairment, weakness, fatigue, and weight loss. A CT-scan shows lymphadenopathy and hepatosplenomegaly. An excisional biopsy of one of the enlarged lymph nodes demonstrates a diffuse, variably dense infiltrate of lymphocytes, plasma cells and plasmacytoid lymphocytes. PAS-positive inclusions are present in nuclei and the cytoplasm of the tumor cells. In addition, the infiltrate is accompanied by reactive hyperplasia of mast cells. The neoplastic cells most commonly secrete which immunoglobulin?
    A. IgD
    B. IgA
    C. IgG
    D. IgM
    E. Free light chains

49. Which of the following viral infections is most commonly associated with lymphoplasmacytic lymphoma?
    A. HIV
    B. HCV
    C. EBV
    D. CMV
    E. HHV-8

50. Which of the following immunophenotype is consistent with a diagnosis of hairy cell leukemia?
    A. CD19+, CD20+, CD5+, CD23+, CD10–, FMC7–
    B. CD19+, CD20+, CD25+, CD11c+, CD103+, FMC7+
    C. CD19+, CD20+, CD5+, CD23–, CD10–, FMC7+
    D. CD19–, CD4+, CD11c+, CD10–, FMC7–
    E. CD19+, CD22+, CD25-, CD11c+, CD103+, FMC7+

51. Which of the following is more common in hairy cell-variant disease than hairy-cell leukemia?
    A. Monocytopenia
    B. Expression of CD123
    C. Expression of annexin A1
    D. Leukocytosis
    E. Dense marrow fibrosis

52. The following cells can be seen in Plasma cell neoplasms EXCEPT:
    A. Mott cell
    B. Flame cell
    C. Hallmark cell
    D. Cells with Dutcher bodies
    E. Cells with Russell bodies

53. The immunophenotype of the neoplastic cells in plasma cell dyscrasias is:
    A. CD19+, CD20+, CD38–, CD138–, CD45+
    B. CD19+, CD20–, CD38+, CD138–, CD45–
    C. CD19–, CD20–, CD38+, CD138+, CD45–
    D. CD19–, CD20+, CD38+, CD138+, CD45+
    E. CD19+, CD20–, CD38–, CD138+, CD45–

14: Lymph Node Questions

54. Which of the following concerning symptomatic myeloma is FALSE?
    A. Can express cyclin D-1
    B. Most have translocations involving 14q32
    C. Demonstrates end organ damage
    D. Rouleaux formation on peripheral smear
    E. Serum protein of >30 g/dL is diagnostic.

55. Which of the following is true of extranodal marginal zone (MALT) lymphoma?
    A. Immunohistochemical staining for CD20 and CD10 is positive.
    B. No characteristic translocations or other genetic alterations have yet been described.
    C. A localized gastric MALT lymphoma is potentially curable with triple antibiotic therapy.
    D. CD23 expression is frequently present.
    E. After the GI tract, the thyroid is the most common site.

56. Aside from *H pylori*, which other infections have been associated with development of MALT lymphoma?
    A. *Chlamydia psittaci*
    B. *Campylobacter jejuni*
    C. *Borrelia burgdorferi*
    D. All the above
    E. A and C

57. Which of the following conditions does NOT demonstrate clonal immunoglobulin gene rearrangement?
    A. Angioimmunoblastic T-cell lymphoma
    B. Plasmablastic lymphoma
    C. Lymphomatoid granulomatosis
    D. Blastic plasmacytoid dendritic cell neoplasm
    E. T-cell lymphoblastic leukemia

58. Which of the following processes is not related to an EBV infection?
    A. Anaplastic large cell lymphoma
    B. Hodgkin lymphoma
    C. Post-transplant lymphoproliferative disorders
    D. Angioimmunoblastic T-cell lymphoma
    E. Extranodal natural killer T-cell lymphoma

59. Cells with various morphologies are seen infiltrating the marginal zone and interfollicular areas of lymph nodes in nodal marginal zone B-cell lymphoma, including which of the following (list all that apply)?
    A. Centrocyte-like B-cells
    B. Monocytoid B-cells
    C. Small B-lymphocytes
    D. Scattered centroblast and immunoblast-like cells
    E. Cells with plasma cell differentiation

60. Extranodal marginal zone lymphomas are usually negative for all the following, EXCEPT?
    A. BCL-2
    B. CD10
    C. CD5
    D. CD23
    E. Negative for all the above markers

14: Lymph Node Questions

61. A 54-year-old man is referred to a hematologist for massive splenomegaly and leukocytosis. A bone marrow biopsy is noncontributory. A splenectomy is performed for relief of abdominal pain as well as for diagnosis. Which of the following is true of splenic marginal zone lymphoma?
    A. The white pulp is primarily infiltrated by small round lymphocytes, with sparing of the red pulp by definition.
    B. The germinal centers of the splenic hilar lymph nodes are often enveloped and replaced by the tumor cells.
    C. By definition, bone marrow biopsies will demonstrate normal marrow elements with no tumor cell infiltration in all cases.
    D. Splenectomy is only for symptomatic relief and diagnosis, and confers no increased survival in these patients.
    E. This type of lymphoma is somewhat common, representing 5%-8% of all lymphoid neoplasms.

62. Which of the following conditions does NOT demonstrate clonal TCR rearrangements?
    A. T-cell lymphoblastic leukemia
    B. B-cell lymphoblastic leukemia
    C. Lymphomatoid papulosis
    D. Aggressive NK-cell leukemia
    E. Sézary syndrome

63. Which of the following is true of splenic marginal zone lymphoma?
    A. Patients will sometimes present with autoimmune thrombocytopenia.
    B. Cytogenetic studies demonstrate a common, unique translocation.
    C. This lymphoma is aggressive, with most patients succumbing within 1 year of diagnosis.
    D. The presence of villous lymphocytes in the peripheral blood would take splenic marginal zone lymphoma out of the differential.
    E. The tumor cells are, by definition, negative for CD20 and surface immunoglobulins.

64. A diagnosis of follicular lymphoma is rendered. Careful histologic examination of 10 neoplastic follicles at 40× reveals 12 centroblasts. Which of the following is true?
    A. This is a grade 1 follicular lymphoma. Flow cytometry will demonstrate CD10 and CD19 expression.
    B. This is a grade 2 follicular lymphoma. Flow cytometry will demonstrate CD19 expression, with no evidence of CD10 expression.
    C. This is a grade 2 follicular lymphoma. Flow cytometry will demonstrate CD10 and CD19 expression.
    D. This is a grade 3 follicular lymphoma. Flow cytometry will demonstrate CD19 expression, with no evidence of CD10 expression.
    E. This is a grade 3 follicular lymphoma. Flow cytometry will demonstrate CD10 and CD19 expression.

65. Which of the following molecular alterations is associated with follicular lymphoma?
    A. t(11;14) involving the *BCL-1* gene
    B. t(14;18) involving the *BCL-2* gene
    C. t(11;18) involving the *API2* gene
    D. t(8;14) involving the *c-Myc* gene
    E. t(12;21) involving the *TEL1* and *AML1* genes

66. Mantle cell lymphoma can be distinguished from follicular lymphoma based on all of the following features EXCEPT:
    A. MCL more commonly presents with peripheral blood lymphocytosis.
    B. MCL commonly has nonparatrabecular as well as paratrabecular aggregates.
    C. MCL more commonly demonstrates extranodal disease, such as lymphomatoid polyposis of the small bowel and colon.
    D. MCL typically expresses CD5 and cyclin-D1 and is negative for CD10 and bcl-6.
    E. MCL demonstrates splenic expansion of the white pulp, and periportal infiltration may be present in the liver.

14: Lymph Node Questions

67. Which of the following is FALSE regarding mantle cell lymphoma?
    A. Splenic involvement is common, with expansion of the white pulp by the neoplastic cells.
    B. Proliferation centers, by definition, are present in the lymph nodes.
    C. Bone marrow is often involved, with either paratrabecular or nonparatrabecular lymphoid aggregates occurring.
    D. Extranodal disease occasionally takes the form of lymphomatoid polyposis of the lower GI tract.
    E. Mantle cell lymphoma occurs more commonly in adult males than females.

68. Which of the following flow cytometry results is most consistent with a diagnosis of mantle cell lymphoma?
    A. CD19+, CD5+, CD23+, CD10+, FMC7+
    B. CD19+, CD5−, CD23−, CD10+, FMC7−
    C. CD19+, CD5+, CD23+, CD10−, FMC7−
    D. CD19+, CD5−, CD23−, CD10+, FMC7+
    E. CD19+, CD5+, CD23−, CD10−, FMC7+

69. Which of the following translocations is found in approximately 30% of diffuse large B-cell lymphomas?
    A. t(8;14)
    B. t(14;18)
    C. t(8;22)
    D. t(11;14)
    E. t(4;18)

70. Which of the following statements is true regarding diffuse large B-cell lymphoma (DLBCL)?
    A. Diffuse large B-cell lymphoma is considered an incurable lymphoma, with almost all patients ultimately dying from the disease.
    B. Approximately 20% of patients who receive aggressive chemotherapy are able to achieve complete remission.
    C. In addition to CD20, diffuse large B-cell lymphomas can frequently be positive for CD10.
    D. Multiple nucleoli in the lymphoma cells would remove diffuse large B-cell lymphoma from the differential.
    E. The tumor cells are approximately the size of small lymphocytes.

71. All of the following statements are true regarding mediastinal (thymic) large B-cell lymphoma EXCEPT:
    A. Generally demonstrate light chain restricted surface immunoglobulin.
    B. Prognosis is related to initial stage of disease at presentation.
    C. The immunoprofile is typically CD10−/CD19+/CD45+.
    D. Histologically, there is a diffuse infiltrate of large cells with abundant cytoplasm separated by variably dense bands of fibrosis.
    E. It is a subtype of diffuse large B-cell lymphoma originating from thymic B cells.

72. The typical patient with mediastinal (thymic) diffuse large B-cell lymphoma would be which of the following?
    A. 74-year-old male
    B. 55-year-old woman with history of breast cancer with radiation therapy
    C. 35-year-old woman
    D. 12-year-old boy
    E. 2-month-old girl

73. Which of the following is NOT a common translocation seen in typical Burkitt lymphoma?
    A. t(8;14)
    B. t(2;8)
    C. t(8;22)
    D. t(8;9)
    E. All the above are common translocations.

14: Lymph Node Questions

74. Which of the following statements regarding Burkitt lymphoma is FALSE?
    A. Commonly involves the GI tract in sporadic cases
    B. Often presents with leukemic involvement
    C. Involvement of the jaw often associated with EBV
    D. Will often involve the CNS
    E. Cytology preps of the cells demonstrate deeply basophilic cytoplasm that frequently contains lipid vacuoles.

75. Which of the following markers are most often lost in T-cell lymphoma/leukemias?
    A. CD2
    B. CD3
    C. CD4
    D. CD5
    E. CD7

76. Which T-cell lymphoma is thought to be derived from intrafollicular T-cells?
    A. Prolymphocytic T-cell lymphoma
    B. Peripheral T-cell lymphoma, unspecified
    C. Adult T-cell lymphoma
    D. Angioimmunoblastic T-cell lymphoma
    E. Sézary syndrome

77. Which of the following is the most important prognostic factor for Adult T-cell Leukemia/lymphoma?
    A. WBC count
    B. Hypercalcemia
    C. LDH
    D. Skin involvement
    E. Decreased β2-microglobulin

78. A 38-year-old graduate student from Panama is referred to a hematologist for leukocytosis and splenomegaly. Physical examination reveals prominent cervical adenopathy. Following clinical work-up, one of these lymph nodes is excised and sent to surgical pathology. The case is discussed with a hematopathologist, who makes the diagnosis of probable adult T-cell lymphoma. Which of the following viruses is strongly associated with this type of lymphoma?
    A. EBV
    B. CMV
    C. HSV-1
    D. HTLV-1
    E. HPV

79. Which of the following statements regarding the variants of adult T-cell leukemia/lymphoma is/are TRUE?
    A. The smoldering variant is frequently associated with hypercalcemia .
    B. The chronic variant is notable for frequent hypercalcemia as well as a lack of the exfoliative rash seen in the acute variant.
    C. The acute variant is notable for frequent hypercalcemia, opportunistic infections, and skin rash.
    D. Approximately 80% of the smoldering and chronic variants ultimately progress to the acute variant.
    E. Patients with the lymphomatous and acute variants have a mean survival of 4.2 and 2.6 years following diagnosis, respectively.

14: Lymph Node Questions

80. Which of the following features best describes extranodal NK/T-cell lymphoma of nasal type?
    A. An angiocentric infiltrate composed of small lymphocytes with accompanying mixed inflammation
    B. Sheets of pleomorphic cells with abundant pale cytoplasm and multiple nucleoli
    C. Diffuse infiltrate of small, cleaved lymphocytes admixed with plasma cells, monocytoid lymphocytes, and immunoblasts
    D. Intermediate-sized lymphoid cells with numerous tingible-body macrophages and a high mitotic index
    E. Variable numbers of large cells containing eccentric kidney-shaped nuclei with surrounding eosinophilic cuffs

81. All of the following are true of extranodal NK/T-cell lymphoma, nasal type EXCEPT:
    A. More prevalent in Asia, Mexico and Central and South America; EBV associated
    B. Demonstrates angiocentric, angioinvasive, and angiodestructive pattern
    C. Heterogeneous: tumor cells may be small and irregular to large and anaplastic
    D. Cytologic grade helps predict the prognosis.
    E. Overlying epithelium may show changes of pseudoepitheliomatous hyperplasia.

82. Which of the following T-cell processes typically does NOT express CD4?
    A. Adult T-cell leukemia/lymphoma
    B. Enteropathy-type T-cell lymphoma
    C. Angioimmunoblastic T-cell lymphoma
    D. Peripheral T-cell lymphoma, unspecified
    E. Anaplastic large cell lymphoma

83. Which of the following best describes the prognosis for enteropathy-type T-cell lymphoma (refractory sprue)?
    A. Treatment of the celiac sprue resolves the disease.
    B. Prognosis for patients with child onset celiac disease is much better than for patients with adult onset celiac disease.
    C. The disease is aggressive and prognosis is typically poor.
    D. Surgical resection alone is often curative.
    E. The disease is indolent and usually does not need to be treated.

84. Which of the following statements regarding mycosis fungoides is FALSE?
    A. The neoplastic, infiltrating lymphocytes often demonstrate prominent infolding of their nuclear membranes.
    B. Rarely, transformation to a large T-cell lymphoma will occur.
    C. The detection of a Pautrier microabscess is not required for diagnosis.
    D. Immunohistochemical staining for CD3, CD4, CD5, and CD2 is characteristically positive.
    E. The tumor cells are never detected in the peripheral blood.

85. Which of the IHC markers can help differentiate the neoplastic cells of angioimmunoblastic T-cell lymphoma from peripheral T-cell lymphoma, NOS?
    A. CXCL13
    B. FoxP3
    C. CD4
    D. CD7
    E. CD25

86. Which of the following T-cell lymphomas is thought to be derived from T-regulatory cells?
    A. Prolymphocytic T-cell lymphoma
    B. Peripheral T-cell lymphoma, unspecified
    C. Adult T-cell leukemia/lymphoma
    D. Angioimmunoblastic T-cell lymphoma
    E. Sézary syndrome

14: Lymph Node Questions

87. All of the following are common clinical features of peripheral T-cell lymphoma, unspecified EXCEPT:
    A. Eosinophilia
    B. Hypercalcemia
    C. Generalized lymphadenopathy
    D. Pruritus
    E. Splenomegaly

88. Which of the following choices correctly lists features of peripheral T-cell lymphoma, unspecified?
    A. Diffuse effacement of the node; pleomorphic malignant T cells of varying size; prominent polymorphic infiltrate of reactive cells; majority are CD4+ and CD8−; complex karyotype
    B. Diffuse effacement of the node; fairly uniform large T cells; prominent polymorphic infiltrate of reactive cells; majority are CD4+ and CD8−; complex karyotype
    C. Diffuse effacement of the node; pleomorphic malignant T cells of varying size; accompanying infiltrate of predominantly histiocytes; majority are CD4+ and CD8−; complex karyotype
    D. Focal/partial nodal effacement; pleomorphic malignant T cells of varying size; prominent polymorphic infiltrate of reactive cells; majority are CD4 CD4+ and CD8−; complex karyotype
    E. Focal/partial nodal effacement; pleomorphic malignant T-cells of varying size; accompanying infiltrate of predominantly histiocytes; majority are CD4+ and CD8−; complex karyotype

89. Which T-cell lymphoma is characterized by "hallmark cells" and is positive for CD30?
    A. Angioimmunoblastic T-cell lymphoma
    B. Adult T-cell leukemia/lymphoma
    C. Mycosis fungoides
    D. Anaplastic large cell lymphoma
    E. Peripheral T-cell lymphoma, unspecified

90. Which is the most common genetic alteration seen in anaplastic large cell lymphoma?
    A. t(2;5)
    B. t(2;8)
    C. Integrated HTLV-1
    D. Trisomy 3
    E. inv(2p)

91. The tumor cells of anaplastic large cell lymphoma stain for all the following markers EXCEPT:
    A. CD30
    B. ALK
    C. EMA
    D. EBV
    E. CD43

92. All of the following are characteristic for this small-cleaved B-cell lymphoma that is positive for CD10, *BCL-6* and *BCL-2*, EXCEPT:
    A. Transformation is most commonly to diffuse large B-cell lymphoma
    B. t(11;14)(q13;q32)
    C. Paratrabecular aggregates in bone marrow
    D. Splenic involvement with expansion of white pulp and involvement of liver portal tracts
    E. High stage at presentation

14: Lymph Node Questions

93. The tumor cells of the entity shown in the image below stain for CD21 and CD35 and are associated with what other pathologic entity?

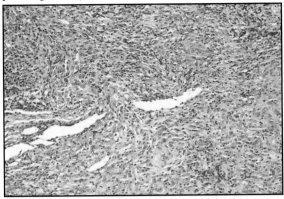

    A. Castleman disease
    B. Measles
    C. Interdigitating dendritic cell sarcoma/tumor
    D. Chemotherapy effect
    E. Postvaccination

94. The images shown below demonstrate features of lymphadenitis that could be associated with all of the following EXCEPT?

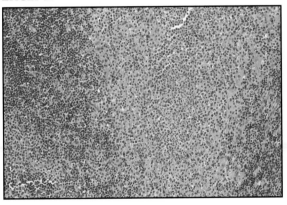 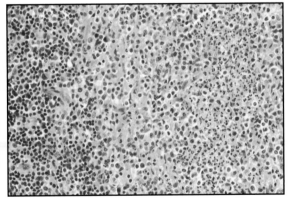

    A. Staphylococcal infections
    B. Cat-scratch disease
    C. Mesenteric lymphadenitis
    D. Lymphogranuloma venereum
    E. Toxoplasmosis

14: Lymph Node Questions

95. A young Asian woman presents with fever, leukopenia, and painless cervical lymphadenopathy. An excisional lymph node biopsy is performed, and representative sections are shown below. This process is most consistent with which of the following?

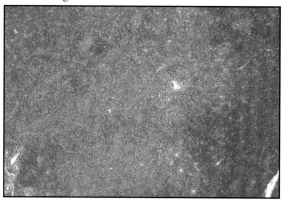 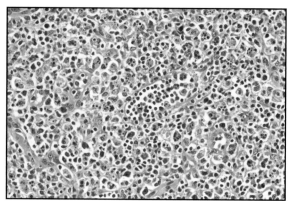

A. Diffuse large B-cell lymphoma
B. Cat-scratch disease
C. Stroma-rich Castleman disease
D. Histiocytic-necrotizing lymphadenitis (Kikuchi-Fujimoto disease)
E. Infectious mononucleosis

96. Which of the following statements concerning the disease process shown in the images shown below is FALSE?

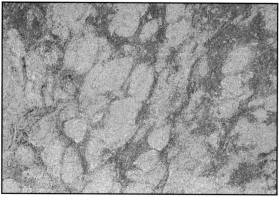 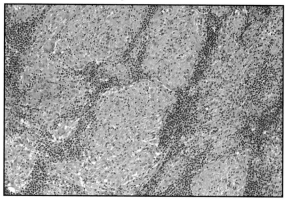

A. In the US, it is more common in African-Americans than in Caucasians.
B. The most commonly involved organs are lung, lymph nodes, eyes, skin, and liver.
C. It is a diagnosis of exclusion.
D. Typical lymph node appearance is one of total effacement of the nodal architecture by epithelioid granulomas and extensive necrosis.
E. Functional hypothyroidism is typically present.

14: Lymph Node Questions

97.   A 22-year-old veterinary student presents to his primary care doctor with enlarged posterior cervical lymph nodes. One of his lymph nodes was excised, and representative sections are shown below. Which is the most likely diagnosis?

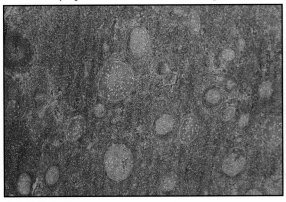 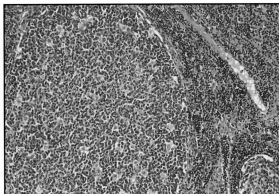

A.   Sarcoidosis
B.   Cat-scratch disease
C.   Histiocytic necrotizing lymphadenitis
D.   Toxoplasmosis
E.   Infectious mononucleosis

98.   A 15-year-old boy with a history of a skin papule 2-3 weeks ago presents with axillary lymphadenopathy. An excisional lymph node biopsy is performed. The process identified in the images shown below is most consistent with which of the following?

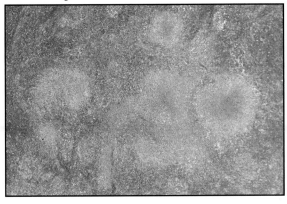 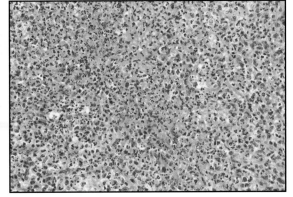

A.   Kikuchi-Fujimoto disease
B.   Cat-scratch disease
C.   Infectious mononucleosis
D.   Diffuse large B-cell lymphoma
E.   AIDS-related lymphadenopathy

99. A 26-year-old woman presents to her primary care doctor with a 3-week history of enlarged inguinal nodes. The day before she saw her doctor, the skin above her nodes started to drain. The sinus tract and nodes were excised, and representative sections are shown below. What is the diagnosis?

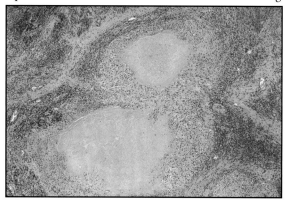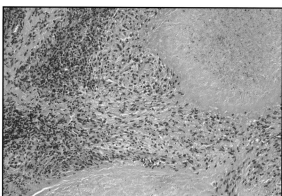

A. AIDS-related lymphadenopathy
B. Lymphogranuloma venereum
C. Sarcoidosis
D. Follicular hyperplasia
E. Cat-scratch disease

100. A 40-year-old man presents with *Pneumocystis (carinii) jiroveci* pneumonia. He had several enlarged lymph nodes, one that was removed, and the H&E- and IHC-stained sections are shown below. What is the diagnosis?

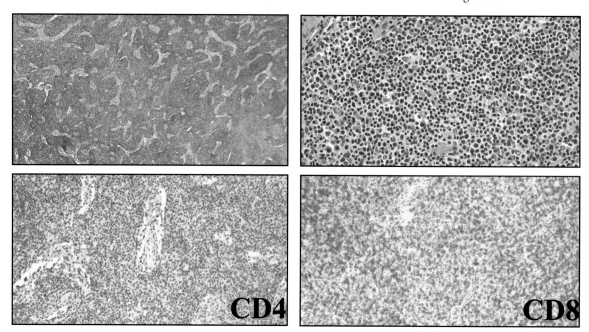

A. *Toxoplasma gondii*
B. Tularemia
C. HIV
D. *Bartonella henselae*
E. *Yersinia* infection

14: Lymph Node Questions

101. A 15-year-old patient presented with several days of a sore throat and fever, now with axillary lymphadenopathy. One of the lesions was biopsied, and representative sections are shown in the images below. While the large cells are CD30+, they are ALK–. Which test would most likely be positive in this patient?

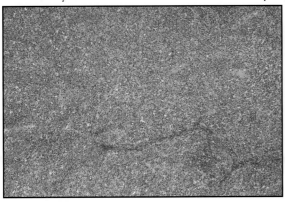 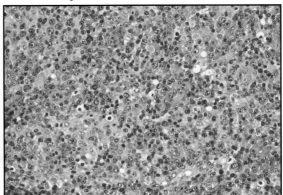

    A. Heterophile antibody
    B. PPD
    C. FTA-ABS
    D. Elevated *Rochalimaea henselae* titers
    E. LAP

102. The following are all TRUE of this type of Castleman disease shown in the images below EXCEPT?

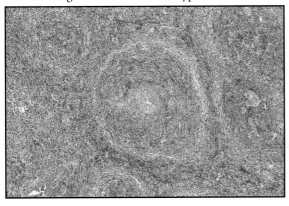 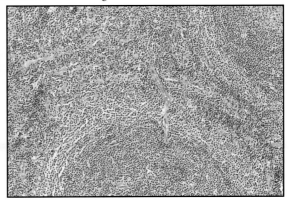

    A. It usually presents as a single mass.
    B. It is the least common subtype of Castleman disease.
    C. It consists of small follicles surrounded by an extensive network of capillaries, which show hyalinized walls and penetrate the germinal center.
    D. It is a clonal disorder of dendritic cells.
    E. All of the above

14: Lymph Node Questions

103. Which of the following statements regarding the disease process depicted in these images is TRUE?

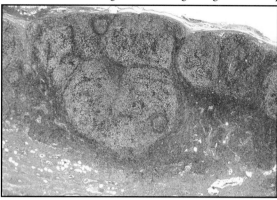 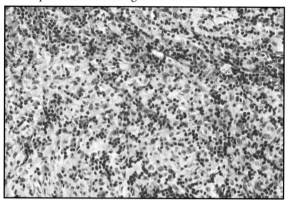

    A.   Patients usually have concomitant reactive or neoplastic skin disorders.

    B.   The bone marrow is a frequent site of involvement.

    C.   The nodules are composed of germinal center-type B cells.

    D.   The presence of melanophages is consistent with metastatic malignant melanoma.

    E.   It is commonly seen in association with acute EBV infection.

104. A 19-year-old black male presents with greatly enlarged cervical lymph nodes that are painless to palpation. One of the nodules was excised, and the images are shown in the images below. These cells are positive for S100 and negative for CD1a. What is the most likely diagnosis?

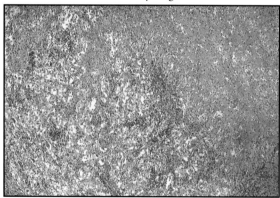 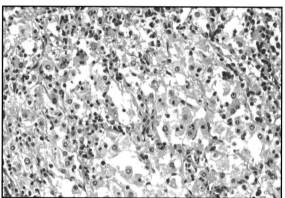

    A.   Rosai-Dorfman (histiocytosis with massive lymphadenopathy)

    B.   Langerhans histiocytosis

    C.   Hemophagocytic lymphohistiocytosis

    D.   Reticulohistiocytoma

    E.   Follicular dendritic cell sarcoma

14: Lymph Node Questions

105. The vascular lesion depicted in the images below can be caused by which 2 organisms? (H&E above and Warthin-Starry below).

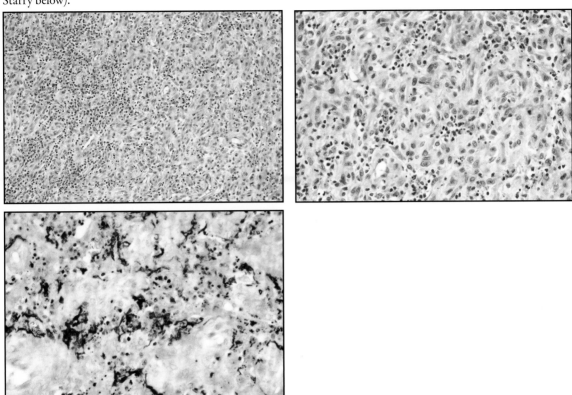

    A.   *Rochalimaea henselae*
    B.   HHV-8
    C.   HHV6
    D.   *Bartonella quintana*
    E.   HIV

106. A 44-year-old man with HIV (CD4 count of 80) presents to his primary care physician with several anterior thigh nodules. Photomicrographs of one of these nodules are shown below. Which of the following viruses is associated with this lesion?

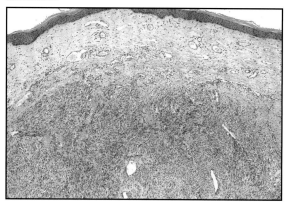 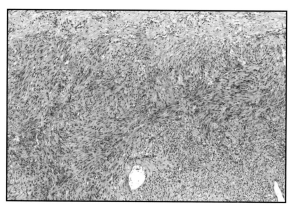

    A. EBV
    B. HHV-8
    C. Adenovirus
    D. CMV
    E. HSV-1

107. All of the following are features of the disease process depicted in these images EXCEPT? (The large neoplastic cells are positive for PU.1.)

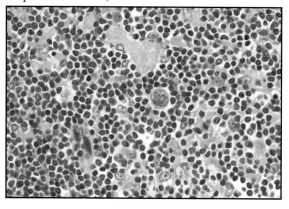 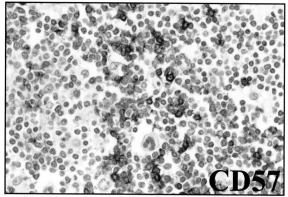

    A. Male predominance
    B. Low clinical stage at presentation
    C. Presence of L&H (lymphohistiocytic) cells
    D. Frequent detection of EBV-specific RNA transcripts
    E. Association with progressive transformation of germinal centers

14: Lymph Node Questions

108. Which of the following statements concerning the images shown below is FALSE?

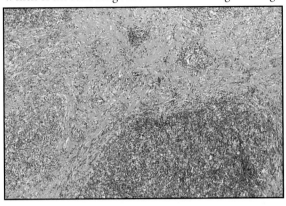 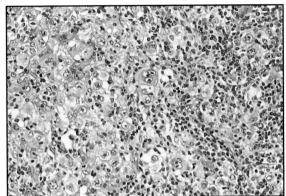

    A.   Typically affects young of adults
    B.   Mediastinal involvement common at presentation
    C.   Large cells express CD30 and CD15
    D.   About 25% of patients present with Pel-Ebstein fever
    E.   Large cells positive for OCT2

109. A 45-year-old male presents with enlarging cervical nodule. The nodule was biopsied, and representative sections are shown below. The larger cells are CD45– and CD30+, and are encircled by CD3 T cells. Which of the following statements is most likely FALSE?

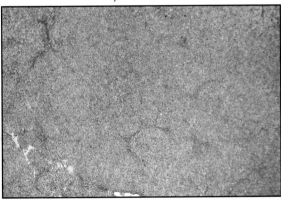 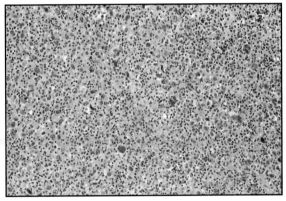

    A.   The encircling T cells express CD57.
    B.   B cells in the nodules express IgM and IgD.
    C.   It is usually without B symptoms.
    D.   Large cells demonstrate IGH rearrangements.
    E.   5-year survival is usually >90%.

14: Lymph Node Questions

114. Which immunoprofile is most consistent with the disease process shown in the images below?

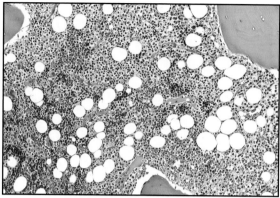 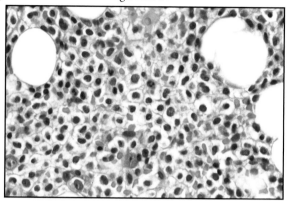

    A.   CD5+/CD19+/CD23+

    B.   CD5+/CD19+/CD23–

    C.   CD11c+/CD25+/CD103+

    D.   CD10+/CD19+/bcl-2+

    E.   CD5–/CD19+/CD23–

115. A 70-year-old man comes to his primary care physician with the complaint of back pain. He was found to have multiple degenerative joints along with multiple lesions in his vertebrae. The biopsy of the lesion is shown in the image below. Which of the following statements concerning his diagnosis is FALSE?

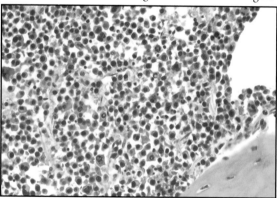

    A.   It is associated with decrease in polyclonal IgG.

    B.   It is heavy chain disease associated with renal failure.

    C.   There is absence of M protein by immunofixation in approximately 3%.

    D.   M protein is usually >30g/L of IgG or >20g/L IgA.

    E.   It often apparently expresses CD56.

14: Lymph Node Questions

116. Where is the most common location for the disease process shown in the images below? The lesion is positive for CD19, CD20, and CD22, and negative for CD5, CD10, and CD23.

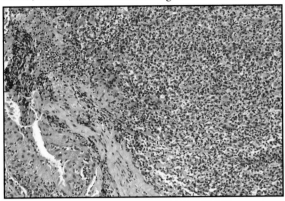 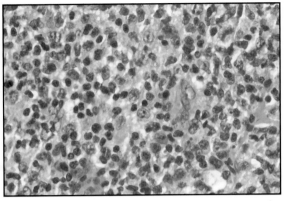

    A.   Skin
    B.   Eye
    C.   Lung
    D.   Gastrointestinal tract
    E.   Lymph node

117. A 68-year-old man was in an automobile accident and suffered a splenic laceration requiring a splenectomy. It was found to be enlarged, and a representative H&E-stained image and associated IHC-stained sections are shown below. Which of the following statements is FALSE?

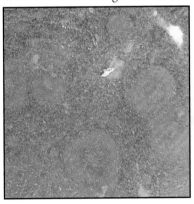 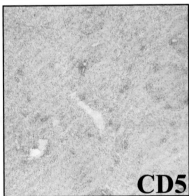 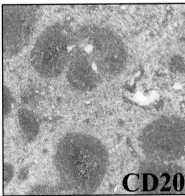

    A.   It usually expresses IgM and IgD.
    B.   It demonstrates a t(11;18).
    C.   Annexin A1 is negative.
    D.   It has circulating lymphoma cells known as villous lymphocytes.
    E.   It responds poorly to chemotherapy.

118. A 47-year-old man is referred to a hematologist for prominent cervical adenopathy. Following clinical work-up, one of these lymph nodes is excised and sent to surgical pathology. A portion of the node is placed in RPMI and sent for flow cytometry. A photomicrograph of the lymph node is shown below. Which of the following is TRUE?

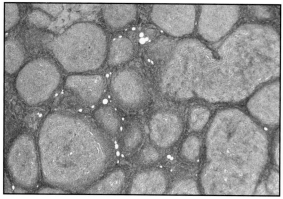

A. This represents the 3rd most common non-Hodgkin lymphoma in the United States, with only diffuse large B-cell lymphoma and Burkitt lymphoma being more common.

B. This lymphoma is diagnosed approximately 3 times more frequently in middle-aged men compared to middle-aged women.

C. The bone marrow is only rarely involved by this lymphoma.

D. Transformation to diffuse large B-cell lymphoma ultimately occurs in 75% of patients.

E. When involved, the bone marrow demonstrates primarily paratrabecular aggregates of lymphoma cells.

119. A 63-year-old man is referred to a hematologist for prominent cervical lymphadenopathy and lymphocytosis. Following clinical work-up, one of these lymph nodes is excised and sent to surgical pathology. The node is depicted in the photomicrograph below. Immunohistochemical stains for CD20, cyclin-D1, and CD5 were positive, with negative CD23 expression. Which of the following translocations is associated with this lymphoma?

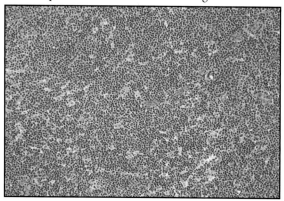

A. t(8;14)
B. t(8,22)
C. t(11;22)
D. t(11;14)
E. t(14;18)

14: Lymph Node Questions

120. A 73-year-old woman presents to her primary care physician complaining of a large swelling on the right side of her neck. Physical examination reveals prominent cervical adenopathy. Abdominal imaging reveals a large, destructive mass in the liver as a well as a mass around the psoas muscle. A cervical node is excised and sent to surgical pathology. A photomicrograph of the node is shown below. The surgical pathologist strongly suspects diffuse large B-cell lymphoma (DLBCL). Which of the following is TRUE?

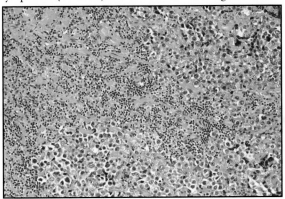

    A.   DLBCL is always seen in patients over the age of 40.

    B.   Most patients initially present with a rapidly enlarging extranodal mass.

    C.   The most common extranodal site at presentation is the spleen.

    D.   Patients with p53 mutations have a better prognosis.

    E.   Patients with BCL-6 rearrangements have a better prognosis.

121. The image shown below is from a biopsy taken from the mediastinum of a 38-year-old female. The lesion is CD5−, LCA+, and CD30+. Which of the following statements is FALSE?

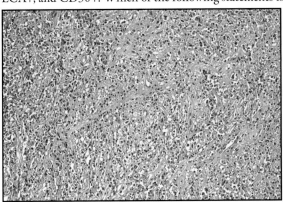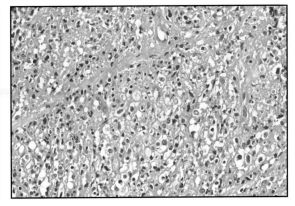

    A.   It has a *c-Myc* translocation.

    B.   Spread into infradiaphragmatic organs predicts an unfavorable outcome.

    C.   It has expressed MAL.

    D.   It often lacks surface immunoglobulin.

    E.   It can express CD10.

14: Lymph Node Questions

122. A 28-year-old male presents with an enlarging mass under his arm that has been growing rapidly. A biopsy was performed, and representative sections are shown in the images below. A touch prep of the biopsy was made and demonstrates vacuolated neoplastic cells that are oil red O+. Which of the following findings would be LEAST likely in the case below?

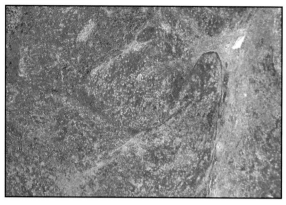 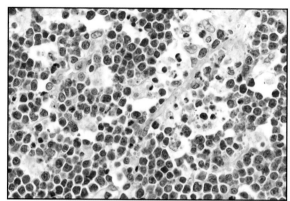

    A. Strong BCL-2 staining with BCL-2 translocation
    B. MYC translocation
    C. 99% staining for Ki67
    D. EBER negative
    E. CD77+

123. A 63-year-old female presented for her annual check-up and was found to have cervical lymphadenopathy. When asked about it, she stated that the swelling comes and goes. An excision biopsy was performed, and representative sections are shown in the images below. The neoplastic cells are CD19+ and CD20+, but CD5–, CD10–, CD23– and cyclin-D1–. What is the diagnosis?

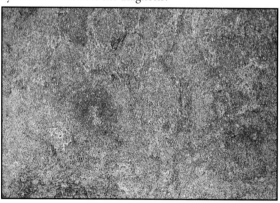 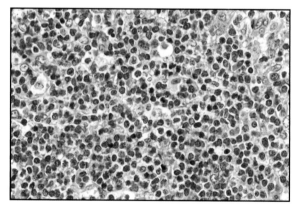

    A. Mantle cell lymphoma
    B. Follicular lymphoma
    C. Small lymphocytic lymphoma
    D. Hairy cell leukemia
    E. Marginal zone lymphoma

14: Lymph Node Questions

124. A 67-year-old man presented with sinus pressure and recurrent nosebleeds. It started several weeks before, but he blamed it on Coumadin. He finally presented to his primary care physician, who saw a mass partially obstructing the nasopharynx. A biopsy was performed and demonstrated an ulcerative lesion, and representative sections are shown below. Flow cytometry was performed and demonstrated a prominent population of cells that express surface CD56 but lack surface CD3. Which of the following statements about this process is FALSE?

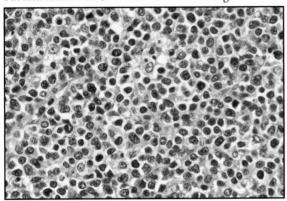 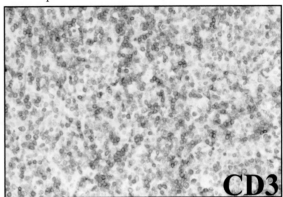

    A.   It expresses TIA-1.
    B.   It is negative for EBER.
    C.   It has *TCR* genes in germline configuration.
    D.   It often demonstrates pseudoepitheliomatous hyperplasia.
    E.   It is more common in Asia, and Central and South America than in the United States.

125. A 53-year-old male presents with long-term abdominal pain and reports several pounds of weight loss. Barium swallow demonstrates circumferential narrowing of the jejunum. The lesion was resected and images from the resection are shown below. Gene rearrangement studies demonstrate germline IGH but clonal rearrangement of the *TCR* γ gene. Which of the following statements regarding this lesion is FALSE?

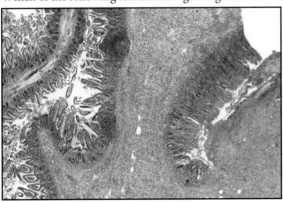 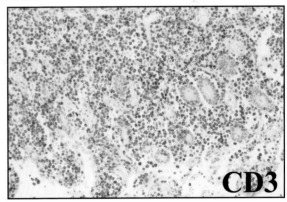

    A.   It is associated with HLA-DQ2 and HLA-DQ8.
    B.   It is CD8− and CD3+.
    C.   It is CD103+.
    D.   It can be treated with gluten avoidance.
    E.   It often presents with perforation.

14: Lymph Node Questions

129. A 26-year-old male presented with an enlarging inguinal lymph node and recent night sweats. After a course of antibiotics, his condition did not improve, so a biopsy was taken of the inguinal mass. The images are shown below. The lesion contains cells that are LCA+ and keratin–. Which of the following is least likely to be TRUE?

 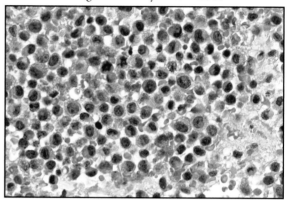

A.   It expresses CD3.
B.   It contains a t(2;5).
C.   It expresses CD30.
D.   It expresses TIA1.
E.   It expresses EMA.

130. A 62-year-old white woman presents to the doctor with recurrent bouts of nosebleeds and blurry vision and was found to have anemia. In the work-up for an etiology a bone marrow biopsy was performed, and representative sections are shown below. The cells are positive for PAX5, CD20, and CD138. Which of the following statements regarding the diagnosis is most likely to be FALSE?

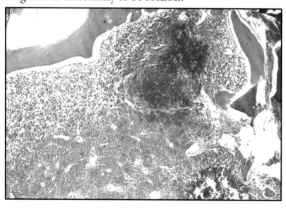 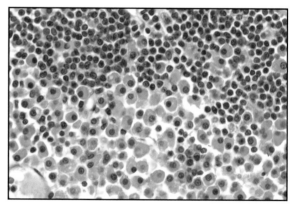

A.   It is associated with hepatitis C.
B.   It is rarely associated with t(9;14).
C.   There is rouleaux formation on blood smear.
D.   There is expression of IgM and IgD.
E.   Symptoms are relieved by plasmapheresis.

14: Lymph Node Answers

1. **B. INTRAABDOMINAL**

   Follicular dendritic cell sarcoma/tumor occurs in both lymph nodes (50%-65% present in nodes, cervical most common) and extranodal sites, and tends to have an indolent clinical course. While local recurrence can be seen in 40%-50%, metastases are seen less commonly in approximately 25% of patients. The metastasis can occur distant from the original site of the tumor, such as to the lung and liver. Around 10%-20% of patients die of their disease and the intraabdominal tumors tend to act more aggressive.

   QCSP, **Follicular Dendritic Cell Sarcoma,** p 468-469.

2. **A. CD21+/CD35+/CD79a–**

   Follicular dendritic cell sarcoma expresses an immunophenotype similar to nonneoplastic follicular dendritic cells (CD21+/CD35+, choices A and B), which are more likely related to true dendritic cells. B-cell specific markers, such as CD19, CD20 (choice C and E), and CD79a (choice B) are typically negative. Additionally, choice D is unlikely, since both dendritic cell markers are negative.

   QCSP, **Follicular Dendritic Cell Sarcoma,** p 468-469.

3. **E. A AND C**

   The absence of granulocytes in the areas of necrosis and the absence of follicular hyperplasia differentiates cases of histiocytic necrotizing lymphadenitis from cat-scratch disease and other bacterial infections. Clinical history is also helpful, as young Asian women are commonly affected and usually demonstrate cervical lymphadenopathy and may have fever and/or leukopenia.

   QCSP, **Suppurative Lymphadenitis,** p 470.

4. **B. *TROPHERYMA WHIPPELII***

   The most common causes of suppurative lymphadenitis, particular of the cervical lymph nodes, are staphylococcal and streptococcal infections (choice D), usually seen in the pediatric population. Other organisms inciting a suppurative response include *Bartonella henselae*, *Chlamydia trachomatis*, and *Yersinia enterocolitica*, the causative agents of cat-scratch disease, lymphogranuloma venereum, and mesenteric lymphadenitis, respectively (choices A, C, E). *Tropheryma whippelii*, although most commonly seen in the intestines, has also been identified in lymph nodes as well as other organs, such as the brain (choice B). The organisms are typically identified as PAS+, diastase-resistant inclusions in foamy macrophages. Suppurative inflammation is not a feature.

   QCSP, **Suppurative Lymphadenitis,** p 470.

5. **A. PATIENT TYPICALLY PRESENTS WITH ELEVATED WBC COUNT**

   Patients with Kikuchi-Fujimoto disease are typically young Asian men or women (slightly more common in women) whom often present with painless lymphadenopathy, often with leukopenia. The most characteristic feature is the large discrete areas of eosinophilic necrosis with lack of granulocytes.
   Necrotizing lymphadenitis has been seen following diffuse large B-cell lymphoma as we all in cases of stroma-rich Castleman disease and lupus erythematous.

   QCSP, **Histiocytic Necrotizing Lymphadenitis (Kikuchi-Fujimoto Disease),** p 470.

6. **C. SARCOIDOSIS**

   Schaumann bodies, as described above, tend to be round and have concentric laminations of calcium and are associated with sarcoidosis. Asteroid bodies (composed of radiating filaments enveloped by "myeloid" membranes) and calcium oxalate crystals are also seen. These are not features of the remaining inflammatory/hyperplastic diseases listed.

   QCSP, **Sarcoidosis,** p 470-471.

7.   B.   **EFFACEMENT OF NODAL ARCHITECTURE**
Nodal architecture in toxoplasmosis is typically preserved. Marked follicular hyperplasia with intense mitotic activity and phagocytosis of nuclear debris, irregular clusters of epithelioid histiocytes (invasion of follicular centers, if seen, is very specific) and distention of marginal and cortical sinuses by parafollicular monocytoid B cells that distort or encroach the subcapsular peritrabecular architecture make up the triad.
QCSP, **Toxoplasmosis,** p 471-472.

8.   D.   *BARTONELLA*
Cat-scratch fever is caused by the bacteria *Bartonella henselae,* which is a small gram-negative bacterium with pleomorphic morphology. Histologically, bartonella infection is associated with a necrotizing lymphadenitis. Additionally, infections with *Francisella tularensis, Chlamydia trachomatis, Listeria monocytogenes, Hemophilus ducreyi,* and *Yersinia enterocolitica* can demonstrate a necrotizing lymphadenitis.
QCSP, **Cat-Scratch Disease,** p 472.

9.   B.   **WARTHIN-STARRY**
The Warthin-Starry stain is a silver nitrate-based staining method that can be useful in highlighting small bacteria such as *Bartonella,* spirochetes, and *Helicobacter.* Even though the special stain in useful, serology and/or PCR are more sensitive and specific.
QCSP, **Cat-Scratch Disease,** p 472.

10.   C.   *CHLAMYDIA TRACHOMATIS*
The condition known as lymphogranuloma venereum is caused by *Chlamydia trachomatis.* Lymph nodes are enlarged with suppurative inflammation and/or necrosis. While Brown-Hopps and Warthin-Starry stains can be used to help identify the organism in tissue sections, serologic testing or PCR testing are more sensitive and specific. The reactive condition regresses with proper treatment of the chlamydial infection. Choices A, B, and D are the infectious agents for chancroid, granuloma inguinale, and atypical pneumonia, respectively.
QCSP, **Lymphogranuloma Venereum,** p 472-473.

11.   A.   **FLORID REACTIVE HYPERPLASIA**
Typically, lymph nodes from HIV infection can demonstrate florid reactive hyperplasia. The follicles contain numerous tingible-body macrophages and plasma cells. One can also see scant or absent mantle zones with intrafollicular areas with vascular proliferation resembling Castleman disease.
QCSP, **AIDS-Related Lymphadenopathy,** p 473-474.

12.   A.   **FOLLICULAR DENDRITIC CELL**
Interestingly, even after treatment with HAART therapy patients with HIV associated lymphadenopathy demonstrates the presence of the virus in follicular dendritic cells (even when virus is not detectable in the blood). The HIV stain also co-localizes with CD21 and CD23. However, HAART therapy will often reverse some of the histological changes seen in this process as well as improve the CD4/CD8 ratio.
QCSP, **AIDS-Related Lymphadenopathy,** p 473-474.

13.   E.   **SUPPURATIVE LYMPHADENITIS**
AIDS-related lymphadenopathy may display a spectrum of changes including florid follicular hyperplasia composed of peculiar dumbbell or serpentine follicles containing numerous plasma cells and tingible-body macrophages (choices A, B, and C). The mantle zone is typically scant or absent (choice C). Suppurative changes are not typically present and would point towards other etiologies, most commonly bacterial (choice E).
QCSP, **AIDS-Related Lymphadenopathy,** p 473-474.

14: Lymph Node Answers

14. **D.** **EXTRANODAL MARGINAL ZONE B-CELL LYMPHOMA**

HIV infections can be associated with a wide range of neoplastic and non-neoplastic disorders. Out of the choices, MALT lymphomas (Extranodal marginal zone B-cell lymphomas) are the least likely to associated with HIV. Specifically, primary effusion lymphoma and Kaposi sarcoma are HHV-8 related neoplasms primarily seen in HIV infected or immunodeficient patients. Plasmablastic lymphomas are primarily oral cavity lymphomas occurring in patients with HIV. Patients with HIV can develop several non-neoplastic tumorlike lesions including mycobacterial spindle cell tumors as well as multicentric Castleman disease, salivary lymphoid hyperplasia, bacillary angiomatosis and pneumocystic lymphadenopathy. HIV patients can also develop lymphomas that also occur in immunocompetent patients, such as Burkitt and diffuse large B-cell lymphoma; however, they will often demonstrate signs of plasmacytic differentiation.
QCSP, **AIDS-Related Lymphadenopathy,** p 473-474.

15. **C.** **CD8+ CYTOTOXIC T CELLS**

EBV infects B cells via the CD21 receptor (complement receptor 2), which is present on B cells and dendritic cells. The CD8 cytotoxic T cells become activated by the infected B cells and takes on atypical/reactive morphology seen on peripheral blood smear.
QCSP, **Infectious Mononucleosis,** p 474.

16. **E.** **PARACORTICAL DISTRIBUTION OF THE LARGE LYMPHOID CELLS**

Lymph nodes from patients with infectious mononucleosis (IM) typically demonstrate a polymorphic population of cells with a mixture of small and large lymphocytes. These larger cells tend to be in a paracortical distribution. The reactive immunoblast in IM are positive for CD30 and negative for CD15. Additionally, while there are several EBV infected cells in IM lymph nodes, lymphomas can also demonstrate EBV positivity. Necrosis can be seen in a variety of reactive and neoplastic processes.
QCSP, **Infectious Mononucleosis,** p 474.

17. **D.** **ENLARGED FOLLICLES**

All of the statements are true except for D. In hyaline-vascular type Castleman disease the follicles tend to be small and numerous while they are large and hyperplastic in the plasma cell type of Castleman disease.
QCSP, **Castleman Disease,** p 474-475.

18. **A.** **HHV-8**

Multicentric Castleman disease is assocated with infection by human herpes virus 8 (also known as Kaposi sarcoma associated virus).
QCSP, **Castleman Disease,** p 474-475.

19. **A.** **POEMS SYNDROME**

A portion of patients with Castleman disease will have a monotypic plasma cell proliferation that can be associated with POEMS syndrome.
POEMS syndrome: polyneuropathy (peripheral neuropathy, papilledema), organomegaly (hepatosplenomegaly, lymphadenopathy), endocrinopathy (amenorrhea, gynecomastia, impotence, adrenal insufficiency, hypothyroidism, glucose intolerance), monoclonal gammopathy (plasmacytosis, paraproteinemia, bone lesions), and skin lesions.
WAGR: increased susceptibility for Wilms tumor, aniridia, genital anomalies, retardation.
Coffin-Siris: medulloblastoma, mental and growth retardation, joint laxity, brachydactyly of 5th digit.
Carney syndrome: myxomas, lentiginous and blue nevi, endocrine tumors.
Carney triad: gastrointestinal stromal tumor (GISTs), pulmonary chondroma, extra-adrenal paraganglioma.
QCSP, **Castleman Disease,** p 474-475.

20.   D.   **ALL OF THE ABOVE ARE ASSOCIATED WITH CASTLEMAN DISEASE**

Castleman disease is associated with the development of follicular dendritic cell tumors as well as non-Hodgkin lymphomas. Additionally these patients, who are co-infected with HIV, have a higher incidence of Kaposi sarcoma.

QCSP, **Castleman Disease,** p 474-475.

21.   D.   **IL-6**

Patients with Castleman disease have elevated levels of IL-6 that correspond to the systemic manifestations of the disease such as fatigue, fever, weight loss, and/or night sweats. The elevation of IL-6 is partly due to virally encoded IL-6 as well as the host response to the infection. Elevated IL-6 seen more commonly in multicentric and plasma cell types.

QCSP, **Castleman Disease,** p 474-475.

22.   E.   **A PRECURSOR LESION FOR MYCOSIS FUNGOIDES**

Dermatopathic lymphadenitis is associated with dermatitis. Dermatopathic lymphadenitis can be associated with mycosis fungoides but is not considered a precursor lesion. This reactive condition is thought to occur secondary to skin antigens presented by Langerhans cells and interdigitating dendritic cells (both are S100+). Histologically, they have pale areas with collections of histiocytes/dendritic/Langerhans cells and a mixed lymphocytic infiltrate and plasma cells. Often there is also the presence of pigment within these cells.

QCSP, **Dermatopathic Lymphadenitis,** p 476.

23.   E.   **CHOICES B AND D**

Choices B and D are characteristic of histiocytosis with massive lymphadenopathy (Rosai-Dorfman disease), while choices A and C are characteristic of Langerhans cell histiocytosis.

QCSP, **Rosai-Dorfman Disease,** p 476-477.

24.   D.   **BIRBECK GRANULES BY ELECTRON MICROSCOPY**

The key histologic features of sinus histiocytosis with massive lymphadenopathy include plasma cells, histiocytes, and emperipolesis (lymphocytes migrating through histiocytes) (choices A, B, and C). Laboratory findings typically are significant for polyclonal hypergammaglobulinemia, anemia and leukocytosis (choice E). Birbeck granules, such as those seen in Langerhans cell histiocytosis, are not present (choice D).

QCSP, **Rosai-Dorfman Disease,** p 476-477.

25.   C.   **10% OF PATIENTS PRESENT WITH SOFT TISSUE INVOLVEMENT.**

Sinus histiocytosis with massive lymphadenopathy typically presents with bilateral painless lymphadenopathy (choice E). 10% of patients present with soft tissue involvement and may or may not exhibit concomitant lymphadenopathy (choice C). Males and females are equally affected (choice B). Histiocytes comprising the lesion are S100+ and CD68+ and CD1a– (choice A). There is no known association with viral organisms (choice D).

QCSP, **Rosai-Dorfman Disease,** p 476-477.

26.   C.   **AN INCIDENTAL FINDING CHARACTERIZED BY ATYPICAL FOLLICULAR HYPERPLASIA AND MANTLE ZONE EXPANSION WITH MIGRATION OF SMALL LYMPHOCYTES INTO GERMINAL CENTERS**

Progressive transformation of germinal centers is usually an incidental finding in lymph nodes excised for other reasons and carries no known adverse prognosis (choice A and E). There is no evidence that progressive transformation of germinal centers is a precursor lesions of classical Hodgkin lymphoma. (choice B). Choice D describes the hyaline-vascular type of Castleman disease.

QCSP, **Progressive Transformation of Germinal Centers,** p 477-478.

14: Lymph Node Answers

27. **B.** **Nodular lymphocyte-predominant Hodgkin lymphoma**

    Progressive transformation of germinal centers has been associated with nodular lymphocyte-predominant Hodgkin lymphoma. These changes are can be seen either before, after, or concurrent with nodular lymphocyte-predominant Hodgkin lymphoma.

    QCSP, **Progressive Transformation of Germinal Centers,** p 477-478.

28. **B.** *Bartonella henselae*

    Both *Bartonella henselae* and *Bartonella quintana* have been shown to cause bacillary angiomatosis in immunocompromised patients. Historically, *Bartonella* was known as *Rochalimaea* and some reference refer to *Bartonella henselae* as *Rochalimaea henselae.* These organisms can be visualized on a Warthin-Starry stain. HHV-8 is the causative agent of Kaposi sarcoma and primary pleural effusion lymphoma (choice A). Choices C, D, and E are not associated with this disease process. In HIV cases, may be EBV related.

    QCSP, **Bacillary Angiomatosis,** p 478.

29. **A.** **Extracellular and cytoplasmic hyaline globules are present in a minority of these tumors**

    Histologically, Kaposi sarcoma is characterized by the presence of proliferating spindle cells with scattered vascular spaces containing erythrocytes. When lymph nodes become involved, the subcapsular and trabecular sinuses are affected first, with possible extension into perinodal soft tissue later. Hyaline globules, whether cytoplasmic or extracellular in location, are present in the great majority of Kaposi sarcomas. These globules are accentuated with the use of a PAS stain. Immunohistochemical nuclear staining for FLI-1 and HHV-8 is generally present, in addition to positivity for CD34 and CD31. Factor VIII staining is uniformly negative. To date, no specific chromosomal abnormalities have been described in Kaposi sarcoma.

    QCSP, **Kaposi Sarcoma,** p 479.

30. **D and E**

    Mixed cellularity and lymphocyte-depleted types most frequently demonstrate classic Reed-Sternberg cells: a large binucleate cell with a huge, round, inclusion-like nucleolus that may have an "owl's eye" appearance. The cytoplasm is usually acidophilic and abundant. Prominent parachromatin clearing produces a paranucleolar halo with a thickened nuclear membrane. Hodgkin cells are mononuclear variants of Reed-Sternberg cells. Lacunar cells have a delicate, folded or multilobulated nucleus with smaller nucleoli and pale cytoplasm and characterize nodular sclerosis Hodgkin lymphoma. By artifact of fixation, the cytoplasm may retract, creating the lacunae. L&H cells contain a polypoid nucleus with small, usually multiple nucleoli and are called "popcorn cells" and are typically found in nodular lymphocyte-predominant Hodgkin lymphoma.

    QCSP, **Hodgkin Lymphoma,** p 479-482.

31. **D.** **Nodular Sclerosing HL**

    The obliterative "syncytial variant" of nodular sclerosing Hodgkin lymphoma is characterized by lacunar cells and other Reed-Sternberg-like cells that occur in sheets and cohesive clusters reminiscent of metastatic carcinoma, sarcoma, non-Hodgkin lymphoma, thymoma, or germ-cell tumors. (Like other classical Hodgkin lymphomas, these cells are CD30+, so they mimic those found in germ-cell tumors.)

    QCSP, **Hodgkin Lymphoma,** p 479-482.

32.   C.   **LYMPHOCYTE-DEPLETED HODGKIN LYMPHOMA**
The Reed-Sternberg cells in the lymphocyte-depleted type of HL tend to be very pleomorphic and sarcomatoid. Nodular sclerosing HL has lacunar cells. These RS cells are located in lacunar spaces (fixation artifact) and show a delicate, folded or multilobated nucleus surrounded by pale cytoplasm. Mixed cellularity HL and lymphocyte-rich HL have classic RS cells as well as Hodgkin cells. These cells are large, binucleated cells with round, inclusion-like nucleoli with an "owl's eye" appearance. Hodgkin cells are mononuclear variants of RS cells.
QCSP, **Hodgkin Lymphoma,** p 479-482.

33.   B.   **ABSENCE OF B SYMPTOMS**
Adverse prognostic factors include stage III/IV disease, old age, presence of B symptoms, presence of bulky disease, extensive splenic involvement, and multiple extranodal sites of involvement.
QCSP, **Hodgkin Lymphoma,** p 479-482.

34.   D.   **MIXED CELLULARITY HODGKIN LYMPHOMA**
In general classical Hodgkin disease is more often assocated with EBV infection. Within classical Hodgkin lymphoma, the mixed cellularity subtype is most commonly associated with EBV, followed by nodular sclerosis, then the rest of the classical subtypes. Nodular lymphocyte-predominant Hodgkin lymphoma is not associated with EBV.
QCSP, **Hodgkin Lymphoma,** p 479-482.

35.   E.   **CD15**
Unlike the neoplastic population in classical Hodgkin lymphoma, L&H cells from nodular lymphocyte-predominant Hodgkin lymphoma are negative for CD15 and CD30. They do, though, express CD45 (choice A). CD20 and PAX5 are typically positive, reflecting B-cell differentiation (choices B and C). Interestingly, EMA may also be expressed and can be very helpful in making the diagnosis (choice D).
QCSP, **Hodgkin Lymphoma,** p 479-482.

36.   D.   **NODULAR LYMPHOCYTE-PREDOMINANT HODGKIN LYMPHOMA**
Nodular lymphocyte-predominant Hodgkin lymphoma (NLPHL) is the variant associated with T-cell/histiocyte-rich B-cell lymphoma (THRBL). It is thought that these 2 entities might represent the opposite spectrum of the same disease process. Some suggest that THRBL might represent the transformation of NLPHL.
QCSP, **Hodgkin Lymphoma,** p 479-482.

37.   B.   **T(12;21)(P13;Q22) TEL1/AML1**
All answers (A-D) are molecular alterations seen in association with precursor B-cell ALL. The most common rearrangement is t(12;21)(p13;q22) involving *TEL1* and *AML1* genes. This rearrangement carries a favorable prognostic implication. All other choices (A, C, D) carry an unfavorable prognosis.
QCSP, **Precursor B-Lymphoblastic Leukemia/Lymphoma,** p 483.

38.   A.   **HYPERDIPLOID (>50)**
Favorable molecular alterations for pre-B-cell leukemia/lymphoma include hyperdiploidy (thus, A is the correct answer for this "except" question), t(12;21)(p13;q22) involving *TEL1* and *AML1* genes (the most common rearrangement) and t(1;19)(q23;p13.3) *PBX/E2A*. The remainder of the choices are unfavorable prognostic factors. The MLL-rearranged leukemias (both pediatric and adult) have a particularly poor prognosis.
QCSP, **Precursor B-Lymphoblastic Leukemia/Lymphoma,** p 483.

39.   E.   **t(12;21)(p13;q22).**
The prognostic parameters of precursor B-cell lymphoblastic leukemia/lymphoma including clinical demographics and cytogenetics are very important, since the rate of complete remission is high among patients with favorable findings. The most common molecular alteration is t(12;21)(p13;q22) involving the *TEL1* and *AML1* genes, which confers a favorable prognosis (choice E). The other choices are all associated with an unfavorable prognosis.
QCSP, **Precursor B-Lymphoblastic Leukemia/Lymphoma,** p 483.

40.   D.   **SURFACE IMMUNOGLOBULIN LIGHT CHAIN**
The leukemic cells in B-lymphoblastic leukemia typically express B-cell markers CD19, CD79a, CD24 and cCD22 but are often negative for CD20 (or it is weakly expressed). Unique to B-cell lymphoblastic leukemia, as compared to other B-cell neoplasms, is the expression of CD34 and/or TdT. Theses cells also often expression CD10 and HLA-DR. Additionally, they can express myeloid markers CD13, CD15, or CD33. Usually B-ALL is negative for surface immunoglobulins; however, those that carry the t(1;19) often express the IgM heavy chain without light chain.
QCSP, **Precursor B-Lymphoblastic Leukemia/Lymphoma,** p 483.

41.   E.   **CD19+ TDT+ CD9+ CD10– CD15+**
B-ALL with the MLL translocations usually has a specific phenotype. Specifically, they have a high peripheral WBC count and demonstrate typical B-ALL markers CD19, CD22, CD79a and TdT but they lack CD10 and often CD24 expression (choice E). They also often express CD15. Those cases with the *BCR-ABL* express B-cell makers CD19, CD22, CD79a and TdT. They express CD10 and also have aberrant expression of CD25 and CD66c (choice B). Those with the t(1;19) also have a characteristic phenotype that includes CD19+ CD22+, CD10+, TdT+, and CD9+ with partial CD20 and lacks CD34 (choice D). B-ALL with hyperdiploidy demonstrates markers typical of B-ALL such as CD19, CD22, CD10, CD34; however, they can lack CD45 (choice C).
QCSP, **Precursor B-Lymphoblastic Leukemia/Lymphoma,** p 483.

42.   A.   **THE GREAT MAJORITY OF CHILDREN TREATED WITH AGGRESSIVE CHEMOTHERAPY WILL ACHIEVE COMPLETE REMISSION.**
Approximately 90% of children treated with an aggressive chemotherapeutic regimen will have a complete remission, with about 2/3 of children being cured. Children under the age of two have a worse prognosis, as do individuals diagnosed in adolescence and adulthood. A deletion of 9p (CDKN2A) is found in roughly 30% of cases of precursor T-cell lymphoblastic lymphoma. While almost all cases have a clonal rearrangement of the TCR genes, about 1/3 of cases are found to be associated with a translocation involving the T-cell receptor genes.
QCSP, **Precursor T-Lymphoblastic Leukemia/Lymphoma,** p 483.

43.   B.   **CD117**
The expression of CD117 in T-ALL is associated with expression of CD135 and activated FLT3 mutations.
QCSP, **Precursor T-Lymphoblastic Leukemia/Lymphoma,** p 483.

44. B. **CLONAL TCR-γ CHAIN PCR IS SPECIFIC FOR T-CELL LINEAGE.**

Clonal TCR-γ rearrangements can be in T-cell lineage neoplasms along with some myeloid neoplasms and up to 70% of B-ALL. Similarly, clonal IGH rearrangements are not entirely specific B cells as they can be seen in T-ALL. MPO expression is considered lineage specific for myeloid. TdT expression can be seen in T- and B-cell lymphoblastic lymphoma/leukemia as well aberrant expression in AMLs. T-cell lineage is demonstrated by cytoplasmic CD3 (CD3-ζ chain). Other T-cell markers (CD2, CD4, CD5, CD7, and CD8) are not specific for T cells. No single marker is specific of B-cell lineage and required strong CD19 with 1 other B-cell markers (CD22, CD79a, CD10) or weak CD19 and 2 other B-cell markers (CD22, CD79a, CD10).

QCSP, **Precursor T-Lymphoblastic Leukemia/Lymphoma,** p 483.

45. C. **CD19+, CD5+, CD23+, CD10−, FMC7−**

The typical flow findings for CLL/SLL is CD19+, CD5+, CD23+, CD10−, and FMC7−. The primary differential for a CD19+ CD5+ neoplasm is CLL/SLL vs mantle cell lymphoma.

QCSP, **Chronic Lymphocytic Leukemia (CLL)/Small Lymphocytic Lymphoma (SLL),** p 484.

46. E. **ALL CAN BE SEEN IN CLL/SLL**

All of the above alterations can been seen in SLL/CLL as well as deletions of 6q21.

QCSP, **Chronic Lymphocytic Leukemia (CLL)/Small Lymphocytic Lymphoma (SLL),** p 484.

47. E. **ALL THE ABOVE INDICATE A POOR PROGNOSIS**

All the above indicate a poor prognosis in CLL/SLL. Specifically, CLL with unmutated IGHV is indicative of a pre-germinal center CLL/SLL and generally have poor outcomes. Expression of Zap70 is used as a surrogate to indicate an unmutated CLL/SLL without the need for molecular studies. However, there is a 20% discordant between the two. In addition, expression of CD38 is a poor prognostic indicator. CLL/SLL can transform into diffuse large B-cell lymphoma (Richter syndrome/transformation) as well as Hodgkin lymphoma and rarely B-cell prolymphocytic leukemia, all with a worse prognosis than CLL/SLL without transformation.

QCSP, **Chronic Lymphocytic Leukemia (CLL)/Small Lymphocytic Lymphoma (SLL),** p 484.

48. D. **IGM**

The neoplastic cells in Waldenström macroglobulinemia may secrete sufficient IgM to cause a hyperviscosity syndrome (visual impairment, neurologic symptoms, bleeding, and cryoglobulinemia). While the cells in lymphoplasmacytic lymphoma usually expression IgM, they can also express IgG or IgA (rarely)

QCSP, **Lymphoplasmacytic Lymphoma/Waldenström Macroglobulinemia,** p 485.

49. B. **HCV**

HCV has been associated with lymphoplasmacytic lymphoma. Specifically, HCV has be associated with the development of type II (mixed type) cryoglobulinemia. The other viruses are associated with a variety of lymphoproliferative disorders that are addressed in other questions.

QCSP, **Lymphoplasmacytic Lymphoma/Waldenström Macroglobulinemia,** p 485.

50. B. **CD19+, CD20+, CD25+, CD11C+, CD103+, FMC7+**

Hairy cell lymphoma is a mature B-cell process and would express B-cell markers CD19, CD20, CD22, CD79a and PAX5. Additionally, this population is negative for expression of CD5 and CD10. However, they have a distinctive phenotype including CD103, CD11c and CD25. Hairy cell variant is a closely related disorder but does not express CD25 or have B-RAF mutations.

QCSP, **Hairy Cell Leukemia,** p 485.

14: Lymph Node Answers

51.   **D.**   **LEUKOCYTOSIS**

As compared to hairy cell leukemia (HCL), hairy cell-variant (HCL-v) often has a leukocytosis. Hairy cell leukemia cases usually demonstrate a monocytopenia. The bone marrow biopsies from hairy cell leukemia are often fibrotic leading to dry taps on aspirates and are usually more fibrotic than the HCL-v. While the phenotype is similar between HCL and HCL-v, HCL-v lacks expression of Annexin A1, and CD25. CD123 is brightly expressed on HCL cells but the expression is either lost or only dimly expressed on HCL-v cells.

QCSP, **Hairy Cell Leukemia,** p 485.

52.   **C.**   **HALLMARK CELL**

Hallmark cells are a feature of anaplastic large cell lymphoma, which contains large cells with eccentric kidney-shaped nuclei and abundant cytoplasm. Plasma cells neoplasms can have Mott cells, flame cells, or cells characterized by Dutcher or Russell bodies. Mott cells have multiple grapelike cytoplasmic droplets. Flame cells have a fringe of fiery red cytoplasm. Dutcher bodies are nuclear inclusions and Russell bodies are cytoplasmic inclusions seen in the neoplastic cells.

QCSP, **Plasma Cell Neoplasms,** p 486.

53.   **C.**   **CD19–, CD20–, CD38+, CD138+, CD45–**

Plasma cells typically strongly express CD138 and CD38. However, they are usually negative or only dimly express other markers of B-cell lineage such as CD19, CD20, or CD22. They often retain expression of CD79a. Additionally, they are often CD45 weak or negative. Neoplastic plasma cells can aberrantly co-express markers such as CD56 or CD117 that indicates an abnormal population. They usually do not express surface immunoglobulin but express cytoplasmic immunoglobulin.

QCSP, **Plasma Cell Neoplasms,** p 486.

54.   **E.**   **SERUM PROTEIN OF >30 G/DL IS DIAGNOSTIC**

While symptomatic plasma cell myeloma cases usually demonstrate elevated serum and/or urine protein, no specific level is required for the diagnosis of symptomatic myeloma. Specifically, the 2008 WHO defines plasma cell myeloma as: M protein in serum or urine (no specific amount, and negative is non-secretory variant), bone marrow clonal plasma cells or plasmacytoma (while most have plasma cells of >10%, some have less), related organ or tissue impairment (commonly referred to by the acronym "CRAB": hypercalcemia, renal insufficiency, anemia, and bone lesions (can be lytic lesions or osteoporosis with compression fractures). More than half of myeloma cases have a translocation involving the IGH locus. Additionally, myeloma cases can express cyclin-D1 either with or without t(11:14). The peripheral blood smear often will show rouleaux with increased serum immunoglobulin.

QCSP, **Plasma Cell Neoplasms,** p 486.

55.   **C.**   **A LOCALIZED GASTRIC MALT LYMPHOMA IS POTENTIALLY CURABLE WITH TRIPLE ANTIBIOTIC THERAPY.**

Although somewhat controversial, it is still generally accepted that eradication of *H pylori* with triple antibiotic therapy can cure gastric MALT lymphoma. While approximately 50% of MALT lymphomas arise in the GI tract, less common sites include the lung (15%) and head and neck (15%). Only 4% of MALT lymphomas arise in the thyroid, generally in patients with Hashimoto disease. MALT lymphoma is characterized by CD20 positivity, with no expression of CD10 or CD23. A few characteristic genetic alterations have been described, including trisomy 3 and t(11;18).

QCSP, **Extranodal Marginal Zone B-Cell Lymphoma,** p 487.

56. **D. ALL THE ABOVE**

While *H pylori* has been associated with cases of gastric MALT lymphomas, *Chlamydia psittaci* has been associated with ocular adnexal MALT lymphomas, *Campylobacter jejuni* has been associated with immunoproliferative small intestinal disease (IPSID), and *Borrelia burgdorferi* has been associated with cutaneous MALT lymphoma.

QCSP, **Extranodal Marginal Zone B-Cell Lymphoma,** p 487.

57. **D. BLASTIC PLASMACYTOID DENDRITIC CELL NEOPLASM**

Blastic plasmacytoid dendritic cell neoplasm is an aggressive tumor in which a few cases were found to have clonally rearranged TCR but no reported cases have demonstrated clonal IGH rearrangements. Up to 20% of T-cell lymphoblastic leukemias can also have clonal IgH rearrangements. Lymphomatoid granulomatosis is an angiocentric and angiodestructive EBV positive B-cell proliferation that demonstrates IgH clonal rearrangements. Interestingly plasmablastic lymphomas demonstrates rearrangement of IGH even if they do not express immunoglobulin heavy chain. Up to 25%-50% of angioimmunoblastic T-cell lymphomas can have both TCR and IGH clonal rearrangements.

QCSP, **Lymph Nodes,** p 467-496.

58. **A. ANAPLASTIC LARGE CELL LYMPHOMA**

Infection with Epstein-Barr virus has been associated with a long list of various lymphoproliferative disorders and lymphomas including hodgkin lymphoma, post-transplant lymphoproliferative disorder, angioimmunoblastic T-cell lymphoma, extranodal NK/T-cell lymphomas, plasmablastic lymphoma, senile EBV-associated lymphoproliferative disease and others. However, EBV infection has not been associated with anaplastic large cell lymphoma.

QCSP, **Lymph Nodes,** p 467-496.

59. **A THROUGH E**

All of the above mentioned morphologies (centrocyte-like B cells being equivalent to marginal zone B cells) can be seen in nodal marginal zone B-cell lymphoma. They are seen infiltrating the marginal zone and interfollicular areas of lymph nodes.

QCSP, **Nodal Marginal Zone Lymphoma,** p 487-488.

60. **A. BCL-2**

Marginal zone lymphomas typically express pan-B-cell markers and usually expressed CD43. Additionally, they usually lack expression of CD5, CD10, CD23, BCL-6, and cyclin D-1. However, they often express BCL-2. It is important to remember that BCL-2 expression in a B-cell lymphoma does not equal a follicular lymphoma.

QCSP, **Nodal Marginal Zone Lymphoma,** p 487-488.

61. **B. THE GERMINAL CENTERS OF THE SPLENIC HILAR LYMPH NODES ARE OFTEN ENVELOPED AND REPLACED BY THE TUMOR CELLS.**

Splenic marginal zone lymphoma is a somewhat rare lymphoid neoplasm, representing less than 1% of all lymphomas. The bone marrow, splenic hilar lymph nodes, and peripheral blood are frequently involved, commonly with splenomegaly. Histologically, both the white and red pulp of the spleen is infiltrated by the neoplastic small lymphocytes, while in the lymph nodes they envelop and replace the germinal center. Splenectomy appears to increase patient survival.

QCSP, **Splenic Marginal Zone Lymphoma,** p 488.

14: Lymph Node Answers

62. D. **AGGRESSIVE NK-CELL LEUKEMIA**
To date, no TCR rearrangements have been reported in aggressive NK-cell leukemia. However, clonal TCR rearrangements have been reported in multiple hemopoietic neoplasms including T-cell lymphoma and leukemia, B- and T-cell lymphoblastic leukemias, acute myeloid leukemia, extranodal NK T-cell lymphoma-nasal type (cytotoxic T-cell variety), and even rare cases of myeloid sarcoma and histiocytic sarcoma. Remember that patients with autoimmune disease, status post bone marrow transplant, and PTLD patients often have clonal TCR rearrangements, but this may represent a pseudoclonal population and is not necessarily specific for a T-cell malignancy.
QCSP, **Lymph Nodes**, p 467-496.

63. A. **PATIENTS WILL SOMETIMES PRESENT WITH AUTOIMMUNE THROMBOCYTOPENIA.**
Patients with splenic marginal zone lymphoma, an indolent lymphoma, sometimes will present with autoimmune thrombocytopenia. Generally speaking, the neoplastic cells express surface IgM and IgD along with CD20 and CD79a. While many cases have been shown to be associated with rearrangements of the light and heavy immunoglobulin chains, no single translocation is associated with most cases. Splenic marginal zone lymphoma is noteworthy for frequently having villous, "hairy" projections that are best seen in the peripheral blood. As such, this entity must always be in the differential when hairy cell leukemia is being considered.
QCSP, **Splenic Marginal Zone Lymphoma**, p 488.

64. C. **THIS IS A GRADE 2 FOLLICULAR LYMPHOMA. FLOW CYTOMETRY WILL DEMONSTRATE CD10 AND CD19 EXPRESSION.**
Yes, this is a fairly picky question, but it is helpful for remembering the grading guidelines. The grading of follicular lymphoma is dependent on the number of centroblasts present in neoplastic follicles. Grade 1 follicular lymphoma has 0-5 centroblasts in 10 neoplastic follicles at 40×, while grade 2 has 6-15 centroblasts and grade 3 has >15. As such, this would be a grade 2 follicular lymphoma. By definition, the neoplastic follicular cells express both CD19 and CD10.
QCSP, **Follicular Lymphoma**, p 488-489.

65. B. **t(14;18) INVOLVING THE *BCL-2* GENE**
Follicular lymphoma is most commonly associated with t(14;18), which juxtaposes the *BCL-2* gene on chromosome 14 next to the immunoglobulin heavy chain locus on chromosome 18. Choices A, C, D, and E may be seen in mantle cell lymphoma, extranodal marginal zone lymphoma, Burkitt lymphoma and acute myelogenous leukemia, respectively.
QCSP, **Follicular Lymphoma**, p 488-489.

66. E. **MCL DEMONSTRATES SPLENIC EXPANSION OF THE WHITE PULP AND PERIPORTAL INFILTRATION MAY BE PRESENT IN THE LIVER**
The correct answer is E because this is a feature that is shared by both MCL and follicular lymphoma. 35% of patients with mantle cell lymphoma (MCL) have peripheral blood lymphocytosis at the time of diagnosis (vs 10% in follicular lymphoma). Bone marrow involvement by MCL can consist of aggregates in a non-paratrabecular and paratrabecular distribution whereas follicular lymphoma is typically paratrabecular. MCL not uncommonly arises at extranodal sites—it is the most common non-Hodgkin lymphoma to involve the small bowel and colon as lymphomatoid polyposis, and often presents as splenomegaly (50%). CD5 and cyclin-D1 are characteristically positive, while follicular lymphoma markers CD10 and BCL-6 are typically negative.
QCSP, **Mantle Cell Lymphoma**, p 489.

67. B. **PROLIFERATION CENTERS, BY DEFINITION, ARE PRESENT IN THE LYMPH NODES.**

As compared to small cell lymphoma, no proliferation centers are detected in mantle cell lymphoma. The spleen is frequently involved by the lymphoma, with prominent expansion of the white pulp. Bone marrow, too, is frequently involved, and paratrabecular and non-paratrabecular aggregates of lymphoma cells can be seen. Mantle cell lymphoma more commonly affects men, with a median age of 60 at the time of diagnosis. It is common for this lymphoma to be present in extranodal locations, and it has a predilection for causing lymphomatoid polyposis of the colon and small bowel.

QCSP, **Mantle Cell Lymphoma,** p 489.

68. E. **CD19+, CD5+, CD23–, CD10–, FMC7+**

The typical flow findings for mantle cell lymphoma is CD19+, CD5+, CD23–, CD10–, FMC7+. The primary differential for a CD19+ CD5+ neoplasm is CLL/SLL vs mantle cell lymphoma. Mantle cells usually lack or have weak CD23 expression, while FMC7 is typically on mantle cell lymphoma and negative on CLL/SLL.

QCSP, **Mantle Cell Lymphoma,** p 489.

69. B. **t(14;18)**

Approximately 30% of cases of diffuse large B-cell lymphoma are associated with t(14;18), which creates a *BCL-2*/IgH rearrangement. In addition, rearrangements of the *BCL-6* gene on 3q27 are found in approximately 25%-30% of cases. The (8;14) and (8;22) translocations are associated with Burkitt lymphoma. The (11;14) translocation is associated with mantle cell lymphoma. The (4;18) translocation is not associated with any particular lymphoma.

QCSP, **Diffuse Large B-Cell Lymphoma,** p 490.

70. C. **IN ADDITION TO CD20, DIFFUSE LARGE B-CELL LYMPHOMAS CAN FREQUENTLY BE POSITIVE FOR CD10.**

Diffuse large B-cell lymphoma characteristically expresses pan-B-cell markers CD20, CD79a, CD19, CD22, and/or PAX5. Importantly CD20 is absent is 50%-60% of recurrent cases after rituximab treatment. CD10 can be expressed in approximately 20%-40% of cases and usually denotes a germinal center B-cell pattern and usually have a better prognosis. Approximately 60%-80% of cases undergo complete remission with an aggressive chemotherapeutic regimen with rituximab, with almost half achieving a cure. In addition to frequently having cleaved or multilobulated nuclei, the lymphoma cells sometimes have multiple nuclei. The tumor cells are usually much larger than small lymphocytes (it is even in the name!). Occasional anaplastic cases will have large, multinucleated cells with prominent nucleoli that suspiciously resemble classic Reed-Sternberg cells.

QCSP, **Diffuse Large B-Cell Lymphoma,** p 490.

71. A. **GENERALLY DEMONSTRATE LIGHT CHAIN RESTRICTED SURFACE IMMUNOGLOBULIN.**

Mediastinal (thymic) large B-cell lymphoma is thought to be a subtype of diffuse large B-cell lymphoma originating from thymic B cells (choice E) and is characterized by a diffuse infiltrate of large cells with variably dense bands of fibrosis (choice D). The immunoprofile is typically CD19+/CD20+/CD45+ with no expression of CD10 and CD5 (choice C). This tumor generally has a defect in the production of immunoglobulins (choice A) and as such, expression of light chains cannot be used to demonstrate clonality. Prognosis is typically better with low stage disease (choice B).

QCSP, **Mediastinal (Thymic) Large B-Cell Lymphoma,** p 490-491.

72. C. **35-YEAR-OLD WOMAN**

Most patients with mediastinal (thymic) large B-cell lymphoma are in their 3rd to 5th decade (mean age of 37 years) and females are more commonly affected than males at a ratio of approximately 2:1.

QCSP, **Mediastinal (Thymic) Large B-Cell Lymphoma,** p 490-491.

14: Lymph Node Answers

73.   D.   **t(8;9)**

Classically, Burkitt cases demonstrates disruption of the *MYC* gene typically with the t(8;14) – (*MYC*/IGH) or less commonly t(2;8) (*MYC*/λ light chain) or t(8;22) (*MYC*/κ light chain). Interesting there has been non-IG-*MYC* translocations that have been reported and include t(8;9) and t(3;8). While t(8;9) and t(3;8) have only rarely been reported in typical Burkitt they make up almost half of the *MYC* translocations seen in atypical, intermediate, or grey-zone lymphomas.

QCSP, **Burkitt Lymphoma,** p 491.

74.   B.   **OFTEN PRESENTS WITH LEUKEMIC INVOLVEMENT**

While involvement of the peripheral blood by Burkitt can occur, in most cases the peripheral findings are normal. Instead the disease often presents as a quickly enlarging soft tissue mass. In sporadic cases, presentation often involves the abdominal organs and the endemic cases often involve the jaw or head and neck. Occasionally, Burkitt can present in the leukemic phase only, but such presentations are rare. Generally, the disease will involve the CNS, either at presentation, during treatment or during recurrence, which is why treatment includes CNS prophylaxis.

QCSP, **Burkitt Lymphoma,** p 491.

75.   E.   **CD7**

CD7 is usually the marker that is lost/downregulated in T-cell malignancies. Often T-cell processes can also aberrantly lose expression of CD5.

QCSP, Mature T-Cell Neoplasms, 492-496

76.   D.   **ANGIOIMMUNOBLASTIC T-CELL LYMPHOMA**

T cells from angioimmunoblastic T-cell lymphoma are thought to be derived from intrafollicular T cells and in addition to T-cell markers will express CD10, BCL-6, PD-1 (CD279), and CXCL13.

QCSP, **Angioimmunoblastic T-Cell Lymphoma,** p 494-495.

77.   C.   **LDH**

LDH is usually considered one of the most important prognostic factors for adult T-cell leukemia/lymphoma. However, high β2-microglobulin and low albumin has also associated with a poor prognosis.

QCSP, **Adult T-Cell Leukemia/Lymphoma,** p 492.

78.   D.   **HTLV-1**

Adult T-cell leukemia/lymphoma is a neoplasm strongly associated with HTLV-1 (human T-lymphotropic virus type I), a virus endemic in some parts of the world (examples include Central America, the Caribbean, and Japan). The tumor cells are generally fairly large, with significant nuclear pleomorphism and prominent nucleoli. The nuclei are frequently polylobated giving it the classic "flower" cell appearance.

QCSP, **Adult T-Cell Leukemia/Lymphoma,** p 492.

79. C. **THE ACUTE VARIANT IS NOTABLE FOR FREQUENT HYPERCALCEMIA, OPPORTUNISTIC INFECTIONS, AND SKIN RASH.**

There are four primary variants of adult T-cell leukemia/lymphoma. The acute variant is associated with diffuse lymphadenopathy, rash, hypercalcemia, opportunistic infections, and marked leukocytosis. The lymphomatous variant, on the other hand, is devoid of blood involvement but lymphadenopathy is evident, and hypercalcemia is very rare. The chronic variant is characterized by an exfoliative rash and is not associated with hypercalcemia. Finally, the smoldering variant has a lower WBC; however, pulmonary and dermatologic manifestations may be evident. It is not associated with hypercalcemia. Patients with the acute and lymphomatous variants generally die less than a year after diagnosis, while patients with the chronic and smoldering variants have a more indolent course. However, up to 25% of chronic and smoldering variants will progress to the acute form.

QCSP, **Adult T-Cell Leukemia/Lymphoma**, p 492.

80. A. **AN ANGIOCENTRIC INFILTRATE COMPOSED OF SMALL LYMPHOCYTES WITH ACCOMPANYING MIXED INFLAMMATION**

While the appearance of extranodal NK/T-cell lymphoma of nasal type can be variable, angiocentric growth with accompanying mixed inflammation composed of plasma cells, eosinophils, and histiocytes is typical (choice A). The neoplastic population may exhibit more cytoplasm, but nucleoli are usually inconspicuous (choice B). Choices C and D lie within the histologic spectrum of this entity, but are more commonly seen in extranodal marginal zone B-cell lymphoma and Burkitt lymphoma, respectively. Choice E describes the "hallmark" cells seen in anaplastic large cell lymphoma.

QCSP, **Extranodal NK/T-Cell Lymphoma, Nasal Type (Lethal Midline Granuloma)**, p 492-493.

81. D. **CYTOLOGIC GRADE HELPS PREDICT THE PROGNOSIS.**

This neoplasm is EBV-related and more prevalent in Asia, Mexico and Central and South America. The tumor cells in extranodal NK/T-cell lymphoma, nasal type demonstrate an angiocentric and angiodestructive pattern and do vary greatly in size; some may be small with irregular nuclei and be almost indistinguishable from normal small lymphocytes; others may be of medium size with pale cytoplasm; still others may be large and anaplastic and associated with numerous apoptotic bodies. Inflammatory cells (including small lymphocytes, plasma cells, eosinophils, and histiocytes) may be admixed and overlying epithelium may show changes of pseudoepitheliomatous hyperplasia that may mimic squamous cell carcinoma. Prognosis varies: some patients respond well to therapy while others die of disseminated disease despite therapy. There is, however, no clear evidence that the cytologic grade of the tumor has any prognostic significance (thus "D" is the correct answer to this EXCEPT question).

QCSP, **Extranodal NK/T-Cell Lymphoma, Nasal Type (Lethal Midline Granuloma)**, p 492-493.

82. B. **ENTEROPATHY-TYPE T-CELL LYMPHOMA**

The vast majority of T-cell neoplasms exhibit a helper T-cell phenotype with expression of CD4, including adult T-cell leukemia, angioimmunoblastic T-cell lymphoma, peripheral T-cell lymphoma, unspecified, and anaplastic large cell lymphoma (choices A, C, D, and E). Enteropathy-type T-cell lymphoma is unusual in that it frequently expresses CD8 rather than CD4 (choice B) and often loses CD8 as the disease progresses so that the phenotype of the neoplastic cells are CD3+ CD4– CD8–.

QCSP, **Enteropathy-Type T-Cell Lymphoma (Refractory Sprue)**, p 493-494.

83. C. **THE DISEASE IS AGGRESSIVE AND PROGNOSIS IS TYPICALLY POOR.**

Enteropathy-type T-cell lymphoma (refractory sprue) arises from cytotoxic T cells in the intestinal mucosa, most commonly the jejunum and ileum. Most patients have adult onset celiac disease and present with abdominal pain, often associated with intestinal perforation. The prognosis is typically poor with death secondary to abdominal complications (usually perforation).

QCSP, **Enteropathy-Type T-Cell Lymphoma (Refractory Sprue)**, p 493-494.

14: Lymph Node Answers

84.   E.   **THE TUMOR CELLS ARE NEVER DETECTED IN THE PERIPHERAL BLOOD.**

While mycosis fungoides is primarily a dermal disease, higher-stage disease (Stages III and IV) have a high blood tumor burden (Stage IV>1,000 circulating Sézary cells/μL). These neoplastic cells, whether present in the skin or in the blood, have prominent nuclear membrane infolding, which gives them a very cerebriform appearance ("Sézary cells"). Pautrier microabscesses are aggregates of >3 neoplastic T cells in the epidermis of a biopsied lesion. While these abscesses are frequently found in mycosis fungoides, they are neither necessary nor sufficient for a diagnosis. Immunohistochemical staining for CD3, CD4, CD5, and CD2 is usually positive, while CD staining is negative. Rarely, mycosis fungoides will transform into a large T-cell lymphoma.

QCSP, **Mycosis Fungoides/Sézary Syndrome,** p 494.

85.   A.   **CXCL13**

Angioimmunoblastic T-cell lymphoma (AILT) is thought to be derived from follicular helper T cells, which would express follicular markers BCL-6 and CD10 along with CXCL13. Both AILT and peripheral T-cell lymphoma-unspecified, are generally CD4 and often have decreased or loss of CD7 expression.

QCSP, **Angioimmunoblastic T-Cell Lymphoma,** p 494-495.

86.   C.   **ADULT T-CELL LEUKEMIA/LYMPHOMA**

T cells from adult T-cell leukemia/lymphoma are thought to be derived from the regulatory T cells. As such the neoplastic cells will express CD4, CD25, and FoxP3. CD7 is almost always absent.

QCSP, **Adult T-Cell Leukemia/Lymphoma,** p 492.

87.   E.   **SPLENOMEGALY**

Peripheral T-cell lymphoma, unspecified, is a heterogeneous group of disorders, which do not meet the criteria for inclusion in other T-cell disorder subcategories. Accordingly, the clinical presentation is highly variable; however, generalized lymphadenopathy, eosinophilia, hypercalcemia, and pruritus as well as other cutaneous manifestations are frequently present (choices A, B, C, and D). While splenomegaly has been reported, it is not a common feature of this disease.

QCSP, **Peripheral T-Cell Lymphoma, Unspecified,** p 495.

88.   A.   **DIFFUSE EFFACEMENT OF THE NODE; PLEOMORPHIC MALIGNANT T CELLS OF VARYING SIZE; PROMINENT POLYMORPHIC INFILTRATE OF REACTIVE CELLS; MAJORITY ARE CD4+ AND CD8−; COMPLEX KARYOTYPE**

A paracortical infiltrate diffusely effaces the lymph node architecture. Tumor cells are a pleomorphic mixture of small, intermediate and large malignant T cells with an accompanying prominent polymorphic infiltrate of reactive cells such as eosinophils and macrophages. These tumor cells are mature T cells (no expression of TdT or CD1a) and generally express pan-T-cell markers, although aberrant expression is common, and most nodal cases are CD4+ and CD8−. There are no consistent characteristic molecular abnormalities and they often demonstrate complex karyotypes.

QCSP, **Peripheral T-Cell Lymphoma, Unspecified,** p 495.

89. **D. ANAPLASTIC LARGE CELL LYMPHOMA**

Anaplastic large cell lymphoma contains large cells with eccentric kidney-shaped nuclei and abundant cytoplasm ("hallmark cells"). Tumor cells may have multiple nuclei resembling Reed-Sternberg cells (Hodgkin lymphoma is an important differential diagnosis to consider). The tumor cells are positive for CD30, EMA, CD2, and CD4. ALK positivity is seen in 60%-85% of cases and is virtually diagnostic of anaplastic large cell lymphoma. CD15 expression is rare. EBV is always negative. Adult T-cell leukemia/lymphoma is characterized by cloverleaf/flower cells, which are positive for CD4 and CD25. Mycosis fungoides is represented by an infiltration of the epidermis and upper dermis by neoplastic T cells with cerebriform nuclei, which are positive for CD2, CD3, CD4, and CD5 and negative for CD8.

QCSP, **Anaplastic Large Cell Lymphoma**, p 495-496.

90. **A. t(2;5)**

The common finding in anaplastic large cell lymphoma with *ALK* expression is the t(2;5)(p23;35). The t(2;5) is between the *ALK* gene on chromosome 2 and the nucleophosmin (NPM) gene on chromosome 5. t(2;8) is seen in Burkitt lymphoma. HTLV-1 is associated with adult T-cell leukemia/lymphoma. Trisomy 3 is seen in angioimmunoblastic T-cell lymphoma. The inv(2p) is the *EML4-ALK* translocation seen in *ALK*-rearranged lung cancers.

QCSP, **Anaplastic Large Cell Lymphoma**, p 495-496.

91. **D. EBV**

The tumor cells in anaplastic large cell lymphoma (ALCL) are *always* negative for EBV. If the lesion is EBV+, then rethink the diagnosis. Anaplastic large cell lymphoma is positive for CD30 and ALK. Additionally, these lesions are generally EMA+. This T-cell process usually lacks CD3 and CD5, though expresses CD4 and/or CD2. Up to 2/3 of cases are positive for CD43. ALCL are thought to be derived from a cytotoxic T-cell and are often positive for TIA and granzyme-B but are usually negative for CD8.

QCSP, **Anaplastic Large Cell Lymphoma**, p 495-496.

92. **B. t(11;14)(q13;q32)**

Follicular lymphoma often presents with advanced stage and bone marrow involvement (in 85%) that is characteristically paratrabecular aggregates. Splenic involvement with expansion of the white pulp and characteristic involvement of liver portal tracts is also seen. Transformation to diffuse large B-cell lymphoma heralds aggressive disease and is seen in approximately 25% of cases. The t(11;14) alteration is characteristic of mantle cell lymphoma.

QCSP, **Follicular Lymphoma**, p 488-489.

93. **A. CASTLEMAN DISEASE**

The image represents follicular dendritic cell sarcoma (tumor cells positive for CD21, CD35, CD23 and EMA, and variably positive for S100 protein, CD68, CD45 and CD20), which is associated with Castleman disease in 10%-20% of cases, occurring simultaneously or subsequently. Multinucleated cells, reminiscent of Warthin-Finkeldey cells (seen in measles), may be present, but no association with measles exists. Interdigitating dendritic cell sarcoma/tumor is in the differential diagnosis but usually involves a single node and is negative for markers of follicular dendritic cells, including CD21, CD23, and CD35, but are positive for S100, MHCII and fascin.

QCSP, **Follicular Dendritic Cell Sarcoma**, p 468-469.

94.   E.   **Toxoplasmosis**

The image depicts a suppurative lymphadenitis, which is a feature of staphylococcal infections, mesenteric lymphadenitis, lymphogranuloma venereum, and cat-scratch disease. This case was associated with a *Staphylococcus aureus* infection. Unlike this case, infection with *Toxoplasma gondii* demonstrates preserved nodal architecture with a triad: marked follicular hyperplasia with intense mitotic activity and phagocytosis of nuclear debris; irregular clusters of epithelioid histiocytes; and distension of marginal and cortical sinuses by parafollicular monocytoid B cells that distort or encroach on the subcapsular peritrabecular architecture.

QCSP, **Suppurative Lymphadenitis**, p 470.

95.   D.   **Histiocytic-necrotizing lymphadenitis (Kikuchi-Fujimoto disease)**

This benign self-limiting process is seen in young Asian women and men of all parts of the world. Patients present with fever, leukopenia, and painless cervical lymphadenopathy. The lymph node architecture is effaced by large discrete areas of paracortical necrosis with abundant nuclear debris surrounded by transformed CD8+ lymphocytes, histiocytes, and CD4+ plasmacytoid monocytes. The absence of granulocytes in the areas of necrosis and the absence of a background of follicular hyperplasia differentiates these cases from cat-scratch disease. Necrotizing lymphadenitis can also be seen in association with diffuse large B-cell lymphoma and stroma-rich Castleman disease.

QCSP, **Kikuchi-Fujimoto Disease**, p 470.

96.   D.   **Typical lymph node appearance is one of total effacement of the nodal architecture by epithelioid granulomas and extensive necrosis.**

Sarcoidosis is a diagnosis of exclusion. The lymph node architecture is completely effaced by epithelioid granulomas. Scattered Langhans giant cells and lymphocytes are seen. The cytoplasm of giant cells can contain Schaumann bodies, asteroid bodies, and calcium oxalate crystals. Necrosis is usually absent! Minute foci of fibrinoid necrosis can be seen, but necrosis is never extensive.

QCSP, **Sarcoidosis**, p 470-471.

97.   D.   **Toxoplasmosis**

The biopsy demonstrates the typical triad seen in lymph node infected with *Toxoplasma gondii*, which includes follicular hyperplasia, clusters of epithelioid histiocytes, and an infiltrate of monocytoid B cells that can distend the sinuses. Additionally, the follicular hyperplasia was associated with intense mitotic activity and phagocytosis of nuclear debris. However, there is no necrosis, no large atypical cell infiltrate, and the nodal architecture is preserved.

QCSP, **Toxoplasmosis**, p 471-472.

98.   B.   **Cat-scratch disease**

The lymph nodes in cat-scratch disease are typically enlarged and on sectioning show suppurative foci. Microscopically, reactive hyperplasia with secondary follicular centers is seen. Small aggregates of epithelioid histiocytes fuse and become stellate areas of necrosis, characterized by neutrophils surrounded by palisading histiocytes. In Kikuchi-Fujimoto disease the necrotic areas *lack* the granulocytes and follicular hyperplasia. In AIDS-related lymphadenopathy, the follicular centers fuse to yield dumbbell, serpentine or serrated configurations. Necrosis is not a prominent feature unless related to a secondary infectious process. Diffuse large B-cell lymphoma can have secondary necrosis but often presents differently and demonstrates clearly malignant cells microscopically.

QCSP, **Cat-Scratch Disease**, p 472.

99. **B.** **LYMPHOGRANULOMA VENEREUM**

The image demonstrates suppurative necrosis of follicular centers forming stellate abscesses. Given the location, history, and histologic findings, the most consistent diagnosis is lymphogranuloma venereum, which is caused by *Chlamydia trachomatis*. As in this case, the stellate abscesses can rupture through the lymph node capsule and extend into the perinodal fat/soft tissue resulting in cutaneous sinus tracts.

QCSP, **Lymphogranuloma Venereum**, p 472-473.

100. **C.** **HIV**

The images demonstrate a lymph node with loss of normal architecture with numerous plasma cells. Additionally, compared to the normal lymph node, the image demonstrates a decreased CD4/CD8 ratio. These findings along with the history are consistent with HIV lymphadenopathy.

QCSP, **AIDS-Related Lymphadenopathy**, p 472-473.

101. **A.** **HETEROPHILE ANTIBODY**

The biopsy demonstrates distortion of the lymph node architecture with a diffuse infiltrate of polymorphic leukocytes including immunoblasts. The morphologic findings along with the history are consistent with an infectious mononucleosis and as such should have a positive Monospot (heterophile antibody). The FRA-ABS (fluorescent treponemal antibody absorption test) is used to detect syphilis. Lymph nodes in syphilitic lymphadenitis demonstrate numerous plasma cells along with marked follicular hyperplasia and prominent vascular changes such as phlebitis, and the changes are most pronounced in the inguinal lymph nodes. The PPD is a screening test for TB infection, which demonstrates a mixture of necrotizing (caseating) and nonnecrotizing granulomas. *Bartonella henselae* is one of the causative agents for bacillary angiomatosis. LAP (leukocyte/neutrophil alkaline phosphate) is often elevated in leukemoid reaction and non-CML myeloproliferative disorders but decreased in CML, PNH, neonatal septicemia, and some myelodysplastic syndromes.

QCSP, **Infectious Mononucleosis**, p 474.

102. **B.** **IT IS THE LEAST COMMON SUBTYPE OF CASTLEMAN DISEASE.**

The hyaline-vascular variant is actually more common than the plasma cell type and transitional/intermediate type of Castleman disease. The key morphologic features for the hyaline-vascular variant include the following: (1) small follicles surrounded by an extensive network of capillaries, (2) capillaries penetrating the germinal centers of the follicles (lollipop appearance), (3) capillaries that have hyalinized walls, (4) follicles that can contain >1 germinal center, (5) follicles that can have concentric layering (onion-skinning) of small lymphocytes, (6) dysplastic dendritic cells. Specifically, the image does not demonstrate the sheets of mature plasma cells surrounding the follicle that are seen in the plasma cell type.

QCSP, **Castleman Disease**, p 474-476.

103. **A.** **PATIENTS USUALLY HAVE CONCOMITANT REACTIVE OR NEOPLASTIC SKIN DISORDERS.**

This image is an example of dermatopathic lymphadenitis ,with the proliferation of large, pale cells and associated with concomitant reactive or neoplastic skin disorders. This entity is not neoplastic itself, although metastatic disease may also be present within the lymph node. Accordingly, there is no involvement of the bone marrow (choice B). The nodules seen in the lymph node are predominantly composed of T cells (choice C). The pale cells in the background consist of Langerhans cells, interdigitating dendritic cells, and macrophages, the latter of which commonly contain melanin and hemosiderin, which should not be interpreted as metastatic malignant melanoma (choice D). Acute lymphadenitis due to EBV infection is characterized by marked distortion of the nodal architecture, and a polymorphic lymphocytic infiltrate including immunoblasts. It would not contain the characteristic pale staining population of cells seen here (choice E).

QCSP, **Dermatopathic Lymphadenitis**, p 476.

14: Lymph Node Answers

104. **A.** **ROSAI-DORFMAN (HISTIOCYTOSIS WITH MASSIVE LYMPHADENOPATHY)**

The above excision demonstrates infiltration by a sheet of histiocytes along with plasma cells. Several of the histiocytes demonstrate the distinctive feature of emperipolesis. The best diagnosis here is Rosai-Dorfman disease. In Rosai-Dorfman Disease mature lymphocytes, plasma cells, neutrophils and erythrocytes can emperipolesis the histiocytes (enter and go through the histiocytes). This is in contrast to hemophagocytic lymphohistiocytosis where the WBC and RBCs are engulfed. Langerhans histiocytosis is typically S100+ and CD1a+ and plasma cells are rare, while eosinophils are more often seen. Follicular dendritic cell sarcomas are more spindle-shape and are S100 and CD1a negative, but CD21, CD35, CD23, CD68, and fascin positive. Reticulohistiocytomas demonstrate large histiocytes without emperipolesis and are negative for S100 and CD1a.

QCSP, **Rosai-Dorfman Disease,** p 476-477.

105. **A AND D**

The lesion depicted is bacillary angiomatosis, which demonstrates pale nodules of plump epithelioid endothelial cells with interspersed neutrophils. This lesion is caused by *Bartonella henselae* and *Bartonella quintana*, which can be seen with a Warthin-Starry silver stain. HHV-8 is associated with Kaposi sarcoma and multicentric Castleman disease. Both bacillary angiomatosis and Kaposi sarcoma are commonly seen in patients with HIV infection.

QCSP, **Bacillary Angiomatosis,** p 478.

106. **B.** **HHV-8**

The history and histologic section are consistent with a nodular Kaposi sarcoma. Human herpesvirus-8, also known as Kaposi sarcoma-associated herpesvirus, is strongly associated with Kaposi sarcoma in immunocompromised patients. Immunohistochemical nuclear staining for HHV-8 is generally positive in Kaposi sarcoma.

QCSP, **Kaposi Sarcoma,** p 479.

107. **D.** **FREQUENT DETECTION OF EBV-SPECIFIC RNA TRANSCRIPTS**

This image is an example of nodular lymphocyte-predominant Hodgkin lymphoma in which the larger neoplastic cells are positive for B-cell lineage markers (CD20, CD79a, PAX5, and PU.1). This type of lymphoma typically affects young males (choice A). The vast majority of patients present with localized peripheral lymphadenopathy (choice B). The biopsy shows effacement of the nodal architecture by small lymphocytes and larger cells with polypoid nucleoli known as L&H, or "popcorn," cells (choice C). EBV transcripts are typically not detected in this entity and are more commonly seen in classical Hodgkin, particularly the mixed cellularity and nodular sclerosing types. An association with progressive transformation of germinal centers has been reported, although there is no evidence of causation (choice E).

QCSP, **Hodgkin Lymphoma,** p 479-482.

108. **E.** **LARGE CELLS POSITIVE FOR OCT2**

The image represents the nodular sclerosing variant of classical Hodgkin disease. As with other cases of classical Hodgkin lymphoma, the large neoplastic cells (Reed-Sternberg and lacunar cells) are CD45–, but CD30+ and CD15+. It typically occurs in younger adults, and about 25% of patients will present with cyclic bouts of fevers (known as Pel-Ebstein fevers), which can be mistaken as infections. OCT2 is a B-cell transcription factor and, along with its cofactor BOB1, is absent in >90% of cases of classical Hodgkin lymphoma cases.

QCSP, **Hodgkin Lymphoma,** p 479-482.

109. A. **THE ENCIRCLING T CELLS EXPRESS CD57.**
The images demonstrate a lymph node with vague nodularity, with primarily small lymphocytes and RS cells. Specifically, there is no increase in plasma cells, neutrophils, and eosinophils. While the histology would raise the possibility of a nodular lymphocyte-predominant lymphoma, the RS cells are CD45 negative, which is more consistent with a nodular lymphocyte-rich classical Hodgkin lymphoma. The nodules in the lymphocyte-rich classic Hodgkin lymphoma are B cells that express IgM and IgD, while the RS cells are encircled by T cells that are usually negative for CD57 (unlike in nodular lymphocyte-predominant lymphoma). This lymphoma is usually asymptomatic and stage I or II at presentation, with a 5-year survival rate of 90%. The RS cells have IGH rearrangements.
QCSP, **Hodgkin Lymphoma,** p 479-482.

110. D. **PROGNOSIS SIMILAR TO NODULAR SCLEROSING HODGKIN LYMPHOMA**
This case is an example of a mixed cellularity Hodgkin lymphoma, which is the most common subtype to occur in HIV-infected patients, and is associated with EBER in 70% of cases. With the current chemotherapy regiments, the subtypes of classical Hodgkin have the same prognosis when compared at the same stage. However, mixed cellularity classical Hodgkin lymphoma typically presents in stage III or IV, while NS Hodgkin usually is lower stage, thus mixed cellularity usually has a worse prognosis. This subtype is also the most common subtype to involve the spleen. While the neoplastic cells in classical Hodgkin do not express typical B cell transcription factors OCT2, BOB.1, or PU-1, it does express PAX5, but at reduced levels as compared to normal/reactive B cells.
QCSP, **Hodgkin Lymphoma,** p 479-482.

111. E. **T(9;22)(Q34;Q11.2) BCR/ABL**
The images demonstrate a monomorphic population of lymphocytes with somewhat finely dispersed chromatin and inconspicuous nucleoli. Additionally the cells are positive for CD79a and TdT, supporting the diagnosis of a precursor B-lymphoblastic leukemia. The following factors or molecular changes are associated with an unfavorable prognosis: t(9;22)(q34;q11.2) *BCR/ABL*, t(4;11)(q21;q23) AF4/MLL, hypodiploidy, age under 2 years or older than 10, and high WBC. 3 factors or molecular changes are associated with favorable prognosis: t(12;21)(p13;q22) *TEL1/AML1*, t(1;19)(q23;p13.3) *PBX/E2A*, between ages 2-10 years, and hyperdiploidy (>50 chromosomes).
QCSP, **Precursor B-Lymphoblastic Leukemia/Lymphoma,** p 482-483.

112. D. **PRECURSOR T-LYMPHOBLASTIC LEUKEMIA/LYMPHOMA**
Precursor T-lymphoblastic leukemia/lymphoma is a neoplastic process composed of precursor T-lymphocytes. The normal nodal architecture is replaced by these lymphoblasts, which are generally small to intermediate in size. The cells have delicate nuclear chromatin with frequent grooving of the nuclear membranes. Nucleoli are inconspicuous. Mitotic figures are frequently seen. The neoplastic pre-T cells are notable for expressing TdT, CD1a, and pan-T-cell markers to variable extent (CD8, CD7, CD5, CD4, CD3, CD2). Histologically, pre-T lymphoblasts and pre-B lymphoblasts are indistinguishable from one another.
QCSP, **T-Lymphoblastic Leukemia/Lymphoma,** p 483-484.

14: Lymph Node Answers

113. A. **t(9;14)(p13;q32)**

The neoplasm depicted is small lymphocytic leukemia. Lymph nodes are diffusely effaced by a population of small lymphocytes with little cytoplasm and round to slightly irregular nuclei with condensed chromatin. Proliferation centers consisting of small aggregates of larger prolymphocytes (<55%) and paraimmunoblasts may be present. The immunohistochemical profile distinguishes it from other mature B-cell neoplasms. Translocations of (9;14) (p13;q32) are characteristic of lymphoplasmacytic lymphoma/Waldenström macroglobulinemia (seen in 50%), thus this is the exception. The remaining alterations are seen, and they are listed in order of most to least frequent. Deletion of 13p14 is the most common, seen in up to 50%, and portends a good prognosis. Trisomy 12 and deletions of 11q22-23 are seen in about 20% and impart an intermediate/poor and poor prognosis, respectively. Deletions of 17p13 (p53 locus) are seen in 10% and are a poor prognostic indicator. Deletions of 6q21 are also seen in CLL/SLL but only in about 5%. Expression of CD38 and Zap70 are also poor prognostic factors (expression defined by >30% and >20%, respectively, of cells expressing the marker).

QCSP, **T-Lymphoblastic Leukemia/Lymphoma,** p 483-484.

114. C. **CD11c+/CD25+/CD103+**

The disease process depicted in this image is hairy cell leukemia. The leukemic infiltrate is diffuse and predominantly interstitial and is composed of cells with clear cytoplasm, imparting a "fried egg" appearance. The typical immunophenotype associated with this disease in CD11c+/CD25+/CD103+ (also CD123+ and annexin A1+). Choices A, B, D, and E would be consistent with small lymphocytic lymphoma/chronic lymphocytic leukemia, mantle cell lymphoma, follicular lymphoma, and mucosa-associated lymphoma, respectively, none of which would impart this architectural and cytologic appearance.

QCSP, **Hairy Cell Leukemia,** p 485-486.

115. B. **THIS IS A HEAVY CHAIN DISEASE ASSOCIATED WITH RENAL FAILURE.**

The biopsy demonstrates a plasma cell neoplasm. While if this lesion was solitary, it could be considered a plasmacytoma, the multifocality would suggest a multiple myeloma. Symptomatic plasma cell myeloma is defined with the acronym CRAB: hypercalcemia, renal insufficiency, anemia, and bone lesions. The M protein can be found in approximately 97% of cases with the subtypes IgG (50%), IgA (20%), light chain (20%), and IgD, IgE, IgM and biclonality (<10%). Renal failure is typically associated with monoclonal light-chain proteinuria and not heavy-chain proteinuria. The increased serum/urine clonal IgG is associated with a decrease in polyclonal IgG and an associated increase risk of recurrent infections. These lesions can express CD56 in around 70%-80% of cases. They can also occasionally express CD20, CD52, CD117, and CD10.

QCSP, **Plasma Cell Neoplasms,** p 486-487.

116. D. **GASTROINTESTINAL TRACT**

The disease process shown here is extranodal marginal zone B-cell MALT lymphoma. The gastrointestinal tract is the most common site involved in 50% of cases. In decreasing order, other common sites include lung (choice C), head and neck including the eye (choice B), skin (choice A), and breast. Nodal marginal zone B-cell lymphoma may be associated with MALT lymphoma, but is considered a distinct entity (choice E). These lesions will often demonstrate the following genetic alterations: trisomy 3 and t(11;18).

QCSP, **Extranodal Marginal Zone B-Cell Lymphoma,** p 487.

117. **B.** **IT DEMONSTRATES A T(11;18).**

The lesion occurred in the spleen, with small lymphocytes replacing the germinal center, and is a CD20+, CD5– neoplasm. This would be consistent with splenic marginal zone lymphoma. This neoplasm is usually positive for B-cell markers CD20 and CD79a and surface immunoglobulin IgM and IgD, but negative for CD5 CD10, and CD23. Even though these cells can have a villous appearance in the peripheral blood, they are negative for the hairy cell marker annexin A1 and usually negative for CD103. The neoplasm lacks the t(11;18) typically seen in MALT lymphomas. The neoplasm usually has an indolent course often with long-term survival after splenectomy. However, splenic marginal zone lymphomas do not typically respond well to chemotherapy treatment.

QCSP, **Splenic Marginal Zone Lymphoma,** p 488.

118. **E.** **WHEN INVOLVED, THE BONE MARROW DEMONSTRATES PRIMARILY PARATRABECULAR AGGREGATES OF LYMPHOMA CELLS.**

The photomicrograph is consistent with a diagnosis of follicular lymphoma, with an abnormal proliferation of neoplastic follicular cells recapitulating germinal centers. Not all cases of follicular lymphoma have such a classic, nodular growth pattern. Both centrocytes (small cells with scant cytoplasm) and centroblasts (larger cells with frequent nucleoli and moderate cytoplasm) are seen. Follicular lymphoma is the most common non-Hodgkin lymphoma in the United States, with males and females diagnosed with equal frequency. Bone marrow is involved in >80% of cases, with primarily paratrabecular involvement. Transformation to diffuse large B-cell lymphoma occurs in approximately 25% of patients. Following transformation, the average patient lives for approximately 1 year.

QCSP, **Follicular Lymphoma,** p 488-489.

119. **D.** **T(11;14)**

The photomicrograph depicts mantle cell lymphoma, with this case representing a diffuse pattern of growth. The individual tumor cells closely resemble the normal lymphocytes inhabiting the mantle zone that surrounds the follicular centers of a normal lymph node. In addition to the diffuse growth pattern, other mantle cell lymphomas demonstrate a weakly nodular or "mantle zone" growth pattern. Proliferation centers are usually absent. The (11;14) translocation is classically associated with mantle cell lymphoma, which creates a *BCL-1*/IgH rearrangement. The (8;14) and (8,22) translocations are associated primarily with Burkitt lymphoma, while the (14;18) translocation is usually seen in follicular lymphoma and sometimes in diffuse large B-cell lymphoma. The (11;22) translocation is associated with Ewing sarcoma and desmoplastic small round cell tumor.

QCSP, **Mantle Cell Lymphoma,** p 489.

120. **E.** **PATIENTS WITH BCL-6 REARRANGEMENTS HAVE A BETTER PROGNOSIS.**

Patients with diffuse large B-cell lymphoma with an underlying *BCL-6* rearrangement have a better prognosis than those patients without the rearrangement present. A p53 mutation, on the other hand, confers a worse prognosis. While diffuse large B-cell lymphoma is more common in adults, it can present, albeit much more rarely, in the pediatric population. Approximately 60% of patients present with a rapidly enlarging nodal mass, with a minority of patients presenting with an extranodal lesion. When the lymphoma presents extranodally, it most commonly occurs in the GI tract. Even more rare sites include, the spleen, liver, skin, urinary tract, brain, bone, and Waldeyer ring.

QCSP, **Diffuse Large B-Cell Lymphoma,** p 490.

121. **A.** **IT HAS A C-MYC TRANSLOCATION.**

The lesion shown above demonstrates fibrosis with neoplastic cells that are large with clear cytoplasm. Histologically this is consistent with a (thymic) primary mediastinal diffuse large B-cell lymphoma. While Hodgkin lymphoma is the most common mediastinal lymphoma, the neoplastic cells are CD45+. While the majority of thymic DLBCL (80%) express CD30 and pan-B-cell markers, they are negative for surface immunoglobulin. Unlike nodal based DLBCL, they express MEL and have increased *c-Rel* gene. Spread beyond the thymus predicts an unfavorable outcome. There are no known translocations of the *c-Myc*, *BCL-2*, or *BCL-6* genes.

QCSP, **Mediastinal (Thymic) Large B-Cell Lymphoma,** p 490-491.

14: Lymph Node Answers

122. A. **STRONG BCL-2 STAINING WITH BCL-2 TRANSLOCATION**
The case represents a Burkitt lymphoma with intermediate-sized cells with clumpy chromatin and a starry sky pattern. The touch prep description is also consistent with Burkitt lymphoma, in which the neoplastic cells are vacuolated with lipids. These cells are positive for the B-cell antigens CD19, CD20, and CD22 as well as CD10, BCL-6, CD38, CD71, CD77, and CD43. The majority of endemic cases are positive for EBV, and 30%-40% of the sporadic and immunodeficiency-associated cases are also positive. Classically, Burkitt cases demonstrate disruption of the *MYC* gene typically with the t(8;14)-(*MYC*/IGH) or less commonly t(2;8)-(*MYC*/κ light chain) or t(8;22)-(*MYC*/λ light chain). While there can be weak scattered positivity of BCL-2 in up to 20% of cases, true Burkitt cases do NOT strongly express BCL-2 nor do they have the *BCL-2* translocation.
QCSP, **Burkitt Lymphoma,** p 491.

123. E. **MARGINAL ZONE LYMPHOMA**
The biopsy demonstrates a lymph node biopsy with trabecular fibrosis giving the low-power impression of nodularity. There is the expansion of the pale zones. The morphology and the immunophenotype are consistent with nodal marginal zone B-cell lymphoma. Specifically, mantle cell lymphomas are typically also CD5 and cyclin-D1 positive, while small lymphocytic lymphomas are usually CD5+ and CD23+. Follicular lymphomas have a different low-power morphology appearance as well as are usually CD10+/BCL-6+.
QCSP, **Nodal Marginal Zone Lymphoma,** p 487-488.

124. B. **NEGATIVE FOR EBER**
The histology and clinical findings are consistent with the diagnosis of extranodal NK/T-cell lymphoma, nasal type. Specifically, the lesion demonstrates a diffuse infiltrate of atypical lymphocytes with various sizes. The cells express the NK marker CD56, and while it lacks surface expression of CD3, it demonstrates cytoplasmic expression of CD3. These lesions typically express CD2, CD56, cytoplasmic CD3, and cytotoxic granule-associated proteins, TIA-1, granzyme B and perforin. This lesion is EBV-associated with expression of LMP-1 and EBER (in situ expression more sensitive), and if the lesion lacks evidence of EBV, then the diagnosis should be questioned. When the lesion occurs in the naso/oral pharynx, it is often associated with a pseudoepitheliomatous hyperplasia that can be mistaken for invasive squamous cell carcinoma (with a dense infiltrate). The lack of surface CD3 expression is more consistent with the NK variant that have the TCR and IGH genes in the germline configuration. This rare tumor occurs mostly in older males and occurs most often in Asia and Central/South America.
QCSP, **Extranodal NK/T-Cell Lymphoma,** Nasal Type (Lethal Midline Granuloma, p 492-493.

125. D. **IT CAN BE TREATED WITH GLUTEN AVOIDANCE.**
The lesion above is an enteropathy-type T-cell lymphoma, which is often associated with refractory celiac disease. Similarly to celiac disease, they are associated with the presence of HLA-DQ2 and HLA-DQ8. These cases are CD3+ but lack CD4 and CD8 and are not responsive to gluten avoidance. However, celiac cases that are CD3+ and CD8+ will generally respond to antigen avoidance. These lesions also demonstrate expression of the integrin associated with intramucosal trafficking CD103. These lymphomas often form masses in the jejunum and ilium and present with abdominal pain and often perforation. This diagnosis has an overall poor prognosis.
QCSP, **Enteropathy-Type T-Cell Lymphoma (Refractory Sprue),** p 493-494.

126. D. **THE NEOPLASTIC CELLS INFILTRATE THROUGH THE UPPER DERMIS AND EPIDERMIS OF THE SKIN.**
Mycosis fungoides is a process characterized by the presence of atypical T-lymphocytes that infiltrate throughout the upper dermis and epidermis. Several sequential biopsies are often needed for a definitive diagnosis, with the diagnosis of mycosis fungoides often rendered months or years after initial presentation. As such, PCR of these biopsies can be very helpful to determine if a clonal rearrangement of the T-cell receptor is present. Sézary syndrome, characterized by exfoliative erythroderma, is found more commonly in males and is caused by the presence of the neoplastic T cells in the peripheral blood. Fortunately, most cases of mycosis fungoides are not aggressive, and the average patient survives >8 years after initial presentation.
QCSP, **Mycosis Fungoides,** p 494.

14: Lymph Node Answers

127. B. **ANGIOIMMUNOBLASTIC T-CELL LYMPHOMA**

The neoplastic cells are positive for CD3 and CD10. The H&E section demonstrates a proliferation of the arborizing high endothelial venules surrounded by a polymorphic infiltrate. These are all classic features of angioimmunoblastic T-cell lymphoma. One of the most telling features is the disruption of the follicular dendritic cell network as evident by CD21 and CD35 staining. The neoplastic CD4 cells are thought to develop from T-follicular helper cells and as such also express BCL-6, CD3, CD2, CD5, CXCL13 and PD-1.
QCSP, **Angioimmunoblastic T-Cell Lymphoma,** p 494-495.

128. B. **IT EXPRESSES TdT.**

The lesion is a peripheral T-cell lymphoma, unspecified. Specifically, there is a medium to large cell population with expression of CD3 and loss of CD7. Additionally, there is an associated eosinophilia. These cases can also present with pruritus and, in some rare instances, a hemophagocytic syndrome. This is a malignancy of mature T cells, primarily CD4, although cases of CD8 have been reported. As they are a malignancy of mature T cells, they do not express TdT. These lesions do have a normally intact follicular dendritic cell network (useful in separation from angioimmunoblastic T-cell lymphoma) and typically have a poor prognosis.
QCSP, **Peripheral T-Cell Lymphoma, Unspecified,** p 495.

129. A. **IT EXPRESSES CD3.**

The lesion represents an anaplastic large cell lymphoma, ALK+ in this case. While there is a broad morphologic spectrum, the lesion demonstrates a mixture of pleomorphic large cells with hallmark features along with tumor cells with a more monomorphic-rounded nucleus. Tumor cells are positive for CD30 and demonstrate membrane and dot-like (Golgi) staining. Additionally, the neoplastic cells are positive for TIA1, EMA, and CD45. While the lesion demonstrates clonal rearrangement of the TCR γ gene, it will often has loss of CD3 expression, but retention of other T-cell markers such as CD2, CD4, and CD5. The t(2;5), which is seen in approximately 85% of cases, leads to an ALK-NPM translocation that leads to increased ALK expression.
QCSP, **Anaplastic Large Cell Lymphoma,** p 495-496.

130. D. **THERE IS EXPRESSION OF IgM AND IgD.**

The lesion demonstrates infiltration of the bone marrow by a mixture of small lymphocytes and plasma cells. There are plasma cells with large cytoplasmic inclusions/globules of immunoglobulin. These findings and the clinical scenario are consistent with the diagnosis of lymphoplasmacytic lymphoma. In this case, the patient's symptoms are caused by an elevated serum IgM (a IgM paraprotein of >3 g/dL), which results in hyperviscosity of the blood. Additionally, this can induce neurological symptoms such as headaches, blurred vision, and neuropathies. Often these symptoms can be relieved (not cured) with plasmapheresis. This increased immunoglobulin also results in the formation of rouleaux on blood smear, positive Coombs test (10% of cases), and coagulopathy from direct interactions with platelets, inhibition of fibrin polymerizations and probably other interactions. The lymphoplasmacytic lymphomas usually express surface IgM without IgD, but there are rare reported cases of IgG and IgA variants. While the text states that the t(9;14) translocation is located in up to 50% of cases, larger (more recent) studies have shown that this IgH/PAX5 translocation only occurs in a minority of cases and is not specific to the diagnosis.
QCSP, **Lymphoplasmacytic Lymphoma/Waldenström Macroglobulinemia,** p 485.

Chapter 15

Male Reproductive System

1. Which of the following tumors is most frequently associated with granulomatous inflammation in the testis?
   A. Teratoma
   B. Leydig cell tumor
   C. Sertoli cell tumor
   D. Seminoma
   E. Gonadoblastoma

2. All of the following are associated with intratubular germ cell neoplasia EXCEPT:
   A. Cryptorchidism
   B. Infertility
   C. Androgen insensitivity syndrome
   D. Postpubertal yolk sac tumor
   E. Spermatocytic seminoma

3. Which of the following findings support the diagnosis of nonneoplastic spermatogonia over intratubular germ cell neoplasia?
   A. PAS positive, diastase resistant
   B. PAS positive, diastase susceptible
   C. PLAP negative
   D. PLAP positive
   E. Absence of gross findings

4. All of the following are significantly associated with seminoma EXCEPT:
   A. HLA types DR5 and Bw41
   B. Down syndrome
   C. Tall stature
   D. Cryptorchidism
   E. Acquired immunodeficiency syndrome (AIDS)

5. Which of the following choices correctly lists testicular neoplasms occurring in elderly men in order of DECREASING incidence?
   A. Lymphoma > spermatocytic seminoma > classic seminoma
   B. Lymphoma > classic seminoma > spermatocytic seminoma
   C. Classic seminoma > spermatocytic seminoma > lymphoma
   D. Classic seminoma > lymphoma > spermatocytic seminoma
   E. Spermatocytic seminoma > lymphoma > classic seminoma

6. All of the following features support the diagnosis of spermatocytic seminoma over classic seminoma EXCEPT:
   A. Absence of intratubular germ cell neoplasia
   B. Absence of admixed germ cell tumors
   C. Absence of stainable glycogen
   D. Polymorphous cell population
   E. Prominent mitotic activity

7. Which of the following immunohistochemical stains is positive in spermatocytic seminoma?
    A. PLAP
    B. hCG
    C. AFP
    D. All of the above
    E. None of the above

8. All of the following features in metastatic embryonal carcinoma are associated with a poor prognosis EXCEPT:
    A. Elevated serum AFP (>1,000 IU/L)
    B. Elevated serum β-hCG (>10,000 IU/L)
    C. Age <2 years
    D. Metastasis to brain, liver, or bone
    E. Mediastinal mass >5 cm

9. Which of the following features distinguishes prepubertal from postpubertal yolk sac tumors?
    A. Presence of other germ cell components
    B. Association with cryptorchidism
    C. Serum AFP level
    D. A and B
    E. All of the above

10. Which of the following is the most important determinant of prognosis in patients with yolk sac tumor?
    A. Age
    B. Stage
    C. Presence of other germ cell components
    D. Elevated serum AFP level
    E. Presence of isochromosome (i)12p

11. All of the following statements regarding testicular choriocarcinoma are TRUE EXCEPT:
    A. The tumor is almost never seen before puberty.
    B. Tumors composed entirely of choriocarcinoma are exceedingly rare.
    C. Patients may present with symptoms of thyrotoxicosis.
    D. The typical patient presents with a palpable testicular mass.
    E. Serums levels of hCG may be higher than 100,000 IU/L.

12. All of the following morphologic features are characteristic of choriocarcinoma EXCEPT:
    A. Dual population composed of syncytiotrophoblasts and cytotrophoblasts
    B. Brisk mitotic activity involving predominantly syncytiotrophoblasts
    C. Angioinvasion
    D. Extensive necrosis
    E. Minimal residual viable tumor concentrated at tumor periphery

13. What percentage of testicular germ cell tumors are mixed?
    A. 10%
    B. 30%
    C. 50%
    D. 70%
    E. 90%

15: Male Reproductive System Questions

14. Which of the following best describes polyembryoma?
    A. An orderly mixture of embryonal carcinoma and yolk sac tumor in equal parts
    B. A mixture of embryonal carcinoma and yolk sac tumor arranged in a pattern resembling the presomatic embryo with embryoid bodies in myxoid mesenchyme
    C. A mixture of embryonal carcinoma and teratoma
    D. A mixture of seminoma-like and Sertoli-like cells arranged in nests
    E. A mixture of embryonic tissue from all 3 germ cell layers including blastematous, neuroblastic-type, or neuroepithelial tissue

15. All of the following components of mixed germ cell tumors are correctly paired with prognostic implications EXCEPT:
    A. Embryonal carcinoma – worse overall prognosis
    B. Teratoma – less aggressive disease course
    C. Teratoma – lower rate of metastasis
    D. Yolk sac tumor – lower rate of metastasis
    E. Yolk sac tumor – better response to chemotherapy

16. What is the most common testicular sex-cord stromal tumor?
    A. Leydig cell tumor
    B. Sertoli cell tumor
    C. Sertoli-Leydig cell tumor
    D. Gonadoblastoma
    E. Large cell calcifying Sertoli cell tumor

17. Which of the following features is NOT predictive of malignant behavior in Leydig cell tumors?
    A. Age >60 years
    B. Absence of endocrine manifestations
    C. Tumor >6 cm
    D. Infiltrative margins
    E. Presence of Klinefelter syndrome

18. Which of the following is NOT a morphologic feature of Sertoli cell tumors?
    A. Tubules and cords surrounded by basement membrane
    B. Oval nuclei with inconspicuous nucleoli
    C. Abundant eosinophilic or pale cytoplasm
    D. Dense microcalcifications
    E. Low mitotic activity

19. Which of the following immunohistochemical stains is negative in Sertoli cell tumors?
    A. EMA
    B. Vimentin
    C. Cytokeratin
    D. Inhibin
    E. NSE

20. Which of the following disorders is/are associated with Sertoli cell tumors?
    A. Androgen insensitivity syndrome
    B. Peutz-Jeghers syndrome
    C. Carney syndrome
    D. A and B
    E. A, B, and C

15: Male Reproductive System Questions

21. Which of the following is NOT a feature of Sertoli-Leydig cell tumors?
    A. Broad age range at presentation
    B. Negative oil red O stain
    C. Association with gynecomastia
    D. Diffuse immunoreactivity for inhibin
    E. Presence of Reinke crystals

22. The presence of bilateral large cell calcifying Sertoli cell tumors is suggestive of which of the following disorders?
    A. Peutz-Jeghers syndrome
    B. Carney syndrome
    C. Androgen insensitivity syndrome
    D. Cryptorchidism
    E. Acquired immunodeficiency syndrome (AIDS)

23. Which of the following morphologic features is NOT characteristic of large cell calcifying Sertoli cell tumors?
    A. Large tumor cells with abundant eosinophilic cytoplasm
    B. Round to oval nuclei with small nucleoli
    C. Prominent lymphocytic infiltrate
    D. Prominent foci of laminated calcifications
    E. Scant mitotic activity

24. Which of the following findings on electron microscopy is associated with Sertoli cells?
    A. Reinke crystals
    B. Charcot-Leyden crystals
    C. Charcot-Böttchen filaments
    D. Tubuloreticular inclusions
    E. Desmosomes

25. Which of the following patient populations is typically affected by gonadoblastoma?
    A. Phenotypic female, genotypic male
    B. Phenotypic male, genotypic female
    C. Phenotypic and genotypic female
    D. Phenotypic and genotypic male
    E. Turner syndrome

26. Which of the following is NOT a morphologic feature of gonadoblastoma?
    A. Reinke crystals
    B. Calcifications
    C. Immature Sertoli cells
    D. Invasive germ cell tumors
    E. Hyaline deposits of basement membrane

27. Which of the following invasive tumors is most likely to occur in the setting of gonadoblastoma?
    A. Embryonal carcinoma
    B. Yolk sac tumor
    C. Teratoma
    D. Seminoma
    E. Choriocarcinoma

28. All of the following are features of the lesion depicted in this image EXCEPT:

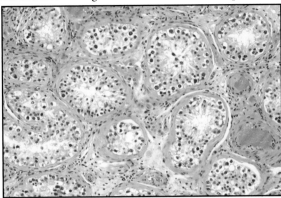

A. Enlarged and dilated seminiferous tubules
B. Large, polygonal cells with abundant clear cytoplasm and prominent nucleoli
C. Frequent mitotic figures
D. Increased Leydig cells
E. Intratubular calcifications

Questions 29 and 30 are based on the following image:

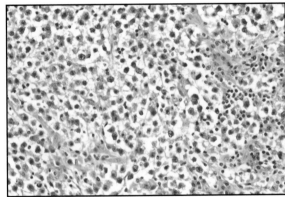

29. Which of the following clinical and laboratory findings are NOT characteristic of the lesion depicted in this image?
A. Hypercalcemia
B. Elevated serum AFP
C. Elevated hCG
D. Exophthalmos
E. Increased incidence in right testis

30. Which of the following markers is typically NOT expressed in this lesion?
A. Vimentin
B. PLAP
C. CD117
D. NSE
E. CD30

Questions 31 and 32 are based on the following image:

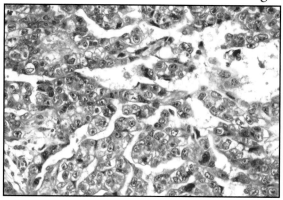

31. Which of the following tumors (depicted in this image) is a component of approximately 90% of all nonseminomatous germ cell tumors?
    A. Embryonal carcinoma
    B. Yolk sac tumor
    C. Choriocarcinoma
    D. Teratoma
    E. Spermatocytic seminoma

32. Which of the following immunohistochemical stains are typically positive in this lesion?
    A. CD30
    B. PLAP
    C. Cytokeratin
    D. A and B
    E. All of the above

33. The most common testicular tumor in prepubescent children, depicted in this image is:

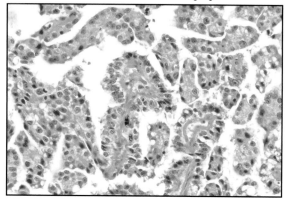

    A. Seminoma
    B. Embryonal carcinoma
    C. Yolk sac tumor
    D. Choriocarcinoma
    E. Teratoma

15: Male Reproductive System Questions

34. The most common site of metastasis in the lesion depicted in this image is:

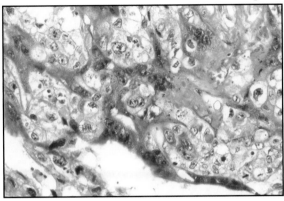

    A. Lung
    B. Liver
    C. Brain
    D. Adrenal gland
    E. Lymph node

Questions 35-37 are based on the following image:

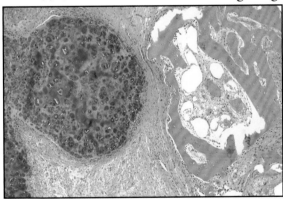

35. All of the following are features of the lesion depicted in this image EXCEPT:
    A. Second most common germ cell tumor of childhood
    B. Present in 50% of mixed germ cell tumors
    C. Enlarged testis on presentation
    D. Frequent extratesticular extension
    E. Treatment differences between prepubertal and postpubertal tumors

36. Which of the following is the most common secondary malignant neoplasm arising in association with this lesion?
    A. Rhabdomyosarcoma
    B. Adenocarcinoma
    C. Squamous cell carcinoma
    D. Leiomyosarcoma
    E. Chondrosarcoma

15: Male Reproductive System Questions

37. Which of the following has NOT been associated with the prepubertal form of this lesion?
     A. Down syndrome
     B. Klinefelter syndrome
     C. Hemihypertrophy
     D. Hemophilia
     E. All of the above are associated with this lesion.

38. All of the following are features of the lesion depicted in this image EXCEPT:

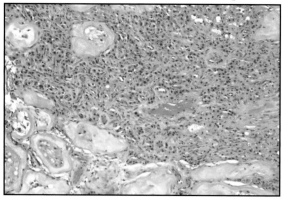 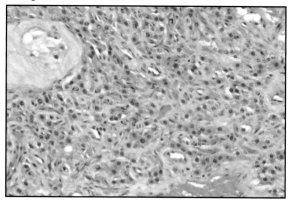

     A. Broad age range at presentation
     B. Endocrine manifestations
     C. Strong immunoreactivity for EMA
     D. Strong immunoreactivity for inhibin
     E. Reinke crystals

15: Male Reproductive System Questions

Questions 39-41 are based on the following image:

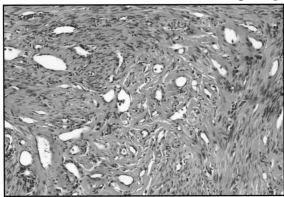

39. Which of the following is the most common neoplasm of the epididymis (depicted in this image)?
    A. Seminoma
    B. Mesothelioma
    C. Rhabdomyosarcoma
    D. Adenomatoid tumor
    E. Gonadoblastoma

40. Which of the following immunohistochemical markers are typically expressed in the lesion depicted in this image?
    A. EMA
    B. Calretinin
    C. Cytokeratin
    D. CEA
    E. A, B, and C

41. Which of the following sites has NOT been described as a common site of the lesion depicted in this image?
    A. Epididymis
    B. Urinary bladder
    C. Thyroid gland
    D. Adrenal gland
    E. Uterus

15: Male Reproductive System Answers

1. **D.** **SEMINOMA**

    Granulomatous inflammation involving the testis and sparing the epididymis has been associated with seminoma (choice D). This is an important consideration in the rare event of a diagnostic incisional biopsy, which may have inadequately sampled the neoplasm.

    QCSP, **Intraoperative Consultation,** p 498.

2. **E.** **SPERMATOCYTIC SEMINOMA**

    Intratubular germ cell neoplasia (IGCN) has been associated with a variety of risk factors including cryptorchidism (choice A), infertility (choice B) and androgen insensitivity syndrome (choice C). IGCN is almost always present in postpubertal yolk sac tumors and teratomas (choice D), unlike in the prepubertal varieties, where it is considered rare. IGCN is not associated with spermatocytic seminoma (choice E).

    QCSP, **Intratubular Germ Cell Neoplasia,** p 498-499.

3. **C.** **PLAP NEGATIVE**

    Unlike intratubular germ cell neoplasia (IGCN), nonneoplastic spermatogonia lining the seminiferous tubules are usually PLAP negative (choice C). IGCN is typically PLAP positive (choice D). Both entities may appear grossly unremarkable (choice E) and contain abundant intracellular glycogen, resulting in PAS positivity with diastase susceptibility (choice B). Neither entity exhibits diastase-resistant PAS staining (choice A).

    QCSP, **Intratubular Germ Cell Neoplasia,** p 499.

4. **B.** **DOWN SYNDROME**

    An increased incidence of seminoma has been seen in patients with HLA types DR5 and Bw41, tall stature, cryptorchidism, and acquired immunodeficiency syndrome (choices A, C, D, and E). No association with Down syndrome has been reported (choice B).

    QCSP, **Seminoma,** p 500.

5. **A.** **LYMPHOMA > SPERMATOCYTIC SEMINOMA > CLASSIC SEMINOMA**

    The most common testicular tumor in elderly men is lymphoma, followed by spermatocytic seminoma (choice A), which is rare under the age of 30 years. Classic seminoma is the most common pure testicular germ cell tumor with a peak incidence in the 4th decade (choices C and D).

    QCSP, **Spermatocytic Seminoma,** p 500.

6. **E.** **PROMINENT MITOTIC ACTIVITY**

    Due to the excellent prognosis associated with spermatocytic seminoma, differentiating these tumors from classic seminoma is important. Unlike classic seminoma, spermatocytic seminoma is not associated with intratubular germ cell neoplasia (choice A), cryptorchidism, or other germ cell tumors (choice B). Additionally, PAS staining confirms the absence of glycogen in spermatocytic seminoma (choice C), which would be positive in classic seminoma. Morphologically, the lesion is composed of a diffuse polymorphous tumor cell population, which is not associated with a prominent lymphoid or granulomatous inflammatory infiltrate (choice D). Mitotic activity may be prominent in either entity and is typically not helpful in differentiation between the 2 (choice E).

    QCSP, **Spermatocytic Seminoma,** p 501 (see also QCSP, Seminoma, p 500.).

7. **E.** **NONE OF THE ABOVE**

    Unlike classic seminoma, PLAP expression is typically not seen in spermatocytic seminoma (choice A). hCG and AFP are also negative, which are more typically associated with choriocarcinoma and yolk sac tumor, respectively (choices B and C).

    QCSP, **Spermatocytic Seminoma,** p 501.

15: Male Reproductive System Answers

8.   C.   **AGE <2 YEARS**

All of the choices have been associated with a poor prognosis in metastatic embryonal carcinomas except for age <2 years (choice C). In fact, elderly patients appear to have a poorer prognosis.

QCSP, **Embryonal Carcinoma,** p 503.

9.   D.   **A AND B**

Unlike prepubertal yolk sac tumors, which are nearly all pure tumors, postpubertal yolk sac tumors usually form a component of a mixed germ cell tumor (choice A). Prepubertal tumors are furthermore not associated with cryptorchidism (choice B), suggesting that they may be etiologically distinct from postpubertal yolk sac tumors. Serum AFP levels have not been demonstrated to differ between the 2 populations (choice C).

QCSP, **Yolk Sac Tumor,** p 503.

10.   B.   **STAGE**

Although there is some controversy over whether prepubertal tumors have a better prognosis than postpubertal tumors (choice A), it is clear that stage is the most important prognostic factor (choice B). Prepubertal tumors typically do not contain other germ cell components or the i(12p) marker chromosome seen in postpubertal tumors, but the significance of these differences is still unknown (choices C and E). Elevated serum AFP levels are present in the vast majority of patients and do not reliably predict outcome (choice D).

QCSP, **Yolk Sac Tumor,** p 504-505.

11.   D.   **THE TYPICAL PATIENT PRESENTS WITH A PALPABLE TESTICULAR MASS.**

Choriocarcinoma is somewhat unique among testicular germ cell tumors in that it is typically widely disseminated prior to forming a palpable testicular mass (choice D). The tumor is virtually never seen before puberty (choice A), and pure tumors comprise <0.5% of testicular neoplasms (choice B). When pure, tumors may be accompanied by levels of hCG higher than 100,000 IU/L (choice E). Because of the similarity in amino acid sequence between hCG and thyroid-stimulating hormone, such patients in particular may present with symptoms of thyrotoxicosis (choice C).

QCSP, **Choriocarcinoma,** p 505.

12.   B.   **BRISK MITOTIC ACTIVITY INVOLVING PREDOMINANTLY SYNCYTIOTROPHOBLASTS**

Choriocarcinoma is typically consists of a biphasic population composed of sheets of cytotrophoblasts surrounded by syncytiotrophoblasts (choice A). It is important to note that cytotrophoblasts are essential to the diagnosis of choriocarcinoma. Syncytiotrophoblasts may be seen in other types of germ cell tumors and should not be misinterpreted as representing a choriocarcinoma component. Accordingly, mitotic activity is not prominent in these cells (choice B). Angioinvasion and extensive necrosis are the rule in choriocarcinoma; small amounts of residual tumor are best visualized at the periphery of the lesion (choices C, D and E).

QCSP, **Choriocarcinoma,** p 505.

13.   B.   **30%**

When taking into account all testicular germ cell tumors, approximately 30% are mixed (choice B). This percentage is much higher when referring only to nonseminomatous germ cell tumors, at 70%-90% (choices D and E).

QCSP, **Mixed Germ Cell Tumors,** p 507.

14.   B.   **A MIXTURE OF EMBRYONAL CARCINOMA AND YOLK SAC TUMOR ARRANGED IN A PATTERN RESEMBLING THE PRESOMATIC EMBRYO WITH EMBRYOID BODIES IN MYXOID MESENCHYME**

Polyembryoma is a variant of mixed germ cell tumor characterized by a mixture of embryonal carcinoma and yolk sac tumor arranged in a pattern resembling the presomatic embryo with scattered embryoid bodies surrounded by a myxoid mesenchyme (choice B). Choice A is a description of diffuse embryoma, a different variant of mixed germ cell tumor. Mixtures of embryonal carcinoma and teratoma may also be known as teratocarcinoma (choice C). Choices D and E are descriptions of gonadoblastoma and immature teratoma, respectively. *QCSP*, **Mixed Germ Cell Tumor**, p 508.

15.   E.   **YOLK SAC TUMOR – BETTER RESPONSE TO CHEMOTHERAPY**
Extensive sampling of mixed germ cell tumors is critical to adequately characterize the proportion of each component present, which markedly affects prognosis. Higher proportions of embryonal carcinoma are associated with worse prognosis (choice A), while the presence of teratoma is associated with a less aggressive disease course and a decreased incidence of metastasis (choices B and C). The presence of yolk sac tumor does predict a decreased incidence of metastasis (choice D); however, yolk sac tumor is also typically resistant to chemotherapy (choice E).
QCSP, **Mixed Germ Cell Tumor**, p 508.

16.   A.   **LEYDIG CELL TUMOR**
Leydig cell tumors are the most common testicular sex-cord stromal tumors, comprising approximately 2% of all testicular tumors and presenting at all ages (choice A). The others are less common.
QCSP, **Leydig Cell Tumor**, p 508.

17.   E.   **PRESENCE OF KLINEFELTER SYNDROME**
All of the choices presented are possible indications of malignancy except for the presence of Klinefelter syndrome (choice E). In the setting of Klinefelter syndrome, Leydig cell hyperplasia is a particularly important diagnostic consideration in the differential diagnosis of a Leydig cell tumor, as hyperplasia is considerably more common in this population.
QCSP, **Leydig Cell Tumor**, p 509.

18.   D.   **DENSE MICROCALCIFICATIONS**
Sertoli cell tumors have a spectrum of morphologic appearances, but are typically composed of tubules and cords surrounded by basement membrane (choice A). Nuclei may be round or oval without prominent nucleoli and with moderate to abundant cytoplasm (choices B and C). Minor microcalcifications are present in 10% of cases, but dense microcalcifications are not typical (choice D). Mitotic activity and pleomorphism are not prominent (choice E).
QCSP, **Sertoli Cell Tumor**, p 510.

19.   A.   **EMA**
The majority of Sertoli tumors are immunoreactive for vimentin, cytokeratin, and NSE (choices B, C and E). Inhibin is positive in <1/2 of cases (choice D). EMA is the only marker listed which is consistently negative (choice A).
QCSP, **Sertoli Cell Tumor**, p 510.

20.   E.   **A, B, AND C**
The androgen insensitivity syndrome is associated with classic Sertoli tumors (choice A), while Peutz-Jeghers and Carney syndromes are associated with the sclerosing and large cell-calcifying variants of Sertoli cell tumor, respectively (choices B and C). Peutz-Jeghers syndrome is characterized by hamartomatous gastrointestinal polyps and hyperpigmented macules of the lips and oral mucosa. Carney syndrome is characterized by pituitary adenoma, bilateral primary adrenocortical hyperplasia, cardiac myxomas, lentigines, blue nevi, and psammomatous melanotic schwannomas. The sclerosing variant of Sertoli cell tumor represents 15% of all Sertoli cell tumors and is clinically benign.
QCSP, **Sertoli Cell Tumor**, p 510.

15: Male Reproductive System Answers

21. **B. NEGATIVE OIL RED O STAIN**

Like its monomorphic counterparts, Sertoli-Leydig cell tumors are composed of cells with copious lipid droplets, highlighted on an oil red O stain (choice B). These tumors occur in all age groups (choice A) and may be associated with gynecomastia (choice C). Both Sertoli and Leydig cells are strongly positive for inhibin (choice D), and Reinke crystals may be present in association with the Leydig cell component (choice E).

QCSP, **Sertoli-Leydig Cell Tumor,** p 511.

22. **B. CARNEY SYNDROME**

Bilateral large cell calcifying Sertoli cell tumors are associated with Carney syndrome (pituitary adenoma, bilateral primary adrenocortical hyperplasia, cardiac myxomas, lentigines, blue nevi, psammomatous melanotic schwannomas) and are typically benign in this setting (choice B). Peutz-Jeghers and androgen insensitivity syndrome are associated with sclerosing and classic Sertoli cell tumor, respectively (choices A and C). Cryptorchidism is associated with Leydig cell tumors (choice D), while AIDS is associated with seminoma (choice E).

QCSP, **Large Cell Calcifying Sertoli Cell Tumor,** p 511.

23. **C. PROMINENT LYMPHOCYTIC INFILTRATE**

All of the choices presented are morphologic features of large cell calcifying Sertoli cell tumors except prominent lymphocytic infiltrate (choice C). Prominent neutrophilic infiltrates, on the other hand, are not uncommon.

QCSP, **Large Cell Calcifying Sertoli Cell Tumor,** p 511.

24. **C. CHARCOT-BÖTTCHEN FILAMENTS**

Cytoplasmic bundles of Charcot-Böttchen filaments are typically seen in association with the Sertoli cells comprising large cell calcifying Sertoli cell tumors (choice C). Intracytoplasmic Charcot-Böttchen crystalloids can be seen on H&E-stained slides as a filamentous structure located in the basal portion of mature Sertoli cells; however, they are best appreciated on electron microscopy where they appear to merge with vimentin intermediate filaments. Reinke crystals are associated with postpubertal Leydig cells (choice A) and are composed of an unknown material that stains negatively for actin, vimentin, and desmin. Charcot-Leyden crystals are composed of breakdown products of eosinophils (choice B). Tubuloreticular inclusions are electron microscopy findings in diseases associated with high levels of α-interferon (HIV, treated hepatitis C, lupus) (choice D) and are commonly seen in the kidney but may be observed in various tissues throughout the body, while desmosomes are junctional complexes specializing in cell-to-cell adhesion seen in squamous epithelium (choice E).

QCSP, **Large Cell Calcifying Sertoli Cell Tumor,** p 512, Histology for Pathologists, p 945, 949.

25. **A. PHENOTYPIC FEMALE, GENOTYPIC MALE**

Gonadoblastoma is a disease which primarily affects phenotypic females; however, the Y chromosome is typically present (choice A). Remaining cases are comprised of phenotypic and genotypic males (choice D).

QCSP, **Gonadoblastoma,** p 512.

26. **A. REINKE CRYSTALS**

Gonadoblastoma is composed of a mixture of seminoma-like and immature Sertoli-like cells, often arranged in nests containing hyaline deposits of basement membrane (choices C and E). Calcifications are common (choice B), as are invasive germ cell tumors (choice D). While Leydig-like cells may also be seen, particularly at the periphery of the tumor, Reinke crystals are not a feature (choice A).

QCSP, **Gonadoblastoma,** p 512.

15: Male Reproductive System Answers

differentiating them from epithelioid hemangiomas, which are immunoreactive for both immunohistochemical stains.

QCSP, **Adenomatoid Tumor,** p 513.

41. C. **THYROID GLAND**

Of the choices listed, only thyroid gland is not considered a common location for adenomatoid tumor (choice C).

QCSP, **Adenomatoid Tumor,** p 513-514.

Chapter 16

Urinary Tract

1. The most common indication(s) for an intraoperative consultation on specimens from the urinary tract is/are:
    A. Margin evaluation
    B. Diagnosis
    C. Adequacy of tissue for ancillary testing
    D. Evaluation for lymph node metastasis
    E. All of the above

2. Which of the following treatments is/are particularly known to compromise the pathologist's ability to reliably diagnose prostatic carcinoma on frozen section?
    A. Nonsteroidal antiandrogens
    B. Luteinizing hormone-releasing hormone (LHRH)
    C. Prior surgery
    D. A and B
    E. All of the above

3. All of the following are TRUE regarding mesoblastic nephroma EXCEPT:
    A. It is commonly bilateral.
    B. It is typically diagnosed within the first 3 months of life.
    C. It may present with hyperreninism due to entrapped renal elements.
    D. It may present with hypercalcemia due to paraneoplastic production of prostaglandin E.
    E. It may be grossly indistinguishable from nephroblastoma.

4. Which of the following is the most common location of mesoblastic nephroma?
    A. Upper renal pole – cortex
    B. Lower renal pole – cortex
    C. Hilum
    D. Upper renal pole – medulla
    E. Lower renal pole – medulla

5. Which of the following variants of mesoblastic nephroma is/are morphologically and cytogenetically related to infantile fibrosarcoma?
    A. Classic variant
    B. Cellular variant
    C. Atypical variant
    D. A and B
    E. None of the above

6. Which of the following histologic features is typically seen with nearly all variants of clear cell sarcoma?
    A. Angioinvasion
    B. Intracytoplasmic vesicles
    C. Prominent nucleoli
    D. High mitotic activity with multipolar mitotic figures
    E. Stromal hyalinization

16: Urinary Tract Questions

7. Which of the following is NOT a histologic pattern of clear cell sarcoma?
    A. Epithelioid pattern
    B. Spindled pattern
    C. Sclerosing pattern
    D. Cystic pattern
    E. Rhabdoid pattern

8. All of the following statements regarding clear cell sarcoma of the kidney are TRUE EXCEPT:
    A. Treatment typically includes surgery and chemotherapy with doxorubicin.
    B. Late recurrence is common.
    C. Bone metastases occur in 15%-20% of patients.
    D. 75% of patients exhibit the chromosomal translocation t(12;22)(q13;q12).
    E. Survival approximates 70%.

9. Which of the following patients is most likely to present with rhabdoid tumor of the kidney?
    A. 1-year-old male
    B. 10-year-old male
    C. 3-year-old female
    D. 15-year-old female
    E. 29-year-old female

10. Which of the following microscopic features is NOT characteristic of rhabdoid tumor?
    A. Infiltrative growth pattern
    B. Large polygonal tumor cells with distinct cell borders
    C. Clusters of cells with eosinophilic, fibrillary cytoplasmic inclusions
    D. Finely granular chromatin with multiple inconspicuous nucleoli
    E. Immunoreactivity with EMA

11. Which of the following molecular alterations is found in 80% of patients with rhabdoid tumors of the kidney?
    A. t(12;22)(q13;q12)
    B. Loss of heterozygosity on 22q11-12
    C. Deletion of chromosome 3p
    D. Translocation involving Xp11.2
    E. Monosomy of chromosome 22

12. Which of the following features is/are NOT a part of the "classic triad" of symptoms seen in renal cell carcinoma?
    A. Scrotal varicocele
    B. Flank pain
    C. Palpable flank mass
    D. Hematuria
    E. All of the above

13. Which of the following laboratory findings is NOT associated with renal cell carcinoma?
    A. Normochromic normocytic anemia
    B. Polycythemia
    C. Erythrocytosis
    D. Hypercalcemia
    E. Increased serum creatinine

16: Urinary Tract Questions

14. Which of the following features is correctly paired with the papillary renal cell carcinoma subtype?
    A. Type 1: single layer of cells with bland nuclear features and scant basophilic cytoplasm, presentation with advanced disease
    B. Type 1: stratified layer of cells with atypical nuclear features and abundant eosinophilic cytoplasm, presentation with localized disease
    C. Type 2: single layer of cells with bland nuclear features and scant basophilic cytoplasm, presentation with advanced disease
    D. Type 2: stratified layer of cells with atypical nuclear features and abundant eosinophilic cytoplasm, presentation with localized disease
    E. Type 2: stratified layer of cells with atypical nuclear features and abundant eosinophilic cytoplasm, presentation with advanced disease

15. Which of the following features is NOT characteristic of carcinoma of the collecting ducts of Bellini?
    A. Involvement of the renal medulla
    B. Abundant hemorrhage and necrosis
    C. High-grade, hobnail nuclear features
    D. Death due to metastasis in 50% of patients
    E. Infiltration with pronounced desmoplastic stromal response

16. Which of the following disorders is associated with renal medullary carcinoma?
    A. von Hippel-Lindau syndrome
    B. Beckwith-Wiedemann syndrome
    C. Sickle cell trait
    D. Li-Fraumeni syndrome
    E. End stage renal disease

17. Expression of which of the following immunohistochemical stains is most helpful in supporting the diagnosis of Xp11.2 translocation carcinoma?
    A. CD10
    B. EMA
    C. INI1
    D. TFE3
    E. CK7

18. Which of the following is NOT a risk factor for renal cell carcinoma?
    A. Obesity
    B. Smoking
    C. Heavy alcohol consumption
    D. Hypertension
    E. Heavy metal exposure

19. Which of the following features is a key difference between classic angiomyolipoma and the epithelioid variant?
    A. Presence of extrarenal tumors with similar morphology
    B. Immunoreactivity with HMB45
    C. Appearance of vasculature
    D. Prognosis
    E. None of the above

16: Urinary Tract Questions

20. Renal cortical adenomas may be an incidental finding in what percentage of individuals?
    A.   2%
    B.   5%
    C.   20%
    D.   40%
    E.   60%

21. Which of the following histologic features is/are commonly seen with renal cortical adenoma?
    A.   Lipid-laden macrophages
    B.   Densely packed tubules and papillae
    C.   Cellular atypia
    D.   A and B
    E.   All of the above

22. Which of the following conditions is NOT associated with renal cortical adenoma?
    A.   von Hippel-Lindau syndrome
    B.   Beckwith-Wiedemann syndrome
    C.   Renal cell carcinoma
    D.   Chronic pyelonephritis
    E.   Renal vascular disease

23. Which of the following stains is particularly helpful in distinguishing oncocytoma from chromophobe renal cell carcinoma?
    A.   CK7
    B.   Hale colloidal iron
    C.   CD10
    D.   PAS with diastase
    E.   Vimentin

24. Which of the following is NOT a feature of medullary fibroma?
    A.   Amyloid
    B.   Electron-dense lipid droplets
    C.   Association with hypertension
    D.   Association with renal cell carcinoma
    E.   Mucopolysaccharide matrix

25. All of the following features are worrisome for multilocular cystic renal cell carcinoma EXCEPT:
    A.   Solid, expansile mural nodules
    B.   Hemorrhage
    C.   Necrosis
    D.   Cellular atypia
    E.   Foci of cartilage

26. Which of the following laboratory findings support(s) the diagnosis of acute proliferative glomerulonephritis?
    A.   Low serum complement levels
    B.   Elevated anti-streptococcal antibody
    C.   Red cell casts
    D.   Azotemia
    E.   All of the above

16: Urinary Tract Questions

27. All of the following types of rapidly progressive glomerulonephritis are correctly paired with their corresponding diseases EXCEPT:
    A. Type I: Goodpasture syndrome
    B. Type II: Henoch-Schönlein purpura
    C. Type II: systemic lupus erythematosus
    D. Type III: IgA nephropathy
    E. Type III: Wegener granulomatosis

28. Which of the following approaches has/have been useful in the treatment of rapidly progressive glomerulonephritis?
    A. Plasmapheresis
    B. Steroids
    C. Cytotoxic agents
    D. Transplantation
    E. All of the above

29. Which of the following factors have been associated with secondary membranous glomerulonephritis:
    A. Hepatitis B
    B. Hepatitis C
    C. Malignancy
    D. Drugs
    E. All of the above

30. Which of the following factors is NOT associated with minimal change disease?
    A. NSAID use
    B. Eczema
    C. Human immunodeficiency virus
    D. Hodgkin lymphoma
    E. Prophylactic immunizations

31. Which of the following genes has NOT been associated with familial focal segmental glomerulosclerosis?
    A. NPHS
    B. PLCE1
    C. TSC2
    D. ACTN4
    E. TRPC6

32. Which of the following factors is NOT associated with focal segmental glomerulosclerosis?
    A. Human immunodeficiency virus
    B. Smoking
    C. Sickle cell disease
    D. Obesity
    E. Nephrin mutation

33. Which of the following is not a common setting for secondary membranoproliferative glomerulonephritis?
    A. Hereditary complement deficiency
    B. Systemic lupus erythematosus
    C. Amyloidosis
    D. Lymphoma
    E. Hepatitis C

16: Urinary Tract Questions

34. Which of the following features is typically associated with type I rather than type II membranoproliferative glomerulonephritis?
    A. C3 deposition on both sides of the basement membrane
    B. Linear intramembranous electron-dense deposits
    C. Partial lipodystrophy
    D. Granular subendothelial deposits of C3 and IgG
    E. "Tram-track" glomerular capillary walls

35. The most common presenting symptom in patients with IgA nephropathy is:
    A. Bilateral lower extremity edema
    B. Fatigue
    C. Oliguria
    D. Hematuria
    E. Hypertension

36. Which of the following electron microscopy findings is characteristic of IgA nephropathy?
    A. Linear intramembranous deposits
    B. Subepithelial "humps" of immune complexes
    C. Mesangial deposits of immune complexes
    D. Granular subendothelial deposits
    E. Irregular intramembranous deposits enveloped by spikes of basement membrane

37. Chronic renal failure develops in what percentage of patients with IgA nephropathy?
    A. 1%
    B. 10%
    C. 30%
    D. 60%
    E. 75%

38. Which of the following features is characteristic of focal proliferative and necrotizing glomerulonephritis?
    A. Microcalcifications
    B. Arteriosclerosis
    C. Segmental necrosis
    D. Lymphocytic infiltrate
    E. Glomerular crescents

39. Which of the following correctly lists the percentage of patients progressing to chronic glomerulonephritis from lowest to highest?
    A. Acute proliferative glomerulonephritis < IgA nephropathy < focal segmental glomerulosclerosis < rapidly progressive glomerulosclerosis
    B. IgA nephropathy < acute proliferative glomerulonephritis < focal segmental glomerulosclerosis < rapidly progressive glomerulosclerosis
    C. Acute proliferative glomerulonephritis < focal segmental glomerulosclerosis < IgA nephropathy < rapidly progressive glomerulosclerosis
    D. IgA nephropathy < focal segmental glomerulosclerosis < acute proliferative glomerulonephritis < rapidly progressive glomerulosclerosis
    E. Acute proliferative glomerulonephritis < IgA nephropathy < rapidly progressive glomerulosclerosis < focal segmental glomerulosclerosis

16: Urinary Tract Questions

40. Which of the following is NOT a histologic feature of chronic glomerulonephritis?
    A. Hyalinized glomeruli
    B. Arteriosclerosis
    C. Tubular atrophy
    D. Interstitial fibrosis
    E. Neutrophilic infiltrate

41. The term "malakoplakia" is reserved for lesions exhibiting which of the following findings?
    A. Lipid-laden macrophages
    B. Michaelis-Gutmann bodies
    C. Gamna-Gandy bodies
    D. Asteroid bodies
    E. Microabscesses

42. Which of the following is NOT a feature of Ask-Upmark kidney?
    A. Congenital hypoplasia
    B. Hypertension
    C. Association with neoplasia
    D. Stenosis of arcuate and interlobular arteries
    E. Reduction in number of medullary pyramids

43. Which of the following is associated with an elevated PSA level?
    A. Prostatic adenocarcinoma
    B. Nodular hyperplasia
    C. Prostate biopsy
    D. Digital rectal examination
    E. All of the above

44. Helpful features differentiating prostatic adenocarcinoma from normal glands include all of the following EXCEPT:
    A. Cellular pleomorphism
    B. Absence of a basal layer
    C. Enlarged nuclei with prominent nucleoli
    D. Intraluminal blue-tinged mucinous secretions
    E. Small, haphazardly arranged glands

45. Prostatic adenocarcinoma consisting of occasional fused glands or irregular, large, cribriform masses of neoplastic glands describes which of the following Gleason grades?
    A. Gleason grade 1
    B. Gleason grade 2
    C. Gleason grade 3
    D. Gleason grade 4
    E. Gleason grade 5

46. Which of the following prostatic adenocarcinoma variants is NOT correctly paired with its typical grading pattern?
    A. Mucinous adenocarcinoma: Gleason grade 4
    B. Signet-ring adenocarcinoma: Gleason grade 5
    C. Adenosquamous cell carcinoma: Gleason grade 5
    D. Prostatic duct adenocarcinoma: Gleason grade 4
    E. Basaloid carcinoma: not graded

16: Urinary Tract Questions

47. The most common benign mesenchymal lesion of the prostate is:
    A. Capillary hemangioma
    B. Leiomyoma
    C. Neurofibroma
    D. Schwannoma
    E. Rhabdomyoma

48. Which of the following differential diagnoses for prostatic adenocarcinoma is NOT correctly paired with a helpful distinguishing feature?
    A. Atrophy: preserved lobular architecture
    B. Seminal vesicle epithelium: prominent lipofuscin granules
    C. Basal cell hyperplasia: expression of high molecular weight cytokeratin
    D. Partial atrophy: presence of micronucleoli
    E. Adenosis: presence of scattered basal cells

49. Prostatic adenocarcinoma involving the seminal vesicles warrants which of the following clinical stages?
    A. T1a
    B. T1b
    C. T1c
    D. T2
    E. T3

50. Which of the following organisms is NOT commonly seen in mycotic prostatitis?
    A. *Mycobacterium tuberculosis*
    B. *Blastomyces dermatitides*
    C. *Coccidioides immitis*
    D. *Cryptococcus neoformans*
    E. *Aspergillus fumigatus*

51. Which of the following are types of metaplastic lesions in the urinary bladder?
    A. Squamous
    B. Intestinal
    C. Nephrogenic
    D. A and B
    E. All of the above

52. Which of the following types of metaplasia is associated with neoplasia?
    A. Vaginal squamous metaplasia
    B. Nonkeratinizing squamous metaplasia
    C. Intestinal metaplasia
    D. Nephrogenic metaplasia
    E. Cystitis cystica

53. Which of the following organisms is associated with squamous cell carcinoma of the urinary bladder?
    A. *Proteus mirabilis*
    B. *Schistosoma haematobium*
    C. *Schistosoma japonicum*
    D. *Schistosoma mansoni*
    E. BK virus

16: Urinary Tract Questions

54. The majority of urinary bladder lesions occur in this location:
    A. Dome
    B. Trigone
    C. Anterior wall
    D. Bladder neck
    E. Urethra

55. Which of the following statements regarding urothelial carcinoma and its variants is NOT true?
    A. Urothelial carcinoma in situ is virtually always present in bladders excised for invasive carcinoma.
    B. The majority of urothelial neoplasms are composed of high-grade urothelial carcinoma.
    C. Small cell neuroendocrine carcinoma of the bladder portends a poor prognosis.
    D. Papillary urothelial neoplasm of low malignant potential can be distinguished from urothelial papilloma by the presence of atypical mitotic figures.
    E. Low-grade urothelial carcinoma can typically be diagnosed based on cystoscopic findings.

56. Which of the following immunohistochemical markers is typically NOT positive in urothelial carcinoma?
    A. CK7
    B. CK20
    C. CEA
    D. CD15
    E. CD45

57. Which of the following factors is NOT an independent negative prognostic factor in urothelial carcinoma?
    A. Presence of dysplasia
    B. Presence of muscle invasion
    C. Presence of lymph node metastasis
    D. Presence of vascular invasion
    E. Primary tumor location in bladder neck

58. Which of the following is NOT a feature of inverted papilloma?
    A. Jigsaw pattern composed of cords and nests of urothelial cells invaginating into the lamina propria
    B. Presence of fibrovascular cores
    C. Cellular atypia
    D. Squamous metaplasia
    E. Exophytic growth on gross examination

59. Which of the following histologic features is characteristic of exophytic papilloma?
    A. Cellular atypia
    B. Absence of fibrovascular stalks
    C. Prominent reactive nucleoli
    D. Detrusor muscle invasion
    E. Extension of tumor cells into adjacent urothelium at base of stalk

16: Urinary Tract Questions

Questions 60-64 are based on the following image:

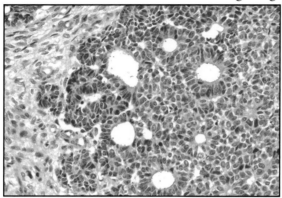

60. The most common genitourinary cancer in children (depicted in this image) is:
    A. Nephroblastoma
    B. Mesoblastic nephroma
    C. Clear cell sarcoma
    D. Angiomyolipoma
    E. Cystic nephroma

61. All of the following are features commonly associated with this lesion EXCEPT:
    A. Bulging, friable cut surface
    B. Scattered hemorrhagic and necrotic foci
    C. Infiltrative edges
    D. Renal vein invasion
    E. Lymph node metastasis

62. Which of the following is NOT a component of this lesion?
    A. Blastema
    B. Epithelium
    C. Stroma
    D. Microcalcifications
    E. None of the above

63. All of the following are TRUE regarding anaplasia in this lesion EXCEPT:
    A. It is defined by the presence of multipolar mitotic figures.
    B. It is defined by marked nuclear enlargement with nuclei being at least 3 times that of nonanaplastic nuclei in other microscopic fields.
    C. It is more common in patients over the age of 6 years.
    D. It is present in approximately 5% of tumors.
    E. It is a sign of more aggressive tumors.

64. Which of the following conditions is NOT associated with this lesion?
    A. Denys-Drash syndrome
    B. Beckwith-Wiedemann syndrome
    C. WAGR syndrome
    D. Klinefelter syndrome
    E. Familial nephroblastoma

16: Urinary Tract Questions

65. All of the following are features of the lesion depicted in this image EXCEPT:

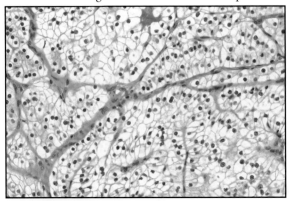

    A.   Association with von Hippel-Lindau syndrome
    B.   May exhibit foci of sarcomatous differentiation
    C.   Network of delicate capillaries supported by thin reticulin fibers
    D.   Immunoreactivity with CD10 and EMA
    E.   Immunoreactivity with CD10 and CK7

66. Which of the following features is NOT associated with the lesion depicted in this image?

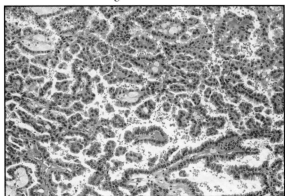

    A.   Fibrovascular stalks lined by neoplastic cells
    B.   Lipid- and hemosiderin-laden macrophages
    C.   Trisomy 17
    D.   von Hippel-Lindau syndrome
    E.   Immunoreactivity with CK7

67. Which of the following statements regarding the lesion depicted in this image is FALSE?

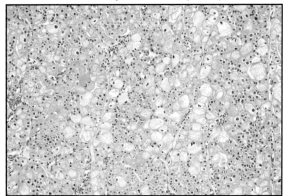 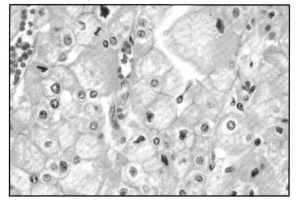

    A.   Pathognomonic gross appearance is characterized by brown cut surface and absence of hemorrhage or necrosis.

    B.   It stains positive with Hale colloidal iron.

    C.   It has a biphasic tumor population composed of acidophilic cells and perivascular transparent cells.

    D.   It has immunoreactivity with CK7.

    E.   Its survival rate exceeds 80%.

Questions 68 and 69 are based on the following image:

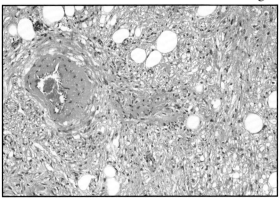

68. Which of the following features is NOT associated with this lesion?
    A.   Predominantly composed of mature adipose tissue
    B.   Delicate capillary network
    C.   PAS positive, diastase resistant intracellular granules
    D.   Immunoreactivity with HMB45 and CD117
    E.   Structures resembling abnormal melanosomes by electron microscopy

69. Which of the following disorders is associated with this lesion?
    A.   MEN type IIB
    B.   Autosomal recessive polycystic kidney disease
    C.   NF2
    D.   von Hippel-Lindau syndrome
    E.   Tuberous sclerosis

Questions 70-72 are based on the following image:

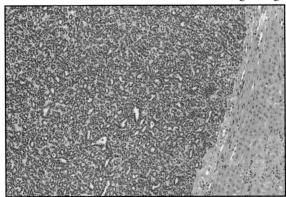

70. Which of the following findings is associated with this lesion?
    A. Hypertension
    B. Hypercalcemia
    C. Hypocalcemia
    D. Polycythemia
    E. Microcytic hypochromic anemia

71. Which of the following histologic features is NOT characteristic of this lesion?
    A. Densely packed, small tubules
    B. Small bland tumor cells with minimal cytoplasm
    C. Lipid-laden macrophages
    D. Glomeruloid and papillary structures
    E. Hyalinized stroma with scattered hemorrhage and necrosis

72. Which of the following tumors is associated with this lesion?
    A. Nephroblastoma
    B. Clear cell (conventional) renal cell carcinoma
    C. Chromophobe renal cell carcinoma
    D. Papillary renal cell carcinoma
    E. Cystic nephroma

16: Urinary Tract Questions

78. The most common cause of nephrotic syndrome in adults (depicted in this light microscopy and immunofluorescence image) is:

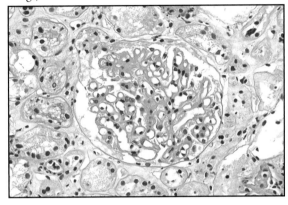 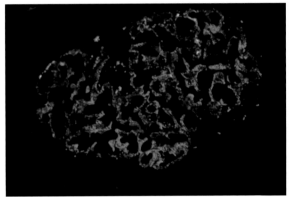

    A. Minimal change disease
    B. Focal segmental glomerulonephritis
    C. Membranous glomerulonephritis
    D. IgA nephropathy
    E. Acute proliferative glomerulonephritis

79. Based on this electron microscopy image, which of the following is the best diagnosis?

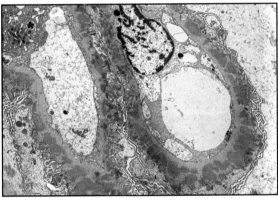

    A. Minimal change disease
    B. Focal segmental glomerulosclerosis
    C. Membranous glomerulonephritis
    D. Rapidly progressive glomerulonephritis
    E. IgA nephropathy

16: Urinary Tract Questions

80.   Which of the following best explains the rapid recurrence of disease seen in transplanted patients with the disease depicted in this image?

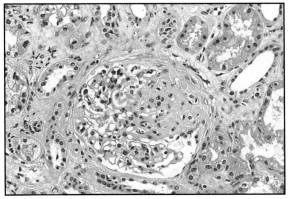

      A.   High incidence of disease in the donor population
      B.   Chronic infection
      C.   HLA antibodies
      D.   ABO incompatibility
      E.   Circulating permeability factor

81.   Which of the following findings is/are depicted in this light microscopy image?

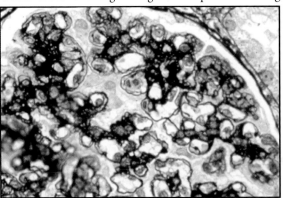

      A.   Type I membranoproliferative glomerulonephritis
      B.   Type II membranoproliferative glomerulonephritis
      C.   Rapidly progressive glomerulonephritis
      D.   Membranous glomerulonephritis
      E.   A and B

16: Urinary Tract Answers

9.   A.   **1-YEAR-OLD MALE**
90% of all rhabdoid tumors are diagnosed in patients less than 3 years of age. There is a slight male predilection. Choice A best represents these demographics.
QCSP, **Rhabdoid Tumor,** p 522.

10.   D.   **FINELY GRANULAR CHROMATIN WITH MULTIPLE INCONSPICUOUS NUCLEOLI**
Rhabdoid tumors typically exhibit an infiltrative growth pattern and are composed of sheets of large polygonal tumor cells with distinct cell borders (choices A, B). Tumor cells contain a single prominent nucleolus, which is usually visible at low power (choice D). Clusters of cells with eosinophilic, fibrillary cytoplasmic inclusions impart a "rhabdoid" appearance on this tumor (choice C). Immunohistochemical staining for EMA is positive (choice E).
QCSP, **Rhabdoid Tumor,** p 522-523.

11.   B.   **LOSS OF HETEROZYGOSITY ON 22Q11-12**
Rhabdoid tumor of the kidney and atypical teratoid/rhabdoid tumor of the central nervous system both share aberrations of chromosome 22 involving the INI1 gene. In the case of rhabdoid tumor of the kidney, the aberration in 80% of patients is a loss of heterozygosity on 22q11-12 (choice B). Immunohistochemistry for INI1 will show absent nuclear staining in tumor cells. The chromosomal translocation t(12;22)(q13;q12) is characteristic of clear cell sarcoma of soft tissue (choice A), while deletion of chromosome 3p may be seen with some clear cell (conventional) renal carcinomas (choice C). Translocations involving Xp11.2 are classified as Xp11.2 translocation carcinoma (choice D). Monosomy of chromosome 22 may be seen in rhabdoid tumors of the kidney, but is not the most common molecular alteration (choice E).
QCSP, **Rhabdoid Tumor,** p 523.

12.   A.   **SCROTAL VARICOCELE**
While scrotal varicocele may be the initial presentation of patients with obstruction of the spermatic vein (choice A), the classic triad of symptoms seen in renal cell carcinoma is comprised of flank pain, palpable flank mass, and hematuria (choices B, C, D).
QCSP, **Renal Cell Carcinoma,** p 523,

13.   E.   **INCREASED SERUM CREATININE**
All of the findings listed are associated with renal cell carcinoma except for choice E.
QCSP, **Renal Cell Carcinoma,** p 523.

14.   E.   **TYPE 2: STRATIFIED LAYER OF CELLS WITH ATYPICAL NUCLEAR FEATURES AND ABUNDANT EOSINOPHILIC CYTOPLASM, PRESENTATION WITH ADVANCED DISEASE**
Papillary renal cell carcinoma may be divided into types 1 and 2 with variable disease presentation and histologic features. Type 1 papillary renal cell carcinomas typically present with localized disease and have a good prognosis. Histologic features include fibrovascular stalks lined by a single layer of bland cells with scant basophilic cytoplasm. Type 2 papillary renal cell carcinomas, on the other hand, may present with advanced disease. The fibrovascular stalks here are lined by stratified atypical nuclei with abundant eosinophilic cytoplasm (choice E).
QCSP, **Renal Cell Carcinoma,** p 525-527.

15.   B.   **ABUNDANT HEMORRHAGE AND NECROSIS**
Carcinoma of the collecting ducts of Bellini most frequently arises in the renal medulla and histologically exhibits an admixture of neoplastic tubules and papillae lined by high-grade nuclei with a hobnail appearance (choices A, C). Not infrequently, the tumor infiltrates the adjacent tissue, inciting a prominent desmoplastic stromal

response (choice E). Despite successful surgical resection, death due to metastasis occurs in about half of patients (choice D). Hemorrhage and necrosis is not typical (choice B).

QCSP, **Renal Cell Carcinoma,** p 524-527.

16. C. **SICKLE CELL TRAIT**
     Renal medullary carcinoma arises almost exclusively in association with sickle cell trait (choice C). The prognosis is abysmal with the vast majority of patients succumbing to their disease due to hematogenous and lymphatic metastases.

     QCSP, **Renal Cell Carcinoma,** p 528.

17. D. **TFE3**
     As implied by the name, Xp11.2 translocation carcinoma is defined by the presence of its characteristic translocation, the gene product of which is TFE3 (choice D). While CD10, EMA, CK7, and INI1 are also variably positive, their presence does not exclusively support the diagnosis of Xp11.2 translocation carcinoma.

     QCSP, **Renal Cell Carcinoma,** p 526.

18. C. **HEAVY ALCOHOL CONSUMPTION**
     All of these have been identified as risk factors for renal cell carcinoma except for heavy alcohol consumption (choice C).

     QCSP, **Renal Cell Carcinoma,** p 528.

19. D. **PROGNOSIS**
     Unlike classic angiomyolipoma, which is a benign lesion typically resected for progressive renal failure or massive hemorrhage, the epithelioid variant is a potentially malignant neoplasm with a significant risk of metastasis (choice D).

     QCSP, **Angiomyolipoma,** p 528-529.

20. C. **20%**
     Based on autopsy data, renal cortical adenomas are incidentally discovered in 20% of individuals.

     QCSP, **Renal Cortical Adenoma,** p 530.

21. D. **A AND B**
     Renal cortical adenoma is composed of densely packed tubules and papillae lined by bland cuboidal cells with uniform nuclei (choice B). Lipid-laden macrophages may be present in the interstitial space (choice A). Cellular atypia, on the other hand, is not common and should raise concern for papillary renal cell carcinoma (choice C).

     QCSP, **Renal Cortical Adenoma,** p 530.

22. B. **BECKWITH-WIEDEMANN SYNDROME**
     All of the choices listed have been associated with renal cortical adenoma except for choice B.

     QCSP, **Renal Cortical Adenoma,** p 531.

23. B. **HALE COLLOIDAL IRON**
     The Hale colloidal iron stain highlights the mucopolysaccharide background as well as a reticular pattern of cytoplasmic staining seen in chromophobe renal cell carcinoma, while oncocytomas are negative (choice B). Both oncocytoma and chromophobe renal cell carcinoma show immunoreactivity for CK7 (choice A) and are negative for vimentin (choice E). PAS with diastase (choice D) will highlight the abundant glycogen component of clear cell renal cell carcinoma and CD10 (choice C) is immunoreactive in clear cell renal cell carcinoma and papillary renal cell carcinoma.

     QCSP, **Oncocytoma,** p 532.

24. D. **ASSOCIATION WITH RENAL CELL CARCINOMA**
     Medullary fibromas are a common incidental finding without clinical significance. The tumor is composed of bland, small cells in a loose collagenized mucopolysaccharide matrix (choice E). Amyloid and neutral lipids are typically present (choices A, B). An association with hypertension has been reported (choice C).
     QCSP, **Medullary Fibroma,** p 532-533.

25. E. **FOCI OF CARTILAGE**
     The differential between multilocular cystic renal cell carcinoma and cystic nephroma may be challenging at times; however, features supporting malignancy include solid mural nodules, hemorrhage, necrosis, and cellular atypia (choices A, B, C, D). Extensive sampling is required to rule out malignancy. Foci of cartilage may be present in cystic nephroma (choice E).
     QCSP, **Cystic Nephroma,** p 533.

26. E. **ALL OF THE ABOVE**
     Acute proliferative glomerulonephritis is an immune-mediated process most commonly due to post-infectious antigen-antibody complex deposition in the kidney with resulting glomerulonephritis. Typical laboratory findings include low complement levels, elevated anti-streptococcal antibody titers (although antecedent nonstreptococcal infections have also been described), red cell casts, and azotemia (choices A, B, C and D).
     QCSP, **Acute Proliferative Glomerulonephritis,** p 533.

27. D. **TYPE III: IgA NEPHROPATHY**
     Type I rapidly progressive glomerulonephritis (RPGN) is characterized by antibodies to the basement membrane, such as those seen in Goodpasture syndrome (choice A). Type II RPGN is characterized by immune complex-deposition and may be associated with multiple diseases, including Henoch-Schönlein purpura, systemic lupus erythematosus (choices B, C), but also IgA nephropathy (choice D). Type III RPGN is characterized by a lack of detectable immune complexes and basement membrane antibodies, and is typified by Wegener granulomatosis (choice E).
     QCSP, **Rapidly Progressive Glomerulonephritis,** p 534.

28. E. **ALL OF THE ABOVE**
     Reflecting the broad spectrum of diseases underlying rapidly progressive glomerulonephritis, multiple approaches have proven useful in treatment including all of the choices listed.
     QCSP, **Rapidly Progressive Glomerulonephritis,** p 535.

29. E. **ALL OF THE ABOVE**
     The prevalence of secondary membranous glomerulonephritis is 20%-25%. Factors associated with secondary membranous glomerulonephritis include drugs, malignancy, metabolic disorders, systemic lupus erythematosus, and a myriad of infectious agents such as hepatitis B and C. It is important to distinguish primary from secondary membranous glomerulonephritis because treatment of the underlying disease or discontinuation of the offending drug can result in remission. A particularly helpful clue is the identification of endothelial tubuloreticular inclusions which are seen in patients with systemic lupus erythematosus and chronic hepatitis patients treated with interferon.
     QCSP, **Membranous Glomerulonephritis,** p 535.

30. C. **HUMAN IMMUNODEFICIENCY VIRUS**
     Of the choices listed, only the human immunodeficiency virus (HIV) has not been shown to be associated with minimal change disease (choice C). However, HIV has been associated with acute proliferative glomerulonephritis and focal segmental glomerulosclerosis.
     QCSP, **Minimal Change Disease,** p 537.

16: Urinary Tract Answers

31. C. **TSC2**

Familial focal segmental sclerosis has been associated with 4 separate genes, including NPHS, ACTN4, TRPC6, and PLCE1 (choices A, B, D, E). TSC2 is one of 2 genes associated with tuberous sclerosis (choice C).

QCSP, **Focal Segmental Glomerulosclerosis,** p 538.

32. B. **SMOKING**

Focal segmental glomerulosclerosis has been associated with all of the choices listed except for smoking (choice B).

QCSP, **Focal Segmental Glomerulosclerosis,** p 538.

33. C. **AMYLOIDOSIS**

Secondary membranoproliferative glomerulonephritis has been described arising in all of the settings listed except for amyloidosis (choice C).

QCSP, **Membranoproliferative Glomerulonephritis,** p 538.

34. D. **GRANULAR SUBENDOTHELIAL DEPOSITS OF C3 AND IGG**

Unlike type II membranoproliferative glomerulonephritis (MPGN), type I MPGN is characterized by granular subendothelial deposits comprised of C3 as well as IgG (choice D). Type II MPGN lacks IgG deposits and has typical linear intramembranous electron-dense deposits, which is why it is sometimes known as "dense deposit disease" (choice A, B). Type II MPGN is associated with partial lipodystrophy (choice C). Both types exhibit "tram-track" glomerular capillary walls (choice E).

QCSP, **Membranoproliferative Glomerulonephritis,** p 538-539.

35. D. **HEMATURIA**

50% of patients with IgA nephropathy present with gross hematuria, which resolves in the majority of cases (choice D). The other symptoms are less common.

QCSP, **Iga Nephropathy,** p 539.

36. C. **MESANGIAL DEPOSITS OF IMMUNE COMPLEXES**

IgA nephropathy is characterized by mesangial deposits of immune complexes by electron microscopy (choice C). Choices A, B, D, and E describe type II membranoproliferative glomerulonephritis, acute proliferative glomerulonephritis, type I membranoproliferative glomerulonephritis, and membranous glomerulonephritis, respectively.

QCSP, **Iga Nephropathy,** p 539.

37. C. **30%**

Chronic renal failure develops over a long period of time in 25%-50% of patients with IgA nephropathy (choice C). This statistic is useful to know, since IgA nephropathy is relatively common in the population.

QCSP, **Iga Nephropathy,** p 539.

38. C. **SEGMENTAL NECROSIS**

As the name implies, segmental necrosis is a key feature of this entity (choice C). The uninvolved portion of glomerulus is typically unremarkable. The other features are not characteristic of focal proliferative and necrotizing glomerulonephritis.

QCSP, **Focal Proliferative and Necrotizing Glomerulonephritis,** p 540.

39. A. **ACUTE PROLIFERATIVE GLOMERULONEPHRITIS < IGA NEPHROPATHY < FOCAL SEGMENTAL GLOMERULOSCLEROSIS < RAPIDLY PROGRESSIVE GLOMERULOSCLEROSIS**
The percentages of patients progressing to chronic glomerulonephritis for acute proliferative glomerulonephritis, IgA nephropathy, focal segmental glomerulosclerosis, and rapidly progressive glomerulosclerosis are 1%, 25%-50%, 50%-80%, and 90%, respectively. Choice A lists these entities in the correct order.
QCSP, **Chronic Glomerulonephritis,** p 540.

40. E. **NEUTROPHILIC INFILTRATE**
While a lymphocytic infiltrate may be present in chronic glomerulonephritis, neutrophils are not a common finding (choice E).
QCSP, **Chronic Glomerulonephritis,** p 540.

41. B. **MICHAELIS-GUTMANN BODIES**
Michaelis-Guttman bodies representing remnants of ingested Gram negative bacteria are required for the diagnosis of malakoplakia (choice B). Lipid-laden macrophages and microabscesses are universal features of xanthogranulomatous pyelonephritis (choices A, E). Gamna-Gandy and asteroid bodies are seen in sickle cell disease and sarcoidosis, among other diseases, respectively (choices C, D).
QCSP, **Xanthogranulomatous Pyelonephritis,** p 541.

42. C. **ASSOCIATION WITH NEOPLASIA**
Ask-Upmark kidney is a type of congenital unilateral renal hypoplasia with is associated with hypertension, possibly because of stenotic arcuate and interlobular arteries (choices A, B, D). The number of medullary pyramids is reduced (choice E). Although the kidney may mimic a renal neoplasm resulting in nephrectomy, there is no definitive association with neoplasia (choice C).
QCSP, **Ask-Upmark Kidney,** p 541.

43. E. **ALL OF THE ABOVE**
When confronted with an elevated PSA, it is important to keep in mind that the differential diagnosis includes nonneoplastic entities such as nodular hyperplasia (choice B), the biopsy itself (choice C), and digital rectal examination (choice E).
QCSP, **Prostate,** Adenocarcinoma, p 542.

44. A. **CELLULAR PLEOMORPHISM**
Cellular pleomorphism is not a characteristic feature of prostatic adenocarcinoma (choice A), although nuclei are frequently enlarged and contain prominent nucleoli (choice C). Intraluminal mucinous secretions, absence of a basal layer, and small, haphazardly arranged glands are features associated with prostatic adenocarcinoma (choices B, D, E).
QCSP, **Prostate,** Adenocarcinoma, p 542.

45. D. **GLEASON GRADE 4**
The presence of fused glands as well as cribriform growth describes a Gleason grade 4 pattern (choice D).
QCSP, **Prostate,** Adenocarcinoma, p 542-543.

46. C. **ADENOSQUAMOUS CELL CARCINOMA: GLEASON GRADE 5**
Squamous differentiation in squamous and adenosquamous carcinoma of the prostate is associated with a poor prognosis and decreased response to hormone therapy. Neither of these variants is graded using Gleason grading (choice C). Mucinous adenocarcinoma frequently exhibits cribriform growth, while signet ring adenocarcinoma typically grows in Indian file, acinar, or single cell pattern, reflecting Gleason grades 4 and 5, respectively (choices A, B). Prostatic duct adenocarcinoma should be graded as Gleason grade 4, unless the presence of comedonecrosis

warrants upgrading (choice D). Basaloid carcinoma of the prostate is not graded using Gleason grading (choice E).

QCSP, **Prostate,** Adenocarcinoma, Variants, p 543-544.

47.   B.   **LEIOMYOMA**

The most common benign mesenchymal tumor of the prostate is a leiomyoma.

QCSP, **Prostate,** Adenocarcinoma, p 544.

48.   D.   **PARTIAL ATROPHY: PRESENCE OF MICRONUCLEOLI**

There are numerous benign mimics of prostatic adenocarcinoma and the differential may be challenging. However, all of the paired features listed may be helpful in distinguishing the two entities from each other except for the presence of micronucleoli (choice D). Although prostatic adenocarcinoma frequently exhibits nucleoli more prominent than the ones seen in partial atrophy, this feature may be concerning and cannot reliably distinguish between the two entities.

QCSP, **Prostate,** Adenocarcinoma, p 544.

49.   E.   **T3**

Prostatic adenocarcinoma involving the seminal vesicles defines clinical stage T3 (Choice E).

QCSP, **Prostate,** Adenocarcinoma, p 545.

50.   E.   *ASPERGILLUS FUMIGATUS*

While mycotic prostatitis in general is not a common entity, the most common offending organisms include *Mycobacterium tuberculosis, Blastomyces dermatitides, Coccidioides immitis,* and *Cryptococcus neoformans* (choices A, B, C and D). Infection with *Aspergillus fumigatus,* although described, is considerably less common (choice E).

QCSP, **Prostatic Infections,** p 546.

51.   E.   **ALL OF THE ABOVE**

Asymptomatic metaplastic lesions of the urinary bladder are of 3 types: squamous, intestinal, and nephrogenic (choice E).

QCSP, **Urinary Bladder,** Metaplastic Lesions, p 546.

52.   C.   **INTESTINAL METAPLASIA**

Nonkeratinizing squamous and nephrogenic metaplasia may be seen as benign reactive lesions which form in response to chronic irritation and have no known association with neoplasia (choices A, B, D). Keratinizing squamous metaplasia, on the other hand, has a low risk of developing subsequent carcinoma and is associated with *Schistosoma haematobium* infection. Cystitis cystica is likewise induced by chronic irritation and has not been shown to be a precursor to malignancy (choice E). Extensive intestinal metaplasia is a precursor lesion in most nonurachal adenocarcinomas (choice C).

QCSP, **Urinary Bladder,** Metaplastic Lesions, p 547.

53.   B.   *SCHISTOSOMA HAEMATOBIUM*

Schistosoma haematobium is associated with squamous cell carcinoma of the urinary bladder and is the only *Schistosoma* species to specifically infect the urinary tract (choice B).

QCSP, **Urothelial Carcinoma,** p 547.

54.   B.   **TRIGONE**

The majority of urinary bladder lesions occur in the trigone. While the bladder neck does form a part of the trigone, the best answer here is choice B, since this includes the ureteral orifices as well.

QCSP, **Urothelial Carcinoma,** p 548.

55. D. **PAPILLARY UROTHELIAL NEOPLASM OF LOW MALIGNANT POTENTIAL CAN BE DISTINGUISHED FROM UROTHELIAL PAPILLOMA BY THE PRESENCE OF ATYPICAL MITOTIC FIGURES.**

Invasive carcinoma of the bladder is virtually always accompanied by an element of urothelial carcinoma in situ (choice A). Approximately half of urothelial neoplasms consist of high-grade urothelial carcinoma (choice B). The small cell variant, in particular, portends a very poor prognosis (choice C). Low-grade, in contrast to high-grade urothelial carcinoma, more commonly presents as small papillary lesions, which are well visualized on cystoscopy, although the diagnosis may be challenging based on urinary cytology (choice E). Papillary urothelial neoplasm of low malignant potential has only rare mitotic figures and can be distinguished from a benign papilloma by the presence of a thicker urothelial layer and larger nuclei (choice D).

QCSP, **Urothelial Carcinoma,** p 548-549.

56. E. **CD45**

While CK7 may be negative, CK7, CK20, CEA, and CD15 are typically expressed in urothelial carcinoma (choices A, B, C, D). CD45 expression is not typically seen (choice E).

QCSP, **Urothelial Carcinoma,** p 549.

57. A. **PRESENCE OF DYSPLASIA**

All of the choices presented are associated with a worse prognosis except for the presence of dysplasia (choice A).

QCSP, **Urothelial Carcinoma,** p 550.

58. B. **PRESENCE OF FIBROVASCULAR CORES**

The inverted variant of urothelial papilloma can be differentiated from the exophytic variant only on the basis of microscopic examination as both types exhibit grossly exophytic growth (choice E). The inverted papilloma is composed of urothelial cells which invaginate into the lamina propria and may exhibit some degree of cellular atypia and squamous metaplasia (choices A, C, D). Fibrovascular cores are not typically present (choice B).

QCSP, **Urothelial Papilloma,** p 551.

59. E. **EXTENSION OF TUMOR CELLS INTO ADJACENT UROTHELIUM AT BASE OF STALK**

Unlike the inverted papilloma, exophytic papillomas exhibit no apparent cellular atypia, but do have fibrovascular stalks (choices A, B). Nucleoli are inconspicuous (choice C). There is no muscle invasion (choice D). The tumor cells do frequently extend into the epithelium immediately adjacent to the papilloma at the base of the stalk (choice E).

QCSP, **Urothelial Papilloma,** p 551.

60. A. **NEPHROBLASTOMA**

Nephroblastoma (Wilms tumor) represents 80% of all genitourinary neoplasms in patients under the age of 15 years (choice A).

QCSP, **Nephroblastoma,** p 517.

61. C. **INFILTRATIVE EDGES**

Nephroblastomas are typically solitary and well-circumscribed, although invasion into the renal vein and lymph node metastasis are common (choices D, E). The tumor is usually bulging and friable and may exhibit hemorrhage and necrosis (choices A, B). The edges are not usually visibly infiltrative (choice C).

QCSP, **Nephroblastoma,** p 517.

62. D. **MICROCALCIFICATIONS**

Although nephroblastomas may exhibit any combination of the components listed, most tumors are triphasic and contain blastemal, epithelial, and stromal elements (choices A-C).

QCSP, **Nephroblastoma,** p 517.

63.   E.   **IT IS A SIGN OF MORE AGGRESSIVE TUMORS.**
      Anaplasia in nephroblastoma is defined as extreme nuclear atypia using the criteria of multipolar mitotic figures and marked nuclear enlargement with nuclei at least 3 times the size of nonanaplastic nuclei (choices A, B). These features are more commonly seen in older patients and represent approximately 5% of tumors (choices C, D). This is a finer point, but it is of minor interest that the presence of anaplasia is not a sign of more aggressive tumors per se, but rather a predictor of lack of response to chemotherapy (choice E).
      QCSP, **Nephroblastoma,** p 518-519.

64.   D.   **KLINEFELTER SYNDROME**
      All of the other listed conditions (choices A-C, E) are associated with an increased risk for the development of nephroblastoma.
      QCSP, **Nephroblastoma,** p 519.

65.   E.   **IMMUNOREACTIVITY WITH CD10 AND CK7**
      The clear cell variant of renal cell carcinoma is the most common variant and is associated with von Hippel-Lindau syndrome (choice A). Sarcomatous differentiation may be present and confers the worst prognosis of all variants (choice B). A network of delicate capillaries is typical (choice C). Immunoreactivity with CD10 supports the diagnosis, although low molecular weight cytokeratins, CK7, and CD20 are negative (choices D, E).
      QCSP, **Renal Cell Carcinoma,** p 524-526.

66.   D.   **VON HIPPEL-LINDAU SYNDROME.**
      Papillary renal cell carcinoma is characterized by fibrovascular stalks lined by neoplastic cells and contains frequent lipid- and hemosiderin-laden macrophages, which may be visualized by special stains and electron microscopy (choices A, B). The tumor is associated with cortical adenomas as well as trisomy 17. Unlike clear cell (conventional) renal cell carcinoma, papillary renal cell carcinoma is immunoreactive with CK7 (choice E). An association with von Hippel-Lindau syndrome has not been described.
      QCSP, **Renal Cell Carcinoma,** p 525-527.

67.   A.   **PATHOGNOMONIC GROSS APPEARANCE IS CHARACTERIZED BY BROWN CUT SURFACE AND ABSENCE OF HEMORRHAGE OR NECROSIS.**
      Chromophobe renal cell carcinoma is a well-circumscribed, solitary tumor typically characterized by a brown cut surface without hemorrhage or necrosis, a gross appearance shared by renal oncocytoma (choice A). Positive staining with Hale colloidal iron as well as the characteristic biphasic tumor population supports the diagnosis of chromophobe renal cell carcinoma (choices B, C). Staining for CK7 is typically positive (choice D), and the prognosis is good (choice E).
      QCSP, **Renal Cell Carcinoma,** p 524-527.

68.   B.   **DELICATE CAPILLARY NETWORK**
      Angiomyolipomas are common renal neoplasms, which have a typical radiographic appearance obviating the need for resection in many instances and therefore are often seen at autopsy. The tumor is typically predominantly composed of mature adipose tissue (choice A) and contains thick, abnormal vessels with aberrant internal elastic laminae (choice B). PAS-positive diastase-resistant granules are the rule, as is immunoreactivity with HMB45 and CD117 (choices C, D). Structures resembling abnormal melanosomes may be seen by electron microscopy (choice E).
      QCSP, **Angiomyolipoma,** p 528-529.

69.   E.   **TUBEROUS SCLEROSIS**
      Tuberous sclerosis (choice E) is an autosomal dominant disorder characterized by hamartomas and benign neoplastic lesions affecting many different organ systems. Neurologic symptoms including epilepsy and mental

retardation are the most frequent and serious manifestations; however, renal angiomyolipomas are a major feature of the disorder, which is caused by a mutation of the *TSC1* gene on 9q or the *TSC2* gene on 16p. von Hippel-Lindau syndrome (choice D) is associated with renal cell carcinoma not angiomyolipoma. Neurofibromatosis type 1 is associated with fibromuscular dysplasia/hyperplasia of the renal artery and angiomyolipomas unlike neurofibromatosis type 2 (choice C), which is not characteristically associated with any renal lesions.

QCSP, **Angiomyolipoma,** p 529, WHO CNS page 205, 218.

70. D. POLYCYTHEMIA

Only choice D has been consistently described with metanephric adenoma (up to 15% of patients).

QCSP, **Metanephric Adenoma,** p 529.

71. C. LIPID-LADEN MACROPHAGES

Metanephric adenoma is a well-circumscribed tumor composed predominantly of densely packed tubules lined by bland tumor cells with minimal cytoplasm (choices A, B). Glomeruloid and papillary structures associated with microcalcifications may be present in 1/2 of cases (choice D). The background stroma exhibits hyalinization, hemorrhage, and necrosis (choice E).

QCSP, **Metanephric Adenoma,** p 530.

72. B. CLEAR CELL (CONVENTIONAL) RENAL CELL CARCINOMA

Approximately 10% of patients with metanephric adenoma have concurrent clear cell renal cell carcinomas (choice B).

QCSP, **Metanephric Adenoma,** p 530.

73. E. STROMAL DESMOPLASIA

Renal oncocytoma is characterized by a classic gross appearance described as a mahogany tumor with well-defined borders and a central scar (choice A). The tumor may contain scattered mitotic figures and clear cells, but the absence of both is typical (choices B, C). Infiltrative growth with stromal desmoplasia is highly unusual and most likely represents a different entity (choice E).

QCSP, **Oncocytoma,** p 531.

74. B. FEMALES

Cystic nephroma exhibits a marked female predilection with a ratio of 8:1 (choice B).

QCSP, **Cystic Nephroma,** p 533.

75. A. ACUTE PROLIFERATIVE GLOMERULONEPHRITIS

This electron microscopy image depicts subepithelial electron-dense "humps" representing deposition of antigen-antibody complexes characteristic of acute proliferative glomerulonephritis (choice A). Occasional cases of rapidly progressive glomerulonephritis may exhibit granular deposits unlike the ones seen here (choice B). Membranous glomerulonephritis and dense deposit disease are also characterized by deposits, although these appear as irregular spikes and continuous intramembranous ribbons, respectively (choices C, E). Minimal change disease lacks deposits (choice D). The only alteration seen by electron microscopy is effacement of the visceral epithelial foot processes.

QCSP, **Acute Proliferative Glomerulonephritis,** p 534.

76. A. ADULTS HAVE A WORSE PROGNOSIS THAN CHILDREN.

Acute proliferative glomerulonephritis is typically a self-limited disease with a particularly good prognosis in children. Rapidly progressive and chronic glomerulonephritis occur in 1% of children (choices B, C). Therapy is conservative and does not require steroids (choice D). Since the disease is usually a consequence of a transient bacterial or viral infection, it does not recur in transplanted organs (choice E). The prognosis is less favorable in adults, 40% of which do not recover full renal function (choice A).

QCSP, **Acute Proliferative Glomerulonephritis,** p 534.

77. E. **GOODPASTURE SYNDROME**
The light microscopy image with Jones stain depicts crescent formation, characteristic of rapidly progressive glomerulonephritis. Additional information is provided by the immunofluorescence (IF) image, which demonstrates linear IgG deposits, characteristic of Goodpasture syndrome (choice E). While crescent formation may be seen with Wegener granulomatosis (choice A) and less commonly IgA nephropathy (choice B), the latter findings support the diagnosis of Goodpasture syndrome. Focal segmental and membranoproliferative glomerulonephritis lack the histologic and IF appearance seen here (choices C, D).
QCSP, **Rapidly Progressive Glomerulonephritis,** p 535.

78. C. **MEMBRANOUS GLOMERULONEPHRITIS**
The most common causes of nephrotic syndrome in adults and children are membranous glomerulonephritis and minimal change disease, respectively (choices C, A). IgA nephropathy and acute proliferative glomerulonephritis typically present with nephritic rather than nephrotic syndrome (choices D, E). The light microscopy image highlights a thickening of the basement membrane, while the immunofluorescence image demonstrates the characteristic beaded appearance of membranous glomerulonephritis.
QCSP, **Membranous Glomerulonephritis,** p 535.

79. C. **MEMBRANOUS GLOMERULONEPHRITIS**
This image demonstrates intramembranous electron-dense deposits surrounded by spikes of basement membrane material, which is diagnostic of membranous glomerulonephritis (choice C). Minimal change disease and focal segmental glomerulosclerosis are characterized by a lack of electron-dense deposits (choices A, B). The deposits seen in IgA nephropathy are mesangial, not intramembranous (choice E). RPGN may present with a variety of findings by electron microscopy; however, this image is more characteristic of membranous glomerulonephritis (choice D).
QCSP, **Membranous Glomerulonephritis,** p 536.

80. E. **CIRCULATING PERMEABILITY FACTOR**
Recurrent proteinuria heralding recurrent disease has been described as early as 24 hours following transplantation in patients with focal segmental glomerulosclerosis. The leading explanation for this phenomenon at this time is that there may be a patient-specific circulating factor responsible for the damage, which is not eliminated at the time of transplantation (choice E).
QCSP, **Focal Segmental Glomerulosclerosis,** p 537.

81. E. **A AND B**
Shown in this image are the homogeneous "tram-track" glomerular capillary walls seen in type I and II membranoproliferative glomerulonephritis (choice E). None of the other entities are characterized by this finding.
QCSP, **Membranoproliferative Glomerulonephritis,** p 539.

82. A. **PRESENTATION IN 2ND DECADE**
Xanthogranulomatous pyelonephritis is typically diagnosed in females in their 4th to 6th decades (choices A, B). The involved kidney is usually nonfunctioning (choice C) and may contain calculi (choice E). Occasionally, this lesion may be mistaken for a neoplastic mass, especially since penetration of the adjacent fascia is not uncommon (choice D).
QCSP, **Xanthogranulomatous Pyelonephritis,** p 541.

83.   D.   **COLLAGENOUS NODULES**

All of the features listed are characteristic of prostatic nodular hyperplasia except for collagenous nodules (choice D). Collagenous nodules are a feature diagnostic of prostatic carcinoma and are often associated with abundant mucin production. The nodules can be found within the stroma adjacent to tumor glands or within the glandular lumina.

QCSP, **Prostatic Nodular Hyperplasia,** p 545-546.

Chapter 17

Mandible and Maxilla

1. Which of the following is NOT a well-recognized variant of ameloblastoma?
    A. Desmoplastic ameloblastoma
    B. Giant cell ameloblastoma
    C. Basal cell ameloblastoma
    D. Acanthomatous ameloblastoma
    E. Papilliferous ameloblastoma

2. Unicystic, peripheral, and desmoplastic ameloblastomas have a higher recurrence rate than the other variants.
    A. True
    B. False

3. Which of the following special stains can be useful for confirming the presence of acellular material between apposing rows of columnar cells in adenomatoid odontogenic tumors?
    A. Trichrome stain
    B. Reticulin stain
    C. Prussian blue iron stain
    D. Periodic acid-Schiff stain
    E. Fontana stain

4. Cementoblastomas histologically resemble osteoid osteomas and osteoblastomas.
    A. True
    B. False

5. Compound odontomas are defined by a chaotic arrangement of pulp, cementum, enamel, and dentin.
    A. True
    B. False

6. Ameloblastic fibromas contain dentin and/or enamel, are generally diagnosed after the age of 30, and generally occur in the maxilla.
    A. True
    B. False

7. Which of the following statements is TRUE regarding squamous odontogenic tumors?
    A. These tumors are uniformly seen before the age of 20.
    B. The great majority of these tumors develop within the maxilla.
    C. Atypia must be present within the squamous epithelium to make this diagnosis.
    D. 95% of these tumors have microscopic foci of degeneration and calcification within islands of squamous epithelium.
    E. Treatment includes extraction of the involved tooth in addition to conservative excision of the tumor.

8. An 18-year-old male is being seen by a dentist for the first time in several years. A radiograph demonstrates a sharply demarcated radiolucent lesion attached circumferentially to the neck of the patient's partially-erupted left mandibular 3rd molar. The patient denies any pain in this area. The most likely diagnosis is:
    A. Eruption cyst
    B. Dentigerous cyst (follicular cyst)
    C. Nasopalatine duct cyst
    D. Nasolabial cyst
    E. Melanotic neuroectodermal tumor of infancy (melanotic progonoma)

17: Mandible and Maxilla Questions

9. The 18-year-old patient in the question above is confused after reading about odontogenic cysts on the internet. He read about another odontogenic cyst that surrounds the crown of an erupting tooth but is predominantly located in the soft tissue surrounding the bone. According to his reading, this cyst usually presents as a blue swelling in the area of tooth eruption. Which of the following is most consistent with the lesion this patient is describing?
    A. Eruption cyst
    B. Gingival cyst of adults
    C. Nasopalatine duct cyst
    D. Nasolabial cyst
    E. Melanotic neuroectodermal tumor of infancy (melanotic progonoma)

10. Which of the following odontogenic cysts is thought to arise from dental lamina remnants and most commonly presents as a swelling in the canine-premolar area of the mandibular buccal gingiva?
    A. Eruption cyst
    B. Gingival cyst of adults
    C. Nasopalatine duct cyst
    D. Nasolabial cyst
    E. Dentigerous cyst

11. Gingival cysts of infants (Epstein pearls) generally develop around 6 months of age and are treated with simple excision.
    A. True
    B. False

12. Which of the following cysts is associated with a botryoid, or multicystic, variant that is aggressive and frequently recurs?
    A. Lateral periodontal cyst
    B. Gingival cyst of adults
    C. Nasolabial cyst
    D. Radicular cyst
    E. Nasopalatine duct cyst

13. A 28-year-old male presents with a cystic lesion of the anterior maxilla. The cyst is resected, and histologic examination reveals a cyst lined by nonkeratinized stratified squamous epithelium. Occasional intraepithelial hyaline (Rushton) bodies are present, and copious foamy macrophages are present within the cyst cavity. Heavy deposits of cholesterol crystals are seen within the fibrous cyst wall. The most likely diagnosis is:
    A. Giant cell granuloma
    B. Odontoma
    C. Eruption cyst
    D. Melanotic progonoma
    E. Radicular cyst

14. A 57-year-old male is being seen by his new dentist for an initial examination. The dentist notices a pronounced elevation of the anterior portion of the palate. An X-ray is performed, demonstrating a distinct, ovoid lucency in the midline of the anterior maxilla. Which of the following is the most likely diagnosis?
    A. Nasolabial cyst (nasoalveolar cyst)
    B. Nasopalatine duct cyst (incisive canal cyst)
    C. Radicular cyst
    D. Calcifying odontogenic cyst
    E. Dentigerous cyst (follicular cyst)

17: Mandible and Maxilla Questions

15. A 38-year-old female is seen by her new dentist for an initial examination. The dentist notices a pronounced swelling of the soft tissues of the canine fossa beneath the ala of the nose. An X-ray is performed, and the lesion is shown to be entirely extraosseous. Which of the following is the most likely diagnosis?
    A. Nasolabial cyst (nasoalveolar cyst)
    B. Nasopalatine duct cyst (incisive canal cyst)
    C. Radicular cyst
    D. Calcifying odontogenic cyst
    E. Dentigerous cyst (follicular cyst)

16. A 2-year-old boy is brought to a pediatrician by his parents for lower facial swelling that has been present for several months and is increasing in severity. The boy's mother had similar symptoms when she was younger that caused her to seek facial cosmetic surgery after college. Based on the family history and physical exam findings, the pediatrician correctly diagnoses cherubism (familial multilocular cystic disease of the jaws). Which of the following regarding cherubism is TRUE?
    A. Lesions most frequently develop during puberty.
    B. Cherubism tends to affect upper jaw, sparing the lower jaw quadrants.
    C. Surgical intervention is ideally performed before the cessation of bone growth.
    D. Radiotherapy has been shown to be curative in most cases.
    E. The condition usually becomes inactive by the 3rd decade of life.

17. Which of the following lesions is/are histologically indistinguishable from the affected jaw of a patient with cherubism?
    A. Giant cell granuloma
    B. Aneurysmal bone cyst (solid variant)
    C. Brown tumor ("osteoclastoma") of hyperparathyroidism
    D. All of the above
    E. None of the above

18. Which of the following immunohistochemical staining profiles is consistent with the large pigmented cells of melanotic neuroectodermal tumors of infancy?
    A. CD57–, HMB45–, vimentin–, cytokeratin–
    B. CD57+, HMB45+, vimentin+, cytokeratin–
    C. CD57–, HMB45+, vimentin+, cytokeratin+
    D. CD57–, HMB45–, vimentin+, cytokeratin–
    E. CD57+, HMB45+, vimentin+, cytokeratin+

17: Mandible and Maxilla Questions

19. A 39-year-old male is referred to an otolaryngologist for resection of a mandibular lesion that is associated with his left impacted mandibular third molar. A partial mandibulectomy is performed, and the pathologist renders a diagnosis. A photomicrograph of this odontogenic tumor is shown below. The most likely diagnosis is:

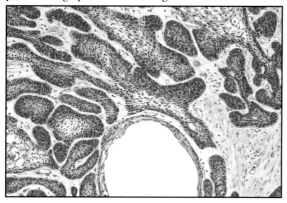

    A.   Pindborg tumor

    B.   Adenomatoid odontogenic tumor

    C.   Odontogenic myxoma

    D.   Cementoblastoma

    E.   Ameloblastoma

20. Photomicrographs of an intraosseous mandibular lesion are shown below. Which of the following statements regarding this lesion is TRUE?

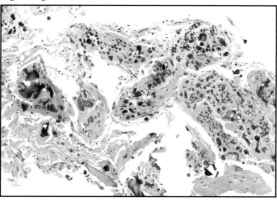 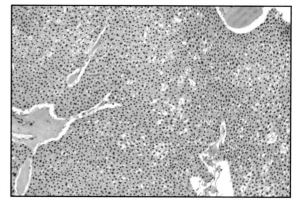

    A.   These tumors are typically less aggressive than ameloblastomas.

    B.   These tumors represent approximately 15% of all odontogenic tumors.

    C.   Most of these lesions occur in the maxilla.

    D.   Multinucleated giant cells are characteristically absent in these lesions.

    E.   There is no known association between these tumors and adenomatoid odontogenic tumors.

17: Mandible and Maxilla Questions

21. A 19-year-old female presents with a slowly enlarging, painless mass involving her maxilla. Radiographic studies demonstrate a distinct, unilocular lesion surrounding an impacted tooth. There are focal calcifications identified. The lesion is resected, and the pathologist notes that the tumor is composed of 2 types of epithelial cells: polyhedral cells arranged in large nodular aggregates, and columnar cells surrounding ductlike spaces. A photomicrograph of the lesion is shown below. The most likely diagnosis is:

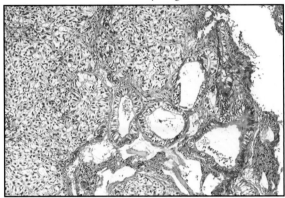

A. Odontogenic fibroma
B. Adenomatoid odontogenic tumor
C. Ameloblastoma
D. Pindborg tumor
E. Odontoma

22. A photomicrograph of an odontogenic myxoma is shown below. Which of the following is TRUE of this lesion?

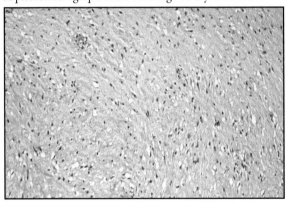

A. Margins are consistently well-defined.
B. Radiographically, these lesions can be indistinguishable from ameloblastoma.
C. 60% of these tumors occur in the 5th and 6th decades of life.
D. 65% occur in the maxilla.
E. The myxoma cells are positive for S100 and neuron-specific enolase, and negative for vimentin.

17: Mandible and Maxilla Questions

23. A 28-year-old female undergoes surgical resection of a maxillary mass anterior to the molars. Gross examination of the specimen reveals a smooth, well-defined, firm, white mass with a homogeneous cut surface. A photomicrograph of the lesion is shown below. The most likely diagnosis is:

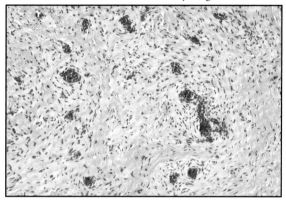

    A.   Odontogenic myxoma
    B.   Pindborg tumor
    C.   Cementoblastoma
    D.   Odontogenic fibroma
    E.   Dentigerous cyst

24. A photomicrograph of a complex odontoma is shown below. During which decades of life are these tumors usually diagnosed?

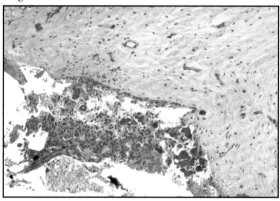

    A.   1st and 2nd decades
    B.   3rd and 4th decades
    C.   5th and 6th decades
    D.   7th and 8th decades
    E.   Equal incidence across all ages

17: Mandible and Maxilla Questions

25. A patient is diagnosed with multiple cysts of the jaw. A photomicrograph of one of these lesions is shown below. Which of the following syndromes is associated with the presence of multiple odontogenic keratocysts?

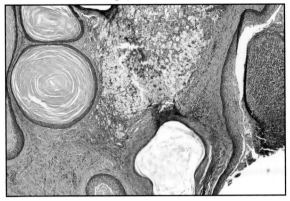

    A.   Neurofibromatosis type I
    B.   Neurofibromatosis type II
    C.   Crouzon syndrome
    D.   Gorlin-Goltz syndrome
    E.   Xeroderma pigmentosum

26. A 29-year-old female is referred to an otolaryngologist for a gingival mass that has been present for several months and that is increasing in size. A radiograph demonstrates a large lesion with a lobulated border and an interior that contains bony septa. A complete resection is performed, and a photomicrograph of the lesion is shown below. The most likely diagnosis is:

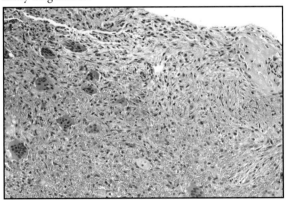

    A.   Radicular cyst
    B.   Calcifying odontogenic cyst
    C.   Giant cell granuloma (giant cell reparative granuloma)
    D.   Odontogenic keratocyst (primordial cyst)
    E.   Nasopalatine duct cyst (incisive canal cyst)

17: Mandible and Maxilla Questions

27. A 9-month-old boy is found to have a prominent, exophytic gingival mass by his pediatrician during a clinic visit. Radiologic studies demonstrate focal bone destruction. The lesion is biopsied by a pediatric otolaryngologist, and a diagnosis is rendered by the pediatric pathologist. A local excision is performed, with gross examination revealing a mass with a heterogeneous appearance with a few foci of dark black pigmentation. A photomicrograph of the lesion is shown below. The most likely diagnosis is:

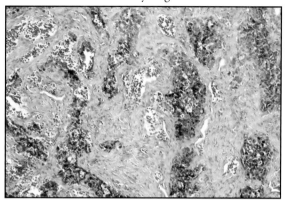 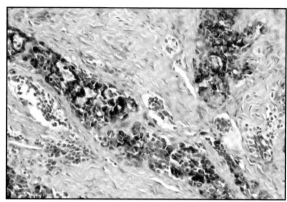

- A. Rhabdomyosarcoma
- B. Melanoma
- C. Gingival cyst of infants (Epstein pearls)
- D. Melanotic neuroectodermal tumor of infancy (melanotic progonoma)
- E. Odontogenic keratocyst (primordial cyst)

17: Mandible and Maxilla Answers

1. **B.** **GIANT CELL AMELOBLASTOMA**
   There are several well-recognized variants of ameloblastoma. Desmoplastic ameloblastoma is a characterized as having a prominent acellular, hyalinized stroma adjacent to the neoplastic epithelium (this variant is usually seen in conjunction with the follicular pattern). Basal cell ameloblastoma is characterized by a prominent basaloid pattern. Acanthomatous ameloblastoma is characterized by exuberant keratinization within the central tumor islands. Papilliferous ameloblastoma (rare!) is characterized by microcysts that are lined by parakeratinized epithelium and contain keratin. Other well-recognized variants include sinonasal ameloblastoma, malignant ameloblastoma, and peripheral ameloblastoma. Malignant ameloblastoma is a designation reserved for a classic appearing ameloblastoma that has metastasized, most commonly to the lung or cervical lymph nodes. Giant cell ameloblastoma is not a recognized variant.
   QCSP, **Ameloblastoma,** p 554.

2. **B.** **FALSE**
   Compared to the other variants of ameloblastoma, unicystic, peripheral, and desmoplastic lesions have a lower rate of recurrence. Ameloblastomas are treated with surgical excision and removal of 1.0 cm of surrounding medullary bone. The simple unicystic ameloblastomas can be treated with simple enucleation. Ameloblastomas, in general, tend to spread along cancellous bone and cause resorption of compact bone without involving the Haversian canals.
   QCSP, **Ameloblastoma,** p 554.

3. **D.** **PERIODIC ACID-SCHIFF STAIN**
   Periodic acid-Schiff (PAS) stains can be useful for confirming the presence of acidophilic material that lies between apposing rows of columnar cells in adenomatoid odontogenic tumors.
   QCSP, **Adenomatoid Odontogenic Tumor,** p 556.

4. **A.** **TRUE**
   Cementoblastomas are very rare tumors that most commonly arise in the posterior segment of the mandible alveolus adjacent to roots of erupted permanent teeth. They are most commonly diagnosed during the 3rd decade of life, are somewhat more common in women, and characteristically present with pain. Radiographic findings include the presence of an expansile mass of opaque tissue with a radiolucent rim associated with roots of teeth. Grossly, these lesions appear as hard, round masses that are fused to tooth roots. These tumors histologically resemble osteoid osteomas and osteoblastomas. Histologic examination reveals tissue with accentuated basophilic, acellular cementumlike lines and irregular lacunae with a background of cellular fibrovascular stroma. Large cementoblasts are present, surrounding the masses of cementum (which is composed of random, unorganized arrays of collagen fibers). Cementocytes are present as well, but occupy lacunae and are smaller than the peripherally located cementoblasts. In addition, the periphery is characterized by dilated vessels and radially oriented bony spicules between the cementum nodules and the fibrovascular stroma. Osteoclast-type giant cells may be present. These lesions are treated with removal of the affected tooth in addition to the mass, and incompletely excised lesions may recur.
   QCSP, **Cementoblastoma,** p 558.

5. **B.** **FALSE**
   Compared to complex odontomas, compound odontomas more closely resemble normal teeth, with pulp, cementum, dentin, and enamel arranged in a more normal manner. These tumors are composed of the above tissue types surrounded by a loose myxoid stroma. Both compound and complex odontomas are treated with conservative local excision, and both may recur if incompletely excised.
   QCSP, **Odontoma,** p 559.

17: Mandible and Maxilla Answers

6. **B.   FALSE**

    Ameloblastic fibromas are rare, benign odontogenic tumors that are usually diagnosed before the age of 20 and generally occur in the mandible (80%). Radiographically, these lesions are well-defined unilocular or multilocular lucencies in the premolar-molar region of the mandible that are associated with unerupted teeth. These lesions can be radiographically identical to ameloblastomas. Grossly, these lesions are well-defined, solid or cystic masses that are tan to white and translucent. Histologically, these lesions are characterized by strands or islands of cuboidal or columnar epithelial cells that are similar to the findings seen in early enamel development. The stroma is composed of a loose stellate proliferation rather than the dense collagen formation that is seen in ameloblastoma. Importantly, hard tooth structures such as dentin and enamel are absent.

    QCSP, **Ameloblastic Fibroma,** p 559.

7. **E.   TREATMENT INCLUDES EXTRACTION OF THE INVOLVED TOOTH IN ADDITION TO CONSERVATIVE EXCISION OF THE TUMOR.**

    Squamous odontogenic tumors are rare tumors that may occur between the 2nd and 7th decades of life. The maxilla and mandible are affected equally, although lesions of the anterior maxilla are generally more aggressive. These tumors usually present as localized loosening of tooth/teeth, and radiographic studies demonstrate a unilocular radiolucency in the alveolar segment of bone involving the tooth root. Histologically, these tumors are characterized by cords and islands of well-differentiated stratified squamous epithelium surrounding vascularized connective tissue. There should be no atypia or mitotic activity within the squamous epithelium. Approximately half of these tumors have microscopic foci of degeneration and calcification within the islands of squamous epithelium. These tumors are treated by conservative excision of the lesion in addition to extraction of the involved tooth/teeth. The more aggressive anterior maxillary tumors may require wider excisions.

    QCSP, **Squamous Odontogenic Tumor,** p 560.

8. **B.   DENTIGEROUS CYST (FOLLICULAR CYST)**

    Developmental odontogenic cysts include dentigerous cysts, gingival cysts of infants, odontogenic keratocysts, eruption cysts, lateral periodontal cysts, gingival cysts of adults, calcifying odontogenic cysts, and botryoid odontogenic cysts. The key to the correct diagnosis is *location* of the cyst, gleaned from both the physical exam and radiograph findings. The case above describes an asymptomatic lesion that is closely attached to the cervical portion of a partially erupted mandibular 3rd molar. These findings are classically associated with a dentigerous (or follicular) cyst, which surrounds the crown of a tooth (usually unerupted or partially erupted) and attached to the tooth neck. These cysts are most commonly found in association with the mandibular third molars or the maxillary cuspids. Radiographs will demonstrate a well-defined lucency in close proximity to the crown of the involved tooth. The cyst forms when fluid is retained between the attenuated enamel epithelium and the crown or between the layers of the attenuated enamel epithelium. These cysts are most commonly detected in patients between the 2nd and 4th decades of life, and are somewhat more common in men. Histologically, the cyst wall consists of connective tissue lined by epithelium 1 or 2 cells thick. In some cysts, foci of keratinization, ciliated cells, and mucus-producing cells are identified. If inflammation is present in the cyst, the normally thin epithelium can become thickened, and it can assume a more squamous appearance. Inflammatory cells can infiltrate the cyst and produce a radicular cyst-like appearance, with cholesterol and Rushton body deposition. Dentigerous cysts are treated by enucleation and extraction of the associated tooth. In rare cases, ameloblastoma, mucoepidermoid carcinoma, and squamous cell carcinoma have been associated with these cysts and therefore it is important to sample any areas of nodularity or thickening of the cyst wall observed on gross examination.

    QCSP, **Dentigerous Cyst,** p 561.

17: Mandible and Maxilla Answers

9. **A.** **ERUPTION CYST**

Eruption cysts are variants of dentigerous cysts, which develop in the soft tissue surrounding teeth facing imminent eruption. They can occur prior to eruption of either permanent or deciduous ("baby") teeth. Unlike dentigerous cysts, which develop within the actual mandible or maxilla around unerupted or partially erupted teeth, eruption cysts develop in the soft tissue overlying the bone. Eruption cysts, not unexpectedly, are most common in the 1st decade of life, when most tooth eruption occurs. Physical examination reveals a blue, translucent swelling in the region of tooth eruption. Histologically, these cysts are lined by nonkeratinizing stratified squamous epithelium that, when inflamed, can thicken significantly. In some cases, the eruption cyst can impede the tooth eruption; as such, cyst marsupialization can be performed to prevent this complication.

QCSP, **Eruption Cyst**, p 561.

10. **B.** **GINGIVAL CYST OF ADULTS**

Gingival cysts of adults are odontogenic cysts that appear to arise from the dental lamina remnants of the gingiva in adults and generally appear as well-circumscribed, small swellings in the canine-premolar area of the mandibular buccal gingiva. These lesions can be confused with lateral periodontal cysts (see question 12), which also arise from odontogenic epithelial remnants but are intraosseous and intimately associated with the periodontium. Gingival cysts of adults can have significant histologic heterogeneity, ranging from thin epithelial cyst walls one cuboidal cell layer thick to thickened, prominent squamous epithelium. In rare cases, plaques of clear or fusiform cells can be present (similar to those seen in lateral periodontal cysts). These cysts are treated with simple excision, and recurrence is quite rare.

QCSP, **Gingival Cyst of Adults**, p 562.

11. **B.** **FALSE**

Gingival cysts of infants are odontogenic cysts that develop from cystic degeneration of dental lamina remnants of the alveolar mucosa. Physical examination will reveal small (1.0-3.0 mm) yellow-white nodules overlying future tooth-bearing regions of the alveolar mucosa. Histologically, these cysts are lined by stratified squamous epithelium and are filled with keratinaceous debris, giving the cysts their yellow hue. These lesions are generally present at birth, and rarely persist after 3 months of age. Since these cysts characteristically rupture or involute within the first few months of life, no surgical treatment is required.

QCSP, **Gingival Cyst of Infants**, p 562.

12. **A.** **LATERAL PERIODONTAL CYST**

Lateral periodontal cysts are odontogenic cysts that arise from odontogenic epithelial remnants and that lie lateral to or between the roots of vital teeth. They most commonly develop in the premolar area of the mandible. These cysts are lined by thin, nonkeratinizing squamous or cuboidal epithelium <5 cells thick. These cysts are treated with enucleation without extraction of adjacent teeth. The multicystic variant (botryoid odontogenic cyst) is more aggressive and tends to recur.

QCSP, **Lateral Periodontal Cyst**, p 563.

13. **E.** **RADICULAR CYST**

Radicular cysts are cysts that generally arise from the epithelial odontogenic remnants (rests of Malassez) in the periodontal ligament as a result of inflammation and necrosis of the dental pulp (from caries or trauma, usually). These lesions are most commonly diagnosed in male patients between 20 and 40 years of age. Most of these cysts are lined by nonkeratinized squamous epithelium, with the epithelial thickness associated with the degree of inflammation present. Intraepithelial hyaline (Rushton) bodies are sometimes present, and foamy macrophages are frequently present within the cyst cavity. Large quantities of cholesterol crystals are sometimes seen in the fibrous parts of the cyst wall.

QCSP, **Radicular Cyst**, p 564.

14.   B.   **NASOPALATINE DUCT CYST (INCISIVE CANAL CYST)**
Nasopalatine duct cysts (incisive canal cysts) are the most common nonodontogenic oral cavity cysts and arise from epithelial remnants in the nasopalatine (incisive) canal in the midline of the anterior maxilla between and posterior to the central incisors. The majority of these cysts develop between the 4th and 6th decades of life. Males are 3 times more likely to develop these midline cysts. The characteristic findings on X-ray include a well-defined round, ovoid, or heart-shaped lucency in the midline of the maxilla. Surgical enucleation of the cyst is performed for treatment. Histologic examination of the cyst lining reveals pseudostratified ciliated columnar epithelium, stratified squamous epithelium, or a combination. Rarely, transitional epithelium can be seen in addition to small cartilage islands. The connective tissue surrounding the cyst frequently contains prominent vessels and nerves in addition to adipose tissue and mucous glands. Rarely, squamous cell carcinoma can arise from these cysts. Nasolabial cysts are located in the tissues of the canine fossa beneath the ala of the nose. Radicular cysts are closely associated with teeth, not midline maxilla. Dentigerous cysts enclose the crowns of teeth and would not be found in the midline of the anterior maxilla. Calcifying odontogenic cysts may occur in the anterior maxilla; however, the lesion is more common in teenagers.
QCSP, **Nasopalatine Duct Cyst,** p 565.

15.   A.   **NASOLABIAL CYST (NASOALVEOLAR CYST)**
The location is the key to the diagnosis. Nasolabial cysts are rare soft tissue cysts that most commonly occur in the 4th and 5th decades of life. Unlike nasopalatine duct cysts, females are far more likely than males to develop nasolabial cysts. These cysts are characteristically found in the soft tissues of the canine fossa beneath the ala of the nose. They are characteristically extraosseous, and therefore will not be readily identifiable on radiographs. That being said, some of these cysts can minimally erode the surrounding maxillary surface. These lesions most likely arise from the remnants of the embryonic nasolacrimal ducts.
QCSP, **Nasolabial Cyst,** p 565.

16.   E.   **THE CONDITION USUALLY BECOMES INACTIVE BY THE 3RD DECADE OF LIFE.**
Cherubism is marked by symmetrical mandibular and maxillary enlargement that results from bony destruction secondary to cyst formation. These lesions typically begin in early childhood, and there is often a family history of the disorder. Indeed, some cases are believed to be inherited in an autosomal dominant fashion, with involvement of chromosome 4p16.3. Cherubism usually affects all 4 jaw quadrants symmetrically, with resultant malocclusion of teeth. Boys are overall twice as likely to be affected. The lesions of cherubism tend to be most active in young patients, with activity decreasing during puberty. The progression tends to halt after puberty, with some regression of the lesions by the beginning of the 3rd decade of life. Radiographic studies demonstrate multilocular foci of radiolucency with bony expansion. A "soap bubble" appearance is sometimes present. The cortical surface of bone is intact, but teeth are frequently absent or significantly displaced. The lytic foci are replaced by bone as the lesion activity decreases with age. Cosmetic surgery, if performed, should be performed only after the cessation of bony growth, since many cases will regress over time. Radiotherapy has not been shown to be beneficial in cherubism. As a side note, patients with Noonan syndrome frequently have numerous giant cell granulomas of the jaws, which can appear histologically identical to cherubism.
QCSP, **Cherubism,** p 566.

17.   D.   **ALL OF THE ABOVE**
The lesions of cherubism consist of reactive-appearing fibrovascular stroma with multinucleated giant cells, frequent foci of hemosiderin, and infrequent foci of woven bone and osteoid. These findings are nonspecific and are found in giant cell granulomas, the solid variants of aneurysmal bone cysts, and osteoclastomas resulting from hyperparathyroidism. As the disease activity wanes, these lesions are characterized by increasing fibrosis and a relative loss of giant cells with new bone deposition.
QCSP, **Cherubism,** p 566.

18. E. **CD57+, HMB45+, VIMENTIN+, CYTOKERATIN+**
The large pigmented cells of melanotic neuroectodermal tumors of infancy are classically positive for cytokeratin, vimentin, HMB-45 and CD57. In addition, they frequently stain for epithelial membrane antigen (EMA) and S100. The small neuroblastic-type cells are immunopositive for synaptophysin, GFAP, and S100. Both cell types stain for CD57.
QCSP, **Melanotic Neuroectodermal Tumor of Infancy,** p 567.

19. E. **AMELOBLASTOMA**
Ameloblastomas are benign, locally invasive tumors composed of proliferating odontogenic epithelium. The name is derived from the old French word for enamel (*amelo*); however, enamel deposition is not seen in this tumor. They are usually diagnosed during the 3rd and 4th decades. Males and females are affected equally, and these tumors tend to be associated with either impacted or unerupted teeth (particularly the mandibular third molars). Approximately 80% of these tumors arise within the mandible, and most of these appear in the molar region and ascending ramus (80%). Histologically, most of these tumors are multicystic/solid with 6 common patterns described. The image shown represents the most common pattern, the follicular variant, which is characterized by discrete islands of tumor cells with a central area resembling primitive stellate reticulum. Mitotic activity is scant. The other common variants include basal cell, granular cell, acanthomatous, plexiform, and desmoplastic types. Unicystic ameloblastomas can also occur, which have lining, luminal, or mural growth patterns.
QCSP, **Ameloblastoma,** p 554.

20. A. **THESE TUMORS ARE TYPICALLY LESS AGGRESSIVE THAN AMELOBLASTOMAS.**
Calcifying epithelial odontogenic tumors (Pindborg tumors) are very rare lesions that represent <1% of all odontogenic tumors. They appear with equal frequency in male and females throughout the 3rd to 7th decades of life. Approximately 65% of these lesions occur in the mandible, with the remaining cases occurring in the maxilla. They most commonly present as painless masses that are associated with embedded or unerupted teeth. The great majority are intraosseous, and they are commonly found in the molar region. Radiographically, these tumors appear as irregular radiolucent lesions that contain radiopaque masses and are generally localized adjacent to the crown of an unerupted tooth. Histologically, these tumors are composed of polyhedral tumor cells with well-defined cell borders and prominent intercellular bridges. The individual cells are generally pleomorphic and have large lobulated nuclei and distinct nucleoli. Multinucleated cells are frequently present in addition to droplet-type calcifications with concentric lamellar appositional rings (Liesegang ring calcifications). Amyloid-like material (which can be identified with Congo red and thioflavine T staining) often is present within the tumor sheets, and it is unclear if this material is secreted by the tumor cells or results from tumor cell degeneration. The intraosseous tumors tend to have less calcification present. While these lesions can be locally invasive and can recur 15% of the time, they are generally less aggressive than ameloblastomas. Around 6% of these tumors are associated with adenomatoid odontogenic tumors.
QCSP, **Calcifying Epithelial Odontogenic Tumor (Pindborg Tumor),** p 555.

17: Mandible and Maxilla Answers

21.   B.   **ADENOMATOID ODONTOGENIC TUMOR**

Adenomatoid odontogenic tumors more frequently develop in young women (2:1) around the 2nd decade of life. The maxilla is involved twice as often as the mandible, and the area around the canines in the anterior maxilla is the most common single site of involvement. These tumors are most commonly associated with an unerupted tooth, and they may resemble a dentigerous cyst radiographically. Grossly, these tumors are encapsulated soft tissue masses surrounding the crown of an unerupted tooth, and may be solid or have prominent cyst formation. Histologically, these tumors are composed of 2 types of epithelial cells. First, polyhedral or spindled cells are present and arranged in nodular aggregates in swirling patterns reminiscent of salivary gland tumors. Second, columnar or cuboidal cells are present surrounding microcystic or ductlike spaces with resultant glandlike structures. It is important to differentiate this tumor from ameloblastoma because the prognosis and treatment differs. Unlike ameloblastoma, adenomatoid odontogenic tumor tends not to recur and conservative surgical enucleation is therapeutic.

QCSP, **Adenomatoid Odontogenic Tumor,** p 556.

22.   B.   **RADIOGRAPHICALLY, THESE LESIONS CAN BE INDISTINGUISHABLE FROM AMELOBLASTOMA.**

Odontogenic myxomas are benign tumors that usually develop in the tooth-bearing areas of the mandible (65%) and maxilla (35%). Approximately 60% of these tumors occur in the 2nd and 3rd decades of life. Grossly, these lesions may have well-defined or poorly defined margins, and cut sections are homogeneous, gelatinous, and somewhat translucent. Radiographically, these lesions consist of multiple variably sized radiolucent foci separated by either curved or straight bony septa, creating a "soap bubble" appearance. These lesions may be radiographically indistinguishable from ameloblastoma, central giant cell granuloma, aneurysmal bone cyst, and odontogenic keratocyst. Histologically, these tumors are composed of stellate or bipolar cells with a background of abundant myxoid stroma that is rich in chondroitin sulfate and hyaluronic acid and that will stain with alcian blue. The myxoma cells are positive for vimentin and are negative for S100 and neuron-specific enolase.

QCSP, **Odontogenic Myxoma,** p 557.

23.   D.   **ODONTOGENIC FIBROMA**

Odontogenic fibromas are uncommon benign tumors that usually occur in the maxilla, anterior to the molars and are associated with an impacted tooth. They have been reported to be more common in women. Grossly, these tumors are well-defined, firm, solid white masses that have homogeneous cut surfaces. Histologically, these tumors can be fibroblastic and myxoid to densely hyalinized, and cellular or acellular. In addition, calcifications are frequently present and odontogenic epithelium is sometimes identified. Histologically, odontogenic fibromas most closely mimic odontogenic myxomas; however, the latter tumors show scant collagen fibrils and abundant myxoid substance.

QCSP, **Odontogenic Fibroma,** p 557.

24.   A.   **1ST AND 2ND DECADES**

Complex odontomas are composed of a chaotic mixture of various dental tissues, including pulpal tissue, tubular dentin, and enamel matrix. While these individual components may be well formed, these tissue types are "arranged" in a haphazard pattern. These can sometimes be difficult to differentiate from ameloblastic fibromas and fibroodontomas. Complex (and compound) odontomas are most commonly diagnosed during the first 2 decades of life.

QCSP, **Odontoma,** p 559.

17: Mandible and Maxilla Answers

25.   **D.**   **GORLIN-GOLTZ SYNDROME**

Gorlin-Goltz syndrome (or autosomal dominant basal cell nevus syndrome) is characterized by the presence of numerous basal cell carcinomas, cysts of the jaw (particularly odontogenic keratocysts), skeletal abnormalities, cutaneous epidermoid cysts, and calcifying ovarian fibromas. This syndrome is associated with mutations of the PTCH gene on chromosome 9q. Odontogenic keratocysts are unilocular or multilocular and have cyst walls with well-defined basal layers beneath layers of squamous cells that mature to a parakeratotic surface. The mandible is most commonly involved.

QCSP, **Odontogenic Keratocyst,** p 563.

26.   **C.**   **GIANT CELL GRANULOMA**

Giant cell granulomas are composed of fibrous tissue with plentiful giant cells, spicules of woven bone, and hemorrhagic foci. A granulation tissue-like appearance can sometimes be seen due to endothelial-lined vascular spaces associated with fibroblasts. Mitotic figures can sometimes be seen. While these aggressive lesions somewhat resemble giant cell tumors of bone, the multinucleated giant cells that are present are smaller and with fewer nuclei than those seen in a usual giant cell tumor. Areas of fresh hemorrhage and fibrinoid deposits are frequently present. These lesions most commonly develop in the 3rd decade of life and are 50% more common in women. They tend to occur in the anterior tooth-containing areas of the mandible. The lesions are locally aggressive, with bony expansion and cortical penetration sometimes seen. While the smaller, less aggressive lesions appear as small, well-defined lucencies on radiographs, the larger, more aggressive lesions are characterized by focal destruction with smooth or lobulated outlines along with narrow bony septa within the lesion. These lesions are treated with curettage for small, nonaggressive lesions and complete resection for larger, more aggressive lesions.

QCSP, **Giant Cell Granuloma,** p 565.

27.   **D.**   **MELANOTIC NEUROECTODERMAL TUMOR OF INFANCY (MELANOTIC PROGONOMA)**

Melanotic neuroectodermal tumors of infancy are very rare tumors that generally develop before the age of 1 and affect boys and girls with equal frequency. These lesions most commonly develop in the craniofacial region (70%), particularly in the anterior portion of the maxilla. Extremely rarely, these can occur in the mandible, skull, long bones, uterus, mediastinum, epididymis, and soft tissues. While most of these tumors are nonfunctional, a few have been reported to be catecholamine secreting. Radiologic studies will often demonstrate osteolytic destruction of the affected bone. Grossly, the lesions can be either entirely contained within bone or can present as an exophytic gingival mass, as in this case. Adjacent teeth can be displaced. Sectioning through the mass will often reveal heterogeneous pigmentation. Histologically, the tumors are composed of alveolar nests and tubules with 2 cell types: small neuroblastic-type cells and large peripheral pigmented cells. These cells are present in a fibrous stroma. The larger cells are pale staining, and contain various quantities of melanin granules. These cells are arranged in sheets or cords and surround the small neuroblastic-type cells, which look similar to small lymphocytes with dense nuclei and scant cytoplasm. These tumors are treated by local excision; however, many cases recur (up to 50% of cases), and rare metastases have been described (5%-7% of cases).

QCSP, **Melanotic Neuroectodermal Tumor of Infancy,** p 567.

Chapter 18

Salivary Glands

1. Which of the following benign neoplasms requires a slightly more extensive excision to avoid local recurrence?
   A. Pleomorphic adenoma
   B. Myoepithelioma
   C. Warthin tumor
   D. Canalicular adenoma
   E. Basal cell adenoma

2. Which of the following carcinomas is NOT considered low grade?
   A. Epithelial-myoepithelial carcinoma
   B. Acinic cell carcinoma
   C. Myoepithelial carcinoma
   D. Salivary duct carcinoma
   E. Basal cell adenocarcinoma

3. Mycobacterial infection is thought to be the primary cause of necrotizing sialometaplasia.
   A. True
   B. False

4. Which of the following is TRUE regarding necrotizing sialometaplasia?
   A. Women are twice as likely to develop this lesion.
   B. The average age at diagnosis is approximately 45 years.
   C. The lesion generally persists for 1-2 years before healing.
   D. A specific mutation on chromosome 17 is associated with the development of this lesion.
   E. Patients never present with bilateral palatal lesions.

5. Which of the following statements is TRUE regarding acinic cell carcinoma?
   A. It is the most common salivary gland malignancy.
   B. Approximately 20% of these tumors occur in the sublingual gland.
   C. It is the most common malignant salivary gland tumor to occur bilaterally.
   D. The majority of these patients present with preauricular pain and facial muscle weakness.
   E. Approximately 75% of these tumors occur in males.

6. Which of the following statements is FALSE regarding acinic cell carcinoma?
   A. A PAS stain with diastase is helpful for accentuating the cytoplasmic secretory granules of the tumor cells.
   B. Electron microscopy will usually demonstrate numerous mitochondria within tumor cells as well as electron-dense cytoplasmic secretory granules.
   C. The papillary cystic variant has a worse prognosis, and approximately 10% of these tumors are associated with regional lymph node metastases.
   D. Survival at 5 years is highly indicative of a cure.
   E. Overall mortality associated with this malignancy is around 15%.

7. Which of the following is TRUE regarding mucoepidermoid carcinoma?
   A. This is the second most common malignant salivary gland tumor in adults, behind adenoid cystic carcinoma.
   B. This is the most common malignant salivary gland tumor in children.
   C. These tumors have never been reported to occur in the lacrimal sac, lungs, or esophagus.
   D. The palate is the most common site of origin for this tumor.
   E. The upper lip is a more common site of origin than the lower lip.

8. All of the following are useful features for distinguishing necrotizing sialometaplasia from mucoepidermoid carcinoma EXCEPT:
   A. Strong and mixed inflammatory reaction
   B. Mucous cells
   C. Lobular architecture
   D. Coagulative necrosis of acini and/or lobules
   E. Bland cytology of surface epithelium

9. Which of the following is FALSE regarding the grading and staging of mucoepidermoid carcinoma?
   A. Grading is determined by the presence of anaplasia (4 points), 4 mitotic figures/10 HPFs (3 points), necrosis (3 points), neural invasion (2 points), and prominent intracystic component (2 points).
   B. Low-grade tumors (0-4 points) are associated with a 98% 5-year survival, with only 5% of cases metastasizing to regional lymph nodes.
   C. High-grade tumors (≥7 points) are associated with a 75% 5-year survival, with only 25% of cases metastasizing to regional lymph nodes.
   D. Tumors of the submandibular gland require radiation therapy in addition to surgical excision.
   E. Stage I tumors of the parotid gland are treated by conservative excision alone.

10. Which of the following statements regarding mucoepidermoid carcinoma is FALSE?
    A. t(11;19)(q21;p13) and p53 mutations have been shown to be associated with this malignancy.
    B. Intermediate and epidermoid tumor cells are positive for cytokeratin.
    C. Prior exposure to ionizing radiation is associated with this tumor.
    D. Extracellular mucus can sometimes incite an inflammatory response with granulation tissue resulting over time, making diagnosis difficult.
    E. Prominent nuclear atypia, mitotic figures, and extensive necrosis are common findings.

11. Which of the following is FALSE regarding adenoid cystic carcinoma?
    A. Grossly well-circumscribed lesions frequently demonstrate microscopic perineural or intraneural invasion.
    B. The cystic structures seen histologically in this tumor are pseudocysts.
    C. Tumors with predominantly solid growth patterns have a better prognosis compared to those with cribriform or tubular patterns.
    D. Chemotherapy with melphalan and cisplatin may be efficacious.
    E. The neoplastic cells are generally positive for S100.

12. Which of the following statements is TRUE regarding adenoid cystic carcinoma?
    A. Survival at 5 years is highly indicative of a cure.
    B. Adenoid cystic carcinoma is far more likely to metastasize to regional lymph nodes than to invade and spread along nerve tracts.
    C. These neoplasms frequently appear cystic on gross examination.
    D. Mutations in 6q and 9p are associated with this neoplasm.
    E. The solid pattern of growth frequently resembles a benign salivary neoplasm.

13. Which of the following is TRUE regarding epithelial-myoepithelial carcinoma?
    A. This is most commonly a tumor of young adulthood, with a median age of 28 at presentation.
    B. This is a fairly common lesion, representing 10% of all salivary gland tumors (benign and malignant combined).
    C. Recurrent tumors are usually more hemorrhagic, necrotic, and multinodular than the primary.
    D. Most of these tumors are >5.0 cm in greatest dimension at the time of resection.
    E. Only one case of this tumor arising in an intraoral minor salivary gland has been reported.

18: Salivary Glands Questions

14. Which of the following statements is FALSE regarding the staining profile of epithelial-myoepithelial carcinoma?
    A. The myoepithelial (clear) cells are usually reactive for S100.
    B. The myoepithelial (clear) cells stain strongly with muscle-specific actin and p63 and sometimes stain with glial fibrillary acidic protein (GFAP).
    C. The lumens of the ductal structures formed by the epithelial tumor cells contain mucicarmine-positive, PAS-negative basophilic material.
    D. A PAS stain can be helpful for confirming the presence of glycogen in myoepithelial cells and demonstrating the hyalinized stroma present between neoplastic cells.
    E. The hyalinized stroma is positive for staining of type IV collagen.

15. A diagnosis of clear cell adenocarcinoma is rendered. The patient is concerned about the diagnosis of this rare tumor, and has numerous questions. The otolaryngologist, fresh out of residency training, has never encountered a patient with this tumor before. Which of the following do you tell the otolaryngologist regarding the grading, treatment, and/or prognosis of this neoplasm?
    A. Following resection, the patient must be treated with chemotherapy for presumed metastases.
    B. This a low-grade neoplasm that is locally infiltrative, but rarely metastasizes.
    C. Most patients that develop this tumor ultimately die from the disease.
    D. Perineural invasion has never been reported.
    E. Herceptin has been shown to be highly effective in patients with metastatic disease and HER-2/neu amplification.

16. Radiation has been shown to be highly effective for cases of adenocarcinoma, not otherwise, specified of the parotid gland.
    A. True
    B. False

17. Which of the following statements is FALSE regarding pleomorphic adenoma?
    A. While many of these tumors have a normal karyotype, some demonstrate rearrangements of 12q13-15 or 8q12.
    B. An excessive proliferation of either the myoepithelial or epithelial cells can result in a highly cellular, malignant appearing neoplasm.
    C. Pleomorphic adenomas of the major salivary glands are much less likely to recur.
    D. A superficial parotidectomy or an extracapsular dissection with a rim of normal tissue is the preferred surgical procedure.
    E. A subtotal excision will likely lead to recurrence.

18. Which of the following syndromes is most strongly associated with membranous basal cell adenomas?
    A. Neurofibromatosis type I
    B. Tuberous sclerosis
    C. Brooke-Spiegler syndrome
    D. Xeroderma pigmentosum
    E. Neurofibromatosis type II

19. Which of the following immunohistochemical stains is most helpful in differentiating a canalicular adenoma from a myoepithelioma or epithelial-myoepithelial carcinoma?
    A. Cytokeratin
    B. Muscle-specific actin
    C. S100
    D. Estrogen receptor
    E. Ki-67

18: Salivary Glands Questions

20. Which of the following stains can be helpful for confirming a diagnosis of oncocytoma?
    A.   Ki-67
    B.   Trichrome
    C.   Reticulin
    D.   Bielschowsky silver
    E.   Phosphotungstic acid-hematoxylin

21. Which of the following statements regarding Warthin tumors is FALSE?
    A.   Heavy smokers are at an 8-fold increased risk.
    B.   The recurrence rate following excision is <2%.
    C.   The median age at diagnosis is 39 years.
    D.   Approximately 5%-10% of patients present with bilateral tumors.
    E.   African-American men are far less likely to develop this tumor compared to Caucasians.

22. A 53-year-old man is referred to an otolaryngologist for a painful ulcer of the hard palate. The lesion developed quickly and has been present for 2 weeks. The patient has never used tobacco, uses dentures, and has frequent upper respiratory infections. A biopsy of the lesion is performed, with findings shown in the photomicrograph below. The most likely diagnosis is:

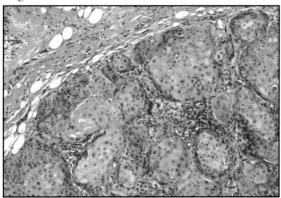

    A.   Mucosal squamous cell carcinoma
    B.   Low-grade mucoepidermoid carcinoma
    C.   Necrotizing sialometaplasia
    D.   Salivary duct carcinoma
    E.   Basal cell adenoma

18: Salivary Glands Questions

23. A 47-year-old woman is referred to an otolaryngologist for a left preauricular mass that has been present for 6 months and is increasing in size. An FNA is performed, which is nondiagnostic. The patient undergoes a left parotidectomy, and gross examination reveals a circumscribed, yellow-white mass measuring 1.6 cm in greatest dimension. A photomicrograph of the lesion is shown below. The most likely diagnosis is:

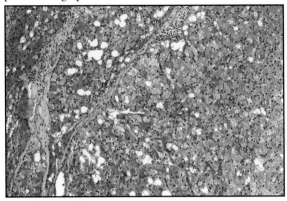

    A.   Mucoepidermoid carcinoma
    B.   Acinic cell carcinoma
    C.   Adenoid cystic carcinoma
    D.   Basal cell adenoma
    E.   Clear cell adenocarcinoma

24. A 55-year-old woman is referred to an otolaryngologist for a mildly painful swelling of the palate that has increased in size over the past 4 months. A biopsy is performed. A photomicrograph of the lesion is shown below. The most likely diagnosis is:

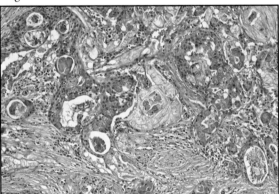

    A.   Mucoepidermoid carcinoma
    B.   Pleomorphic low-grade adenocarcinoma
    C.   Adenoid cystic carcinoma
    D.   Pleomorphic adenoma
    E.   Necrotizing sialometaplasia

25.   A 48-year-old woman is referred to an otolaryngologist for a nonpainful, right preauricular mass that she first noticed 4 weeks ago. An FNA is performed by the cytopathologist, and is diagnostic. A right parotidectomy is performed, revealing a firm, tan-white mass that is 1.6 cm in greatest dimension. A photomicrograph of the lesion is shown below. The most likely diagnosis is:

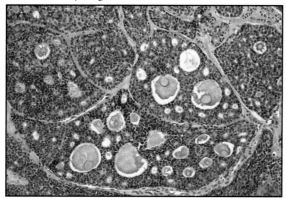

    A.   Mucoepidermoid carcinoma
    B.   Salivary duct carcinoma
    C.   Adenoid cystic carcinoma
    D.   Epithelial-myoepithelial carcinoma
    E.   Clear cell adenocarcinoma

26.   A 62-year-old woman is referred to an otolaryngologist for an ulcerated lesion of the soft palate that has been present for 2 months and is slowly increasing in size. The patient has noted bleeding from the site over the past 2 weeks, which prompted her initial visit to her PCP. The lesion is biopsied and is consistent with carcinoma. A wide excision is performed, and a diagnosis of polymorphous low-grade adenocarcinoma (PLGA) is rendered. A photomicrograph of the lesion is shown below. Which of the following is FALSE regarding PLGA?

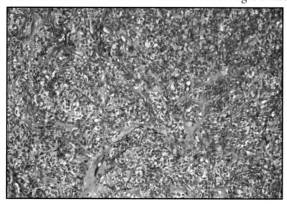

    A.   This tumor can assume a host of architectural patterns, including ductular, tubular, trabecular, and solid, with foci of papillary-cystic, cribriform, and cystic architecture sometimes seen.
    B.   It is most common to see invasive features at the periphery, with linear invasive growth frequently seen.
    C.   Perineural invasion is seldom identified.
    D.   Mitotic figures are rare, and focal oncocytic change is sometimes identified.
    E.   The tumor is often composed of small tubules lined by cuboidal cells.

18: Salivary Glands Questions

27. A 56-year-old man is referred to an otolaryngologist for a painless right parotid mass that was first noticed 1 month ago while the patient was shaving. The mass has increased in size over the past 4 weeks. A right parotidectomy is performed. Gross examination of the specimen reveals a well-circumscribed 2.7 cm solid, white mass. Histologic examination of the mass reveals a biphasic cell population, with a photomicrograph of the lesion shown below. The most likely diagnosis is:

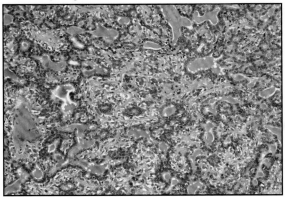

    A.   Pleomorphic adenoma
    B.   Myoepithelioma
    C.   Hyalinizing clear cell adenocarcinoma
    D.   Metastatic renal cell carcinoma
    E.   Epithelial-myoepithelial carcinoma

28. A 71-year-old presents to an otolaryngologist with a painful, ulcerated lesion of the hard palate that has been present for 6 weeks. The mass is resected. Gross examination reveals a poorly circumscribed, gray, firm mass that is 2.2 cm in greatest dimension. A photomicrograph of the lesion is shown below. The most likely diagnosis is:

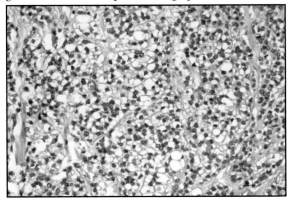

    A.   Acinic cell carcinoma
    B.   Metastatic renal cell carcinoma
    C.   Mucoepidermoid carcinoma
    D.   Clear cell adenocarcinoma
    E.   Epithelial-myoepithelial carcinoma

29. A 65-year-old man is referred to an otolaryngologist for a left preauricular mass as well as left cervical lymphadenopathy. An FNA of the left parotid mass is performed, with a subsequent left parotidectomy and left neck dissection. 17 out of 31 dissected left cervical lymph nodes are involved by tumor. Gross examination of the left parotid gland reveals a solid, gray unencapsulated mass. A photomicrograph of the lesion is shown below. The most likely diagnosis is:

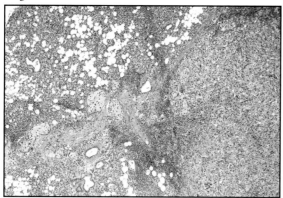

    A.   Salivary duct carcinoma
    B.   Clear cell adenocarcinoma
    C.   Oncocytic carcinoma
    D.   Epithelial-myoepithelial carcinoma
    E.   Polymorphous low-grade adenocarcinoma

30. A 53-year-old man is referred to an otolaryngologist for a right parotid mass that has rapidly increased in size over the past 2 months. The patient also has marked right cervical lymphadenopathy. An FNA that was performed 2 weeks ago was nondiagnostic. A right parotidectomy and a right neck dissection are performed. Gross examination of the parotid gland reveals a yellow, necrotic mass that is poorly-circumscribed and unencapsulated. 61 of 65 lymph nodes are involved by tumor. A diagnosis of salivary duct carcinoma is rendered. A photomicrograph of the lesion is shown below. Which of the following statements regarding salivary duct carcinoma is TRUE?

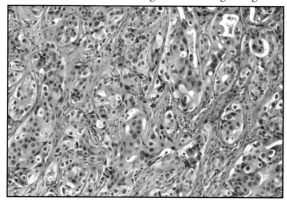

    A.   Most cases arise in the intraoral minor salivary glands.
    B.   Women are far more commonly affected by this neoplasm.
    C.   Despite frequent metastases, only 20% of patients ultimately die due to the cancer.
    D.   Histologic examination will often reveal areas of tumor that are reminiscent of invasive ductal carcinoma of the breast.
    E.   Radiation has no role in therapy.

18: Salivary Glands Questions

31.   A 47-year-old woman returns to her otolaryngologist 5 years after a superficial left parotidectomy for pleomorphic adenoma. She has noticed a firm, painless mass in the area of the prior surgery. The surgeon suspects a recurrence and schedules the patient for surgery. The left deep lobe is removed and sent to pathology. Gross examination reveals a poorly circumscribed, infiltrative lesion with a white cut surface and scattered foci of necrosis. The pathologist strongly suspects carcinoma ex pleomorphic adenoma, and this is confirmed on histologic examination. A photomicrograph of the lesion is shown below. Which of the following is TRUE regarding carcinoma ex pleomorphic adenoma?

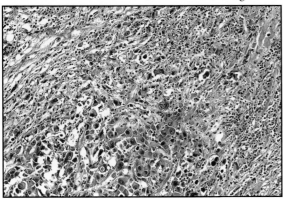

   A.   Pleomorphic adenomas that have been present for 5 years without malignant transformation to carcinoma ex pleomorphic adenoma have a negligible chance to transform in the future.
   B.   Only 1% of patients with this diagnosis report having prior operations for pleomorphic adenomas.
   C.   The malignant transformation and subsequent carcinomatous element always arises from the epithelial component of the pleomorphic adenoma.
   D.   Perineural and vascular invasion are only rarely identified.
   E.   Immunohistochemical stains for S100 and muscle-specific actin are uniformly negative in these tumors.

32.   A 45-year-old woman is referred to an otolaryngologist for a painless preauricular mass that has been present for several years. An FNA is performed, with diagnostic material obtained. A left superficial parotidectomy is performed, and gross examination of the lesion reveals a well-circumscribed white, shiny mass. A photomicrograph of the lesion is shown below. The most likely diagnosis is:

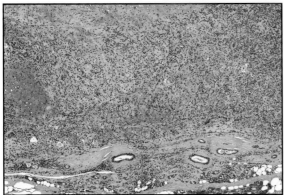

   A.   Basal cell adenoma
   B.   Myoepithelioma
   C.   Pleomorphic adenoma
   D.   Oncocytoma
   E.   Adenoid cystic carcinoma

18: Salivary Glands Questions

33. A 42-year-old man is referred to an otolaryngologist for a slowly-growing left preauricular mass that has been present for 3 months. An FNA is performed, with a subsequent left parotidectomy. Gross examination reveals a well-circumscribed, solid yellow mass with a prominent fibrous capsule. Histologic examination of the tumor reveals a tumor composed predominantly of spindle cells arranged in tight fascicles with minimal stroma present. Immunohistochemical stains for cytokeratin, muscle-specific actin, and p63 are positive. A photomicrograph of the lesion is shown below. The most likely diagnosis is:

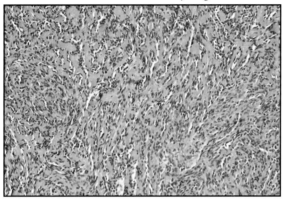

A. Basal cell adenoma
B. Myoepithelioma
C. Pleomorphic adenoma
D. Oncocytoma
E. Adenoid cystic carcinoma

34. A 62-year-old woman is referred to an otolaryngologist for a right preauricular mass. An FNA is performed by the cytopathologist, with a subsequent right parotidectomy. Gross examination reveals a circumscribed, solitary mass with a prominent fibrous capsule. The mass is sectioned to reveal a homogenous gray cut surface. A diagnosis of basal cell adenoma is rendered. A photomicrograph of the lesion is shown below. Which of the following architectural patterns is most associated with the worst prognosis?

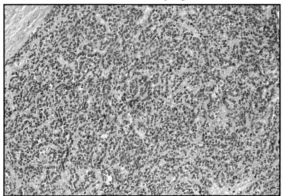

A. Solid
B. Trabecular
C. Trabecular-tubular
D. Tubular
E. Membranous

18: Salivary Glands Questions

35. Canalicular adenomas (see photomicrograph of the lesion below) most commonly occur at which of the following sites?

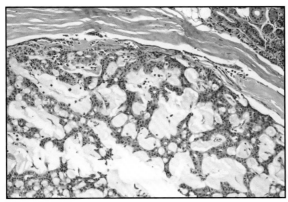

    A. Submandibular gland
    B. Sublingual gland
    C. Hard palate
    D. Upper lip
    E. Parotid gland

36. An 81-year-old woman is referred to an otolaryngologist for a painless preauricular mass. Following FNA, a left parotidectomy is performed. Gross examination reveals a well-circumscribed, red-brown mass measuring 3.2 cm in greatest dimension. A single, small cyst is identified within the lesion. A photomicrograph of the lesion is shown below. The most likely diagnosis is:

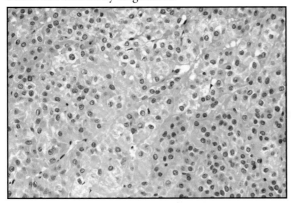

    A. Oncocytoma
    B. Canalicular adenoma
    C. Adenoid cystic carcinoma
    D. Follicular lymphoma
    E. Warthin tumor

18: Salivary Glands Questions

37. A 61-year-old man is referred to an otolaryngologist for bilateral preauricular masses, one of which been present for approximately 12 months. An FNA of the left parotid mass is performed, with diagnostic material obtained. As the left lesion is larger, a left parotidectomy is performed. Gross examination reveals a 2.4 cm well-circumscribed lesion with cysts containing thin, brown fluid. A photomicrograph of the lesion is shown below. The most likely diagnosis is:

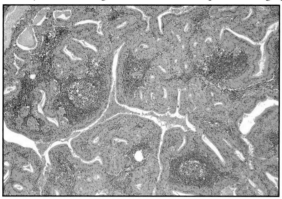 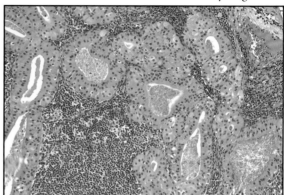

- A. Oncocytoma
- B. Canalicular adenoma
- C. Adenoid cystic carcinoma
- D. Follicular lymphoma
- E. Warthin tumor

18: Salivary Glands Answers

1. A. **PLEOMORPHIC ADENOMA**

   While each of these benign salivary neoplasms are treated with local excision, pleomorphic adenomas commonly have small, irregular surface protuberances that can extend into surrounding normal gland tissue. As such, wider excisions are generally preferred for pleomorphic adenomas to ensure removal of these protuberances, thereby avoiding local recurrence.

   QCSP, **Intraoperative Consultation,** p 570.

2. D. **SALIVARY DUCT CARCINOMA**

   Salivary duct carcinoma is a highly aggressive neoplasm, associated with local invasion, angiolymphatic metastases, and a poor prognosis.

   QCSP, **Intraoperative Consultation,** p 570.

3. B. **FALSE**

   Ischemic insult appears to be the primary etiology of necrotizing sialometaplasia. Trauma, abscess, poorly fitting dentures, oral surgery, and bulimia as well as allergies and upper respiratory infections have all been shown to be associated with this entity. According to a model proposed by Anneroth and Hansen in 1982, necrotizing sialometaplasia histologically develops and evolves through 5 stages: infarction, sequestration, ulceration, repair, and healing. The progression and duration of these stages depends on the magnitude of the initial ischemic insult.

   QCSP, **Necrotizing Sialometaplasia,** p 571.

4. B. **THE AVERAGE AGE AT DIAGNOSIS IS APPROXIMATELY 45 YEARS.**

   Necrotizing sialometaplasia occurs twice as frequently in men as compared to women. These lesions develop rapidly, but usually resolve with 3-12 weeks. Although patients usually present with a unilateral lesion, bilateral and midline ulcers can occur. There is no mutation associated with this benign entity. The average age at presentation is approximately 45 years.

   QCSP, **Necrotizing Sialometaplasia,** p 571.

5. C. **IT IS THE MOST COMMON MALIGNANT SALIVARY GLAND TUMOR TO OCCUR BILATERALLY.**

   Acinic cell carcinoma is the 3rd most common epithelial malignancy of salivary glands, behind mucoepidermoid carcinoma and adenocarcinoma, not otherwise specified. Approximately 85% of these tumors occur in the parotid glands, with 5% occurring in the submandibular glands. Almost all of the remaining 10% involve the minor salivary glands (particularly intraoral). Involvement of the sublingual gland is very rare. These are the most common malignant salivary gland tumors to occur bilaterally (3% of cases). A minority of patients present with either pain (30%) or facial muscle weakness (5%). These tumors occur 1.5 times more frequently in women. The average age at diagnosis is 45; however, there is a relatively even distribution in patients between the 2nd and 7th decades of life. Interestingly, acinic cell carcinoma is one of the most common salivary gland malignancies to affect the pediatric population (although it is still extremely rare).

   QCSP, **Acinic Cell Carcinoma,** p 572.

6. D. **SURVIVAL AT 5 YEARS IS HIGHLY INDICATIVE OF A CURE.**

   Several studies have indicated that survival at 5 years is not a strong indicator of a cure, as local recurrence and metastases can frequently occur a decade or more after the initial surgical excision. A PAS stain with diastase is helpful for highlighting the cytoplasmic secretory granules (the granules are resistant to diastase digestion). Electron microscopy will demonstrate the electron-dense cytoplasmic secretory granules as well as an abundance of mitochondria. The papillary cystic variant appears to have the worst prognosis, with 10% of these cases having regional lymph node metastases. Mortality is cited as approximately 15%.

   QCSP, **Acinic Cell Carcinoma,** p 572.

7.   B.   **THIS IS THE MOST COMMON MALIGNANT SALIVARY GLAND TUMOR IN CHILDREN.**
While malignant salivary gland tumors are quite rare in children, mucoepidermoid carcinomas are the carcinomas that most frequently occur (more commonly than acinic cell carcinoma). These lesions generally develop in the 2nd decade of life. Mucoepidermoid carcinomas are also the most common malignant salivary gland tumors of adults (15% of all tumors, malignant or benign). Women are 50% more likely than men to be affected. While the parotid is the most common site of involvement (45% of cases), the palate is the site of origin 20% of the time. An additional 20% of these tumors occur in the buccal mucosa, retromolar region, tongue, and lips. The lower lip is more frequently involved than the upper lip. Although very rare, these tumors have been reported in the bronchial tree, lacrimal sac, breast, thyroid, thymus, esophagus, and skin.
QCSP, **Mucoepidermoid Carcinoma,** p 573.

8.   B.   **MUCOUS CELLS**
Necrotizing sialometaplasia must be included in the differential when considering a diagnosis of mucoepidermoid carcinoma, as these lesions both frequently present as painful swellings of the palate. Necrotizing sialometaplasia is distinguished by its retained, lobular architecture of the involved salivary gland and bland cytology of the surface epithelium and metaplastic ducts. In addition, coagulative necrosis of the acini and lobules is seen along with a frequent mixed inflammatory reaction. These features are not characteristic of mucoepidermoid carcinoma. Mucous cells, however, are frequently present in necrotizing sialometaplasia and are often present in the metaplastic squamous areas. In addition, areas of necrosis within necrotizing sialometaplasia are often surrounded by mucin pools left by necrotic cells. This is important to remember when examining the histology of a palatal lesion. Regarding mucoepidermoid carcinoma, a predominance of epidermoid cells always includes squamous cell carcinoma in the differential. A large proportion of intermediate cells would include pleomorphic adenoma in the differential, while a predominance of clear cells would be reminiscent of clear cell carcinoma or epithelial-myoepithelial carcinoma.
QCSP, **Mucoepidermoid Carcinoma,** p 573.

9.   C.   **HIGH-GRADE TUMORS (≥7 POINTS) ARE ASSOCIATED WITH A 75% 5-YEAR SURVIVAL, WITH ONLY 25% OF CASES METASTASIZING TO REGIONAL LYMPH NODES.**
Mucoepidermoid carcinomas are graded based on the presence of an intracystic component of >20% (2 points), the presence of neural invasion (2 points), the presence of necrosis (3 points), the presence of at least 4 mitotic figures/10 hpf (3 points), and prominent anaplasia (4 points). A score of 4 or less is consistent with a low-grade tumor and is associated with a 98% 5-year survival and only a 5% risk of metastases to regional lymph nodes. On the other hand, a tumor with a score of 7 or more is a high-grade lesion and is associated with a 56% 5-year survival and a 55% risk of metastasizing to regional lymph nodes. An intermediate-grade tumor (5 or 6 total points) has, not surprisingly, an intermediate prognosis compared to the low- and high-grade lesions. Tumors of the parotid gland (stage I and II) are treated with conservative excision. A tumor in a submandibular gland, however, requires both excision and radiation therapy. Tumors of the minor salivary glands are treated with wide excision. For either high-grade tumors or low-grade tumors with extraparenchymal extension or >4 cm (T3 disease), a radical neck dissection is indicated.
QCSP, **Mucoepidermoid Carcinoma,** p 573.

18: Salivary Glands Answers

10. E. **PROMINENT NUCLEAR ATYPIA, MITOTIC FIGURES, AND EXTENSIVE NECROSIS ARE COMMON FINDINGS.**

It is rare to find significant nuclear atypia, necrosis, and mitotic figures within mucoepidermoid carcinomas. Approximately 25% of these tumors are associated with p53 mutations, and many mucoepidermoid carcinomas have been shown to have a translocation involving chromosomes 11 and 19. Not unexpectedly, the epidermoid and intermediate cells within these tumors are positive for cytokeratin, as are some scattered clear cells. A prior exposure to ionizing radiation does appear to significantly increase the risk of developing this malignancy. Extracellular mucus sometimes results in the formation of granulation tissue within these lesions. This must be remembered when considering the diagnosis.

QCSP, **Mucoepidermoid Carcinoma,** p 573.

11. C. **TUMORS WITH PREDOMINANTLY SOLID GROWTH PATTERNS HAVE A BETTER PROGNOSIS COMPARED TO THOSE WITH CRIBRIFORM OR TUBULAR PATTERNS.**

Solid growth is associated with a worse prognosis compared to those tumors with primarily tubular or cribriform patterns. Indeed, tumors with predominantly solid architecture are considered grade III malignancies. Peripheral nerve invasion is histologically identified in over 50% of these tumors, even in lesions that grossly appear well circumscribed. The tumor cells are suspended by a collagenous stroma that is continuous with the cystic lumens that are present in the cribriform and tubular architectural growth patterns. As such, these "cysts" so characteristic of this tumor are in actuality pseudocysts (which stain positively with alcian blue). High-dose melphalan and cisplatin appear to confer a benefit when included in the treatment regimen of wide or radical surgical excision followed by radiation therapy. The tumor cells are positive for S100.

QCSP, **Adenoid Cystic Carcinoma,** p 574.

12. D. **MUTATIONS IN 6Q AND 9P ARE ASSOCIATED WITH THIS NEOPLASM.**

A recurrent mutation seen in adenoid cystic carcinoma is a translocation involving chromosomes 6q and 9p (t(6;9)(q22-23;p23-24)), with a resultant fusion of the transcription factor gene *NFIB* to the oncogene *MYB*. This translocation has been found to be a recurring finding, regardless of the site of origin of the adenoid cystic carcinoma. Loss of both 12q and 19q has also been associated with this tumor. While survival rates at 5 years are good, survival at 20 years is rather abysmal. These tumors are indolent and frequently recur over a decade after the initial excision. While adenoid cystic carcinoma can metastasize to regional lymph nodes, this neoplasm is far more likely to invade and spread via peripheral nerves. The "cystic" in the name of this tumor is derived from the pseudocysts seen on histologic examination. Grossly, the tumor is solid and usually gray to tan-white in color. The tubular pattern of growth is the architectural pattern most likely to be confused for a benign neoplasm (such as a monomorphic adenoma).

QCSP, **Adenoid Cystic Carcinoma,** p 574.

13. C. **RECURRENT TUMORS ARE USUALLY MORE HEMORRHAGIC, NECROTIC, AND MULTINODULAR THAN THE PRIMARY LESION.**

Epithelial-myoepithelial carcinoma is a tumor of older adults, with a peak incidence in the 7th decade of life. It is quite rare, representing only about 1% of all salivary gland tumors. While most of these neoplasms arise in the parotid glands or other salivary glands, up to 15% of cases occur in the intraoral minor salivary glands. At the time of resection, these tumors usually measure 2.0-3.0 cm in greatest dimension. Although a primary lesion is usually solid and homogeneous, recurrent tumors are frequently hemorrhagic, focally necrotic, and/or multinodular.

QCSP, **Epithelial-Myoepithelial Carcinoma,** p 576.

18: Salivary Glands Answers

14. C. **THE LUMENS OF THE DUCTAL STRUCTURES FORMED BY THE EPITHELIAL TUMOR CELLS CONTAIN MUCICARMINE-POSITIVE, PAS-NEGATIVE BASOPHILIC MATERIAL.**

The lumens of the ductal structures formed by the epithelial tumor cells contain eosinophilic material that is PAS positive and mucicarmine negative. The myoepithelial cells are positive for MSA, P63, and S100, with occasional staining for GFAP. The hyalinized stroma is usually positive for type IV collagen. PAS stains are frequently helpful for identifying the glycogen present within the myoepithelial cells as well as identifying the eosinophilic hyalinized stroma.

QCSP, **Epithelial-Myoepithelial Carcinoma,** p 576.

15. B. **THIS IS A LOW-GRADE NEOPLASM THAT IS LOCALLY INFILTRATIVE, BUT RARELY METASTASIZES.**

Clear cell adenocarcinoma is considered to be a low-grade malignancy. It is locally infiltrative and histologic examination frequently reveals perineural invasion. However, metastases are rare, and there have been no reported deaths directly due to clear cell carcinoma in the literature. Adjuvant radiotherapy is sometimes given following surgical excision, but chemotherapy is never used in the absence of obvious metastases. Salivary duct carcinoma is the salivary gland neoplasm associated with HER-2/neu amplification and treatment with Herceptin.

QCSP, **Clear Cell Adenocarcinoma,** p 577.

16. B. **FALSE**

Adenocarcinoma, not otherwise specified, is the 2nd most common malignant salivary gland tumor behind mucoepidermoid carcinoma (15% of all carcinomas). The tumors are somewhat more common in women and are very rare in children. Approximately 60% of these tumors arise in the major salivary glands (particularly the parotid glands), and the lesions usually present as a hard, asymptomatic mass. Grossly, these lesions are usually partially circumscribed with a white-yellow cut surface and may have focal necrosis or hemorrhage. Histologic examination reveals glandular or ductal differentiation without morphologic features that would allow classification as one of the other salivary gland carcinomas. Infiltrative growth into surrounding tissue frequently occurs, and a large assortment of architectural patterns can be present. The prototypical tumor cell is cuboidal or oval, but rare clear cells and oncocytic cells may be seen in addition to small pools of extracellular mucin and eosinophilic acellular material. The tumors are classified as having low-grade, intermediate-grade, or high-grade histology based on the level of ductal differentiation, pleomorphism, and mitotic rate. Interestingly, some of these tumors will demonstrate immunoreactivity with an immunohistochemical stain for prostate specific antigen. The carcinomas are treated with aggressive excision. Radiation has not been shown to be effective. While prognosis is related to tumor grade, the carcinomas that arise in the minor salivary glands generally have better prognoses.

QCSP, **Adenocarcinoma, Not Otherwise Specified,** p 580.

17. C. **PLEOMORPHIC ADENOMAS OF THE MAJOR SALIVARY GLANDS ARE MUCH LESS LIKELY TO RECUR.**

Pleomorphic adenomas that arise in the major salivary glands are actually far more likely to recur. A subtotal excision also increases the chance of a recurrence. These tumors frequently have small, irregular surface protuberances that can extend into surrounding normal gland tissue. As such, superficial parotidectomies or extracapsular dissections with margins of normal salivary gland are performed to ensure removal of these protuberances, thereby avoiding local recurrence.

QCSP, **Pleomorphic Adenoma,** p 582.

18. C. **BROOKE-SPIEGLER SYNDROME**

Brooke-Spiegler syndrome is an autosomal dominant disease characterized by the development of numerous skin adnexal tumors such as spiradenomas, trichoepitheliomas, and cylindromas, in addition to membranous basal cell adenomas of the salivary glands. It is believed that mutations in the cylindromatosis (CYLD) tumor-suppressor gene located at chromosome 16q12-q13 are responsible for this syndrome.

QCSP, **Basal Cell Adenoma,** p 585.

18: Salivary Glands Answers

19. **B. MUSCLE-SPECIFIC ACTIN**

Muscle-specific actin is useful for differentiating a canalicular adenoma from both myoepithelioma and epithelial-myoepithelial carcinoma. Canalicular adenomas are negative for muscle-specific actin, which is indicative of the lack of myoepithelial differentiation in these lesions. Cytokeratin and S100 would be positive in all 3 of these tumors.

QCSP, **Canalicular Adenoma,** p 586.

20. **E. PHOSPHOTUNGSTIC ACID-HEMATOXYLIN**

Phosphotungstic acid-hematoxylin (PTAH) has strong affinity for mitochondria. As such, the cytoplasm of mitochondria-rich oncocytic cells will stain dark blue, helping to confirm the diagnosis.

QCSP, **Oncocytoma,** p 586.

21. **C. THE MEDIAN AGE AT DIAGNOSIS IS 39 YEARS.**

Warthin tumors are strongly associated with smoking, with heavy smokers having an 8× increased risk compared to nonsmokers. Given proper excision, the recurrence risk should be <2%. Interestingly, 5%-10% of patients present with bilateral parotid masses. African-Americans rarely present with this tumor. The median age at diagnosis is 62 years. It is very rare for an individual under 40 to develop this lesion.

QCSP, **Warthin Tumor,** p 587.

22. **C. NECROTIZING SIALOMETAPLASIA**

Necrotizing sialometaplasia presents as either an ulcerated or nonulcerated area of swelling that is generally painful and develops rapidly. Approximately 75% of cases involve the minor salivary glands of the palate, with predilection for the hard palate or hard/soft junction. More rarely, the lesion can involve the parotid gland, retromolar mucosa, tongue, buccal mucosa, and lower lip. Histologically, necrotizing sialometaplasia is characterized by squamous metaplasia of salivary gland ducts, lobular coagulative necrosis of individual salivary gland acini, surrounding inflammation, and pseudoepitheliomatous hyperplasia of adjacent mucosal epithelium.

QCSP, **Necrotizing Sialometaplasia,** p 571.

23. **B. ACINIC CELL CARCINOMA**

Acinic cell carcinoma is a low-grade carcinoma of the salivary glands composed of large, polygonal tumor cells with cytoplasm that is usually basophilic and granular. In some cases, the tumor cells can be quite clear, depending on the glycogen content of the cells. In general, the nuclei are small, round, and uniform and are located eccentrically within the cells. These tumor cells can grow in solid, papillary-cystic, follicular, or microcystic patterns. Tumors growing in a papillary-cystic pattern have branching papillae with extension into cystic lumens. The follicular pattern consists of variably sized cystic structures containing proteinaceous debris. It is not uncommon to find lymphoid follicles with well-formed germinal centers around the tumor edge. Rarely, psammoma bodies can be identified.

QCSP, **Acinic Cell Carcinoma,** p 572.

18: Salivary Glands Answers

24.   A.   **MUCOEPIDERMOID CARCINOMA**

Mucoepidermoid carcinoma is a malignant salivary gland tumor that is composed of 4 cell types in various configurations: intermediate (basal) cells, mucus-producing cells, epidermoid cells, and clear cells. The intermediate cells are generally larger than lymphocytes are present in solid sheets or clusters within the tumor. The mucus-producing cells characteristically contain epithelial mucin and may appear as epidermoid, clear, columnar, or intermediate cells in morphology. These cells can be present either individually in the tumor or in clusters. The epidermoid cells generally form nests. In some cases, epidermoid differentiation may be hard to find within the tumor. It is rare to find individual cell keratinization or keratin pearling, although inflamed mucoepidermoid carcinomas more commonly have these features. The clear cells contain glycogen and generally represent about 10% of the tumor cells. A prominent fibrous hyalinized stroma is common, with surrounding lymphoid proliferations seen commonly.

QCSP, **Mucoepidermoid Carcinoma,** p 573.

25.   C.   **ADENOID CYSTIC CARCINOMA**

Adenoid cystic carcinoma is composed of bland tumor cells with a basaloid, myoepithelial appearance. The individual tumor cells generally have clear or basophilic cytoplasm and indistinct cell borders. The nuclei are usually round and hyperchromatic. Nucleoli are very inconspicuous. These cells grow in 3 primary architectural patterns: cribriform (most common), tubular, and solid (least common). Grossly, these tumors are usually solid and well circumscribed, but are rarely encapsulated. Overall, adenoid cystic carcinoma represents 5% of all salivary gland tumors and approximately 8% of salivary gland carcinomas. These tumors occur more commonly in women, and peak incidence is in the 4th and 5th decades of life. Over 50% of these tumors occur in either the parotid glands or submandibular glands. If the tumor occurs in a minor salivary gland, the palate is the most common site (over 50%).

QCSP, **Adenoid Cystic Carcinoma,** p 574.

26.   C.   **PERINEURAL INVASION IS SELDOM IDENTIFIED.**

Polymorphous low-grade adenocarcinoma is an uncommon salivary gland malignancy that is generally felt to be limited to the minor salivary glands. Approximately 60% occur in the palate (hard or soft), with 15% arising in the buccal mucosa and 12% developing in the upper lip. Women are more commonly affected than men. While overall quite rare, PLGAs are the 2nd most common salivary gland malignancy to occur in the palate, the most common being adenoid cystic adenocarcinoma. These tumors are recognized to assume a huge variety of architectural patterns, including solid, trabecular, tubular, and ductular patterns in varying ratios, with foci of cribriform, cystic, and papillary-cystic architecture sometimes identified. Frequently, the tumor cells form small tubules with clear lumens lined by cuboidal cells. The individual tumor cells are generally uniform in appearance, with round nuclei, inconspicuous nucleoli, and stippled chromatin. It is common to see invasive features in the periphery of the lesion, with occasional linear-pattern invasion resembling an invasive lobular carcinoma of the breast. Perineural invasion is classically present, and in this regard this tumor is similar to adenoid cystic carcinoma. Mitotic figures are difficult to identify, and when seen, are characteristically typical mitoses. Foci of oncocytic change may be present, and there is usually some degree of collagenous stroma present. Grossly, these tumors are usually well circumscribed and have a tan, firm cut surface. These tumors are treated with wide excision. There is no evidence that chemoradiation has a benefit.

QCSP, **Polymorphous Low-Grade Adenocarcinoma (PLGA),** p 575.

18: Salivary Glands Answers

27.   E.   **EPITHELIAL-MYOEPITHELIAL CARCINOMA**

Epithelial-myoepithelial carcinoma is a salivary gland tumor with biphasic differentiation, with glandular lumens containing eosinophilic material that are lined by cuboidal cells of epithelial differentiation. A single layer of cells with abundant clear cytoplasm surrounds these glandular structures (myoepithelial differentiation). The myoepithelial and epithelial cells are generally present in a ratio of 3:1, with myoepithelial cells being the predominant cell type. The myoepithelial cells are generally large, with glycogenated (clear) cytoplasm. These cells often have irregularly shaped nuclei and have indistinct cell borders. The epithelial cells, on the other hand, are usually cuboidal, with prominent, regular nuclei and eosinophilic cytoplasm. The tumor cells are generally arranged in sheets, nests, or organoid architecture with surrounding hyalinized eosinophilic or myxoid stroma. In some cases, there may be a cystic portion of tumor. Perineural invasion is sometimes seen, but cytologic atypia is generally absent. Mitotic figures can be identified.

QCSP, **Epithelial-Myoepithelial Carcinoma**, p 576.

28.   D.   **CLEAR CELL ADENOCARCINOMA**

Clear cell adenocarcinoma is a rare tumor that represents approximately 1% of all salivary gland neoplasms. Most cases (60%) involve the minor salivary glands, with the palate being the most common site of origin. Males and females are equally affected, and most cases occur between the 5th and 7th decades of life. These tumors are usually <3.0 cm in greatest dimension at the time of resection and are generally poorly circumscribed with invasion throughout adjacent mucosa or bone. The cut surface is generally white or gray. Histologically, the tumor is composed of round or polygonal cells with clear or faintly eosinophilic cytoplasm. The nuclei are usually round and contain inconspicuous nucleoli. Mitotic figures are rare. Architectural arrangements include sheets, cords, and nests of cells, with intervening connective tissue stroma. This stroma can be highly variable in appearance and can be hyalinized, thick, or fine. In rare instances, microcysts may be detected. The micrograph above depicts a hyalinizing clear cell carcinoma, a variant found more commonly in women.

QCSP, **Clear Cell Adenocarcinoma**, p 577.

29.   C.   **ONCOCYTIC CARCINOMA**

Oncocytic carcinoma is a rare salivary gland tumor found predominantly in the parotid glands (80%) that represents only 1% of all salivary gland neoplasms. Patients usually present with painful, enlarging masses that are sometimes associated with facial paralysis. Men are twice as likely to be affected, and the average age at diagnosis is 63. These tumors frequently have local recurrences and can metastasize to either cervical lymph nodes or distant sites such as the lungs, liver, mediastinum, and bone. Lesions are treated with aggressive excision, and radiation has not been shown to be useful. Grossly, these lesions present as firm tan to gray unencapsulated masses that sometimes contain necrosis. Histologically, the tumor cells are large and either round or polygonal and are arranged as sheets, cords, or individual cells. The tumor cells frequently invade surrounding nerves, muscle, and lymphatics. The cells have granular eosinophilic cytoplasm secondary to the copious mitochondria within the cells. A PTAH stain will stain the mitochondria-rich cytoplasm dark blue.

QCSP, **Oncocytic Carcinoma**, p 578.

18: Salivary Glands Answers

30. **D.** **HISTOLOGIC EXAMINATION WILL OFTEN REVEAL AREAS OF TUMOR THAT ARE REMINISCENT OF INVASIVE DUCTAL CARCINOMA OF THE BREAST.**

Salivary duct carcinoma is a highly aggressive salivary gland carcinoma that represents 4% of all salivary gland malignancies. Approximately 85% of these carcinomas arise in the parotid glands, with the remainder occurring in the submandibular glands and intraoral minor salivary glands. These neoplasms are 3 times more common in men, and most commonly present in the 5th and 6th decades of life. These lesions typically grow rapidly, and can cause facial nerve dysfunction in 25% of patients. Palpable cervical lymphadenopathy is seen in around 35% of patients. Grossly, these lesions are grey to yellow in color, multinodular, unencapsulated, and poorly circumscribed. The cut surface is often necrotic and cystic. Histologic examination reveals foci of polygonal tumor cells with eosinophilic cytoplasm. Nuclei are usually round and large. Mitotic activity can be brisk. Cystic nodules, when present, have epithelium arranged in cribriform, papillary, and bandlike patterns. Comedonecrosis as well as perineural and lymphatic infiltration is frequently seen. Some areas are histologically similar to invasive ductal carcinoma of the breast. Salivary duct carcinoma is treated with wide surgical excision in addition to radical neck dissection and radiation therapy. Approximately 60% of patients succumb to their carcinoma, most of these within 5 years of diagnosis. Many of these tumors demonstrate HER-2/neu amplification and respond to therapy with trastuzumab (Herceptin).
QCSP, **Salivary Duct Carcinoma**, p 579.

31. **C.** **THE MALIGNANT TRANSFORMATION AND SUBSEQUENT CARCINOMATOUS ELEMENT ALWAYS ARISES FROM THE EPITHELIAL COMPONENT OF THE PLEOMORPHIC ADENOMA.**

Carcinoma ex pleomorphic adenoma represents the malignant transformation of a benign pleomorphic adenoma. Importantly, for this diagnosis to be rendered, at least a focus of pleomorphic adenoma must be present. In some cases the carcinomatous element is clearly separated from the benign element, while in other examples the foci of malignant transformation are scattered throughout the benign element. The incidence of the malignant transformation increases with the length of time a pleomorphic adenoma has been present. While only 2% of pleomorphic adenomas transform in the first 5 years, this number greatly increases to 10% after 15 years. Up to 20% of patients who report prior surgeries for pleomorphic adenoma resection are ultimately diagnosed with carcinoma ex pleomorphic adenoma, presumably due to incomplete resection during the original surgeries. The carcinomatous element in these malignancies always arises from the epithelial component of the pleomorphic adenoma. Perineural and vascular invasion are frequently present, and immunohistochemical stains for S100 and muscle-specific actin can be positive if the carcinomatous cells have a myoepithelial component. If these lesions are encapsulated, complete surgical excision with preservation of the facial nerve can be performed; however, unencapsulated, large, or recurrent lesions are best treated with radical parotidectomy.
QCSP, **Carcinoma ex Pleomorphic Adenoma**, p 581.

32. **C.** **PLEOMORPHIC ADENOMA**

Pleomorphic adenoma (benign mixed tumor) is the most common neoplasm of the salivary glands, with up to 85% of these lesions arising in the parotid glands. These tumors most commonly occur in patients between the 3rd and 5th decades of life. Approximately 50% of these tumors arise in the lower pole of the superficial parotid glands. Grossly, these tumors are well-circumscribed, partially encapsulated white to tan masses that frequently have a shiny cut surface. Histologic examination reveals both epithelial and mesenchymal-like tissue. The epithelial component of the tumor includes epithelial and myoepithelial cells that can be arranged in a large variety of architectural patterns. The background stroma contains large quantities of mucopolysaccharides and frequently contains chondroid and osseous tissue. A large variety of extracellular substances may be present, including amyloid, calcium oxalate crystals, collagenous spherules, and tyrosine-rich crystalloids.
QCSP, **Pleomorphic Adenoma**, p 582.

18: Salivary Glands Answers

33.   B.   **MYOEPITHELIOMA**

Myoepitheliomas are rare, benign salivary gland tumors that typically present in the 5th decade of life and are found with equal frequency in men and women. They most commonly arise in the parotid glands (40%). Grossly, these tumors are usually well circumscribed with a yellow-tan, solid cut surface. While fibrous capsules are usually present, the tumors may occasionally push through the capsule, creating a nodular tumor boundary. Histologically, these tumors can be marked by impressive heterogeneity. Most tumors are composed predominantly of spindle cells arranged in tight intertwined fascicles with minimal surrounding stroma. The spindle cell nuclei are typically vesicular with inconspicuous nucleoli. These cells have eosinophilic and finely granular cytoplasm with indistinct cell borders. These tumors composed primarily of spindle cells can still have pockets of polygonal epithelioid cells present. These tumors can also be composed primarily of epithelioid or plasmacytoid cells. The tumor cells are positive for cytokeratin, muscle-specific actin, and p63, and negative for desmin staining. The spindle cells are more reactive for muscle-specific actin than either epithelioid cells or plasmacytoid cells. These tumors are treated with complete surgical excision, and recurrence is quite rare.
QCSP, **Myoepithelioma**, p 583.

34.   E.   **MEMBRANOUS**

Basal cell adenomas are benign salivary gland tumors that most frequently arise in the superficial lateral lobe of parotid glands (70% of the time). The mean age at diagnosis is 58, and women are twice as likely as men to be affected. Grossly, these tumors are usually circumscribed, gray to tan on cut surface, and have a prominent fibrous capsule present. The membranous type, however, is often multifocal and unencapsulated. Histologically, the tumors are composed of nests of basaloid epithelial cells with peripheral palisading. The individual tumor cells vary widely from light to dark in appearance, with the lighter cells having faint nuclei, pale cytoplasm, and a more central location within the tumor. The tumor cells can assume a large variety of architectural growth patterns, including solid, trabecular, trabecular-tubular, tubular, and membranous patterns. A solid growth pattern is most common, with nests of cells with conspicuous palisading of nuclei along stromal surfaces. The trabecular pattern is composed of interlacing bands of cells, with less collagenous stroma present. The tubular pattern is characterized by small lumens formed by lining basaloid cells. Finally, the membranous pattern is characterized by cell nests that approximate each other closely, forming a "jigsaw" pattern typically seen in cylindromas of the skin. The nests of cells can also possess droplets of membrane and are frequently surrounded by prominent hyaline bands. The membranous-type tumors have a worse prognosis, due to their frequent multifocality and lack of encapsulation. These membranous-pattern tumors have recurrence rates as high as 25%. Treatment of basal cell adenomas includes a total excision, including a small rim of normal salivary gland. Malignant transformation can occur in all architectural patterns; however, the membranous type is far more likely to undergo this transformation (25% vs 4%). Histologic features of malignant transformation include perineural involvement, marked cytologic atypia, and angiolymphatic invasion in addition to local infiltration.
QCSP, **Basal Cell Adenoma**, p 585.

35.   D.   **UPPER LIP**

The majority of canalicular adenomas arise within the minor salivary glands of the upper lip. Histologically, these tumors are characterized by dual rows of columnar epithelial cells arranged in cords. These rows frequently bifurcate, creating canaliculi. Nuclei are round with finely stippled chromatin. Loose stroma is present, with small quantities of collagen and rare fibroblasts present. Grossly, these lesions are well circumscribed and yellow-tan in color. The cut surface is usually homogeneous and gelatinous. These lesions are more common in women and usually present in the seventh decade of life. Canalicular adenomas represent approximately 1% of all salivary gland neoplasms.
QCSP, **Canalicular Adenoma**, p 586.

18: Salivary Glands Answers

36. **A.** **ONCOCYTOMA**

Oncocytomas are rare salivary gland neoplasms that usually occur in the parotid glands (90% of cases). The peak incidence is between the 7th and 9th decades of life, with a mean age of 58 at diagnosis. Women are slightly more likely than men to develop this lesion. Grossly, these tumors are well circumscribed and red-brown to tan in color. Sometimes cysts are present within the lesion, as in this case. Histologically, the tumors are composed of oncocytes with copious granular, eosinophilic cytoplasm. The cells are large and have large nuclei with prominent nucleoli. The tumor cells are usually arranged in an organoid pattern. While there can be mild cellular and nuclear pleomorphism, mitotic figures are almost never identified. Glycogenated clear cells may also be present in the lesion. Besides oncocytic carcinoma, oncocytic metaplasia and nodular oncocytosis must be included in the differential diagnosis.

QCSP, **Oncocytoma,** p 586.

37. **E.** **WARTHIN TUMOR**

Warthin tumors are the 2nd most common benign tumors of the parotid glands (next to pleomorphic adenoma), with nearly all of these tumors occurring in the parotid glands or periparotid tissue. Most of the lesions involve the parotid tails. Grossly, these tumors are well circumscribed with a cut surface characterized by cysts containing brown, mucoid, or clear fluid. These cysts are separated by fibrous septa. Histologically, these tumors are composed of cystic spaces lined by a double layer of oncocytic epithelial cells with surrounding lymphocytes, with germinal centers sometimes present. The luminal epithelial cells are characterized by eosinophilic cytoplasm and oval nuclei. Squamous metaplasia can sometimes be identified within areas of epithelial proliferation. The cystic lumens often contain cellular debris mixed with secretions. The proportion of epithelial to lymphoid cells within these tumors can vary greatly.

QCSP, **Warthin Tumor,** p 587.

Chapter 19

Bones and Joints

___

1. Which of the following are epiphyseal tumors?
    A. Giant cell tumor of bone
    B. Chondroblastoma
    C. Clear cell chondrosarcoma
    D. Osteomyelitis
    E. All of the above are epiphyseal lesions.

2. Which of the following statements about chondroblastoma is FALSE?
    A. It primarily occurs in patients with an open growth plate.
    B. Neoplastic cells are S100+.
    C. It often shows true lung metastasis.
    D. There is an approximately 10%-15% recurrence rate after treatment.
    E. It can demonstrate aneurysmal bone cyst.

3. Which of the following would be most likely to present as a sclerotic lesion?
    A. Fibrous dysplasia
    B. Osteomyelitis
    C. Myeloma
    D. Chondrosarcoma
    E. Giant cell tumor

4. Which of the following would most likely present as a permeative lesion?
    A. Ewing sarcoma
    B. Langerhans histocytosis
    C. Fibrosarcoma
    D. Osteomyelitis
    E. All of the above

5. Which of the following is least likely to demonstrate a chondroid matrix?
    A. Mesenchymal chondrosarcoma
    B. Chondromyxoid fibroma
    C. Enchondroma
    D. Chondroblastoma
    E. Osteochondroma.

6. Which of the following syndromes is/are associated with multiple enchondromas and soft tissue angiomas?
    A. Ollier disease
    B. Metachondromatosis
    C. Ehlers-Danlos
    D. Maffucci syndrome
    E. Marfan syndrome

19: Bones and Joints Questions

7. Which of the following syndromes is/are associated with cartilaginous lesions and juvenile granulosa cell tumors?
    A. Ollier disease
    B. Metachondromatosis
    C. Maffucci syndrome
    D. A & C
    E. All the above

8. Which of the following syndromes generally demonstrates a slow-growing progressive disease that tends to stabilize at puberty?
    A. Ollier disease
    B. Metachondromatosis
    C. Ehlers-Danlos
    D. Maffucci syndrome
    E. Marfan syndrome

9. Which lesions are associated with hereditary multiple exostoses?
    A. Periosteal chondroma
    B. Osteochondroma
    C. Enchondroma
    D. Osteoma
    E. Chondroblastoma

10. Which is the most common area for an osteochondroma?
    A. Pelvic bones
    B. Distal femur
    C. Sternum
    D. Scapula
    E. Patella

11. Which of the following statements regarding periosteal chondroma is FALSE?
    A. It is usually found incidentally.
    B. It extends from the medullary cavity.
    C. There are occasional atypical chondrocytes.
    D. Treatment is with surgical excision or curettage.
    E. Cortex under the lesion demonstrates saucerization.

12. Which of the following lesions most closely resembles an osteoblastoma histologically?
    A. Osteochondroma
    B. Chondroblastoma
    C. Osteoid osteoma
    D. Aneurysmal bone cyst
    E. Fracture callus

13. Which of the following statements regarding aggressive osteoblastoma is FALSE?
    A. It progresses to osteosarcoma in approximately 45% of cases.
    B. It generally consists of epithelioid osteoblasts.
    C. It is typically larger than standard osteoblastoma.
    D. It contains thicken bony trabeculae.
    E. It has increased risk of recurrence as compared with conventional osteoblastoma.

19: Bones and Joints Questions

14. Which of the following lesions typically presents with pain that is worse at night?
    A. Enchondroma
    B. Osteoid osteoma
    C. Aneurysmal bone cyst
    D. Giant cell tumor of bone
    E. Langerhans cell histiocytosis

15. The associated reactive sclerosis of osteoid osteoma is thought to be secondary to prostaglandin E2 and prostacyclin released by which cell type(s)?
    A. Osteoclasts
    B. Endothelium
    C. Osteoblasts
    D. A&B
    E. All the above

16. What are the typical radiologic findings of an aneurysmal bone cyst?
    A. Moth-eaten lesion
    B. Solitary cystic lesion
    C. Sharply demarcated, round, lytic lesion
    D. Sclerotic lesion
    E. Expansive soap-bubble lytic lesion

17. Which of the following lesions can demonstrate features of aneurysmal bone cyst?
    A. Osteoblastoma
    B. Chondroblastoma
    C. Fibrous dysplasia
    D. Giant cell tumor of bone
    E. All of the above

18. Which translocation is seen in primary aneurysmal bone cyst but not in secondary aneurysmal bone cyst?
    A. t(12;16) FUS-ATF1
    B. t(16;17) CDH11-USP6
    C. t(12;16) FUS-CHOP
    D. t(11;22) EWS-FLI
    E. t(11;22) EWS-WT1

19. Which patient and clinical situation is most typically of patients with solitary (unicameral) bone cysts?
    A. 7-year-old girl with an epiphyseal lesion of the distal femur
    B. 38-year-old woman with phalangeal lesion
    C. 20-year-old man with vertebral lesions
    D. 55-year-old woman with scapular lesion
    E. 10-year-old boy with lesion in the proximal femur metaphysis

20. Which of the following statements concerning fibrosarcoma of bone is FALSE?
    A. It usually presents between ages 40 and 50.
    B. It can demonstrate osteoid production.
    C. Low-grade lesions have an 80% 10-year survival.
    D. It can demonstrate a permeative pattern.
    E. It can demonstrate a moth-eaten pattern.

19: Bones and Joints Questions

21. Fibrous dysplasia can be associated with all the following syndromes or conditions, EXCEPT:
    A. Tuberous sclerosis
    B. McCune-Albright syndrome
    C. Mazabraud syndrome
    D. Multiple endocrinopathies
    E. It can be associated with all of the above.

22. Which of the following statements regarding fibrous dysplasia is FALSE?
    A. It usually presents prior to age 30.
    B. These lesions are most often found incidentally.
    C. It can be associated with somatic GNAS1 mutations.
    D. After an average of 5 years, the monostotic form typically progresses to the polyostotic form.
    E. It will often increase in size with pregnancy.

23. Malignant fibrous histiocytomas of bone can be associated with all the following, EXCEPT:
    A. Paget disease
    B. Chronic osteomyelitis
    C. Periosteal osteosarcoma
    D. Fibrous dysplasia
    E. Giant cell tumor of bone

24. All of the following statements regarding the prognosis or treatment of malignant fibrous histiocytomas (MFH) of bone are TRUE, EXCEPT:
    A. Amount of post-chemotherapy necrosis is used as a prognostic factor.
    B. There is a high likelihood of lymph node metastasis.
    C. Those associated with preexisting conditions tend to be more aggressive than a de novo MFH.
    D. Localized disease has a 50% 5-year survival rate.
    E. All the above are true.

25. Which bone-based lesion is associated with Jaffe-Campanacci syndrome?
    A. Osteochondroma
    B. Nonossifying fibroma
    C. Osteoid osteoma
    D. Osteoblastoma
    E. Fibrous dysplasia

26. Which of the characteristics described below is more consistent with a giant cell tumor of bone than a nonossifying fibroma?
    A. Involves both the epiphysis and the metaphysis
    B. Contains a significant number of giant cells
    C. Lytic lesion
    D. Narrow rim of marginal sclerosis
    E. Areas of necrosis

27. Which patient characteristics and bone involvement are most likely to be seen in a patient with osteofibrous dysplasia?
    A. 25-year-old woman with swelling of the jaw
    B. 15-year-old boy with lesion of the distal finger
    C. 10-year-old girl with lesion of the distal femur
    D. 65-year-old woman with proximal tibial lesion
    E. 8-year-old with lesions in both the tibia and fibula

28. Which of the following is more consistent with fibrous dysplasia than osteofibrous dysplasia?
    A.   Spontaneous regression
    B.   Osteoblastic rimming
    C.   Can have a deformity
    D.   Keratin positive cells
    E.   Located intramedullary

29. Which of the following lesions are microscopically indistinct from a giant cell reparative granuloma?
    A.   Brown tumor of hyperparathyroidism
    B.   Giant cell tumor bone
    C.   Nonossifying fibroma
    D.   Osteosarcoma, giant cell variant
    E.   Chondrosarcoma

30. All the following statements are TRUE about giant cell reparative granuloma, EXCEPT:
    A.   Pregnancy increases their size.
    B.   It is most likely related to previous trauma.
    C.   Stromal cells show myofibroblastic differentiation.
    D.   It most frequently occurs in the long bone.
    E.   Patients are usually between the ages of 15 and 25 at the time of diagnosis.

31. Which of the following statements concerning giant cell tumor of bone is TRUE?
    A.   It most often occurs in the metaphysis.
    B.   It is more common in men.
    C.   It has well-defined lytic lesions with sclerotic margins.
    D.   It can have lung lesions.
    E.   It usually requires chemotherapy treatment.

32. Which of the following statements concerning the microscopic appearance of giant cell tumor of bone is FALSE?
    A.   Giant cells have approximately 20 nuclei per cell.
    B.   The mononuclear cells and giant cells have the same morphology.
    C.   It can have infarct-related necrosis.
    D.   It is often mitotically active but without atypia.
    E.   Giant cells are evenly distributed.

33. Which of the following statements is TRUE of a malignant giant cell tumor?
    A.   It is usually limited to the bone.
    B.   It often produces osteoid.
    C.   It is not associated with previous irradiation.
    D.   It occurs at the site of previous giant cell tumor.
    E.   All of the above are true.

34. Which of the following are features of clear cell chondrosarcoma?
    A.   Cells that are PAS+
    B.   Clear cytoplasm
    C.   Woven bone
    D.   Clear cells that are S100+
    E.   All of the above are features.

35. Which of the following statements is FALSE regarding conventional chondrosarcoma?
    A. It is particularly radiation-sensitive.
    B. It most often presents with pain.
    C. It is an intramedullary lesion.
    D. Recurrences can occur may years (decades) after initial diagnosis.
    E. The most helpful diagnostic criteria is the presence of the chondroid lesion infiltrating into laminar bone.

36. Which of the following features is most sensitive for the differentiation of a benign vs malignant growth pattern?
    A. Binucleation of chondrocytes
    B. Endochondral ossification
    C. Spindling of the chondrocytes
    D. Presence of hyaline cartilage
    E. Infiltration of the lesion by hematopoietic cells

37. Which of the following statements concerning dedifferentiated chondrosarcoma is FALSE?
    A. A high-grade lesion often forms a soft tissue mass.
    B. It demonstrates features of a grade 1 chondrosarcoma.
    C. The low-grade and high-grade portions of the lesion are intermixed.
    D. It can produce osteoid.
    E. Long-term survival is <10%.

38. Which of the following statements regarding mesenchymal chondrosarcoma is TRUE?
    A. It generally affects younger patients than conventional chondrosarcoma.
    B. It most frequently involves the jawbones.
    C. It is the most common extraosseous chondrosarcoma.
    D. It has a better prognosis than dedifferentiated chondrosarcoma.
    E. All of the above are true.

39. Which of the following sarcomas are not associated with Paget disease?
    A. Osteosarcoma
    B. Fibrosarcoma
    C. Chondrosarcoma
    D. Malignant giant cell tumor bone
    E. All of the above are sarcomas associated with Paget disease.

40. Which of the following statements concerning Paget disease is FALSE?
    A. In the active phase of the disease, osteoclasts tend to aggregate, forming the irregular scalloped appearance of the trabecula.
    B. It is generally an inherited disease, with an autosomal dominant pattern.
    C. Bowing deformities and fractures most often occur in weight-bearing bones.
    D. The classical radiologic finding is a "cotton wool-like" appearance.
    E. It was recently associated with paramyxovirus.

41. Which of the following combinations are the correct crystal type and polarization pattern/color associated with tophaceous gout?
    A. Calcium pyrophosphate dihydrate crystals, blue parallel to polarized light
    B. Monosodium urate crystals, blue parallel to polarized light
    C. Calcium oxalate, yellow parallel to polarized light
    D. Monosodium urate crystals, yellow parallel to polarized light
    E. Hydroxyapatite, yellow parallel to polarized light

19: Bones and Joints Questions

42. Which of the following is the correct crystal type and polarization pattern associated with tophaceous pseudogout?
    A. Calcium pyrophosphate dihydrate crystals, blue parallel to polarized light
    B. Monosodium urate crystals, blue parallel to polarized light
    C. Calcium oxalate, yellow parallel to polarized light
    D. Monosodium urate crystals, yellow parallel to polarized light
    E. Hydroxyapatite, yellow parallel to polarized light

43. Which of the following immunohistochemical profiles is most consistent with the diagnosis of Ewing sarcoma/PNET?
    A. CD99+, TdT+, NSE+, CD45−, FLI-1−
    B. CD99−, TdT+, NSE−, CD45+, FLI-1−
    C. CD99−, TdT−, NSE+, CD45−, FLI-1−
    D. CD99+, TdT−, NSE−, CD45+, FLI-1+
    E. CD99+, TdT−, NSE+, CD45−, FLI-1+

44. Which of the following translocations are seen in Ewing sarcoma/PNET?
    A. t(11;22)(q24;q12)
    B. t(21;22)(q22;q12)
    C. t(7;22)
    D. t(17;22)
    E. All of the above

45. Which comment about the prognosis of Ewing sarcoma is FALSE?
    A. Patients under 10 years of age typically have a better prognosis.
    B. Approximately 25% of patients with Ewing sarcoma/PNET present with metastatic disease.
    C. Cases with EWS/ERG translocation have a better prognosis.
    D. Tumors of the appendicular skeleton do better than those of the axial skeleton.
    E. Percent of necrosis after neoadjuvant chemotherapy used to predict prognosis.

46. Which of the following syndromes are associated with osteosarcomas?
    A. Li-Fraumeni syndrome
    B. Bloom syndrome
    C. Rothmund-Thompson
    D. Werner
    E. All of the above are associated.

47. Why is it important to extensively sample an osteosarcoma resection specimen?
    A. Number of mitotic figures/HPF
    B. Chemotherapy-induced tumor necrosis
    C. Lymphovascular involvement
    D. Percent of medullary cavity involvement
    E. Determine subtype

48. Which osteosarcoma subtype has the worst prognosis?
    A. Parosteal osteosarcoma
    B. Paget disease associated osteosarcoma
    C. Periosteal osteosarcoma
    D. Chondroblastic variant of conventional osteosarcoma
    E. Intracortical osteosarcoma

19: Bones and Joints Questions

49. Which of the following statements regarding the intracortical osteosarcoma is FALSE?
    A. Radiologic findings are similar to osteoid osteoma.
    B. It acts similarly to the well-differentiated intramedullary osteosarcoma.
    C. There is no evidence of intramedullary involvement.
    D. It primarily involves the tibial diaphysis and femoral shaft.
    E. It demonstrates extensive bone formation with occasional cartilage formation.

50. Which of the following statements concerning parosteal osteosarcoma is FALSE?
    A. 5-year survival is 85%-90%.
    B. It is primarily located on the proximal humerus.
    C. 15% of cases harbor high-grade/dedifferentiated histology.
    D. It demonstrates broad stalk-like attachment to underlying bone.
    E. It does not typically involve the medullary cavity.

51. Histologically, which lesion does periosteal osteosarcoma resemble?
    A. Chondroblastoma
    B. Chondrosarcoma
    C. Intracortical osteosarcoma
    D. Osteoblastoma
    E. Chondromyxoid fibroma

52. Which of the following lesion does telangiectatic osteosarcoma most closely resemble?
    A. Intramedullary osteosarcoma
    B. Giant cell tumor of bone
    C. Clear cell chondrosarcoma
    D. Aneurysmal bone cyst
    E. Periosteal osteosarcoma

53. Which statement regarding telangiectatic osteosarcoma is FALSE?
    A. It demonstrates minimal osteoid production.
    B. Patients usually have elevated alkaline phosphate levels.
    C. It usually presents as an epiphyseal lesion.
    D. Up to 25% of patients present with pathologic fracture.
    E. The most common site is the knee.

54. Which statement regarding well-differentiated intramedullary osteosarcoma is FALSE?
    A. Treatment is primarily surgical excision alone.
    B. Metastasis does not occur.
    C. Histologically it resembles fibrous dysplasia
    D. Typically there is an expansion of the bone and not invasion.
    E. It can have a dedifferentiated component.

55. Which of the following lesion is most closely related to pigmented villonodular synovitis?
    A. Villous lipomatous proliferation of synovial membrane
    B. Hemosiderotic synovitis
    C. Loose bodies
    D. Synovial chondromatosis
    E. Giant cell tumor of tendon sheath

19: Bones and Joints Questions

56. Which of the following statements about pigmented villonodular synovitis (PVNS) is FALSE?
    A. PVNS is a reactive process.
    B. It is a benign lesion that does not metastasize.
    C. Recurrence rate after surgery is around 50%.
    D. It most commonly affects the knee.
    E. Radiation is used in refractory disease.

57. Which of the follow patient characteristics would be most consistent with a patient with primary synovial chondromatosis?
    A. 25-year-old woman with elbow
    B. 16-year-old boy with hip lesions
    C. 68-year-old woman with knee lesions
    D. 42-year-old man with knee lesions
    E. 28-year-old man with elbow lesions

58. What is the typical immunophenotypic pattern for an adamantinoma?
    A. CK14+, CK19+, vimentin+, S100+, EGFR+, NSE+
    B. CK14-, CK19−, vimentin+, S100+, EGFR−, NSE+
    C. CK14-, CK19+, vimentin+, actin+, EGFR−, NSE+
    D. CK14+, CK19+, vimentin+, S100−, EGFR+, NSE−
    E. CK14+, CK19+, vimentin-, S100−, EGFR−, NSE−

59. Which of the following statements concerning adamantinoma is FALSE?
    A. It may be related to osteofibrous dysplasia.
    B. It can have synchronous involvement of both the tibia and fibula.
    C. It has multiple basic growth patterns including basaloid, squaloid, and spindled.
    D. Primary treatment is with resection.
    E. Similar to other bone tumors, it always metastasizes to the lung.

60. Which location is most likely to be involved by chordoma?
    A. Distal femur
    B. Proximal humerus
    C. Sacrococcygeal area
    D. Sternum
    E. Metacarpals

61. What is the classic neoplastic cell of a chordoma?
    A. Chondrocyte
    B. Myocyte
    C. Physaliphorous cell
    D. Osteoblast
    E. Neuroglia

62. Which of the following stains is most specific for the diagnosis of chordoma?
    A. S100
    B. Pan-keratin
    C. CEA
    D. Brachyury
    E. EMA

63.   What is the typical phenotype of the malignant cell in Langerhans cell histiocytosis?
     A.   Langerin+, S100-, CD1a-, CD163+, CD68+
     B.   Langerin+, S100+, CD103+, CD1a–
     C.   Langerin-, S100-, CD123+, CD1+, CD163+
     D.   Langerin-, S100+, CD1a–, CD163+
     E.   Langerin+, S100+, CD1a+, CD45–, vimentin+

64.   Which of the following is more commonly associated with the unifocal Langerhans cell histiocytosis (eosinophilic granuloma) as compared to multifocal Langerhans cell histiocytosis (Hand-Schuller-Christian disease)?
     A.   Typically occurs in younger children usually <3 years of age
     B.   Typically demonstrates cutaneous involvement
     C.   Histologically appears less aggressive
     D.   May heal spontaneously
     E.   Has symptoms of diabetes insipidus

65.   What characteristic electron microscopy finding is associated with Langerhans cell histiocytosis?
     A.   Weibel-Palade
     B.   Birbeck granules
     C.   Phagolysosome
     D.   Microvilli
     E.   Rhomboid crystals

66.   An 11-year-old female presented with shoulder pain. An X-ray and subsequently an MRI was ordered, which is shown below. The lesion was resected, and a section is shown below. What is the diagnosis?

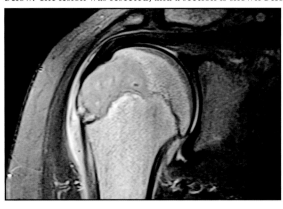 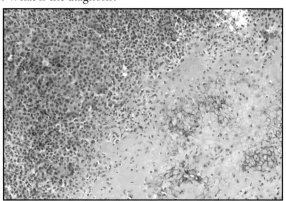

     A.   Osteoblastoma
     B.   Clear cell chondrosarcoma
     C.   Osteoid osteoma
     D.   Chondroblastoma
     E.   Osteochondroma

19: Bones and Joints Questions

67. A 20-year-old man presented to the ER with complaints of right lower quadrant abdominal pain. A CT demonstrated an inflamed appendix. There was also a lesion in the right iliac crest, and plain films were performed, which showed a lobulated lesion with sharply-defined sclerotic scalloped border (shown below). The lesion was curetted and the biopsy is shown below. What is the diagnosis?

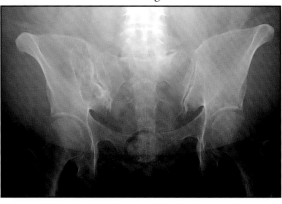 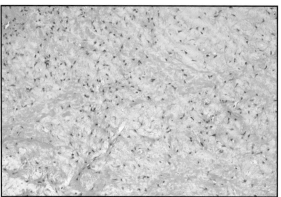

A.   Enchondroma
B.   Chondromyxoid fibroma
C.   Osteosarcoma
D.   Chondroblastoma
E.   Myxoma

68. A 45-year-old woman noticed a painful nodule forming in her left index finger. The lesion was X-rayed and then resected with placement of a bone graft. Given the radiologic and histologic appearance (shown below), what is the diagnosis?

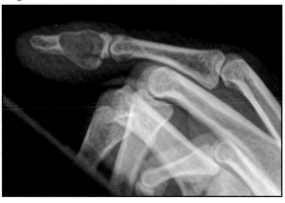 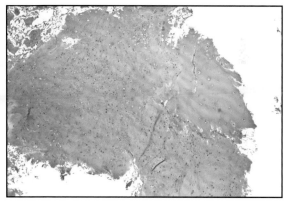

A.   Fibroma
B.   Clear-cell chondrosarcoma
C.   Chondroblastic osteosarcoma
D.   Enchondroma
E.   Conventional chondrosarcoma

19: Bones and Joints Questions

69. A 27-year-old female presented with increase pain on walking. She reports that she has had a bump or knot just below her knee for several years that has only recently begun to hurt. A lesion was seen on X-ray, and is shown below. Additionally the lesion was excised, and a histologic image is shown below. What is the diagnosis?

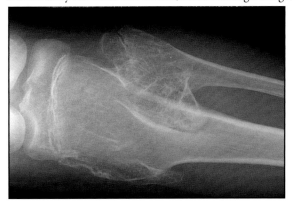 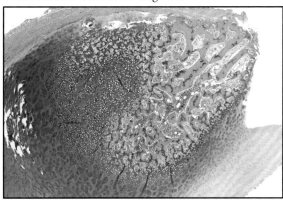

    A.   Osteochondroma
    B.   Enchondroma
    C.   Chondrosarcoma
    D.   Parosteal osteosarcoma
    E.   Juxtacortical myositis ossificans

70. A 24-year-old rugby player presented with a concussion during a game and was transported to an ER. His clearance films demonstrated a proximal humus lesion, which was imaged and is shown below. The lesion was removed and the histologic image is shown below. What is the diagnosis?

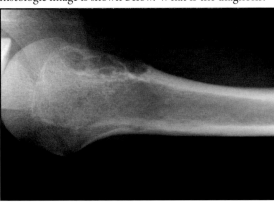 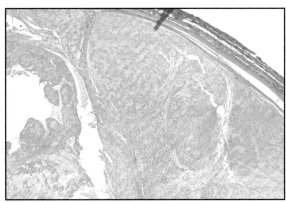

    A.   Enchondroma
    B.   Chondroma
    C.   Chondrosarcoma
    D.   Periosteal osteosarcoma
    E.   Osteochondroma

19: Bones and Joints Questions

71. A 32-year-old female presented after weeks of ankle pain. A nodule was found on her ankle, and a MRI was performed (shown below), which demonstrated a 2.3 cm lesion. The lesion was resected, and the histology is shown below. What is the diagnosis?

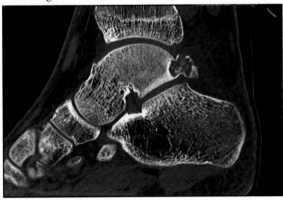 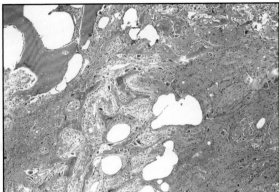

    A.   Osteoid osteoma
    B.   Osteosarcoma
    C.   Osteoblastoma
    D.   Chondroma
    E.   Osteochondroma

72. A 37-year-old male presented with recurrent back pain. MRI (shown below) demonstrates a 5.5 cm lesion developing from the spinous process. Resection of the lesion demonstrates the histology below. At higher power, there are epitheloid osteoblasts. What is the diagnosis?

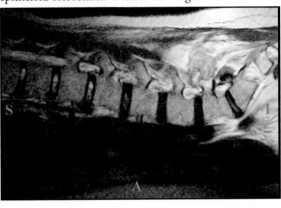 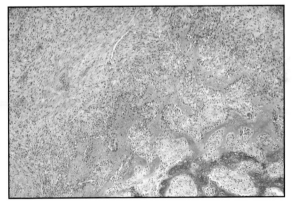

    A.   Aggressive osteoblastoma
    B.   Fibrous dysplasia
    C.   Aneurysmal bone cyst
    D.   Osteosarcoma
    E.   Chondroblastoma

73. A 17-year-old female presented with leg pain that was initially relieved by aspirin. X-ray and CT of the leg demonstrated a 0.8 cm tibial lesion, which was radiolucent with associated cortical thickening. Below are images of the X-ray and CT. A curetting was performed with cementing, and the histology is also shown below. What is the diagnosis?

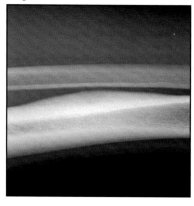 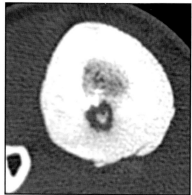 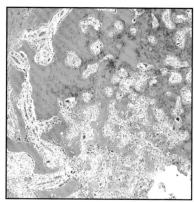

A. Langerhans cell histiocytosis
B. Osteosarcoma
C. Bone island
D. Osteoid osteoma
E. Ewing sarcoma

74. A 13-year-old girl presented with pain in the left arm/shoulder, especially when she tried to raise her arm. The pain has rapidly progressed in the last few weeks. An X-ray is performed and finds a lytic lesion in the metaphysis of the humerus. The lesion was biopsied, and the imaging and histology are shown below. What is the most likely diagnosis?

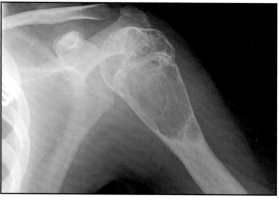 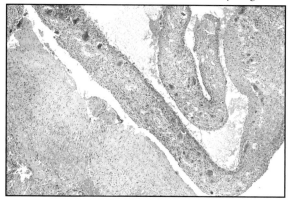

A. Chondroblastoma
B. Aneurysmal bone cyst
C. Osteoblastoma
D. Giant cell tumor of bone
E. Osteosarcoma

19: Bones and Joints Questions

75. A 9-year-old girl fell off a horse and twisted her leg. A MRI demonstrated a cystic lesion in the distal femur (shown below). The lesion was curetted and cemented. The resulting histology is shown below. What is the most likely diagnosis?

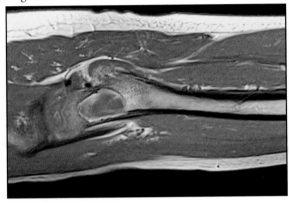 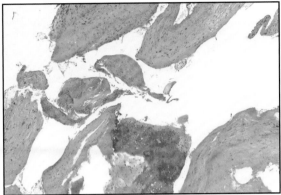

    A. Giant cell reparative granuloma
    B. Aneurysmal bone cyst
    C. Giant cell tumor of bone
    D. Chordoma
    E. Solitary bone cyst

76. A 44-year-old woman presented with facial pain including frequent nosebleeds and congestion. A representative MRI image and histological section are shown below. What is the diagnosis?

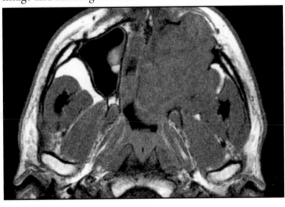 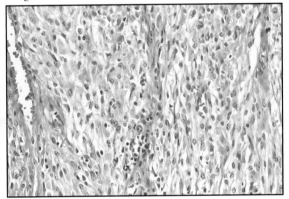

    A. Osteosarcoma
    B. Fibrosarcoma
    C. Fibrous dysplasia
    D. Chondrosarcoma
    E. Nonossifying fibroma

19: Bones and Joints Questions

77. A 28-year-old man presented with symptoms of pneumonia, and an X-ray demonstrated diffuse pulmonary infiltrates and a rib lesion. After resolution of his pneumonia, a CT was performed and the lesion excised. The radiology and histology are shown below. What is the diagnosis?

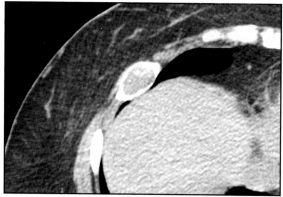 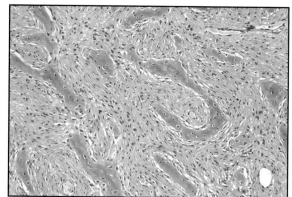

    A.   Giant cell tumor of bone
    B.   Fibrous dysplasia
    C.   Askin tumor
    D.   Osteochondroma
    E.   Osteoid osteoma

78. A 60-year-old patient with peripheral vascular disease and arthritis had swelling in/around her distal femur and knee. She went to stand up, and there was a cracking sound and a sharp intense pain. She was unable to get back up and was transported to the hospital. Imaging (seen below) demonstrates a mass in the distal femur with an associated fracture. The lesion was resected, and a representative image is shown below. What is the diagnosis?

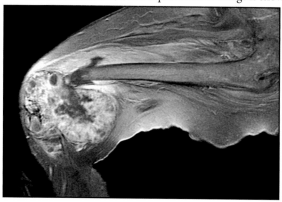 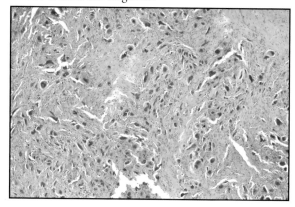

    A.   Osteosarcoma
    B.   Malignant fibrous histiocytoma
    C.   Chondrosarcoma
    D.   Metastatic synovial sarcoma
    E.   Malignant giant cell tumor

79. A 12-year-old girl fell off her bike and complained of pain in her leg. Her leg was imaged, and while no fracture was seen, an eccentric, sharply circumscribed lytic lesion was found. The lesion was biopsied, and both the radiograph and a representative histological image are shown below. What is the diagnosis?

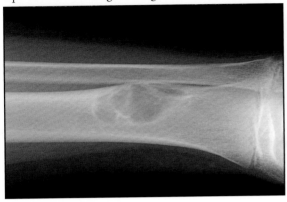 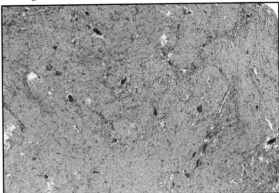

 A. Aneurysmal bone cyst
 B. Osteoid osteoma
 C. Nonossifying fibroma
 D. Chondromyxoid fibroma
 E. Solitary bone cyst

80. A 7-year-old boy presented with swelling of the left lower leg with associated pain. Imaging was performed and demonstrates multiple lytic and sclerotic lesions of the tibia. Which of the following is the best diagnosis?

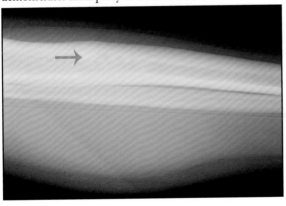 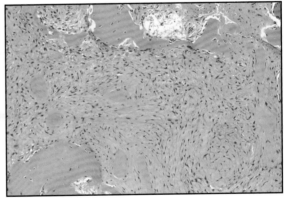

 A. Ossifying fibroma
 B. Fibrous dysplasia
 C. Giant cell tumor of bone
 D. Hemangioma
 E. Fibrosarcoma

19: Bones and Joints Questions

81. A 23-year-old woman presented with pain and swelling of her lower jaw. The lesion was imaged, and the patient was treated with steroids and subsequent curettage with bone graft. Representative radiologic image and histologic section are shown below. What is the diagnosis?

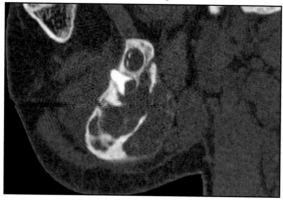 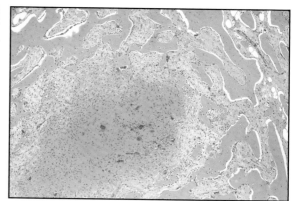

    A.   Odontogenic cyst
    B.   Ameloblastoma
    C.   Giant cell tumor of bone
    D.   Cementoma
    E.   Giant cell reparative granuloma

82. A 22-year-old woman presented with swelling of the right knee with pain on walking. Imaging of her knee demonstrates a metaepiphyseal lesion. The lesion was excised, and representative radiology and histology are shown below. What is the diagnosis?

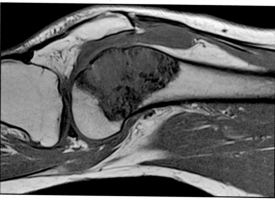 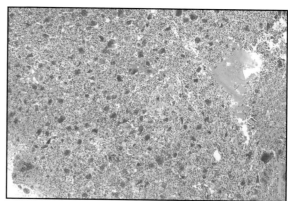

    A.   Nonossifying fibroma
    B.   Osteosarcoma
    C.   Giant cell tumor of bone
    D.   Malignant fibrosis histiocytoma
    E.   Osteomyelitis

19: Bones and Joints Questions

83. A 28-year-old man presented to the ER after several years of hip pain that has suddenly gotten worse. The MRI demonstrated a lesion in the trochanteric epiphysis of the left femur. The lesion was excised, and representative radiology and histology are shown below. What is the diagnosis?

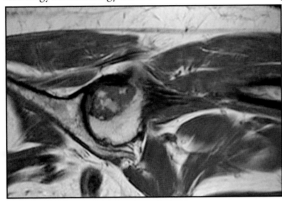 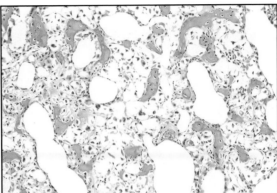

    A.   Metastatic renal cell carcinoma
    B.   Clear cell chondrosarcoma
    C.   PEComa
    D.   Osteoblastoma
    E.   Chondroblastoma

84. A 56-year-old man comes to the doctor after weeks of increasing right leg pain. The pain is described as a dull aching sensation that seems to be worse at night and keeps him awake. His hip and leg was imaged and a lesion as found in the proximal femur. The lesion was excised, and representative radiology and histology are shown below. What is the diagnosis?

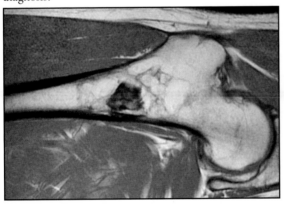 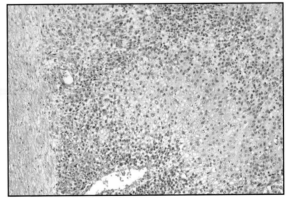

    A.   Conventional chondrosarcoma
    B.   Chondroblastoma
    C.   Osteochondroma
    D.   Chondroblastic osteosarcoma
    E.   Enchondromatosis

19: Bones and Joints Questions

85. A 57-year-old man presented with a nodule on his chest from several months that has suddenly started to enlarge and has become tender. Imaging demonstrates a lesions originating from his rib as shown below. The lesion was excised and demonstrated a well-differentiated chondrosarcoma juxtaposed to the lesion seen below. What is the diagnosis?

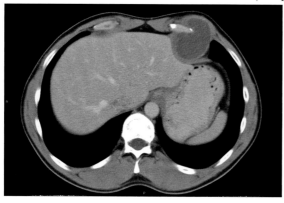 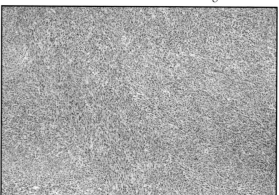

    A. Associated aneurysmal bone cyst
    B. Fibrosarcoma
    C. Synovial sarcoma
    D. Dedifferentiated chondrosarcoma
    E. Plasmacytoma

86. A 17-year-old female presented with complaints of a painful nodule located just behind her knee. A MRI of the lesion is shown below. The lesion was excised, and the histology is shown in 2 images below. What is the best diagnosis?

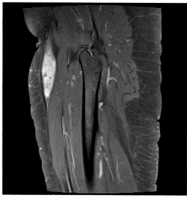 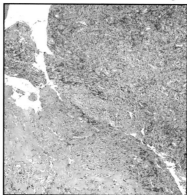 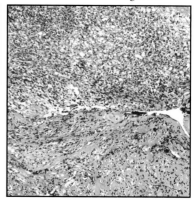

    A. Mesenchymal chondrosarcoma
    B. Nonossifying fibroma
    C. Fibrous dysplasia
    D. Enchondromatosis
    E. Chondroblastic osteosarcoma

19: Bones and Joints Questions

87. A 62-year-old man presented to autopsy after a motor-vehicle crash. He was generally in good health with drug-controlled hypertension and hyperlipidemia. The only other note in the patient's chart was an increase in his hat size in the several years prior. A gross image of the patient's skull and a representative histologic image are shown below. What is the most likely diagnosis?

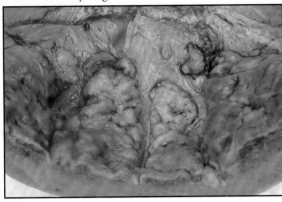 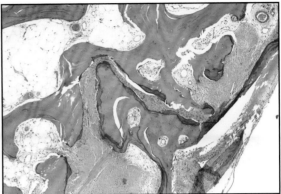

    A.   Fibrous dysplasia
    B.   Paget disease
    C.   Osteochondroma
    D.   Brown tumor of hyperparathyroidism
    E.   Osteomyelitis

88. A 48-year-old man presented to his doctor with a painless nodule on his index finger that is starting to inhibit mobility. The lesion was excised and submitted in 100% ethanol. The X-ray of his finger and histologic section of the excision are shown below. The crystals are blue when perpendicular to polarized light. What is the diagnosis?

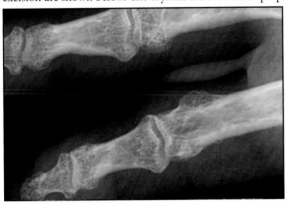 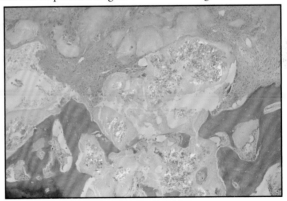

    A.   Rheumatoid arthritis
    B.   Tophaceous gout
    C.   Septic arthritis
    D.   Tophaceous pseudogout
    E.   Pigmented villonodular synovitis

89. A 63-year-old woman presented with pain and small nodular masses of her index finder. Representative imaging and histology are shown below. The biopsy demonstrates yellow crystals when perpendicular to polarized light. What is the diagnosis?

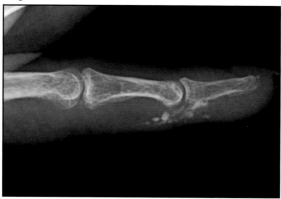 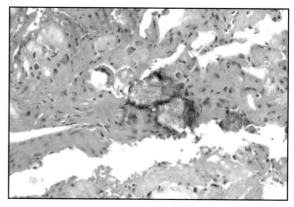

A. Rheumatoid arthritis
B. Tophaceous gout
C. Septic arthritis
D. Tophaceous pseudogout
E. Pigmented villonodular synovitis

90. An 11-year-old girl presented with increasing fatigue and pain in her right chest and back. The imaging of her chest demonstrated a large lesion that appears to originate in the rib with soft tissue extension. The lesion was resected, and representative radiology and histologic images are shown below. The lesion is positive for NSE but negative for CD45 and muscle antigens. What is the best diagnosis?

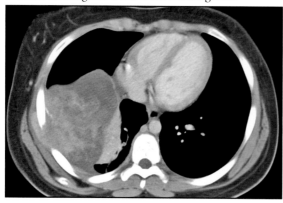 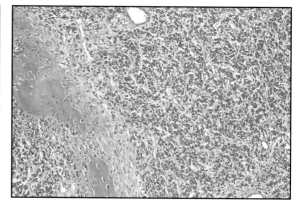

A. Lymphoma
B. Askin tumor
C. Neuroblastoma
D. Small cell osteosarcoma
E. Rhabdomyosarcoma

19: Bones and Joints Questions

91. A 9-year-old boy presents to his doctor with ongoing leg pain that has progressively worsened. His laboratory results demonstrate a mild normocytic normochromic anemia with an elevated white blood cell count. The lesion was imaged and biopsied. Representative radiologic and histologic images are shown below. What is the best diagnosis?

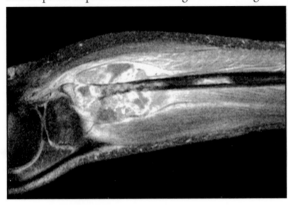 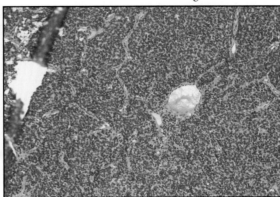

    A.   Chondroblastoma
    B.   Osteoblastoma
    C.   Giant cell tumor of bone
    D.   Ewing sarcoma
    E.   Granulocytic sarcoma

92. A 13-year-old boy presented to his pediatrician with a several-week history of knee pain after a bicycle accident. He now complains of swelling and limited mobility of his knee. Imaging was performed, and the lesion was biopsied to confirm the diagnosis. Representative images of the radiology and histology are seen below. What is the diagnosis?

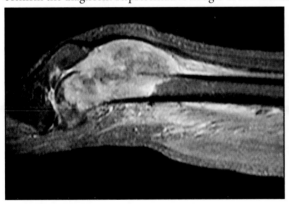 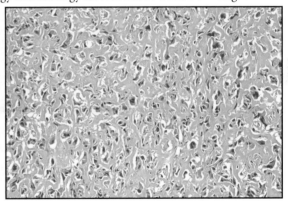

    A.   Fibrosarcoma
    B.   Aggressive osteoblastoma
    C.   Chondrosarcoma
    D.   Osteosarcoma
    E.   Reparative giant cell granuloma

19: Bones and Joints Questions

93. A 36-year-old patient presented with swelling and pain in his wrist. On imaging a lesion was found, and given the probable diagnosis, was excised. There were 2 histologic patterns seen on the excision. The radiology and representative images from both histologic patterns are shown below. What is the diagnosis?

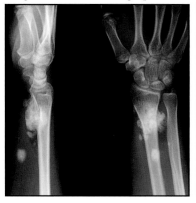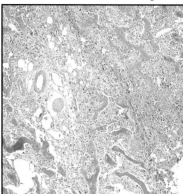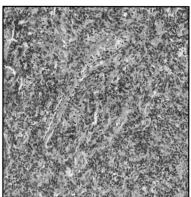

   A. Intracortical osteosarcoma
   B. Ewing sarcoma
   C. Parosteal osteosarcoma
   D. Myositis ossificans
   E. Fibromatosis

94. A 25-year-old man presented with swelling of his knee and pain upon running. There was a questionable palpable mass on exam and an X-ray was performed. The lesion was subsequently excised. The images of the radiology and histology can be seen below. What is the best diagnosis?

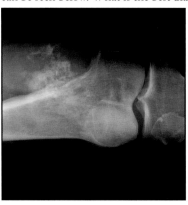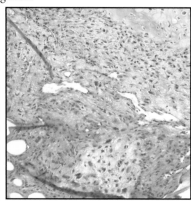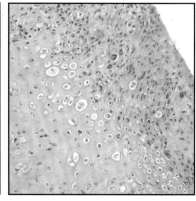

   A. Osteochondroma
   B. Periosteal osteosarcoma
   C. Fracture callus
   D. Chondroblastoma
   E. Chondromyxoid fibroma

19: Bones and Joints Questions

95. A 14-year-old JV football player presented with left knee/thigh pain. An MRI was performed, and there was a lesion involving the metaphysis and extending proximally into the diaphysis (the image below shows the diaphyseal portion of the lesion with the most typical features for the tumor). The T2 lesion demonstrates fluid levels. The lesion was biopsied, and representative images are shown below. What is the best diagnosis?

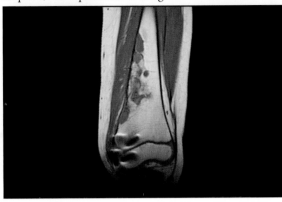 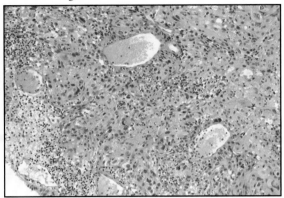

    A.   Telangiectatic osteosarcoma
    B.   Aneurysmal bone cysts
    C.   Giant cell tumor of bone
    D.   Hemangioma
    E.   Nonossifying fibroma

96. A 32-year-old woman presents with knee pain and swelling. She stated that her knee had been giving her problems for several months prior, but most recently she had begun to have a limited range of movement. Imaging was performed, and the lesion is seen below. The lesion was excised, and a representative low- and high-magnification sections are shown below. What is the diagnosis?

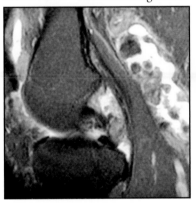 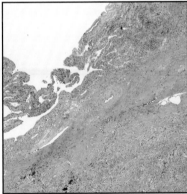 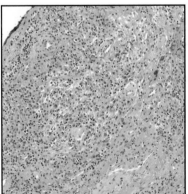

    A.   Loose bodies
    B.   Synovial chondromatosis
    C.   Nonossifying fibroma
    D.   Rheumatoid nodule
    E.   Pigmented villonodular synovitis

97. A 45-year-old man presented with a long-standing history of ankle swelling and pain. Recently he has had problem with his ankle "locking-up" with limited range of motion. Imaging was performed, including a MRI, which is shown below. The lesions were excised and a representative histologic section is shown below. What is the diagnosis?

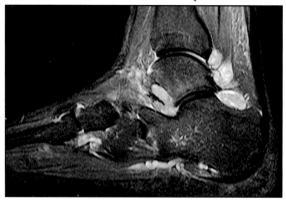 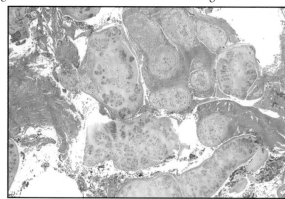

    A.   Chondroblastoma
    B.   Chondroma
    C.   Osteochondroma
    D.   Primary synovial chondromatosis
    E.   Clear cell chondrosarcoma

98. A 21-year-old woman presented with pain on walking and what she describes as a "bowing" of her lower leg. MRI was performed, and a lesion was seen in the proximal tibia (shown below). The lesion was excised, and 2 representative sections are shown below. What is the diagnosis?

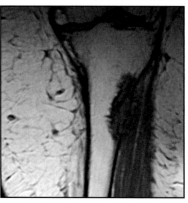 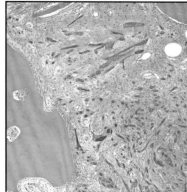 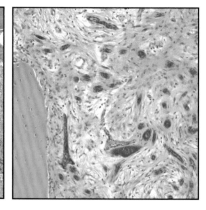

    A.   Osteofibrous dysplasia
    B.   Metastatic carcinoma
    C.   Hemangioendothelioma
    D.   Adamantinoma
    E.   Fibrous dysplasia

19: Bones and Joints Questions

99. A 14-month-old presented after multiple ear infections. On examination he had a diffuse cutaneous eruption involving the scalp, especially around the ear. He has also had increased urination and thirst. Imaging was performed, and an X-ray of the skull is shown below. One of the lesions was biopsied and is shown below. What is the diagnosis?

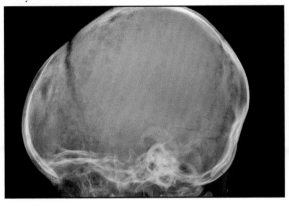 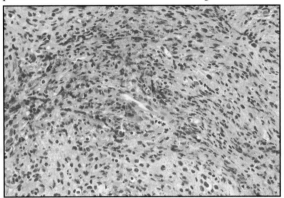

    A.   Langerhans histiocytosis
    B.   Multiple myeloma
    C.   Ewing sarcoma
    D.   Metastatic carcinoma
    E.   Reparative granuloma

19: Bones and Joints Answers

1.   E.   **ALL OF THE ABOVE ARE EPIPHYSEAL LESIONS.**

The location of the lesion and the radiological characteristics are often as important to the diagnosis as the histologic examination. A limited number of lesions are seen centered in the epiphyseal area and include chondroblastoma, giant cell tumor of bone, clear cell chondrosarcoma and osteomyelitis.
QCSP, **Chapter 19.**

2.   C.   **IT OFTEN SHOWS TRUE LUNG METASTASIS.**

Chondroblastoma is a chondroid lesion, and as such the chondrocytes are positive for S100. This lesion is considered benign and often treated with curetting and cement and/or bone graft. There is a recurrence rate of approximately 10%-15%. Like many bone tumors, this one can also be associated with an aneurysmal bone cyst (ABC). These lesions. occur in younger patients with an open epiphysis. While there might be "mets" to the lung, this situation is thought to be secondary to the curetting procedure and not a true metastatic lesion. This "pseudometastasis" can be seen in other bone tumors.
QCSP, **Chondroblastoma,** p 590-592.

3.   A.   **FIBROUS DYSPLASIA**

Of those choices listed, fibrous dysplasia is the most likely to present with a sclerotic border. Those that typically present as a type IA geographic lytic lesion with a sclerotic border include: bone cyst, chondromyxoid fibroma, fibrous dysplasia, chondroblastoma, and enchondroma. Those that have a type IB geographic lytic lesion have well-defined borders without sclerosis. The lesions that can present with IB-type imaging include: giant cell tumor of bone, fibrous dysplasia, chondroblastoma, enchondroma, and chondromyxoid fibroma.
QCSP, **Chapter 19.**

4.   E.   **ALL OF THE ABOVE**

Several lesions (typically aggressive) can have a permeative growth patterns. The typical differential diagnosis for permeative lesions includes: Ewing sarcoma and other small round blue cell tumors, fibrosarcoma/MFH, metabolic disorders, osteomyelitis, osteosarcoma, Langerhans histiocytosis, myeloma, and metastasis,
QCSP, **Chapter 19.**

5.   B.   **CHONDROMYXOID FIBROMA**

Most chondroid lesions have at least some component of true hyaline. However, chondromyxoid fibroma may only have a very small component of true hyaline cartilage or may lack true hyaline cartilage. Additionally, clear-cell chondrosarcoma often lacks true hyaline cartilage.
QCSP, **Chondromyxoid Fibroma,** p 592-593.

6.   D.   **MAFFUCCI SYNDROME**

Ollier disease, metachondromatosis, and Maffucci syndrome are all forms of enchondromatosis. However, only Maffucci syndrome is associated with soft tissue angiomas. The vascular lesions are usually cavernous hemangiomas with frequent thrombosis (which can be calcified). Additionally, it can be associated with arteriovenous aneurysms/fistula, lymphedema, and lymphangiomas.
QCSP, **Enchondroma,** p 593-595.

7.   D.   **A & C**

Both Ollier disease and Maffucci syndrome are forms of enchondromatosis, which have been associated with juvenile granulosa cell tumors. Additionally, both syndromes are associated with increased risk of malignant transformation.
QCSP, **Enchondroma,** p 593-595.

19: Bones and Joints Answers

8. **A. OLLIER DISEASE**
    Ollier disease is an enchondromatosis that is typically a progressive slow-growing disease with multifocal intramedullary proliferation of hypercellular dysplastic cartilage. However, the disease tends to stabilize at puberty.
    QCSP, **Enchondroma,** p 593-595.

9. **B. OSTEOCHONDROMA**
    Hereditary multiple exostoses is an autosomal dominant disorder with multiple osteochondromas. In approximately 90% of patients with multiple osteochondromas, they demonstrate germline mutations in tumor-suppressor genes EXT1 or EXT2. These patients also have an increased rate of malignant transformation (as compared to solitary osteochondromas).
    QCSP, **Osteochondroma,** p 595-596.

10. **B. DISTAL FEMUR**
    The lesion is most commonly found in the metaphysis of the long bones (including the distal femur). It is less commonly found in flat bones and pelvic bones.
    QCSP, **Osteochondroma,** p 595-596.

11. **B. IT EXTENDS FROM THE MEDULLARY CAVITY.**
    Periosteal chondromas typically involve long bones and are well-circumscribed cartilaginous lesions on the surface of the bone that do not involve the intramedullary cavity. The cortex beneath the lesion will typically demonstrate a craterlike appearance (saucerization). Complete excision is generally curative. While these lesions can demonstrate occasional mild atypia, they do not demonstrate the atypica seen in chondrosarcoma. While they can occasionally be symptomatic they are most often incidentally found.
    QCSP, **Periosteal Chondroma (Juxtacortical Chondroma),** p 596-597.

12. **C. OSTEOID OSTEOMA**
    Histologically, osteoid osteoma and osteoblastoma demonstrate similar features. Specifically, there are numerous bony trabeculae of various size and thickness with various degrees of mineralization. These are distributed throughout a cellular and vascular stroma. While the prominent osteoblast rimming is seen more commonly in osteoblastoma, it can also be a feature of osteoid osteomas.
    QCSP, **Osteoblastoma,** p 597-598.

13. **A. IT PROGRESSES TO OSTEOSARCOMA IN APPROXIMATELY 45% OF CASES.**
    Aggressive osteoblastoma can be confused with osteosarcomas; however, the well-defined border as well as the presence of osteoblastic rimming is reassuring of a benign lesion. Even though there is some histologic overlap with osteosarcoma, aggressive osteoblasts (or other variants) do not transform into an osteosarcoma.
    QCSP, **Aggressive Osteoblastoma,** p 598.

14. **B. OSTEOID OSTEOMA**
    The typical presentation of an osteoid osteoma is a painful lesion that worsens at nights and is relieved by NSAIDS.
    QCSP, **Osteoid Osteoma,** p 598-599.

15. **C. OSTEOBLASTS**
    The pain and reactive sclerosis seen in the osteoid osteoma are the results of release of prostaglandin E2 and prostacyclin by osteoblasts.
    QCSP, **Osteoid Osteoma,** p 598-599.

19: Bones and Joints Answers

63. **E.** **LANGERIN+, S100+, CD1A+, CD45−, VIMENTIN+**

    Langerhans cell histiocytosis is a dendritic cell neoplasm and as such is S100+. The specific combination of langerin and CD1a along with S100 is the classical phenotype. Additionally, the lesions can be HLA II, CD68, CD4, and vimentin positive. However, the lesions are generally negative for lysozyme, CD15, CD30, and cytokeratin. Additionally, expression of CD163 has been reported.

    QCSP, **Langerhans Cell Histiocytosis,** p 631-633.

64. **D.** **MAY HEAL SPONTANEOUSLY**

    The unifocal Langerhans cell histiocytosis (LCH) (eosinophilic granuloma) is the most frequent presentation of this uncommon disease, typically occurs in older patients, and is more prevalent than either the multifocal (Hand-Schuller-Christian) or the disseminated (Letterer-Siwe) forms of LCH. All 3 have similar morphologic, immunophenotype and ultrastructural findings, but have different disease presentation and organ involvement. Most cases of the multifocal and disseminated forms of LCH have cutaneous involvement; however, eosinophilic granulomas usually only involves the bone with a minority of cases that demonstrates dermal involvement. Interestingly, unifocal Langerhans cell histiocytosis lesion can spontaneously heal; otherwise, it can be treated with curettage of the osseous lesions with or without intralesional injection of steroids or low-dose radiation. Patients with multifocal (Hand-Schuller-Christian disease) LCH will often have the classic triad of bone involvement (lytic bone lesions), diabetes insipidus, and exophthalmos.

    QCSP, **Langerhans Cell Histiocytosis,** p 631-633.

65. **B.** **BIRBECK GRANULES**

    Birbeck granules are the classic EM finding of LCH. Additionally, the langerin protein has been localized to the Birbeck granules. Additionally, numerous filopodia can be seen on the surface of the cells. Weibel-Palade bodies are storage granules for von Willebrand factor and P-selectin found in cells with an endothelial differentiation. Rhomboid crystals are a typical EM finding of alveolar soft part sarcoma.

    QCSP, **Langerhans Cell Histiocytosis,** p 631-633.

66. **D.** **CHONDROBLASTOMA**

    The case in question is an epiphyseal tumor in a patient with an open epiphyseal. The lesion demonstrates fine "chicken-wire-like" calcification and neoplastic cells that have a coffee bean appearance with grooved nuclei. These are all characteristic findings in a chondroblastoma.

    QCSP, **Chondroblastoma,** p 590-592.

67. **B.** **CHONDROMYXOID FIBROMA**

    The film demonstrated a sharply sclerotic lesion with a scalloped border typical of benign lesions. Histologically this lesion demonstrates a hypocellular myxomatous matrix reminiscent of a myxoid lesion. The cells are spindled and often have a stellate appearance. They can form a lobular growth pattern with increased cellularity at the edge of the lobules. Occasionally the cells can appear hyperchromic and malignant; however, it is important to recognize that there is preserved (low) nuclear-to-cytoplasmic ratio. Generally necrosis and prominent mitotic activity are not seen.

    QCSP, **Chondromyxoid Fibroma,** p 592-593.

68. **D.** **ENCHONDROMA**

    The X-ray demonstrates a lesion with expansile growth and intact cortex with a sclerotic rim. While not as evident in this image, plain films of these lesions often demonstrate "ring-calcifications" with some peripheral calcification/mineralization. The histologic examination of the lesion demonstrates an obvious chondroid lesion. This lesion is a fairly typical example of a phalangeal enchondroma. Some of these cases can demonstrate a fair amount of atypia; however, chondrosarcoma of the phalanges are extremely rare.

    QCSP, **Enchondroma,** p 593-594.

19: Bones and Joints Answers

69. **A.** **OSTEOCHONDROMA**

The X-ray indicates an exophytic and somewhat pedunculated projection. The involvement is both medullary and cortical. The lesion demonstrates normal appear bone marrow with a cartilage cap with normal-appearing chondrocytes. There is normal ossification of the chondrocytes with cancellous bone beneath the cap.

QCSP, **Osteochondroma,** p 595-596.

70. **B.** **CHONDROMA**

The X-ray demonstrates a periosteal lesion with some cortical erosion that does not involve the medullary cavity. The histological examination demonstrates lobular chondroid matrix. There is an increase in cellularity, and histologically it appears similar to an enchondroma; however, enchondromas are intramedullary. Remember that chondroma can show some mild atypica, including binucleation.

QCSP, **Periosteal Chondroma (Juxtacortical Chondroma),** p 596-597.

71. **C.** **OSTEOBLASTOMA**

The imaging demonstrated a 2.3 cm lesion that is radiolucent with scattered areas of mineralization and a well-defined margin. The histology demonstrates an ossifying lesion with woven bone with prominent osteoblastic rimming. These findings are consistent the diagnosis of osteoblastoma. The histologic features are also consistent with an osteoid osteoma. However, osteoid osteomas are <2.0 cm (usually <1.5 cm) and are associated with significant pain at night.

QCSP, **Osteoblastoma,** p 597-598.

72. **A.** **AGGRESSIVE OSTEOBLASTOMA**

This lesion represents an aggressive osteoblastoma. This lesion is most often located in the vertebrate and often involves the spinal process. As compared to standard osteoblastoma, the aggressive variant is typically larger and demonstrates epitheloid osteoblasts that are 2-4 times as large as the osteoblast seen in standard osteoblastoma. While on occasion the histology can be concerning for an osteosarcoma, the well-defined margin is reassuring of a benign lesion.

QCSP, **Aggressive Osteoblastoma,** p 598.

73. **D.** **OSTEOID OSTEOMA**

The lesion represents an osteoid osteoma that will often present with pain that worsens at night and is relieved with aspirin and other NSAIDS. The X-ray demonstrates a sclerotic lesion of the tibia with cortex thickening. As is often typical in these lesions, the sclerosis obscures the lesion on plain film, but the transverse CT demonstrates the nidus. The curettage demonstrates a haphazard arrangement of woven and lamellar bone with a "nidus." The stroma is cellular and fibrous in appearance. This lesion can demonstrate similar histologic features with osteoblastoma.

QCSP, **Osteoid Osteoma,** p 598-599.

74. **B.** **ANEURYSMAL BONE CYST**

The lesion demonstrates an expansive "soap-bubble" lytic lesion centered in the metaphysis of the humerus. This multilocular cystic lesion demonstrates bland fibrous tissue with multinucleated giant cells with extravasated blood. The histologic and radiologic features are most consistent with aneurysmal bone cyst.

QCSP, **Aneurysmal Bone Cyst,** p 599-601.

19: Bones and Joints Answers

75.   E.   **SOLITARY BONE CYST**

The findings are most consistent with the diagnosis of a solitary/unicameral bone cyst. Specifically, the lesion is a solitary cyst in the diaphysis of a skeletally immature patient. Additionally, the curettage of the lesion only demonstrates reactive bone and fibrous tissue. If the lesion is connected with the intramedullary cavity, it will often be filled with a serous fluid.

QCSP, **Solitary Bone Cyst (Unicameral Bone Cyst),** p 601.

76.   B.   **FIBROSARCOMA**

The MRI demonstrates a large, aggressive lesion that has eroded through the maxillary sinus and forms a soft tissue mass. This radiologic appearance would be consistent with an osteosarcoma, fibrosarcoma, or other high-grade lesion. However, the histologic section demonstrates a spindle cell lesion with an arranged "herringbone" pattern with nuclear atypia. The combined radiology and histologic features are consistent with the diagnosis of fibrosarcoma.

QCSP, **Fibrosarcoma of Bone,** p 601-302.

77.   B.   **FIBROUS DYSPLASIA**

This lesion is consistent with the diagnosis of fibrous dysplasia. The imaging demonstrates an expansile lesion of the rib with intact cortex. The histology demonstrates a fibrous lesion without atypia. The reactive woven bone takes on the appearance of "Chinese characters."

QCSP, **Fibrous Dysplasia,** p 603-604.

78.   B.   **MALIGNANT FIBROUS HISTIOCYTOMA**

The MRI shown demonstrates a destructive lytic lesion in the distal femur with an associated fracture. The lesion extends into the surrounding soft tissue. The lesion demonstrates a fibrous lesion with large pleomorphic/anaplastic-appearing cells along with an inflammatory infiltrate. Given the radiology and histologic findings this lesion is best diagnosed as a malignant fibrous histiocytoma (MFH). The lesion does not produce osteoid or a chondroid matrix. There is, however, a myxoid variant of MFH of bone. Remember that this diagnosis is one of exclusion, in which you must rule out muscle, chondroid, osteoid or lipomatous differentiations. Additionally, carcinoma and melanoma should be ruled out.

QCSP, **Malignant Fibrous Histiocytoma of Bone,** p 605-606.

79.   C.   **NONOSSIFYING FIBROMA**

The X-ray demonstrates an eccentrically located and sharply circumscribed lytic lesion in the metaphysis of the tibia. The histology demonstrates a solid cellular spindle lesion in a storiform pattern, which is admixed with multinucleated giant cells. These findings are consistent with the diagnosis of a nonossifying fibroma. These lesions are often self-limited but can occasionally present with pathologic fracture.

QCSP, **Nonossifying Fibroma (Fibrous Cortical Defect; Histiocytic Fibroma),** p 606-607.

80.   A.   **OSSIFYING FIBROMA**

The radiological and histological findings are consistent with the diagnosis of ossifying fibroma/osteofibrous dysplasia. Specifically, this case demonstrates a lesion in the anterior cortex of the tibia diaphysis. These lesions are typically centered in the cortex of the tibial diaphysis and can occasionally involve the fibula. These lesions present in patients younger than 15 (most under 10 years of age). The histology demonstrates a fibrous lesion with a somewhat loose stellate appearance. These lesions also typically demonstrate immature woven bone and lamellar bone with osteoblastic rimming.

QCSP, **Osteofibrous Dysplasia (Ossifying Fibroma of Long Bones),** p 607-608.

19: Bones and Joints Answers

81.   E.   **GIANT CELL REPARATIVE GRANULOMA**

The MRI lesion demonstrates a lytic lesion with trabeculations that can resemble an aneurysmal bone cyst. The lesion demonstrates an area of hemorrhage with spindle cells and multinucleated giant cells that cluster around the areas of hemorrhage. On high power, the multinucleated giant cells often look like siderophage. The nuclei of these giant cells are not the same as the spindle cell component. There is reactive bone, some of which demonstrate osteoblastic rimming (others not). No cartilage is seen.

QCSP, **Giant Cell Reparative Granuloma,** p 608-609.

82.   C.   **GIANT CELL TUMOR OF BONE**

The MRI of the knee demonstrates a nonhomogenous lesion that involves both the epiphysis and the metaphysis of the femur. The lesion demonstrates a 2-cell population with a dense mononuclear cell population with evenly disturbed giant cells. There is no osteoid or chondroid matrix or mineralization. As compared with other lesions with giant cells, both the mononuclear and the giant cells in giant cell tumor of bone lesions have the same nuclei. The giant cells have approximately 50-100 nuclei per cell.

QCSP, **Giant Cell Tumor of Bone,** p 609-611.

83.   B.   **CLEAR CELL CHONDROSARCOMA**

The images demonstrate an epiphyseal lesion. Remember that the femur has multiple physis plates, including the capital and trochanteric physis. This lesion is centered in the trochanteric epiphysis. There are only a few lesions that occur in the epiphysis. The histologic sections demonstrate cells with eosinophilic to clear cytoplasm. There is woven bone but hyaline cartilage is almost completely absent (a typical feature).

QCSP, **Clear Cell Chondrosarcoma,** p 611-612.

84.   A.   **CONVENTIONAL CHONDROSARCOMA**

The MRI demonstrates a nodular/lobulated lesion involving the metaphysis of the right femur. The lesion demonstrates the productions of chondroid matrix by atypical chondrocytes with an increased nuclear to cytoplasmic ratio. Additionally, there are spindled chondrocytes within the lesion. Conventional chondrosarcoma almost always presents with pain and in patients between the ages of 40-60.

QCSP, **Chondrosarcoma (Conventional; Intramedullary),** p 612-614.

85.   D.   **DEDIFFERENTIATED CHONDROSARCOMA**

This lesion represents a dedifferentiated chondrosarcoma. Specifically, the radiology demonstrates an intramedullary component that demonstrates stippled/mineralized area (which, granted, is a little difficult to fully appreciated with the image shown) with an associated soft tissue lesion. The juxtaposition of the well-differentiated chondrosarcoma with the shown high-grade lesion is typical of dedifferentiated chondrosarcomas. The high-grade portion of dedifferentiated chondrosarcomas most often resembles MFH; however, they can demonstrate features of osteosarcoma, fibrosarcoma, and/or rhabdomyosarcoma.

QCSP, **Dedifferentiated Chondrosarcoma,** p 614.

86.   A.   **MESENCHYMAL CHONDROSARCOMA**

This lesion represents a mesenchymal chondrosarcoma. The radiology demonstrates an extraosseous lesion with matrix calcification and a lobular architecture consistent with a chondrosarcoma. Histology of the lesion demonstrates a biphasic tumor with a mixture of more classic malignant chondrocytes with eosinophilic to clear cytoplasm with a small round blue cell component. Just on the histology (without the radiology) one would need to also entertain the possibility of an Ewing sarcoma or lymphoma. While not well here, the small round blue cells can take on a hemangiopericytoma-like pattern. This lesion is the most common of the chondrosarcomas to occur as an extraskeletal lesion and often will present as a meningeal lesion.

QCSP, **Mesenchymal Chondrosarcoma,** p 615.

19: Bones and Joints Answers

87.   **B.   PAGET DISEASE**
The history, gross image, and histology are all representative of a case of Paget disease. The skull demonstrates a nonhomogenous thickening of the skull. The histologic section demonstrates a mosaic disorganization of the bone with the formation of cement lines. There is also occasional osteoblastic rimming. This case is a more advanced case (nonactive) with bone sclerosis; however, the early lesions of Paget disease often have increased lytic activity with fibrous tissue and prominent vascular. The active phase of the disease will demonstrate a mixture of both osteoclastic and osteoblastic activity.
QCSP, **Paget Disease (Osteitis Deformans),** p 616.

88.   **B.   TOPHACEOUS GOUT**
These findings are consistent with the diagnosis of tophaceous gout. Specifically, the X-ray demonstrates a boney lesion with an associated soft tissue swelling. The histology demonstrates a mass of needle-like crystals that have a polarization pattern consistent with monosodium urate crystals. These crystals induce a granulomatous/foreign body response with histiocytes and giant cell formation. The lesion has to be fixed in ethanol in order to see the crystals, as they dissolve in formalin. This lesion is more common in men.
QCSP, **Tophaceous Gout,** p 616-617.

89.   **D.   TOPHACEOUS PSEUDOGOUT**
These findings are consistent with the diagnosis of tophaceous pseudogout. Specifically, the X-ray demonstrates a variable calcified lesion of the index finger. The histology demonstrates a granulomatous lesion with a mass of crystals. While the individual crystal morphology cannot be determined from this biopsy, the polarization pattern is consistent with calcium pyrophosphate dihydrate crystals. There are histiocytes and giant cells through out the lesion. This lesion is more common in women.
QCSP, **Tophaceous Pseudogout (Chondrocalcinosis),** p 617-618.

90.   **B.   ASKIN TUMOR**
This case represents a Ewing sarcoma/PNET of the thoracopulmonary region. The radiology images demonstrate an aggressive lesion with soft tissue expansion. The histology demonstrates a small round blue cell lesion. The expression of NSE without the expression of CD45 would argue against a hemopoietic lesion. Patients with neuroblastoma generally present at much younger age. While there is reactive bone in the lesion, there is no production of osteoid. The lesion is also negative for muscle antigens, which would argue against a rhabdomyosarcoma.
QCSP, **Askin Tumor,** p 618.

91.   **D.   EWING SARCOMA**
This lesion represents a Ewing sarcoma. Specifically, the imaging demonstrates a lesion involving the medullary cavity and extends into the soft tissue with associated edema. The histology demonstrates a homogeneous small round blue cell lesion without matrix production. Additionally, there is no large cell or giant cell component seen in this lesion.
QCSP, **Ewing Sarcoma/Primitive Neuroectodermal Tumor (PNET),** p 618-620.

19: Bones and Joints Answers

92. D. **OSTEOSARCOMA**

This case represents a conventional osteosarcoma. The imaging (MRI) demonstrates a large, aggressive metaphyseal lesion with destruction of the cortex and extension into the soft tissue. There are ill-defined borders and heterogeneous appearance with scattered mineralization of the matrix (seen as a cloudy opacity on X-ray). The histologic images demonstrate an osteoid producing lesion with large neoplastic (sarcomatous tumor) cells. These osteosarcoma cells are usually pleomorphic, but maybe spindled, oval, clear, epithelioid, or plasmacytoid. Additionally, the neoplastic cells can be large and multinucleated. Osteosarcoma is defined as an osteoid-producing tumor, and osteoid can sometimes be in the eye of the beholder and in certain cases can be difficult to identify. Usually osteoid is eosinophilic and glassy with irregular borders and often has a lace-like appearance with variable mineralization.

QCSP, **Conventional (Intramedullary) Osteosarcoma,** p 621-623.

93. C. **PAROSTEAL OSTEOSARCOMA**

This lesion presents a parosteal osteosarcoma. Specifically, the radiology demonstrates an exophytic mass extending from the surface of the bone. As is also typical of parosteal osteosarcoma, the lesion has a broad base attachment to the underlying bone. It is also lobulated and heterogeneously (yet usually densely) mineralized with a somewhat "wrapping" feature. There are 2 histologic components to this lesion. The majority of the lesion demonstrates a low-grade fibroblastic spindle. The other portion is a small cell variant of osteosarcoma. Up to 15% of cases of parosteal osteosarcoma will have foci of high-grade neoplasm present. In cases without a high-grade lesion, the overall appearance is usually more hypocellular without large numbers of atypical cells.

QCSP, **Parosteal (Juxtacortical) Osteosarcoma,** p 623-624.

94. B. **PERIOSTEAL OSTEOSARCOMA**

The lesion represents a periosteal osteosarcoma. Radiographically the lesion involves around 75% of the diaphysis of the femur, wrapping around the bone. The lesion also has the standardly described "hair on end" or "sunburst" pattern. While Codman's triangle is present is this tumor, it may not be readily apparent on the small image shown. The histology demonstrates an atypical/malignant cartilaginous tumor that blends into a smaller cell sarcomatous portion with the production of malignant osteoid. Given the radiologic and morphologic findings, this case is best diagnosed as a periosteal osteosarcoma.

QCSP, **Periosteal Osteosarcoma,** p 624.

95. A. **TELANGIECTATIC OSTEOSARCOMA**

This case best represents a telangiectatic osteosarcoma. The T1 MRI demonstrates a heterogenous lytic lesion with cystic spaces with thickened walls between the cystic areas. Often in T2 MRIs some fluid is seen in the cysts. The lesion consists of cystic spaces with hemorrhage. The cystic lining cells are usually bland, while the cells between the cystic spaces are large and atypical. While there is a possible hint of osteoid formation, there is no definite osteoid formation. Even though this is an osteosarcoma, the production of osteoid is usually minimal. Radiographically there can be overlap with ABC; however, the highly atypical cells and osteoid production suggest the correct diagnosis. While the lesion can have giant cell (both benign and malignant appearing), the lesion lack the nuclear homogeneity seen in giant cell tumor of bone.

QCSP, **Telangiectatic Osteosarcoma,** p 625.

96. E. **PIGMENTED VILLONODULAR SYNOVITIS**

This lesion represents a pigmented villonodular synovitis. The MRI demonstrates a destructive lesion involving the posterior aspect of the joint with extension into the soft tissue. Typically, plain films will be normal or might show some soft tissue swelling. Grossly, the lesion will have a shag-rug appearance with fingerlike excrescences mixed with small nodules. Histologically the lesion demonstrates a mixture of spindled and plump epitheloid cells. There are also hemosiderin-rich cells with a hyaline/collagenous matrix. The low-power image demonstrates overlying hyperplastic synoviocytes. Additionally, the lesion is nodular and demonstrates cleftlike spaces.

QCSP, **Pigmented Villonodular Synovitis (Giant Cell Tumor, Diffuse Type),** p 626-627.

19: Bones and Joints Answers

97.   D.   **PRIMARY SYNOVIAL CHONDROMATOSIS**

These lesions represent a primary synovial chondromatosis. The imaging demonstrates multiple high-signal lesions with sharp margins that involve the ankle. Histologically, there is synovial tissue that contains mature lobulated cartilage. It is important to remember that osseous chondrosarcomas can have soft tissue components and that there are forms of extraosseous chondrosarcoma that can involve the synovium. However, osseous chondrosarcomas have an associated bone lesion. While there might be some atypia in some of the chondrocytes, they do not demonstrate the increased cellularity and atypia seen in chondrosarcomas.

QCSP, **Synovial Chondromatosis,** p 627-628.

98.   D.   **ADAMANTINOMA**

This lesion represents an adamantinoma of the long bones. Specifically, the MRI of the lesion demonstrates a lytic lesion of the anterolateral cortex of the tibia. It has a destructive growth pattern with a cookie-cutter or bite appearance. This can also be a typical radiologic appearance of metastatic carcinoma, except adamantinoma often has a sclerotic margin indicative of slow growth. Histologically, the lesion is a biphasic tumor with spindled fibroblastic-appearing cells in the background with a nest of epithelial cells. While multiple patterns can be seen, this case demonstrates cells with a basaloid cell appearance. These cells are pankeratin+, so a panel of IHC must be performed.

QCSP, **Adamantinoma of Long Bones,** p 628-630.

99.   A.   **LANGERHANS HISTIOCYTOSIS**

This case represents a Langerhans histiocytosis (specifically, Hand-Schuller-Christian disease). This case demonstrates multiple lytic lesions in the skull. The histological image demonstrates a histiocytic lesion with ample eosinophilic cytoplasm. Additionally there is a significant population of eosinophils. The histiocytic cells, Langerhans cells, are oval cells that have a folded (so-called coffee bean) nucleus. There are no mitotic figures seen. As compared to Langerhans cells, normal histiocytes demonstrate phagocytic activity and, in general, lack the nuclear folds/grooves.

QCSP, **Langerhans Cell Histiocytosis,** p 631-633.

Chapter 20

Soft Tissue

1. Which of the following is/are a common indication for intraoperative consultation on soft tissue tumors?
   A. Ensuring the presence of adequate viable, lesional tissue
   B. Evaluating margin status
   C. Obtaining tissue for cytogenetics and electron microscopy
   D. A and B
   E. All of the above

2. Typical clinical findings of extraskeletal mesenchymal chondrosarcoma in young patients on initial presentation include:
   A. Bone pain
   B. Pathologic fracture
   C. Deep-seated painless mass
   D. Changes in vision
   E. History of trauma

3. Which of the following microscopic features is NOT correctly paired with its variant of extraskeletal chondrosarcoma?
   A. Calcifications: well-differentiated extraskeletal chondrosarcoma
   B. Eosinophilic chondroblasts: extraskeletal myxoid chondrosarcoma
   C. Fibrous septa: extraskeletal myxoid chondrosarcoma
   D. Binucleated chondrocytes: extraskeletal mesenchymal chondrosarcoma
   E. Sinusoidal vascular spaces: extraskeletal mesenchymal chondrosarcoma

4. Which of the following short-hand molecular alterations is characteristic of extraskeletal myxoid chondrosarcoma?
   A. t(8;21)
   B. t(9;22)
   C. t(12;15)
   D. t(12;16)
   E. t(X;18)

5. Which of the following entities typically does NOT pose a microscopically difficult differential diagnosis for extraskeletal mesenchymal chondrosarcoma?
   A. Synovial sarcoma
   B. Hemangiopericytoma
   C. Chordoma
   D. Ewing sarcoma
   E. Embryonal rhabdomyosarcoma

6. Which of the following immunohistochemical stains typically does NOT stain extraskeletal osteosarcoma?
   A. Vimentin
   B. Osteocalcin
   C. Smooth muscle actin
   D. EMA
   E. Cytokeratin

20: Soft Tissue Questions

21. Which of the following variants of pleomorphic malignant fibrous histiocytoma is most common in the abdomen?
    A. Storiform variant
    B. Giant cell variant
    C. Inflammatory variant

22. Which of the following is NOT a feature of storiform pleomorphic malignant fibrous histiocytoma?
    A. Atypical mitotic figures
    B. Bony or cartilaginous metaplasia
    C. Pleomorphic, bizarre cells
    D. Thick vessels
    E. Bland fibroblasts

23. Which of the following features is/are found in giant cell pleomorphic malignant fibrous histiocytoma?
    A. Nodular growth pattern
    B. Osteoclast-like giant cells
    C. Presence of keratin staining
    D. A and B
    E. All of the above

24. Which type of tenosynovial giant cell tumor is less common?
    A. Diffuse type
    B. Localized type

25. Which of the following statements regarding tenosynovial giant cell tumor, diffuse type, is TRUE?
    A. Males are more commonly affected than females.
    B. Destruction of adjacent tissue is unusual and should raise concern for malignancy.
    C. The neoplastic population consists of sheets of monomorphic cells with large nuclei admixed with scattered multinucleated giant cells.
    D. The prognosis of this tumor is excellent with minimal chance of recurrence.
    E. High mitotic activity in the absence of atypical mitotic figures is a benign feature.

26. In contrast to the diffuse type, tenosynovial giant cell tumor of localized type demonstrates all of the following EXCEPT:
    A. Decreased risk of recurrence
    B. Higher density of giant cells
    C. An older patient demographic
    D. A preference for the interphalangeal joints of the hand
    E. Stromal hyalinization

27. Which of the following features predicts an increased risk of recurrence in tenosynovial giant cell tumor of localized type?
    A. Incomplete excision
    B. High mitotic activity
    C. Dense cellularity
    D. A and B
    E. All of the above

20: Soft Tissue Questions

28. Which of the following variants of xanthoma is NOT correctly paired with its characteristic location?
    A. Eruptive xanthoma: face
    B. Tuberous xanthoma: elbows
    C. Tendinous xanthoma: Achilles tendons
    D. Xanthelasma: eyelids
    E. Plane xanthoma: palmar creases

29. Which of the following variants typically contains a significant population of nonfoamy histiocytes?
    A. Eruptive xanthoma
    B. Tuberous xanthoma
    C. Tendinous xanthoma
    D. Xanthelasma
    E. Plane xanthoma

30. In the absence of hyperlipidemia, a diagnosis of plane xanthoma should raise concern for which of the following?
    A. Cardiovascular disease
    B. Hepatic dysfunction
    C. Diabetes mellitus
    D. Lymphoma
    E. Liposarcoma

31. Which of the following best describes the clinical presentation of calcifying aponeurotic fibroma?
    A. Painless, slowly enlarging mass involving the fingers of young adults
    B. Small, broad-based nodule involving a single toe of an infant
    C. Painless mass involving the palm of a young child
    D. Painless, slowly enlarging mass involving the trunk of adults
    E. Painless, slowly enlarging mass involving the upper lateral back of older adults

32. Which of the following is NOT a microscopic feature of calcifying aponeurotic fibroma?
    A. Nodular growth pattern
    B. Pseudocapsule
    C. Variable degree of calcification
    D. Cartilage formation
    E. Stromal hyalinization involving center of nodules

33. The fragments of elastic fibers seen microscopically in elastofibroma are referred to as:
    A. Ferruginous bodies
    B. Chenille bodies
    C. Asteroid bodies
    D. Michaelis-Gutmann bodies
    E. Schaumann bodies

34. Which of the following statements regarding fibroma of tendon sheath is TRUE?
    A. It typically occurs in the seventh decade.
    B. There is a striking female predominance.
    C. It is associated with trauma.
    D. It may recur as a fibrosarcoma.
    E. It presents as a painful lesion, which may erode into the adjacent tissue.

35. Which of the following immunohistochemical stains is negative in fibroma of tendon sheath?
    A. Vimentin
    B. Desmin
    C. Smooth muscle actin
    D. Factor XIIIa
    E. CD34

36. Which of the following statements regarding the superficial variant of fibromatosis is TRUE?
    A. This variant occurs predominantly in patients in their 2nd and 3rd decades.
    B. Penile fibromatosis may be treated with excision and chemotherapy.
    C. Plantar fibromatosis typically presents as localized disease, whereas palmar fibromatosis occurs more frequently as multiple bilateral lesions.
    D. Palmar and plantar fibromatosis are also known as Peyronie disease and Ledderhose disease, respectively.
    E. Cartilaginous metaplasia is worrisome for malignant transformation.

37. Which of the following features is NOT characteristic of the extraabdominal form of deep fibromatosis?
    A. Younger patient demographic than superficial fibromatosis
    B. Association with pregnancy
    C. Preference for the trunk
    D. Infiltrative growth into adjacent skeletal muscle
    E. Ill-defined dense white mass on gross examination

38. Which of the following is associated with the abdominal form of deep fibromatosis?
    A. Pregnancy
    B. Gardner syndrome
    C. Mesenteric fibromatosis
    D. A and B
    E. All of the above

39. Which of the following is FALSE regarding fibromatosis?
    A. It shows immunoreactivity with desmin.
    B. It shows immunoreactivity with β-catenin.
    C. Trisomy 8 is present in superficial fibromatosis.
    D. There is deletion of 5q in deep fibromatosis.
    E. Treatment consists of radical excision, radiation, and chemotherapy.

40. Which of the following clinical and laboratory features does NOT distinguish adult-type from juvenile-type fibrosarcoma?
    A. Location of tumor
    B. Patient age
    C. Rate of growth
    D. Presence of associated hypoglycemia
    E. Overlying skin ulceration

41. Which of the following is NOT characteristic of adult-type fibrosarcoma?
    A. "Herringbone" growth pattern
    B. Focal areas of hypocellularity resembling fibromatosis
    C. Immunoreactivity for vimentin and smooth muscle actin
    D. Lymphatic seeding
    E. Absence of a recurrent molecular alteration

42. The molecular alteration characteristic of juvenile-type fibrosarcoma is:
    A. t(12;16)(q13;p11.2)
    B. t(12;22)(q13;q12)
    C. t(12;15)(p13;q25)
    D. t(11;22)(q24;q12)
    E. t(11;22)(q13;q12)

43. Which of the following statements regarding the sclerosing epithelioid variant of adult-type fibrosarcoma is FALSE?
    A. In contrast to classic adult-type fibrosarcoma, it is predominantly hypocellular.
    B. Mitotic figures are less common than in classic adult-type fibrosarcoma.
    C. It has a pattern of immunoreactivity that is distinct from classic adult-type fibrosarcoma.
    D. There is a significant risk of recurrence.
    E. There is a significant incidence of lung metastasis.

44. What percentage of cases of infantile digital fibromatosis is diagnosed at birth?
    A. <5%
    B. 25%
    C. 35%
    D. 50%
    E. 75%

45. The inclusions characteristically seen in infantile digital fibromatosis are:
    A. Eosinophilic and cytoplasmic
    B. Basophilic and cytoplasmic
    C. Eosinophilic and nuclear
    D. Basophilic and nuclear
    E. Amphophilic and cytoplasmic

46. The inclusions characteristic of infantile digital fibromatosis exhibit staining for which of the following?
    A. PAS with diastase
    B. PAS without diastase
    C. Masson trichrome
    D. Alcian blue
    E. None of the above

47. Which of the following features distinguishes low-grade myofibroblastic sarcoma from fibromatosis?
    A. Gross appearance
    B. Diffuse infiltrative growth
    C. Presence of mitotic activity
    D. Cellular atypia
    E. Neoplastic spindle cell population

48. Which of the following immunohistochemical stains is reliably negative in low-grade myofibroblastic sarcoma?
    A. Smooth muscle actin
    B. Desmin
    C. CD34
    D. CD99
    E. S100

49. Which of the following histologic features is NOT characteristic of myofibroma?
    A. Focal necrosis
    B. Dystrophic calcification
    C. Nodular growth pattern
    D. Hemangiopericytoma-like vessels
    E. Diffuse lymphocytic infiltrate

50. Which of the following is an indicator of poor prognosis in myofibroma?
    A. Multicentric disease
    B. Solitary lesions involving the bone
    C. Pulmonary disease
    D. Presence of an inflammatory infiltrate
    E. High mitotic activity

51. The most common location of myxoinflammatory fibroblastic sarcoma is:
    A. Head and neck area
    B. Trunk
    C. Proximal extremities
    D. Distal extremities
    E. Retroperitoneum

52. Which of the following cell types is NOT characteristic of myxoinflammatory fibroblastic sarcoma?
    A. Giant cells
    B. Atypical spindle cells
    C. Ganglion-like cells
    D. Lipoblast-like cells
    E. Lymphocytes

53. Patients with a diagnosis of myxofibrosarcoma are typically in which of the following age ranges?
    A. Infancy
    B. Late childhood
    C. Adolescence
    D. Middle-aged adults
    E. Elderly adults

54. Microscopic features of high-grade myxofibrosarcoma include all of the following EXCEPT:
    A. Necrosis
    B. Atypical mitotic figures
    C. Atypical multinucleated giant cells
    D. Hypocellular areas with prominent myxoid matrix resembling low-grade myxofibrosarcoma
    E. Thick hyalinized vessels

55. In comparison to classic pleomorphic malignant fibrous histiocytoma, the prognosis of myxofibrosarcoma is:
    A. Better
    B. Worse
    C. Identical

20: Soft Tissue Questions

56. Which of the following best describes the natural progression of lipoblastoma (not lipoblastomatosis)?
    A. Infiltration into adjacent tissues
    B. Malignant transformation to liposarcoma
    C. Maturation to lipoma
    D. Hematogenous metastasis
    E. Lymphatic metastasis

57. Which of the following microscopic features is NOT compatible with a diagnosis of lipoma?
    A. Infiltrative growth into skeletal muscle
    B. Cellular atypia
    C. Wide spectrum of cell size
    D. Dense delicate vasculature
    E. Fat necrosis

58. Of the choices below, which exhibit identical molecular alterations and most likely represent ends of the same disease spectrum?
    A. Fibrolipoma
    B. Myxolipoma
    C. Myolipoma
    D. Spindle cell lipoma
    E. Pleomorphic lipoma

59. Which of the following variants typically presents as multiple painful lesions in the forearm of pubescent patients?
    A. Conventional lipoma
    B. Myxolipoma
    C. Chondroid lipoma
    D. Angiolipoma
    E. Myolipoma

60. Which of the following syndromes is NOT associated with multiple lipomas?
    A. Bannayan-Zonana syndrome
    B. Cowden syndrome
    C. Frohlich syndrome
    D. Maffucci syndrome
    E. Proteus syndrome

61. The most common variant of liposarcoma is:
    A. Well-differentiated liposarcoma, adipocytic type
    B. Well-differentiated liposarcoma, sclerosing type
    C. Myxoid liposarcoma
    D. Dedifferentiated liposarcoma
    E. Pleomorphic liposarcoma

62. The distinction between atypical lipomatous tumor and well-differentiated liposarcoma is based on which of the following?
    A. Tumor size
    B. Tumor location
    C. Mitotic activity
    D. Cellular atypia
    E. Presence of lipoblasts

20: Soft Tissue Questions

63. Which of the following features best differentiates lipoma from well-differentiated liposarcoma of adipocytic type?
    A. Tumor size
    B. Tumor location
    C. Variation in size of adipocyte
    D. Cellular atypia
    E. Presence of lipoblasts

64. The variant of liposarcoma with the highest degree of mitotic activity is:
    A. Well-differentiated liposarcoma
    B. Myxoid liposarcoma
    C. Round cell liposarcoma
    D. Pleomorphic liposarcoma
    E. Dedifferentiated liposarcoma

65. Which of the following factors best predicts the risk of dedifferentiation in well-differentiated liposarcoma?
    A. Patient age
    B. Tumor location
    C. Duration of disease
    D. High mitotic activity
    E. Presence of lipoblasts

66. Which of the following statements regarding lymphangiomas is FALSE?
    A. Cystic lymphangiomas are typically well-circumscribed.
    B. Cavernous lymphangiomas commonly exhibit infiltrative growth.
    C. Cutaneous lymphangioma preferentially occurs in the proximal limbs and buttocks.
    D. Most lesions present in patients older than 10 years of age.
    E. It is a malformation which does not communicate with the lymphatic or venous system.

67. Which of the following factors has been associated with malignant transformation of lymphangioma?
    A. High mitotic activity
    B. Cellular atypia
    C. Infiltrative growth
    D. Radiation treatment
    E. Patient age

68. Which of the following syndromes has NOT been associated with cystic lymphangioma?
    A. Turner syndrome
    B. Noonan syndrome
    C. Down syndrome
    D. Fetal alcohol syndrome
    E. Familial pterygium colli

69. Which variant of lymphangiomatosis typically confers the worst prognosis?
    A. Visceral form
    B. Skeletal form

20: Soft Tissue Questions

70. Which of the following is NOT a microscopic feature of lymphangiomatosis?
    A. Stromal hemosiderin
    B. Infiltrative growth
    C. Lymphatic channels lined by bland, attenuated endothelium
    D. Lymphatic channels containing thick, concentric smooth muscle
    E. Scattered lymphoid aggregates

71. The typical patient with lymphangiomyomatosis is:
    A. 1-year-old female infant with multiple cutaneous nodules
    B. 1-year-old female infant with a neck mass
    C. 35-year-old male with shortness of breath
    D. 35-year-old female with shortness of breath
    E. 35-year-old female with multiple cutaneous nodules

72. Which of the following immunohistochemical stains is helpful in identifying lymphangiomatosis?
    A. Smooth muscle actin
    B. Desmin
    C. HMB-45
    D. Cytokeratin
    E. EMA

73. Which of the following immunohistochemical stains is more specific in tumors with vascular and lymphatic differentiation?
    A. CD31
    B. CD34

74. Which of the following microscopic features is NOT characteristic of angiomyoma?
    A. Circumscription
    B. Organized circumferential layering of inner smooth muscle
    C. Organized circumferential layering of outer smooth muscle
    D. Attachment to thick-walled medium-sized vessels
    E. Myxoid change and hyalinization

75. Intravenous leiomyomatosis typically presents as:
    A. A uterine mass in women of reproductive age
    B. A uterine mass in postmenopausal women
    C. Shortness of breath in women of reproductive age
    D. Shortness of breath in postmenopausal women
    E. Shortness of breath in men

76. Leiomyosarcoma arising in the soft tissue of the lower extremities typically occurs in men.
    A. True
    B. False

77. The most common location of epithelioid leiomyosarcoma is:
    A. Uterus
    B. Retroperitoneum
    C. Soft tissue
    D. Mesentery
    E. Testis

78. All of the following statements regarding cutaneous leiomyosarcoma are TRUE EXCEPT:
    A. It is more common in men than in women.
    B. It tends to be multifocal.
    C. It preferentially involves the extensor surfaces of extremities.
    D. It is associated with pain.
    E. It is a lesion which predominantly affects older adults.

79. Which of the following is NOT a feature of cardiac rhabdomyoma?
    A. Association with tuberous sclerosis
    B. Multifocal growth
    C. Spontaneous regression
    D. Ill-defined borders
    E. Predilection for the ventricular myocardium and septum

80. Fetal rhabdomyoma associated with peripheral nerve is also known as:
    A. Neurofibroma
    B. Alveolar rhabdomyosarcoma
    C. Embryonal rhabdomyosarcoma
    D. Askin tumor
    E. Benign triton tumor

81. The most common sarcoma of children is:
    A. Leiomyosarcoma
    B. Liposarcoma
    C. Rhabdomyosarcoma
    D. Clear cell sarcoma
    E. Synovial sarcoma

82. Which variant of rhabdomyosarcoma has the best prognosis?
    A. Embryonal rhabdomyosarcoma, not otherwise specified
    B. Embryonal rhabdomyosarcoma, botryoid type
    C. Embryonal rhabdomyosarcoma, spindle cell type
    D. Embryonal rhabdomyosarcoma, anaplastic type
    E. Alveolar rhabdomyosarcoma

83. All of the following are features of the botryoid variant of embryonal rhabdomyosarcoma EXCEPT:
    A. Polypoid mass arising within hollow organs with mucosal surfaces
    B. Subepithelial layer of increased cellularity
    C. Hyperplastic overlying epithelium
    D. Neoplastic population composed of scattered spindled rhabdomyoblasts with abundant cross-striations
    E. Abundant loose myxoid stroma

84. Which of the following stains is most specific for rhabdomyosarcoma?
    A. Desmin
    B. Muscle-specific actin
    C. Vimentin
    D. Myogenin
    E. PAS without diastase

20: Soft Tissue Questions

85. The most common location of extraskeletal Ewing sarcoma is:
    A. Head and neck
    B. Testis
    C. Ovary
    D. Chest wall
    E. Extremities

86. Which of the following microscopic features is characteristic of extraskeletal Ewing sarcoma?
    A. Prominent basophilic nucleoli
    B. Abundant mitotic figures
    C. Thick-walled, hyalinized vessels
    D. Densely collagenized stroma
    E. Monotonous population of round blue cells

87. Prognostic indicators of extraskeletal Ewing sarcoma include which of the following? (Choose all that apply.)
    A. Tumor size
    B. Tumor location
    C. Degree of mitotic activity
    D. Presence of necrosis
    E. Presence of molecular aberrations

88. Which of the following statements regarding malignant peripheral nerve sheath tumor is FALSE?
    A. Half of cases occur in patients with neurofibromatosis.
    B. It typically presents as a painful, rapidly enlarging mass.
    C. Most lesions arise from major nerve trunks such as the brachial plexus.
    D. On gross examination, the lesion exhibits diffusely infiltrative growth.
    E. The most common locations are the trunk, extremities, and head and neck.

89. Which of the following is NOT a microscopic feature of malignant peripheral nerve sheath tumors?
    A. Alternating hyper- and hypocellular areas
    B. Palisading necrosis
    C. Hyperchromatic, wavy nuclei
    D. Multinucleated, pleomorphic cells
    E. Ganglion-like cells

90. S100 staining in malignant peripheral nerve sheath tumors is typically:
    A. Diffusely and strongly present in all cases
    B. Focally and strongly present in all cases
    C. Diffusely and weakly present in some cases
    D. Focally and weakly present in some cases
    E. Focally and strongly present in some cases

91. Which of the following is not a typical location for melanotic neuroectodermal tumor of infancy?
    A. Jaw
    B. Spine
    C. Brain
    D. Mediastinum
    E. Epididymis

92. Which of the following statements regarding melanotic neuroectodermal tumor of infancy is FALSE?
     A.   It may be associated with elevated levels of vanillylmandelic acid.
     B.   Approximately 1/2 of cases recur.
     C.   Immunohistochemical staining for cytokeratin is negative.
     D.   The neoplastic population is composed of primitive nonpigmented cells resembling the ones seen in neuroblastoma.
     E.   The lesion contains irregular spaces lined by cuboidal pigmented cells.

93. Microscopic features of melanotic schwannoma include all of the following EXCEPT:
     A.   Dense deposits of granular pigment
     B.   Clear intranuclear pseudoinclusions
     C.   Psammoma bodies
     D.   Distinct nuclear palisading
     E.   Admixture of spindled and epithelioid cells

94. The presence of significant mitotic activity in melanotic schwannoma is:
     A.   Common and without prognostic significance
     B.   Uncommon, but without prognostic significance
     C.   Common and indicates malignancy
     D.   Uncommon, but indicates malignancy
     E.   Never seen

95. All of the following are features of Carney syndrome EXCEPT:
     A.   Cardiac myxoma
     B.   Pigmented nodular adrenal disease
     C.   Large-cell calcifying Sertoli cell tumor
     D.   Acromegaly
     E.   Gastrointestinal stromal tumor

96. Which of the following variants of neurofibroma are almost entirely associated with neurofibromatosis? (Choose all that apply.)
     A.   Localized cutaneous neurofibroma
     B.   Diffuse cutaneous neurofibroma
     C.   Localized intraneural neurofibroma
     D.   Plexiform neurofibroma
     E.   Massive soft tissue neurofibroma

97. Which of the following variants of neurofibroma is characterized by particularly prominent mucoid matrix?
     A.   Localized cutaneous neurofibroma
     B.   Diffuse cutaneous neurofibroma
     C.   Localized intraneural neurofibroma
     D.   Plexiform neurofibroma
     E.   Massive soft tissue neurofibroma

98. Which of the following is NOT a criterion for the diagnosis of neurofibromatosis, type I?
     A.   Axillary or inguinal freckles
     B.   Plexiform neurofibroma
     C.   Meningioma
     D.   Optic glioma
     E.   Pigmented iris hamartomas

20: Soft Tissue Questions

99. Which of the following criteria present in isolation is sufficient for the diagnosis of neurofibromatosis, type II?
    A. Bilateral acoustic schwannoma
    B. Plexiform neurofibroma
    C. 1st-degree relative with NF-2
    D. Juvenile cortical cataract
    E. Meningioma

100. The tactoid structures seen in plexiform neurofibroma differ from true Pacinian corpuscles in that:
    A. They are positive for EMA.
    B. They are positive for S100.
    C. They are negative for S100 and EMA.

101. Which of the following correctly matches the genetic locus with its product and syndrome?
    A. Chromosome 22q12: merlin: NF-1
    B. Chromosome 17q11.2: merlin: NF-2
    C. Chromosome 22q12: neurofibromin: NF-2
    D. Chromosome 17q11.2: neurofibromin: NF-1
    E. Chromosome 22q12: neurofibromin: NF-1

102. Mucosal neuromas are associated with which of the following syndromes?
    A. MEN I
    B. MEN IIA
    C. MEN IIB
    D. Gorlin syndrome
    E. Cowden syndrome

103. The term "Morton neuroma" is typically used to describe:
    A. Localized interdigital neuritis
    B. Palisaded encapsulated neuroma
    C. Pacinian neuroma
    D. Mucosal neuroma
    E. Traumatic neuroma

104. The most common location of neurotropic-desmoplastic melanoma is:
    A. Chest
    B. Head and neck area
    C. Upper extremities
    D. Lower extremities
    E. Back

105. The most common precursor lesion of neurotropic-desmoplastic melanoma is:
    A. Superficial spreading melanoma
    B. Acral lentiginous melanoma
    C. Nodular melanoma
    D. Lentigo maligna melanoma
    E. Amelanotic melanoma

106. Which of the following statements regarding neurotropic-desmoplastic melanoma is FALSE?
    A.   It arises from a precursor lesion that is typically amelanotic.
    B.   It does not contain pigment.
    C.   There may be single cell infiltration.
    D.   Immunohistochemical staining for S100 is positive.
    E.   Immunohistochemical staining for HMB-45 is negative.

107. Intraneural perineurioma typically presents with:
    A.   Pain
    B.   Muscle spasticity
    C.   Muscle weakness
    D.   Sensory deficit
    E.   A palpable mass

108. Which of the following statements regarding the characteristic "onion-bulbing" seen in perineurioma is FALSE?
    A.   It is a feature of intraneural perineurioma.
    B.   It is a feature of extraneural perineurioma.
    C.   The "onion bulbs" are formed by concentric layers of perineural cells surrounding a central axon.
    D.   The "onion bulbs" are formed by concentric layers of perineural cells surrounding a Schwann cell.
    E.   It causes fusiform expansion of the affected nerve.

109. The characteristic translocation seen in primitive neuroectodermal tumor is:
    A.   t(11;22)(q24;q12)
    B.   t(11;22)(q13;q12)
    C.   t(X;18)(p11.2;q11.2)
    D.   t(12;22)(q13;q12)
    E.   t(2;13)(q35;q14)

110. The most important prognostic indicators in primitive neuroectodermal tumor include which of the following? (Choose all that apply.)
    A.   Presence of necrosis
    B.   Degree of mitotic activity
    C.   Tumor size
    D.   Tumor location
    E.   Presence of t(11;22)(q24;q12)

111. Which of the following immunohistochemical markers is negative in primitive neuroectodermal tumor?
    A.   CD99
    B.   S100
    C.   Cytokeratin
    D.   GFAP
    E.   CD57

112. The presence of psammoma bodies and melanin pigment in a schwannoma is associated with:
    A.   Malignancy
    B.   Carney syndrome
    C.   Carney triad
    D.   Ancient change
    E.   Peutz-Jeghers syndrome

20: Soft Tissue Questions

113. Schwannoma is typically treated by:
     A. Wide excision
     B. Local excision
     C. Chemotherapy
     D. Radiation
     E. A and D

114. Which of the following immunohistochemical markers is negative in angiomatoid fibrous histiocytoma?
     A. CD34
     B. EMA
     C. CD99
     D. Desmin
     E. CD68

115. The differential diagnosis of epithelioid sarcoma includes all of the following EXCEPT:
     A. Granulomatous inflammation
     B. Epithelioid hemangioendothelioma
     C. Synovial sarcoma
     D. Primitive neuroectodermal tumor
     E. Malignant peripheral nerve sheath tumor

116. Which of the following features has/have prognostic implications in epithelioid sarcoma?
     A. Age
     B. Sex
     C. Tumor size
     D. Tumor location
     E. All of the above

117. Which of the following statements regarding giant cell angiofibroma is FALSE?
     A. It typically involves the eyelids of adults.
     B. There is a male predominance.
     C. The cut surface exhibits a solid, well-demarcated, white cut surface.
     D. Treatment consists of local excision.
     E. The neoplastic population expresses CD34 and CD99.

118. Which of the following is NOT a microscopic feature of hemangiopericytoma?
     A. Large, collapsed vessels surrounding the periphery of the lesion
     B. Inter- and perivascular proliferation of uniform cells with angulated nuclei
     C. Mature adipose tissue
     D. Prominent myxoid matrix
     E. Focal storiform growth

119. Which of the following immunohistochemical stains is negative in hemangiopericytoma?
     A. CD31
     B. CD34
     C. CD99
     D. Factor XIIIa
     E. Vimentin

20: Soft Tissue Questions

120. Which of the following features is/are suggestive of malignancy in hemangiopericytoma?
    A.   Tumor size >5 cm
    B.   Tumor cell necrosis
    C.   Abnormal mitotic figures
    D.   >4 mitotic figures/10 hpf
    E.   All of the above

121. Which of the following is NOT a feature of malignant extrarenal rhabdoid tumor?
    A.   Presentation in childhood
    B.   Unifocal
    C.   Rapid growth
    D.   Intradermal location
    E.   Pain

122. Which of the following is NOT a microscopic feature of malignant extrarenal rhabdoid tumor?
    A.   Discohesive growth
    B.   Dense eosinophilic cytoplasmic inclusions
    C.   Multiple small inconspicuous nucleoli
    D.   Polygonal cells with eccentric round nuclei
    E.   Necrosis

123. Which of the following immunohistochemical markers is typically negative in malignant extrarenal rhabdoid tumor?
    A.   Vimentin
    B.   Desmin
    C.   Keratin
    D.   EMA
    E.   CD99

124. The term "malignant mesenchymoma":
    A.   Refers to sarcomas with greater than 4 lines of differentiation
    B.   Is a synonym for synovial sarcoma
    C.   Is discouraged in favor of itemizing differing lines of differentiation
    D.   Implies a poor prognosis
    E.   Is reserved for metastatic sarcomas

125. The juxta-articular variant of myxoma typically occurs in the:
    A.   Wrist
    B.   Ankle
    C.   Knee
    D.   Hip
    E.   Shoulder

126. Which of the variants of myxoma is NOT associated with a syndrome?
    A.   Intramuscular
    B.   Juxta-articular
    C.   Cutaneous

20: Soft Tissue Questions

127. The most common location of ossifying fibromyxoid tumor is:
    A. Head and neck area
    B. Trunk
    C. Extremities
    D. Pelvis
    E. Mediastinum

128. All of the following features are suggestive of malignancy in ossifying fibromyxoid tumor EXCEPT?
    A. Hypercellularity
    B. Brisk mitotic activity
    C. Incomplete capsule
    D. Central ossification
    E. Thrombotic vasculature

129. The molecular alteration associated with ossifying fibromyxoid tumor is:
    A. Ring chromosome 12
    B. t(9;22)(q22;q12)
    C. Trisomy 8
    D. t(12;15)(p13;q26)
    E. None of the above

130. The most common location of synovial sarcoma is:
    A. Head and neck area
    B. Trunk
    C. Retroperitoneum
    D. Upper extremity
    E. Lower extremity

131. Which of the following immunohistochemical stains is typically negative in synovial sarcoma?
    A. EMA
    B. CD34
    C. CD99
    D. Cytokeratin
    E. Bcl-2

132. Which of the following prognostic factors imparts an improvement in survival for patients with synovial sarcoma?
    A. Presence of extensive calcifications
    B. Age >25 years
    C. Proximal tumor location
    D. Monophasic spindle cell histology
    E. Presence of rhabdoid cells

133. Longstanding lymphedema as may be seen following mastectomy has been associated with:
    A. Squamous cell carcinoma
    B. Malignant peripheral nerve sheath tumor
    C. Angiosarcoma
    D. Kaposi sarcoma
    E. Leiomyosarcoma

148. Which of the following statements regarding lymphadenopathic Kaposi sarcoma is TRUE?
     A. It is associated with HIV infection.
     B. In children, the internal organs are commonly involved.
     C. Lesions may regress spontaneously.
     D. It is associated with transplantation.
     E. Immunohistochemical staining for HHV8 is negative.

149. Which of the following microscopic features is NOT characteristic of Kaposi sarcoma?
     A. Irregular anastomosing vascular channels lined by bland endothelium
     B. Stromal plasma cells
     C. Intracellular hyaline globules
     D. Fascicles of bland, eosinophilic spindle cells
     E. Prominent nuclear atypia

150. Which of the following statements regarding myopericytoma is FALSE?
     A. Males and females are equally affected.
     B. It typically involves the distal extremities.
     C. It typically presents as a rapidly enlarging lesion.
     D. Most tumors are solitary.
     E. It is uncommon in children.

151. Which of the following immunohistochemical stains are negative in myopericytoma (choose all that apply)?
     A. S100
     B. CD34
     C. Desmin
     D. Smooth muscle actin
     E. Cytokeratin

152. Which of the following is NOT a feature of the lesion depicted in the image?

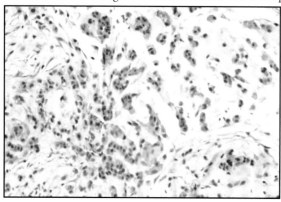

     A. Preferential localization to the head and neck area
     B. Slow, progressive growth
     C. A nodular, lobulated gross appearance
     D. A hemorrhagic, gelatinous cut surface
     E. Male predominance

20: Soft Tissue Questions

153. Which of the following is NOT associated with the lesion depicted in these images?

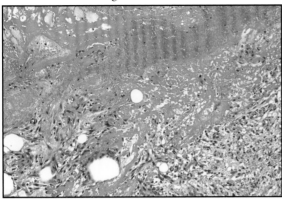 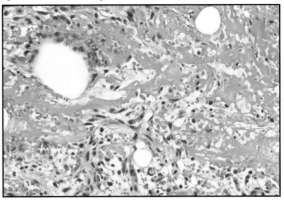

    A. Radiation therapy
    B. Administration of radioactive thorium dioxide (Thorotrast)
    C. High-dose alkylating agents
    D. Trauma
    E. Older patient population

Questions 154 and 155 are based on the following images:

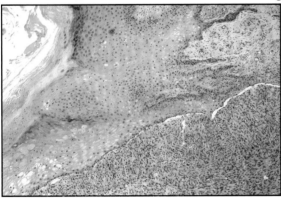 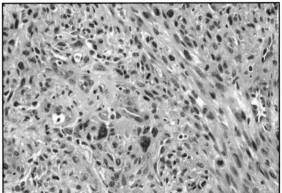

154. The most common location of this lesion is:
    A. Head and neck area
    B. Lower extremities
    C. Upper extremities
    D. Trunk
    E. Retroperitoneum

155. All of the following are common microscopic features of this lesion EXCEPT:
    A. Dermal location
    B. Abundant mitotic activity
    C. Actinic damage involving the surrounding tissue
    D. Necrosis
    E. Marked cytologic atypia

20: Soft Tissue Questions

156. All of the following are features of dermatofibrosarcoma protuberans (seen in this image) EXCEPT:

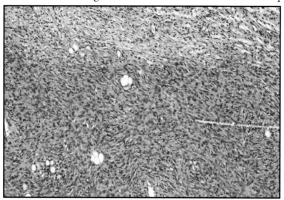

    A.   Male predominance
    B.   Preferential localization to the trunk and proximal extremities
    C.   Fleshy nodule with rim of red or blue discoloration
    D.   Average size of >3 cm on presentation
    E.   Presentation in the 6th decade

157. All of the following are common microscopic features of the lesion depicted in the image EXCEPT:

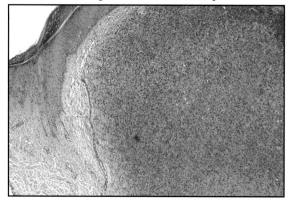 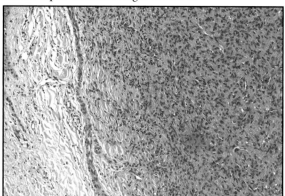

    A.   Touton giant cells
    B.   Stromal hyalinization
    C.   Hemorrhagic cystic change
    D.   Lymphocytic infiltrate
    E.   Mitotic figures

Questions 158 and 159 are based on the following image:

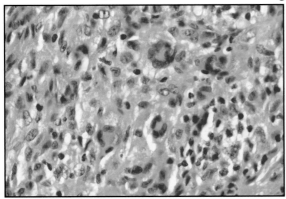

158. Which of the following statements regarding this lesion obtained from the eye of a 2-month-old infant is FALSE?
    A.   It may present at birth.
    B.   The majority of lesions involve the head and neck area.
    C.   Lesions occurring after the age of 20 years are less likely to regress.
    D.   It is associated with underlying lipid abnormalities.
    E.   Lesions may present in internal organs, such as the lung.

159. Which of the following microscopic features is NOT characteristic of this lesion?
    A.   Flattened epidermis with elongated rete ridges
    B.   Infiltration of subcutis and adnexal structures
    C.   Touton and Langerhans cells
    D.   Dermal sheets of histiocytes
    E.   Neutrophilic infiltrate

160. The most common location of tenosynovial giant cell tumor, diffuse type (depicted in this image) is:

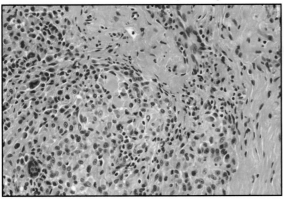

    A.   Ankle
    B.   Foot
    C.   Knee
    D.   Wrist
    E.   Hand

161. Which of the following features is NOT characteristic of elastofibroma (depicted in this image)?

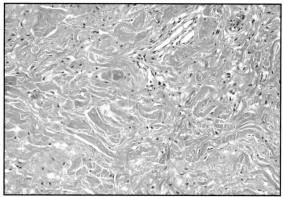

    A.   Predilection for the right scapular area
    B.   Female predominance
    C.   History of repetitive manual labor
    D.   Bilaterality
    E.   Rapid growth

162. Which of the following is NOT a microscopic feature of the lesion depicted in these images?

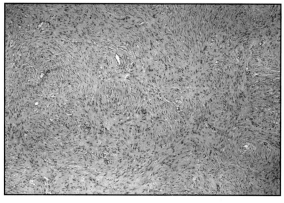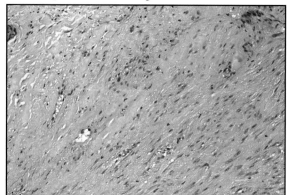

    A.   Hypercellularity
    B.   Occasional mitotic figures
    C.   Infiltrative growth
    D.   Thin-walled vasculature
    E.   Bland fibroblastic proliferation

Questions 163-165 are based on the following image:

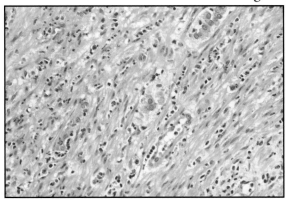

163. Which of the following statements regarding this lesion is FALSE?
    A.   It is predominantly a disease of young children.
    B.   Most cases are localized to the lungs.
    C.   The lesion may be associated with systemic symptoms, such as fever and weight loss.
    D.   Concomitant laboratory abnormalities may include anemia, thrombocytosis, and hypergammaglobulinemia.
    E.   Multiple lesions are present in a third of cases.

164. Which of the following histologic features is NOT characteristic of this lesion?
    A.   Focal psammomatous calcification
    B.   Cellular atypia
    C.   Prominent nucleoli
    D.   Atypical mitotic figures
    E.   Myxoid stroma

165. Which of the following features is/are associated with more aggressive behavior in this lesion?
    A.   Cytologic atypia
    B.   Presence of ganglion-like cells
    C.   Expression of p53
    D.   Chromosomal aneuploidy
    E.   All of the above

Questions 166-168 are based on the following images:

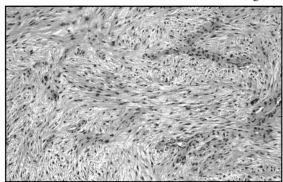 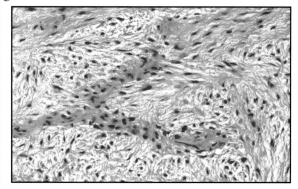

166. Which of the following is NOT a preferred location of this lesion?
    A. Proximal extremities
    B. Trunk
    C. Wrist
    D. Head
    E. Retroperitoneum

167. Which of the following best describes the histologic appearance of this lesion?
    A. Fascicles of bland spindle cells in a background of hypocellular, collagenized areas admixed with myxoid nodules
    B. Elongated myofibroblasts with abundant eosinophilic cytoplasm and scattered mixed inflammatory infiltrate
    C. Sheets of pleomorphic spindle cells with focal necrosis in a myxoid matrix
    D. Bland immature fibroblasts arranged in C-shaped bundles with irregular stromal mucin pools imparting a "feathery" appearance
    E. Infiltrative fascicles of spindle cells exhibiting pleomorphism and hyperchromatism

168. Treatment for this lesion consists of:
    A. Local excision
    B. Radical excision +/– adjuvant chemotherapy
    C. Radical excision +/– adjuvant radiation
    D. Radical excision with lymph node dissection
    E. Chemotherapy

169. The most common location of myofibroma (depicted in this image) is:

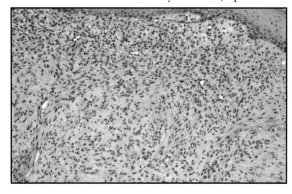

    A. Trunk
    B. Head and neck area
    C. Long bone
    D. Kidney
    E. Liver

20: Soft Tissue Questions

Questions 170-172 are based on the following images:

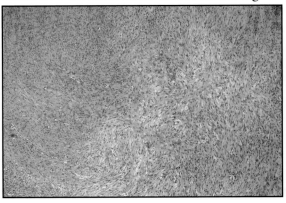 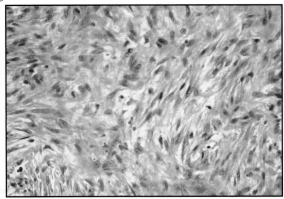

170. All of the following statements regarding the lesion depicted in this image are TRUE EXCEPT:
    A. It is rare in elderly patients.
    B. A significant number of cases may be painful.
    C. There is a slight association with trauma.
    D. Lesions grow rapidly and may measure up to 7 cm on initial presentation.
    E. It occurs most commonly on the upper extremities and trunk.

171. Which of the following microscopic features is NOT characteristic of this lesion?
    A. Fibroblasts arranged in C-shaped bundles
    B. Extravasated red blood cells
    C. Fibroblastic nodules lined by plump myofibroblasts
    D. Thin-walled branching vessels
    E. Keloid-like collagen bands

172. The presence of large, eosinophilic ganglion cell-like myofibroblasts in a lesion arising within the proximal extremity of an older adult describes which of the following variants of this lesion?
    A. Intravascular fasciitis
    B. Cranial fasciitis
    C. Ossifying fasciitis
    D. Proliferative fasciitis
    E. A and B

Questions 173 and 174 are based on the following image:

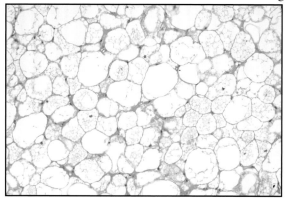

173. Which of the following clinical presentations is most characteristic of this lesion?
    A.   25-year-old male with a painless shoulder mass
    B.   25-year-old female with a painful thigh mass
    C.   50-year-old male with a painful shoulder mass
    D.   50-year-old female with a painless thigh mass
    E.   50-year-old female with a painless shoulder mass

174. The molecular alteration characteristic of this lesion is:
    A.   t(12;16)(q13;p11.2)
    B.   Ring chromosome 12
    C.   Aberration of chromosome 11q13
    D.   Aberration of chromosome 8q11-13
    E.   Aberration of chromosome 16q13

175. The typical patient with lipoblastoma (depicted in this image) is:

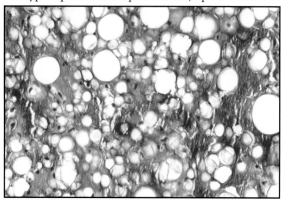

    A.   1-year-old female infant with a lower extremity mass
    B.   1-year-old male infant with a lower extremity mass
    C.   1-year-old male infant with a flank mass
    D.   15-year-old female with a lower extremity mass
    E.   15-year-old male with a flank mass

20: Soft Tissue Questions

176. Which of the following histologic features in a myxoid liposarcoma (depicted in this image) are suggestive of a round cell component? (Choose all that apply.)

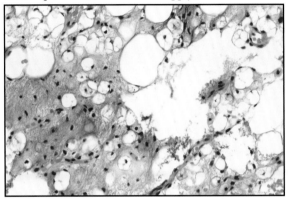

    A.   Sheets of small tumor cells with a high nuclear-cytoplasmic ratio

    B.   High mitotic activity

    C.   Frequent lipoblasts

    D.   Absence of intervening myxoid stroma

    E.   Prominent "chicken-wire" vasculature

177. The eponym given to the lesion depicted in this image arising in the breast or upper extremity following mastectomy with axillary dissection is:

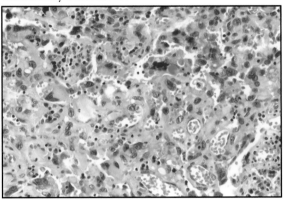

    A.   Stewart-Treves syndrome

    B.   Gorlin syndrome

    C.   Denys-Drash syndrome

    D.   Mazabraud syndrome

    E.   Bourneville disease

178. Which of the following statements regarding cutaneous variants of the lesion depicted in this image is FALSE?

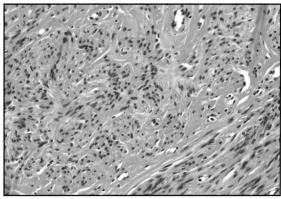

    A.   It arises in association with a pilar erector muscle.

    B.   It is inherited in an autosomal recessive fashion.

    C.   The typical patient is a young adult.

    D.   It is less circumscribed than leiomyomas of the genital tract.

    E.   Exposure to cold may result in pain.

179. All of the following are microscopic features of the lesion depicted in these images EXCEPT:

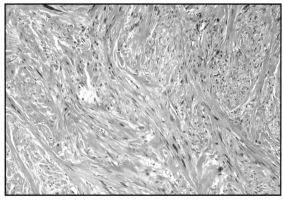 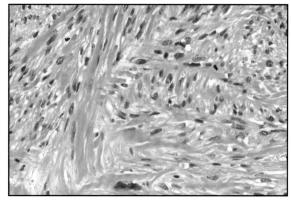

    A.   Prominent nuclear pleomorphism and hyperchromatism

    B.   Spindle cells with wavy nuclei

    C.   Necrosis

    D.   Frequent mitotic figures

    E.   Fascicular growth pattern

180. Based on the microscopic features, the differential diagnosis of adult rhabdomyoma depicted in this image includes all of the following EXCEPT:

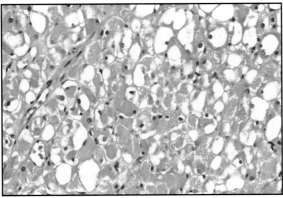

   A.   Granular cell tumor
   B.   Embryonal rhabdomyosarcoma
   C.   Paraganglioma
   D.   Hibernoma
   E.   Oncocytoma

181. The translocation t(2;13)(q35;q14) is associated with which of the following variants of rhabdomyosarcoma (depicted in this image)?

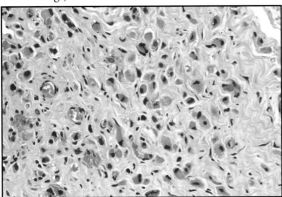

   A.   Embryonal rhabdomyosarcoma, botryoid type
   B.   Embryonal rhabdomyosarcoma, spindle-cell type
   C.   Embryonal rhabdomyosarcoma, anaplastic type
   D.   Alveolar rhabdomyosarcoma
   E.   Pleomorphic rhabdomyosarcoma

Questions 189-191 are based on the following images:

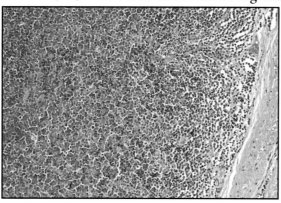 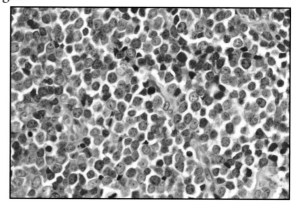

189. Which of the following is NOT a microscopic feature of this lesion, which presented as a firm cutaneous nodule in the neck of an elderly woman?
    A.   Sheets of small, discohesive round blue cells
    B.   Frequent mitotic activity
    C.   Single cell necrosis
    D.   Dense vasculature lined by plump endothelial cells
    E.   Pleomorphic multinucleated giant cells

190. Immunohistochemical staining of this lesion with cytokeratin 20 is:
    A.   Positive in the cytoplasm
    B.   Positive in the nucleus
    C.   Positive in a perinuclear distribution
    D.   Positive in the nucleus and cytoplasm
    E.   Negative

191. Which of the following is NOT associated with this lesion?
    A.   Malignant melanoma
    B.   Basal cell carcinoma
    C.   Adnexal carcinoma
    D.   Bowen disease
    E.   Invasive squamous cell carcinoma

20: Soft Tissue Questions

Questions 192 and 193 are based on the following image:

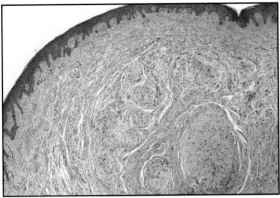

192. The typical location of this lesion is:
    A. Mucosal surface of a child
    B. Mucosal surface of a middle-aged adult
    C. Trunk of a child
    D. Trunk of a middle-aged adult
    E. Trunk of an elderly adult

193. Which of the following microscopic features is NOT characteristic of this lesion?
    A. Benign giant cells
    B. Lobules of uniform round cells
    C. Prominent myxoid matrix
    D. Delicate vasculature
    E. Necrosis

194. All of the following are microscopic features of the lesion depicted in these images, EXCEPT:

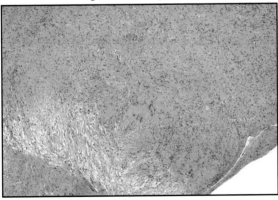 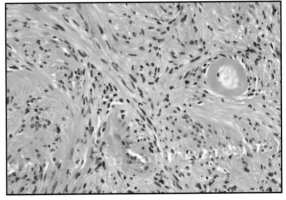

    A. Nuclear palisading
    B. Compact cellular zones
    C. Atypical mitotic figures
    D. Necrosis
    E. Thick hyalinized vessels

Questions 195-197 are based on the following images:

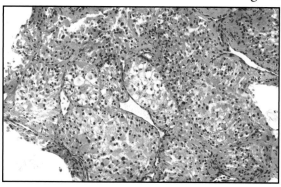 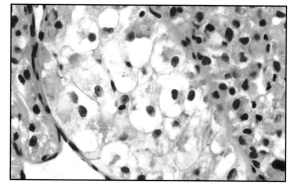

195. Which of the following statements regarding this lesion is FALSE?
    A. It typically occurs in adolescents and young adults.
    B. It is characterized by rapid growth.
    C. The most common location in children is the head and neck area.
    D. The most common location in adults is the lower extremity.
    E. It may be accompanied by bony destruction.

196. Which of the following special stains may be particularly helpful in the diagnosis of this lesion?
    A. PAS with diastase
    B. PAS without diastase
    C. Colloidal iron
    D. Warthin-Starry
    E. GMS

197. Metastases to which of the following locations are more common in this lesion than with any other soft tissue sarcoma?
    A. Lung
    B. Lymph node
    C. Brain
    D. Bone
    E. Liver

198. Which of the following statements regarding angiomatoid fibrous histiocytoma (depicted in these images) is FALSE?

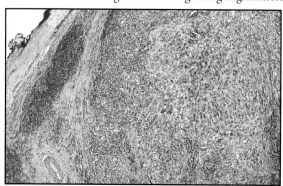 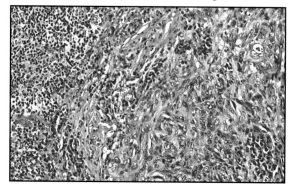

    A. It occurs predominantly in children and young adults.
    B. It may be associated with anemia, fever, and weight loss.
    C. The extremities are the most common location.
    D. It typically presents as a painless mass.
    E. It is characterized by rapid growth.

20: Soft Tissue Questions

Questions 199-201 are based on the following image:

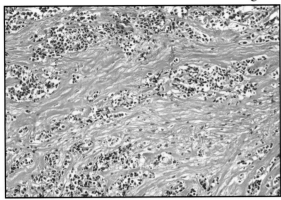

199. The typical presentation of this lesion is:
    A. 2-year-old male with a chest wall mass
    B. 2-year-old female with a chest wall mass
    C. 10-year-old male with an abdominal mass
    D. 10-year-old female with an abdominal mass
    E. 40-year-old male with an abdominal mass

200. Which of the following is NOT a microscopic feature of this lesion?
    A. Rhabdoid cells
    B. Cellular pleomorphism
    C. Necrosis
    D. Mitotic figures
    E. Epithelial differentiation

201. The immunohistochemical profile of this lesion is:
    A. CK+EMA+desmin+
    B. CK–EMA+desmin+
    C. CK–EMA–desmin+
    D. CK–EMA–desmin–
    E. CK+EMA+desmin–

20: Soft Tissue Questions

202. The most common soft tissue sarcoma involving the wrist (depicted in these images) is:

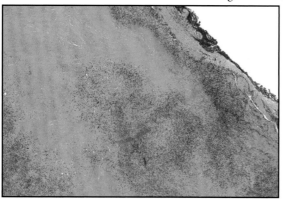 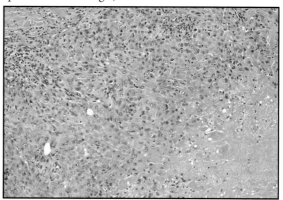

    A. Synovial sarcoma
    B. Malignant peripheral nerve sheath tumor
    C. Epithelioid sarcoma
    D. Extraskeletal chondrosarcoma
    E. Extraskeletal osteosarcoma

Questions 203 and 204 are based on the following image:

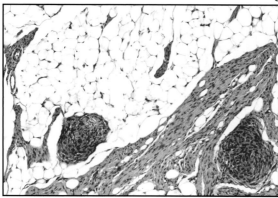

203. Which of the following statements regarding this lesion arising in the posterior axillary fold of a child is TRUE?
    A. It is more common in females.
    B. It frequently involves the hands and feet.
    C. It presents as multiple subcutaneous nodules.
    D. Malignant transformation is a common complication.
    E. Most cases are discovered during the first 2 years of life.

204. Which of the following is NOT a microscopic feature of this lesion?
    A. Intersecting fascicles of spindle cells and collagen
    B. Small stellate cells embedded in a mucoid matrix
    C. Multinucleated giant cells
    D. Islands of mature adipose tissue
    E. Organoid growth pattern

205. Which of the following laboratory anomalies is occasionally seen in association with hemangiopericytoma (depicted in these images)?

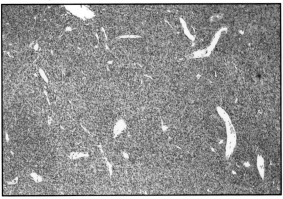 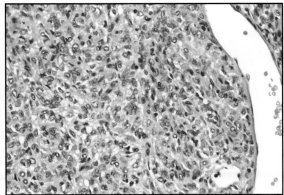

A. Hypercalcemia
B. Hypocalcemia
C. Hyperglycemia
D. Hypoglycemia
E. Hyperlipidemia

206. Which of the following microscopic features can be seen in the lesion depicted in this image?

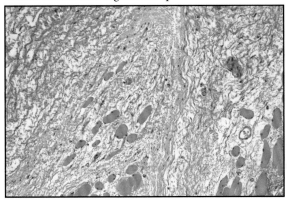

A. Infiltrative growth
B. Nuclear atypia
C. Pleomorphism
D. Multinucleated giant cells
E. Mitotic figures

207. The most common location of the lesion depicted in this image is:

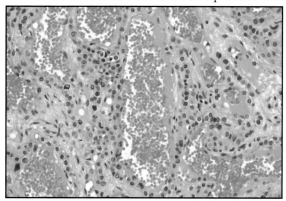

    A.   Tongue
    B.   Toe
    C.   Finger
    D.   Neck
    E.   Scalp

208. Which of the following statements regarding epithelioid hemangioendothelioma (depicted in these images) is FALSE?

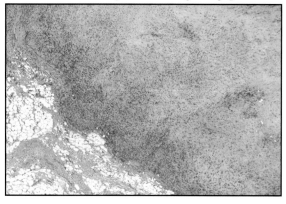 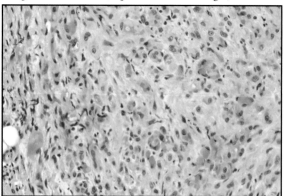

    A.   This variant occurs predominantly in men.
    B.   This variant affects young adults.
    C.   Parenchymal tumors are frequently multifocal.
    D.   Erythrocytes may be seen within intracellular cytoplasmic lumina.
    E.   Approximately 1/2 of cases are associated with vessel walls.

20: Soft Tissue Questions

209. Which of the following viruses is associated with Kaposi sarcoma (depicted in this image?

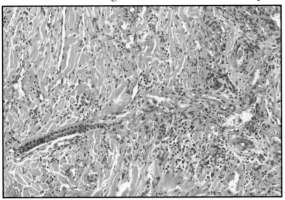

    A.   EBV
    B.   CMV
    C.   HHV6
    D.   HHV8
    E.   BK

20: Soft Tissue Answers

1. **E.** **ALL OF THE ABOVE**

   Intraoperative consultations on soft tissue tumors, although uncommonly requested, are appropriate in all of the situations listed (choice E).

   QCSP, **Intraoperative Consultation,** p 636.

2. **D.** **CHANGES IN VISION**

   Young patients with extraskeletal mesenchymal chondrosarcoma typically develop lesions localized to the head and neck area and present with increased intracranial pressure or changes in vision (choice D). While painless deep-seated masses do occur, these are more common in older patients (choice C). Because of the extraosseous nature of the lesion, bone pain and pathologic fractures are not common (choices A, B). Extraskeletal mesenchymal chondrosarcoma is not associated with a history of trauma (choice E).

   QCSP, **Extraskeletal Chondrosarcoma,** p 637.

3. **D.** **BINUCLEATED CHONDROCYTES: EXTRASKELETAL MESENCHYMAL CHONDROSARCOMA**

   The neoplastic population in extraskeletal mesenchymal chondrosarcoma consists of primitive, uniform spindled cells with minimal cytoplasm, which bear no direct resemblance to chondrocytes, making this lesion challenging to diagnose in the absence of distinct cartilaginous tissue (choice D). Binucleated chondrocytes are more commonly seen in the other 2 variants. The other choices presented are correctly paired with their respective variants.

   QCSP, **Extraskeletal Chondrosarcoma,** p 637.

4. **B.** **t(9;22)**

   The molecular aberration characteristic of extraskeletal myxoid chondrosarcoma is a reciprocal translocation involving chromosomes 9 and 22 creating the EWS/TEC fusion protein, which is unrelated to the Philadelphia chromosome (choice B). The t(8;21), t(12;15), t(12;16), and t(X;18) represent classic aberrations involved in the pathogenesis of acute myeloid leukemia, infantile fibrosarcoma, myxoid liposarcoma, and synovial sarcoma, respectively (choices A, C, D, E). It is important to keep in mind that chromosomes do house a myriad of genes such that separate disease entities may have identical shorthand translocations affecting vastly differing genes.

   QCSP, **Extraskeletal Chondrosarcoma,** p 638.

5. **C.** **CHORDOMA**

   The primitive spindled mesenchymal cells characteristic of extraskeletal mesenchymal chondrosarcoma in the absence of mature hyaline cartilage islands may be misinterpreted as synovial sarcoma, Ewing sarcoma, or embryonal rhabdomyosarcoma (choices A, D, E). The growth pattern in particular may resemble that of a hemangiopericytoma (choice B). Chordoma, on the other hand, is characterized by cells containing vacuolated, distended cytoplasm ("physaliphorous cells"), which may pose more of a problem in the differential diagnosis of more differentiated variants of chondrosarcoma (choice C).

   QCSP, **Extraskeletal Chondrosarcoma,** p 638.

6. **E.** **CYTOKERATIN**

   Although cytokeratin staining is not routinely observed in extraskeletal osteosarcoma, up to 10% of cases may show some immunoreactivity and should not be misinterpreted (choice E). Vimentin, osteocalcin, smooth muscle actin, and EMA stain approximately 100%, 80%, 70%, and 50% of cases, respectively (choices A, B, C, D).

   QCSP, **Extraskeletal Osteosarcoma,** p 639.

7. **B.** **TUMOR SIZE**

   The tumor size in extraskeletal osteosarcoma is considered the most important prognostic indicator, with measurements >5 cm conferring a worse prognosis (choice B).

   QCSP, **Extraskeletal Osteosarcoma,** p 639.

20: Soft Tissue Answers

8. **C.** **25-YEAR-OLD MALE DEFENSIVE LINEMAN**

Myositis ossificans predominates in the 2nd and 3rd decade, typically affecting active men. There is a strong association with trauma. The individual that best fits this description is the 25-year-old defensive lineman (choice C).

QCSP, **Myositis Ossificans**, p 639.

9. **A.** **THE ZONING PATTERN**

Myositis ossificans exhibits a particular zoning pattern characterized by a central proliferation of vascular fibroblastic tissue surrounded by peripheral maturing bony elements (choice A). While extraskeletal osteosarcoma frequently does not exhibit zonation, some cases may demonstrate the reverse pattern with central osteoid and peripheral fibroblastic proliferation. The other choices presented do not reliably differentiate between the 2 entities.

QCSP, **Myositis Ossificans**, p 640.

10. **B.** **OVERLYING EPIDERMAL HYPERPLASIA**

Unlike fibrous histiocytoma, dermatofibrosarcoma protuberans does not exhibit overlying epidermal hyperplasia, which can be helpful (choice B). Additionally, immunohistochemical staining for CD34 can help differentiate between the 2 entities, as dermatofibrosarcoma protuberans typically stains strongly, while fibrous histiocytoma does not. The other microscopic features listed may be seen in either entity.

QCSP, **Dermatofibrosarcoma Protuberans**, p 641-642.

11. **C.** **BEDNAR TUMOR**

Cases of pigmented dermatofibrosarcoma protuberans are also known as Bednar tumors (choice C). Askin tumor is the name given to primitive neuroectodermal tumors involving the thoracopulmonary area (choice A). Warthin tumors are benign salivary gland neoplasms (choice B), while Klatskin tumors are cases of bile duct carcinoma involving the hepatic duct bifurcation (choice E). Malignant mesenchymoma is a term used to describe lesions exhibiting at least 2 different types of sarcomatous differentiation (choice D).

QCSP, **Dermatofibrosarcoma Protuberans**, p 642.

12. **D.** **RADIATION**

All of the factors listed have been associated with dermatofibrosarcoma protuberans except for radiation (choice D).

QCSP, **Dermatofibrosarcoma Protuberans**, p 642.

13. **D.** **EPITHELIOID FIBROUS HISTIOCYTOMA: CELLULAR NECROSIS**

The variants presented are of interest, because they have slightly differing gross appearances and occur in differing patient populations and locations. Cellular fibrous histiocytoma occurs in the head and neck region or extremities of young adult males and microscopically exhibits plump spindle cells with prominent eosinophilic cytoplasm (choices A, B). Necrosis is occasionally present. Epithelioid fibrous histiocytoma typically presents in the lower extremities of adults as a red nodule (choice C). Necrosis is not a prominent feature (choice D). Aneurysmal fibrous histiocytoma occurs in the lower extremities of adults as a blue or brown nodule, due to the hemosiderin present in the lesion (choice E).

QCSP, **Fibrous Histiocytoma**, p 643.

14. **B.** **CD34−, FACTOR XIIIa+**

Fibrous histiocytoma exhibits staining for factor XIIIa, but not for CD34 or S100 (choice B). Staining for factor XIIIa and CD34 is particularly helpful in differentiating this entity from dermatofibrosarcoma protuberans, which shows the opposite immunoreactivity pattern.

QCSP, **Fibrous Histiocytoma**, p 644.

20: Soft Tissue Answers

15.   C.   **THE LESION MAY REPRESENT A JUVENILE ANALOGUE OF DERMATOFIBROSARCOMA PROTUBERANS.**
Giant cell fibroblastoma most commonly occurs in the extremities or chest wall of male children (choice A, B). The lesion may represent a juvenile analogue of dermatofibrosarcoma protuberans, with which it shares recurrent molecular alterations such as ring chromosome 17 and 22 (choice C, E). The immunohistochemical staining pattern is also similar to dermatofibrosarcoma protuberans in that CD34 may be positive, while S100 is typically negative (choice D).
QCSP, **Giant Cell Fibroblastoma,** p 644.

16.   D.   **50%**
Close follow-up for patients with giant cell fibroblastoma is critical, as the recurrence rate approximates 50% (choice D). The lesion may also recur as dermatofibrosarcoma protuberans, underscoring the relationship between these 2 entities.
QCSP, **Giant Cell Fibroblastoma,** p 645.

17.   B.   **FALSE**
There is no evidence at this time to support that juvenile xanthogranuloma is a heritable condition (choice B).
QCSP, **Juvenile Xanthogranuloma,** p 645.

18.   E.   **NUMEROUS GIANT CELLS**
Malignant giant cell tumor of tendon sheath frequently contains large areas of benign giant cell tumor and occurs predominantly in the distal extremities (choices A, B). Both typical as well as atypical mitotic figures may be seen (choices C, D). Giant cells are usually less prominent than in benign giant cell tumors (choice E).
QCSP, **Malignant Giant Cell Tumor of Tendon Sheath,** p 646.

19.   B.   **FALSE**
Surgical resection is the treatment of choice for malignant giant cell tumors of tendon sheath, which are frequently radioresistant (choice B).
QCSP, **Malignant Giant Cell Tumor of Tendon Sheath,** p 646.

20.   D.   **A AND B**
Although the classification of malignant fibrous histiocytoma is somewhat controversial, storiform growth and the presence of giant cells have led some pathologists to categorize these as distinct variants of pleomorphic malignant fibrous histiocytoma (choices A, B). The presence of myxoid matrix in the setting of pleomorphic cells with atypical mitotic figures and other features of malignant fibrous histiocytoma may be more compatible with a diagnosis of myxofibrosarcoma (choice C).
QCSP, **Pleomorphic Malignant Fibrous Histiocytoma,** p 646.

21.   C.   **INFLAMMATORY VARIANT**
Unlike the other 2 variants, which typically occur in the extremities, the inflammatory variant of pleomorphic malignant fibrous histiocytoma is more common in the abdomen (choice C).
QCSP, **Pleomorphic Malignant Fibrous Histiocytoma,** p 646.

22.   D.   **THICK VESSELS**
Storiform malignant fibrous histiocytoma exhibits a bland fibroblastic population arranged in a storiform growth pattern with admixed pleomorphic, bizarre cells and atypical mitotic figures (choices A, C, E). The stroma is remarkable for thin, slit-like vessels and may contain areas of bony or cartilaginous metaplasia (choices B, D).
QCSP, **Pleomorphic Malignant Fibrous Histiocytoma,** p 647.

23. E. **ALL OF THE ABOVE**

Giant cell pleomorphic malignant fibrous histiocytoma is characterized by a proliferation of ovoid fibroblasts arranged in a nodular growth pattern with admixed osteoclast-like giant cells (choices A, B). These giant cells are positive for keratin by immunohistochemistry (choice C).

QCSP, **Pleomorphic Malignant Fibrous Histiocytoma,** p 647.

24. A. **DIFFUSE TYPE**

The diffuse type of tenosynovial giant cell tumor is less common and occurs in a younger patient population (choice A).

QCSP, **Tenosynovial Giant Cell Tumor,** Diffuse Type, p 648.

25. C. **THE NEOPLASTIC POPULATION CONSISTS OF SHEETS OF MONOMORPHIC CELLS WITH LARGE NUCLEI ADMIXED WITH SCATTERED MULTINUCLEATED GIANT CELLS.**

Tenosynovial giant cell tumor of diffuse type shows a female predominance (choice A). The lesion commonly erodes the adjacent tissue, which by itself does not indicate malignancy (choice B). Microscopically, the neoplastic population consists of sheets of monomorphic cells with large nuclei admixed with scattered multinucleated giant cells (choice C). High mitotic activity (even in the absence of atypical mitotic figures) is worrisome and should raise concern for malignant behavior (choice E). While the tumor is considered benign, recurrence is not uncommon, occurring in approximately 1/2 of cases (choice D).

QCSP, **Tenosynovial Giant Cell Tumor,** Diffuse Type, p 648-649.

26. E. **STROMAL HYALINIZATION**

Compared to the diffuse type, tenosynovial giant cell tumor of localized type occurs in an older patient population and exhibits a preference for the tendons of the hand (choices C, D). Microscopically, there is typically a higher density of giant cells (choice B). The localized type recurs less commonly (choice A). Both types may demonstrate prominent stromal hyalinization (choice E).

QCSP, **Tenosynovial Giant Cell Tumor,** Localized Type, p 648-649.

27. E. **ALL OF THE ABOVE**

All of the features listed predict an increased risk of recurrence (choice E).

QCSP, **Tenosynovial Giant Cell Tumor,** Localized Type, p 650.

28. A. **ERUPTIVE XANTHOMA: FACE**

Eruptive xanthoma typically presents as small yellow papules involving the buttocks, not the face (choice A). The other variants are correctly paired. Note that the tuberous variant may also involve fingers, knees, and buttocks as well as elbows (choice B).

QCSP, **Xanthoma,** p 650.

29. A. **ERUPTIVE XANTHOMA**

The majority of histiocytes comprising eruptive xanthoma are of the nonfoamy type (choice A). The other variants are largely composed of foamy histiocytes.

QCSP, **Xanthoma,** p 650.

30. D. **LYMPHOMA**

While all variants of xanthoma are associated with various types of hyperlipidemia to varying degrees, the presence of plane xanthoma in a normolipemic patient is associated with reticuloendothelial malignancies, which include lymphoma (choice D).

QCSP, **Xanthoma,** p 651.

20: Soft Tissue Answers

31. C. **PAINLESS MASS INVOLVING THE PALM OF A YOUNG CHILD**
Calcifying aponeurotic fibroma is a painless lesion, which arises in the tendons or aponeuroses of the hands and feet. The lesion most commonly involved the palm. The patient population includes infants and young children (choice C). Choices A, B, D, E may be good clinical descriptions for fibroma of tendon sheath, infantile digital fibromatosis, low-grade fibromyxoid sarcoma, and elastofibroma, respectively, although the differential of each presentation is broad.
QCSP, **Calcifying Aponeurotic Fibroma,** p 651.

32. B. **PSEUDOCAPSULE**
Calcifying aponeurotic fibroma exhibits a striking nodular growth pattern with infiltration into adjacent muscle and adipose tissue (choice A). The nodules are largely composed of plump fibroblasts, which surround a central area of hyalinized stroma (choice E). The degree of calcification and cartilage formation is variable and highly dependent on the age of the lesion (choice C, D). Although most of the lesion is well-circumscribed and distinct from the adjacent tissue, the portion attached to the tendon is tightly adherent and microscopically infiltrative (choice B).
QCSP, **Calcifying Aponeurotic Fibroma,** p 651-652.

33. B. **CHENILLE BODIES**
The fragments of elastic fibers seen in elastofibroma are typically arranged linearly, creating a "beads on a string" appearance, and are known as chenille bodies (choice B). Ferruginous bodies are asbestos fibers coated with iron and calcium, which are seen in asbestosis (choice A). Asteroid and Schaumann bodies are associated with (but not entirely specific for) granulomatous diseases, such as sarcoidosis or tuberculosis, and consist of cytoskeletal elements and calcium/protein inclusions within Langerhans giant cells, respectively (choices C, E). Michaelis-Guttman bodies are basophilic concentric inclusions representing remnants of Gram-negative bacteria and are a feature of malakoplakia (choice D).
QCSP, **Elastofibroma,** p 652.

34. C. **IT IS ASSOCIATED WITH TRAUMA.**
Fibroma of tendon sheath is a well-circumscribed, painless lesion that occurs predominantly in the fingers of young to middle-aged adults (choices A, E). There is a male predominance (choice B). While lesions do recur, they do not undergo malignant transformation (choice D).
QCSP, **Fibroma of Tendon Sheath,** p 653.

35. B. **DESMIN**
The use of immunohistochemical stains has a very limited role in the diagnosis of fibroblastic and myofibroblastic tumors, as the profiles of many entities overlap. Staining for desmin in fibroma of tendon sheath is usually negative (choice B).
QCSP, **Fibroma of Tendon Sheath,** p 653.

36. C. **PLANTAR FIBROMATOSIS TYPICALLY PRESENTS AS LOCALIZED DISEASE, WHEREAS PALMAR FIBROMATOSIS OCCURS MORE FREQUENTLY AS MULTIPLE BILATERAL LESIONS.**
The superficial variant of fibromatosis occurs predominantly in the penis, palm, and plantar aspect of the foot of patients in the 6th and 7th decades, which are known as Peyronie disease, Dupuytren contracture, and Ledderhose disease, respectively (choices A, D). Peyronie disease may be treated with excision and/or radiation; chemotherapy is typically not useful (choice B). The clinical presentation of palmar and plantar fibromatosis is slightly different in that the former occurs as multiple bilateral lesions, whereas the plantar form is usually more localized (choice C). Cartilaginous metaplasia occurs over time and is not a sign of malignancy (choice E).
QCSP, **Fibromatosis,** p 654.

37. B. **ASSOCIATION WITH PREGNANCY**
The extraabdominal form of deep fibromatosis occurs in patients in their 2nd and 3rd decades (choice A). There is a marked predilection for the shoulder and chest wall, although the proximal lower extremity is also frequently involved (choice C). On gross examination, the lesion appears firm, white, and ill-defined, corroborating its infiltrative microscopic growth (choices D, E). Unlike the abdominal form, the extraabdominal form of deep fibromatosis is not associated with pregnancy (choice B).
QCSP, **Fibromatosis,** p 654.

38. E. **ALL OF THE ABOVE**
All of the conditions listed have been associated with the abdominal form of deep fibromatosis (choice E).
QCSP, **Fibromatosis,** p 655.

39. C. **TRISOMY 8 IS PRESENT IN SUPERFICIAL FIBROMATOSIS**
Fibromatosis exhibits immunoreactivity with desmin and β-catenin (choices A, B). Deep fibromatosis has 2 characteristic molecular alterations, including trisomy 8 in up to 25% of cases and deletion of 5q in 10% of cases (choices C, D). Treatment consists primarily of radical excision, although radiation and chemotherapy have an important adjuvant role (choice E).
QCSP, **Fibromatosis,** p 655.

40. A. **LOCATION OF TUMOR**
Adult- and juvenile-type fibrosarcoma exhibit differing clinical and laboratory presentations. The juvenile-type of fibrosarcoma by definition must occur in patients under the age of 10 years, while the adult-type is more common in the 4th and 5th decades (choice B). The juvenile-type is characterized by rapid growth frequently accompanied by taut, possibly ulcerating overlying skin (choices C, E). In contrast, the adult-form exhibits slower growth and may be accompanied by hypoglycemia due to the elaboration of insulin-like substances from the tumor (choice D). The preferred locations of both types include the trunk, head and neck area, and extremities (choice A).
QCSP, **Fibrosarcoma,** p 656.

41. D. **LYMPHATIC SEEDING**
Adult-type fibrosarcoma is characterized by a "herringbone" growth pattern with easily identifiable mitotic figures, some of which may be atypical (choice A). On the other hand, it is not uncommon for lesions to contain areas of hypocellularity that are indistinguishable from fibromatosis (choice B). Although immunohistochemistry has only limited utility in the diagnosis, the typical staining pattern includes reactivity for vimentin as well as focal smooth muscle actin (choice C). Unlike the juvenile-type of fibrosarcoma, the adult-type does not exhibit a characteristic molecular alteration (choice E). Metastasis is not unusual and occurs hematogenously, most commonly to the lung (choice D).
QCSP, **Fibrosarcoma,** p 656-657.

42. C. **t(12;15)(p13;q25)**
The molecular alteration characteristic of juvenile-type fibrosarcoma is identical to the one seen in congenital mesoblastic nephroma and results in the gene fusion product ETV6-NTRK3 (choice C). Choices A, B, D, and E represent the molecular alterations present in myxoid liposarcoma, clear cell sarcoma, primitive neuroectodermal tumor, and desmoplastic small round cell tumor, respectively.
QCSP, **Fibrosarcoma,** p 657.

43. C. **It has a pattern of immunoreactivity that is distinct from classic adult-type fibrosarcoma.**

The sclerosing epithelioid variant of adult-type fibrosarcoma distinguishes itself from classic adult-type fibrosarcoma by the microscopic features. It is less cellular with a corresponding decrease in mitotic figures (choices A, B). Approximately 1/2 of cases recur and metastasis to the lungs is common (choices D, E). The diagnosis of this variant rests on the identification of epithelioid fibroblasts in hyalinized stroma that do not exhibit the classic "herringbone" pattern. Immunohistochemistry is not helpful in distinguishing between classic adult-type fibrosarcoma and this variant (choice C).
QCSP, **Fibrosarcoma,** p 657.

44. C. **35%**

About 1/3 of cases of infantile digital fibromatosis are diagnosed at birth, while the rest of cases are predominantly identified within the 1st year.
QCSP, **Infantile Digital Fibromatosis,** p 657.

45. A. **Eosinophilic and cytoplasmic**

The inclusions characteristic of infantile digital fibromatosis are typically eosinophilic and cytoplasmic, resembling engulfed red blood cells (choice A).
QCSP, **Infantile Digital Fibromatosis,** p 658.

46. C. **Masson trichrome**

The inclusions characteristic of infantile digital fibromatosis stain deeply with Masson trichrome as well as phosphotungstic acid hematoxylin (choice C). PAS and alcian blue stains are negative (choices A, B, D).
QCSP, **Infantile Digital Fibromatosis,** p 658.

47. D. **Cellular atypia**

There is some overlap in the clinical as well as the histologic features of low-grade myofibroblastic sarcoma and the extraabdominal variant of fibromatosis. Both occur in young adults as a painless mass with predilection for the head and neck area as well as the thigh, although fibromatosis may also involve many other sites. Both entities share an ill-defined firm gross appearance that corroborates their infiltrative growth by a neoplastic spindle cell population (choices A, B, E). Occasional mitotic figures may be present in either entity; however, cellular atypia is not a feature of fibromatosis and supports a diagnosis of low-grade myofibroblastic sarcoma (choices C, D).
QCSP, **Low-Grade Myofibroblastic Sarcoma,** p 660.

48. E. **S100**

In line with its divergent myoid and fibroblastic differentiation, low-grade myofibroblastic sarcoma may express smooth muscle actin, desmin, or CD34, although all 3 of these may also be negative (choices A, B, C). CD99 staining may likewise be present (choice D). Of the choices presented, only S100 is reliably negative in low-grade myofibroblastic sarcoma (choice E).
QCSP, **Low-Grade Myofibroblastic Sarcoma,** p 660.

49. E. **Diffuse lymphocytic infiltrate**

Myofibroma has a distinct histologic pattern, exhibiting a prominent nodular growth pattern (choice C). The periphery of the nodules is lined by plump, mature myofibroblasts, while the center contains primitive round, polygonal cells reminiscent of primitive neuroectodermal tumor that are typically arranged around hemangiopericytoma-like vessels (choice D). A lymphocytic infiltrate, if present, is usually confined to the periphery of the nodules rather than diffuse (choice E). Dystrophic calcification and focal necrosis may be present, but do not confer any changes in prognosis (choices A, B).
QCSP, **Myofibroma,** p 661.

50. C. **PULMONARY DISEASE**

Pulmonary involvement by myofibroma(tosis) is associated with a poor prognosis (choice C). While pulmonary involvement is associated with multicentric disease, it is the respiratory complications in particular that prove fatal in many neonatal and young pediatric patients (choice A). Disease involving the bone is not associated with a change in prognosis (choice B). The presence of an inflammatory infiltrate and the degree of mitotic activity are variable, but appear to have no influence on prognosis (choice D, E).

QCSP, **Myofibroma,** p 661.

51. D. **DISTAL EXTREMITIES**

The location of the tumor as well as the patient demographics and radiologic findings are critical in shaping the differential diagnosis of soft tissue tumors. In regards to myxoinflammatory fibroblastic sarcoma, the most common location is the hand, while the foot is the second most common (choice D).

QCSP, **Myxoinflammatory Fibroblastic Sarcoma,** p 661.

52. A. **GIANT CELLS**

Myxoinflammatory fibroblastic sarcoma exhibits 3 types of neoplastic cells: spindle cells with moderate cellular atypia, ganglion-like cells with prominent nucleoli, and multivacuolated cells reminiscent of lipoblasts (choices B, C, D). True to its name, this lesion typically exhibits a prominent acute and chronic inflammatory infiltrate including lymphocytes (choice E). Giant cells are not a feature of this tumor (choice A).

QCSP, **Myxoinflammatory Fibroblastic Sarcoma,** p 661.

53. E. **ELDERLY ADULTS**

Myxofibrosarcoma, formerly known as myxoid malignant fibrous histiocytoma, is a common sarcoma which typically present in elderly patients (choice E).

QCSP, **Myxofibrosarcoma,** p 662.

54. E. **THICK HYALINIZED VESSELS**

High-grade myxofibrosarcoma exhibits overtly malignant features consisting of focal necrosis, numerous atypical mitotic figures, and bizarre multinucleated giant cells (choices A, B, C). Typically, residual areas of low-grade myxofibrosarcoma can be identified within the lesion (choice D). The vasculature is characteristically thin-walled rather than thick and hyalinized (choice E).

QCSP, **Myxofibrosarcoma,** p 662.

55. A. **BETTER**

Although the recurrence and metastasis rates remain high for myxofibrosarcoma, the prognosis is better than that of classic pleomorphic malignant fibrous histiocytoma (choice A).

QCSP, **Myxofibrosarcoma,** p 663.

56. C. **MATURATION TO LIPOMA**

Unlike lipoblastomatosis, lipoblastoma presents as a localized subcutaneous mass and does not exhibit significant infiltration into adjacent tissues (choice A). Neither malignant transformation nor metastases are features of this benign tumor (choices B, D, E). Serial biopsies of these lesions have shown maturation of the lipoblasts into adipocytes forming a conventional lipoma (choice C).

QCSP, **Lipoblastoma,** p 665.

57.　B.　**CELLULAR ATYPIA**

The microscopic features of lipoma closely resemble those of normal mature adipose tissue. The diagnosis rests predominantly on the clinical impression of a lesion as well as the variation in adipocyte size (choice C). The tumor is typically highly vascular (choice D). Fat necrosis and infarction are not uncommon (choice E); however, cellular atypia is abnormal and points toward a malignant process (choice B). The intramuscular variant of lipoma frequently exhibits an infiltrative growth pattern (choice A).

QCSP, **Lipoma**, p 666.

58.　D AND E　**SPINDLE CELL LIPOMA; PLEOMORPHIC LIPOMA**

Spindle cell and pleomorphic lipoma exhibit similar clinical demographics with a predilection for the shoulder and neck of middle-aged men (choices D and E). Spindle cell lipoma contains bland spindle cells with wavy nuclei admixed with adipocytes in a mucinous background. "Keloid-like" collagen bundles are typically present in the stroma. Pleomorphic lipoma, on the other hand, characteristically contains multinucleated "floret-like" cells and abundant thick collagen fibers. Both variants share aberrations of chromosome 16q13 and may represent opposite ends of the same disease spectrum.

QCSP, **Lipoma**, p 666.

59.　D.　**ANGIOLIPOMA**

The mnemonic "blue ANGEL" can serve as a useful reminder for painful skin lesions and stands for blue rubber bleb nevus, angiolipoma, neuroma, glomus tumor, eccrine spiradenoma, and leiomyoma. Angiolipoma presents as multiple painful nodules in pubescent patients (choice D). The forearm is a classic site. Conventional lipoma is a neoplasm of older adults (choice A). The other variants listed typically are not associated with pain and do not exhibit a predilection for pubescent patients (choices B, C, E).

QCSP, **Lipoma**, p 666.

60.　D.　**MAFFUCCI SYNDROME**

Maffucci syndrome is characterized by cutaneous vascular tumors and enchondromas involving the small and long bones (choice D). Bannayan-Zonana syndrome (hemangiomas, microcephaly), Cowden syndrome (hemangiomas, nodular goiter, lichenoid/papular/papillomatous skin lesions), Frohlich syndrome (obesity, sexual infantilism), and Proteus syndrome (fibroplasia of distal extremities, skeletal hypertrophy, bony exostoses, scoliosis, and linear verrucous epidermal nevi) are all associated with multiple lipomas (choices A, B, C, E)

QCSP, **Lipoma**, p 667.

61.　C.　**MYXOID LIPOSARCOMA**

Myxoid liposarcoma comprises approximately 1/2 of all cases of liposarcoma, making it the most common variant (choice C). Within the category of well-differentiated liposarcoma, the adipocytic type occurs more commonly than the sclerosing type (choices A, B). Dedifferentiation occurs in a subset of well-differentiated liposarcoma, while pleomorphic liposarcoma represents only 5% of cases (choices D, E).

QCSP, **Liposarcoma**, p 668.

62.　B.　**TUMOR LOCATION**

The histologic features (mitotic activity, cellular atypia, presence of lipoblasts) of atypical lipomatous tumor and well-differentiated liposarcoma are identical (choices C, D, E). The difference in nomenclature reflects the divergent prognoses of these 2 entities based on resectability, which is a function of location. Atypical lipomatous tumor is a term typically reserved for lesions occurring in locations amenable to complete resection, such as the extremities, while the term well-differentiated liposarcoma is universally used for identical lesions occurring in the retroperitoneum (choice B). Tumor size does not contribute to the distinction between these entities (choice A).

QCSP, **Liposarcoma**, p 668.

63.   D.   **CELLULAR ATYPIA**
The distinction between conventional lipoma and well-differentiated liposarcoma can be exceptionally difficult. Clinically, both lesions may form large masses (choice A). There is significant overlap in preferred locations of the 2 entities, although certain locations such as the retroperitoneum strongly favor liposarcoma (choice B). Both lesions are characterized by variation in adipocyte size (choice C). The presence of lipoblasts, while frequently associated with liposarcoma, is neither necessary nor sufficient for its diagnosis (choice E). Cellular atypia, however, is not a feature of conventional lipoma and supports a diagnosis of malignancy (choice D).
QCSP, **Liposarcoma,** p 668.

64.   D.   **PLEOMORPHIC LIPOSARCOMA**
Although the pleomorphic variant of liposarcoma typically occurs in the extremities, its resectability based on location offers little in the way of improvement in prognosis due to the prevalence of widespread metastases at the time of diagnosis. Histologically, pleomorphic liposarcoma resembles pleomorphic malignant fibrous histiocytoma with bizarre multinucleated giant cells, marked mitotic activity, and atypical mitotic figures. The distinction between these 2 entities rests on the identification of cells reminiscent of lipoblasts. The mitotic activity is considerably higher than in any other variant of liposarcoma (choice D).
QCSP, **Liposarcoma,** p 668.

65.   C.   **DURATION OF DISEASE**
Dedifferentiation arises in the setting of well-differentiated liposarcoma and appears to be time-dependent (choice C). Patient demographics, tumor location, and the presence of lipoblasts have no impact on the incidence of dedifferentiation (choice A, B, E). High mitotic activity may be associated with rapid tumor growth, but has not been associated with dedifferentiation (choice D).
QCSP, **Liposarcoma,** p 669.

66.   D.   **MOST LESIONS PRESENT IN PATIENTS OLDER THAN 10 YEARS OF AGE.**
Lymphangioma is predominantly thought to be a malformation, which does not communicate with the lymphatic or venous system and affects newborns as well as young children (choices D, E). The cutaneous variant preferentially involves the proximal limbs and buttocks, while the cavernous variant occurs in the head and neck area, inguinal region, and trunk (choice C). Cystic lymphangiomas are usually well-circumscribed, while cavernous lymphangiomas are commonly infiltrative (choices A, B).
QCSP, **Lymphangioma,** p 670.

67.   D.   **RADIATION TREATMENT**
Lymphangioma is a benign lesion and treated surgically. Mitotic activity and cellular atypia are never associated with lymphangioma; thus, they are not harbingers of malignant transformation (choices A, B). Cavernous lymphangioma may present with infiltrative growth, but does not predispose toward malignant transformation (choice C). There is no association with patient age and malignant transformation (choice E). Radiation treatment, however, has been shown to predispose toward the formation of angio- and lymphangiosarcoma (choice D).
QCSP, **Lymphangioma,** p 670.

68.   C.   **DOWN SYNDROME**
All of the choices listed have been associated with cystic lymphangioma except for Down syndrome.
QCSP, **Lymphangioma,** p 671.

69.   A.   **VISCERAL FORM**
The visceral form typically has a considerably worse prognosis compared to the skeletal form due to the presence of widespread disease, which is not amenable to resection in most patients (choice A). The skeletal (somatic) form of lymphangiomatosis is more common in young children and confers a better prognosis, since such lesions tend to stabilize over time (choice B).
QCSP, **Lymphangiomatosis**, p 671.

70.   D.   **LYMPHATIC CHANNELS CONTAINING THICK, CONCENTRIC SMOOTH MUSCLE**
Lymphangiomatosis exhibits infiltrative growth, typically isolating islands of normal tissue (choice B). The stroma contains hemosiderin and scattered lymphoid aggregates (choices A, E). The channels themselves are lined by attenuated endothelium and demonstrate variably thick vessel walls with disorganized smooth muscle (choice C). The smooth muscle within the vessel wall does not exhibit organized concentric growth (choice D).
QCSP, **Lymphangiomatosis**, p 671.

71.   D.   **35-YEAR-OLD FEMALE WITH SHORTNESS OF BREATH**
Lymphangiomyomatosis occurs in women of childbearing age and typically presents as shortness of breath, abdominal pain, or ascites due to a predilection for the lungs, thoracic duct, and mediastinal/retroperitoneal lymph nodes (choice D). It is not a cutaneous disease and does not occur in infants or men (choices A, B, C, E).
QCSP, **Lymphangiomyoma**, p 671-672.

72.   C.   **HMB-45**
Lymphangiomyomatosis is a member of the perivascular epithelioid tumor family that coexpresses muscle and melanocytic markers. This family includes angiomyolipoma as well as clear cell tumors of multiple organs, such as lung, pancreas, and uterus. While the lesion expresses smooth muscle actin and desmin much like other typical smooth muscle tumors, the presence of staining for HMB-45 is helpful in making the diagnosis (choices A, B, C). Cytokeratin and EMA staining is typically negative (choices D, E).
QCSP, **Lymphangiomyoma**, p 672.

73.   A.   **CD31**
CD31 is more specific for angio- and lymphangiosarcoma, while CD34 is typically more sensitive.
QCSP, **Lymphangiosarcoma**, p 673.

74.   C.   **ORGANIZED CIRCUMFERENTIAL LAYERING OF OUTER SMOOTH MUSCLE**
Angiomyoma, also known as vascular leiomyoma, arises from the outer wall of medium-sized vessels (choice D). This well-circumscribed tumor blends in with the outer wall of the vessel, imparting a disorganized appearance to the layering of smooth muscle (choices A, C). In contrast, the inner wall typically retains its organized circumferential layering of smooth muscle (choice B). The lesion may be associated with myxoid change, hyalinization, and calcification (choice E).
QCSP, **Leiomyoma**, p 674.

75.   A.   **A UTERINE MASS IN WOMEN OF REPRODUCTIVE AGE**
Intravenous leiomyomatosis typically presents as a myometrial mass which may involve the uterine and/or pelvic veins in middle-aged women (choice A). Lymphangiomyomatosis has a predilection for the lungs and typically present as shortness of breath in women of reproductive age (choice C).
QCSP, **Leiomyoma**, p 674.

20: Soft Tissue Answers

76. **A. TRUE**

Leiomyosarcoma exhibits a female predominance, especially in locations such as the retroperitoneum. However, leiomyosarcoma arising within the soft tissue of the lower extremities preferentially occurs in men (choice A).

QCSP, **Leiomyosarcoma,** p 675.

77. **D. MESENTERY**

The most common locations of epithelioid leiomyosarcoma are the mesentery and the omentum (choice D).

QCSP, **Leiomyosarcoma,** p 675.

78. **B. IT TENDS TO BE MULTIFOCAL.**

Cutaneous leiomyosarcoma occurs predominantly in men in their 5th to 7th decades (choices A, E). There is a predilection for the extensor surfaces of the extremities and a marked association with pain (choices C, D). The lesion is typically solitary and exhibits ill-defined borders akin to those seen in retroperitoneal leiomyosarcomas (choice B).

QCSP, **Leiomyosarcoma,** p 675-676.

79. **D. ILL-DEFINED BORDERS**

Cardiac rhabdomyoma is a multifocal hamartomatous process involving the ventricular myocardium and septum (choices B, E). The lesion is typically well-demarcated from the adjacent normal cardiac tissue (choice D). Smaller tumors may exhibit spontaneous regression (choice C). There is an association with tuberous sclerosis (choice A).

QCSP, **Rhabdomyoma,** p 677-678.

80. **E. BENIGN TRITON TUMOR**

The correct term for a fetal rhabdomyoma that involves a peripheral nerve is "benign triton tumor" (choice A). The lesion does exhibit some features of skeletal muscle differentiation and should not be classified as a neurofibroma (choice A). In the absence of malignant cytologic features, these lesions are considered benign and do not warrant a diagnosis of rhabdomyosarcoma (choices B, C). "Askin tumor" is the term used to describe a primitive neuroectodermal tumor that involves the chest wall.

QCSP, **Rhabdomyoma,** p 677.

81. **C. RHABDOMYOSARCOMA**

The most common sarcoma of children and adolescents is rhabdomyosarcoma (choice C). Leiomyosarcoma and liposarcoma are tumors of the middle-aged to elderly (choices A, B). Clear cell tumor is an uncommon sarcoma involving young adults, although children are occasionally affected as well (choice D). Synovial sarcoma may occur in children, but is not nearly as common as rhabdomyosarcoma (choice E).

QCSP, **Rhabdomyosarcoma,** p 678.

82. **C. EMBRYONAL RHABDOMYOSARCOMA, SPINDLE CELL TYPE**

The spindle cell variant of embryonal rhabdomyosarcoma is uncommon, representing approximately 5% of all embryonal rhabdomyosarcoma. The most common location is paratesticular, although the head and neck area may be involved as in other variants of embryonal rhabdomyosarcoma. While the botryoid variant of embryonal rhabdomyosarcoma does exhibit a prognostic advantage over the other choices presented, the spindle cell variant has the best prognosis overall (choice C).

QCSP, **Rhabdomyosarcoma,** p 679.

83. D. **NEOPLASTIC POPULATION COMPOSED OF SCATTERED SPINDLED RHABDOMYOBLASTS WITH ABUNDANT CROSS-STRIATIONS**
The botryoid variant, as mentioned in the last answer, has a prognostic advantage over most other types of rhabdomyosarcoma. Its presentation is classic, often described as a "grape-like" mass arising within the urinary bladder, vagina, or other hollow organs lined by mucosal surfaces (choice A). The characteristic histologic findings include a hyperplastic epithelium overlying a loose, myxoid stroma with scattered spindled rhabdomyoblasts (choices C, E). Cross-striations are only rarely identified (choice D). The most striking finding, however, is that of a densely cellular subepithelial layer of small rhabdomyoblasts, also known as the cambium layer (choice B).
QCSP, **Rhabdomyosarcoma,** p 679,

84. D. **MYOGENIN**
Of the stains listed, myogenin is most specific for skeletal muscle differentiation and rhabdomyosarcoma (choice D). Staining for vimentin is useful in evaluating whether the specimen obtained is "stainable," as most tissues do express vimentin strongly (choice C). Desmin and muscle specific actin are also present in smooth muscle and do not provide unambiguous support for skeletal muscle differentiation (choices A, B). PAS without diastase is widely positive in all tissues containing abundant amounts of glycogen, which includes but is certainly not limited to rhabdomyosarcoma (choice E).
QCSP, **Rhabdomyosarcoma,** p 680.

85. D. **CHEST WALL**
The most common location of extraskeletal Ewing sarcoma is the chest wall/paravertebral region (choice D). The extremities may be the primary site in occasional cases as well (choice E). The head and neck area and the gonads are not common locations for this lesion (choices A, B, C).
QCSP, **Extraskeletal Ewing Sarcoma,** p 682.

86. E. **MONOTONOUS POPULATION OF ROUND BLUE CELLS**
Extraskeletal Ewing sarcoma, as well as Ewing sarcoma in other locations, is characterized by sheets of monotonous round blue cells with minimal cytoplasm with extensive hemorrhage and necrosis (choice E). Prominent nucleoli and mitotic activity are not characteristic features of this lesion (choices A, B). The vasculature is typically inconspicuous and delicate, while the stroma exhibits no appreciable collagen (choices C, D).
QCSP, **Extraskeletal Ewing Sarcoma,** p 682.

87. A. **TUMOR SIZE; D. PRESENCE OF NECROSIS**
Large tumor size and the presence of extensive necrosis portend an unfavorable prognosis (choices A, D). The location, degree of mitotic activity, and presence of molecular aberrations do not appear to modify the prognosis (choices B, C, E).
QCSP, **Extraskeletal Ewing Sarcoma,** p 683.

88. D. **ON GROSS EXAMINATION, THE LESION EXHIBITS DIFFUSELY INFILTRATIVE GROWTH.**
Malignant peripheral nerve sheath tumor occurs most commonly in association with neurofibromatosis. Approximately 1/2 of cases are associated with the syndrome (choice A). It typically present as a painful, rapidly enlarging mass in the trunk, extremities, or head and neck, although sensory and motor deficits may also be present (choices B, E). The majority of cases arise from major nerve trunks, such as the brachial and sacral plexi (choice C). While the lesion is clearly infiltrative by microscopic examination, the gross appearance may be deceptively circumscribed (choice D).
QCSP, **Malignant Peripheral Nerve Sheath Tumor,** p 684-685.

89. E. **GANGLION-LIKE CELLS**
This is a difficult question to answer, as malignant peripheral nerve sheath tumors exhibit a wide spectrum of microscopic features. In typical foci of this lesion, there are sharply demarcated hyper- and hypocellular areas populated with cells with hyperchromatic, wavy nuclei (choices A, C). Palisading necrosis is a common feature (choice B). Multinucleated, pleomorphic cells may also be seen (choice D). Ganglion-like cells are not typically a feature of this tumor (choice E). Most importantly, however, malignant peripheral nerve sheath tumors frequently exhibit diffuse heterologous differentiation, mimicking carcinoma, melanoma, or any other sarcoma. The diagnosis may be impossible to render without the presence of adjacent neural tissue.
QCSP, **Malignant Peripheral Nerve Sheath Tumor,** p 685.

90. D. **FOCALLY AND WEAKLY PRESENT IN SOME CASES**
Approximately 1/2 of cases of malignant peripheral nerve sheath tumors exhibit some degree of staining for S100; however, diffuse staining is the exception (choices A, B, C). When present, S100 staining affects only a small number of cells and is typically weak (choice D).
QCSP, **Malignant Peripheral Nerve Sheath Tumor,** p 685.

91. B. **SPINE**
Melanotic neuroectodermal tumor of infancy typically arises from the pigmented epithelium of the neural crest. The most common locations of this tumor are the jaw, brain, anterior fontanelle, mediastinum, and epididymis (choices A, C, D, E). The spine does not usually give rise to this lesion (choice B).
QCSP, **Melanotic Neuroectodermal Tumor of Infancy,** p 686.

92. C. **IMMUNOHISTOCHEMICAL STAINING FOR CYTOKERATIN IS NEGATIVE.**
Melanotic neuroectodermal tumor of infancy occurs in infants under 1 year of age and arises from the pigmented epithelium of the neural crest. The microscopic features are characterized by irregular cystic spaces lined by primitive, pigmented cuboidal cells (choice E). Within these spaces, there is a population of primitive, nonpigmented cells, which strongly resemble the ones seen in neuroblastoma (choice D). The lining cells typically stain with cytokeratin (choice C). The lesion may be associated with elevated levels of vanillylmandelic acid (choice A). Although it is considered benign, approximately 1/2 of cases recur and metastasis has been reported (choice B).
QCSP, **Melanotic Neuroectodermal Tumor of Infancy,** p 686.

93. D. **DISTINCT NUCLEAR PALISADING**
Melanotic schwannoma is associated with Carney syndrome approximately 50% of the time. Microscopic features include a mixed population composed of spindled and epithelioid cells which frequently contain clear intranuclear pseudoinclusions (choices B, E). Dense deposits of granular pigment are a hallmark of this lesion and psammoma bodies are commonly seen (choices A, C). Nuclear palisading characteristic of classic schwannoma, however, is not common (choice D).
QCSP, **Melanotic Schwannoma,** p 687.

94. D. **UNCOMMON, BUT INDICATES MALIGNANCY**
Because of its tendency to recur, melanotic schwannoma is thought to be a low-grade lesion. Significant mitotic activity occurs in 10% of cases associated with Carney syndrome and is considered a sign of frank malignancy (choice D).
QCSP, **Melanotic Schwannoma,** p 687.

20: Soft Tissue Answers

95. **E. GASTROINTESTINAL STROMAL TUMOR**
     Carney syndrome is characterized by an autosomal dominant mutation of PRKAR1A located on chromosome 17 in the majority of cases, although a subtype that involves chromosome 2 has been described. Lesions associated with this syndrome include cardiac, skin, and breast myxomas, lentiginosis, blue nevi, bilateral pigmented nodular adrenal disease (frequently associated with Cushing syndrome), large-cell calcifying Sertoli cell tumors, steroid-type tumors, pituitary adenomas of growth hormone-type, and melanotic schwannomas (choices A, B, C, D). There is a separate entity known as Carney's triad, which consists of gastrointestinal stromal tumor, extraadrenal paraganglioma, and pulmonary chondroma and is completely unrelated to Carney syndrome (choice E).
     QCSP, **Melanotic Schwannoma,** p 687.

96. **D. PLEXIFORM NEUROFIBROMA; E. MASSIVE SOFT TISSUE NEUROFIBROMA**
     The plexiform and massive soft tissue variants of neurofibroma occur almost exclusively in patients with neurofibroma (choices D, E). Only occasional cases of localized cutaneous, localized intraneural, and diffuse cutaneous neurofibroma are associated with the syndrome (choices A, B, C).
     QCSP, **Neurofibroma,** p 689.

97. **D. PLEXIFORM NEUROFIBROMA**
     In addition to its characteristic gross appearance resembling a "bag of worms," plexiform neurofibroma microscopically exhibits a particular prominent mucoid matrix not typically seen in the other variants (choice D).
     QCSP, **Neurofibroma,** p 689.

98. **C. MENINGIOMA**
     Neurofibromatosis, type I, is diagnosed based on the presence of 2 or more of the following findings: >6 café-au-lait macules, >2 neurofibromas, 1 plexiform neurofibroma, axillary or inguinal freckles, optic glioma, >2 pigmented iris hamartomas (Lisch nodules), and 1st-degree relative with NF-1 (choices A, B, D, E). Meningioma may be a feature of neurofibromatosis, type II (choice C).
     QCSP, **Neurofibromatosis,** p 690-691.

99. **A. BILATERAL ACOUSTIC SCHWANNOMA**
     The diagnosis of neurofibromatosis, type II, is frequently more difficult than that of neurofibromatosis, type I. The only criterion that is sufficient in isolation for the diagnosis is the presence of bilateral acoustic schwannomas (choice A). The other choices presented must be accompanied by at least 1 other finding as well as a unilateral acoustic schwannoma (choices B, C, D, E).
     QCSP, **Neurofibromatosis,** p 691.

100. **B. THEY ARE POSITIVE FOR S100.**
     True Pacinian corpuscles, while positive for EMA, should not exhibit staining for S100. The tactoid structures seen in plexiform neurofibroma demonstrate a peripheral rim of EMA staining but are also positive for S100 (choice B).
     QCSP, **Neurofibromatosis,** p 692.

101. **D. CHROMOSOME 17Q11.2: NEUROFIBROMIN: NF-1**
     Neurofibromatosis, type I, is due to a mutation on chromosome 17q11.2, which encodes for neurofibromin (choice D), while neurofibromatosis, type II, involves a mutation on chromosome 22q12, which encodes for merlin.
     QCSP, **Neurofibromatosis,** p 692.

20: Soft Tissue Answers

102. **C. MEN IIB**
Mucosal neuromas are associated with MEN IIB, which also includes C cell hyperplasia, medullary carcinoma, pheochromocytoma, ganglioneuroma, and Marfanoid habitus (choice C). MEN I consists of parathyroid hyperplasia, pituitary adenoma, pancreatic endocrine tumor, and adrenocortical tumor (choice A). MEN IIA consists of medullary carcinoma, pheochromocytoma, and parathyroid hyperplasia (choice B). Gorlin syndrome, also known as nevoid basal cell carcinoma syndrome, is characterized by epidermoid cyst, pits involving the palms and soles, odontogenic keratocyst, ovarian fibroma, and basal cell carcinoma (choice D). Cowden syndrome includes hemangioma, nodular goiter, and lichenoid, papular, and papillomatous lesions of skin and mucosa (choice E).
QCSP, **Neuroma,** p 693.

103. **A. LOCALIZED INTERDIGITAL NEURITIS**
The term "Morton neuroma" is occasionally used synonymously with many different variants of neuroma; however, it typically describes localized interdigital neuritis, most commonly affecting the plantar nerve between the 3rd and 4th toes (choice A).
QCSP, **Neuroma,** p 693.

104. **B. HEAD AND NECK AREA**
The vast majority of cases of neurotropic-desmoplastic melanoma involve the head and neck area (choice B).
QCSP, **Neurotropic-Desmoplastic Melanoma,** p 696.

105. **D. LENTIGO MALIGNA MELANOMA**
Although lentigo maligna melanoma is the most common precursor lesion of neurotropic-desmoplastic melanoma, the superficial spreading and acral lentiginous variants have also been known to give rise to this lesion (choices A, B, D).
QCSP, **Neurotropic-Desmoplastic Melanoma,** p 696.

106. **A. IT ARISES FROM A PRECURSOR LESION THAT IS TYPICALLY AMELANOTIC.**
Neurotropic-desmoplastic melanoma itself does not contain pigment, although it typically arises from pigmented precursor lesions (choices A, B). As the name implies, this lesion exhibits a marked predilection for nerves with frequent involvement of the endo- and perineurium of nerves. Single cell infiltration is common (choice C). Like other variants of melanoma, this lesion is typically positive for S100; however, in contrast to its epithelioid counterparts, HMB-45 staining is negative (choices D, E).
QCSP, **Neurotropic-Desmoplastic Melanoma,** p 696.

107. **C. MUSCLE WEAKNESS**
The most common presentation of intraneural perineurioma is muscle weakness (choice C). Less common symptoms include sensory deficits and pain (choices A, D). Muscle spasticity is not a feature of this lesion (choice B). The lesion is best detected on imaging and not usually palpable (choice E).
QCSP, **Perineurioma,** p 696.

108. **B. IT IS A FEATURE OF EXTRANEURAL PERINEURIOMA.**
The "onion bulbs" of perineurioma are strictly seen in the intraneural variant (choices A, B) and are composed of concentric layers of perineural cells surrounding a central axon and Schwann cell (choices C, D). The layers merge with those of adjacent onion bulbs, creating a fusiform expansion of the affected nerve, which can be seen grossly (choice E).
QCSP, **Perineurioma,** p 696-697.

20: Soft Tissue Answers

109. **A.** **T(11;22)(Q24;Q12)**

The correct answer is A. The remaining choices listed represent the translocations seen in desmoplastic small round cell tumor (choice B), synovial sarcoma (choice C), clear cell sarcoma (choice D), and alveolar rhabdomyosarcoma (choice E).

QCSP, **Primitive Neuroectodermal Tumor,** p 698.

110. **A.** **PRESENCE OF NECROSIS; C. TUMOR SIZE**

The most important prognostic indicators in primitive neuroectodermal tumor are tumor size and the presence of necrosis (choices A, C). The remaining choices presented do not affect the prognosis (choices B, D, E).

QCSP, **Primitive Neuroectodermal Tumor,** p 698.

111. **D.** **GFAP**

Primitive neuroectodermal tumor typically expresses CD99 and variably expresses S100, cytokeratin, and CD57 (choices B, C, E). GFAP, however, is negative (choice D).

QCSP, **Primitive Neuroectodermal Tumor,** p 698.

112. **B.** **CARNEY SYNDROME**

The presence of psammoma bodies and abundant melanin pigment in a schwannoma is suggestive of a psammomatous melanotic schwannoma. 1/2 of these cases are associated with Carney syndrome (myxomas, lentiginous nevi, endocrine tumors) (choice B). Carney triad consists of gastrointestinal stromal tumor, pulmonary chondroma, and extra-adrenal paraganglioma (choice C). Malignancy and ancient change are not characterized by the finding of psammoma bodies or melanin pigment (choices A, D). Peutz-Jeghers syndrome is associated with hamartomatous polyps and hyperpigmented oropharyngeal macules (choice E).

QCSP, **Schwannoma,** p 700.

113. **B.** **LOCAL EXCISION**

Schwannoma is a benign tumor that occasionally recurs. Local excision is typically adequate (choice B).

QCSP, **Schwannoma,** p 700.

114. **A.** **CD34**

All of the stains listed may be positive in angiomatoid fibrous histiocytoma except for CD34 (choice A). The absence of staining with CD34 supports the lack of true vascular differentiation in this lesion.

QCSP, **Angiomatoid Fibrous Histiocytoma,** p 702.

115. **D.** **PRIMITIVE NEUROECTODERMAL TUMOR**

Epithelioid sarcoma exhibits characteristic microscopic features that lead to several differential diagnoses. Because of the central necrosis seen in this lesion in association with epithelioid and spindled cells, there is an architectural and cytologic resemblance to granulomatous inflammation and epithelioid hemangioendothelioma (choices A, B). The epithelioid zones of biphasic synovial sarcoma and epithelioid variants of malignant peripheral nerve sheath tumor may also pose diagnostic difficulties (choices C, E). Primitive neuroectodermal tumor, on the other hand, is composed of monotonous small blue cells with little cytoplasm and single cell necrosis, which do not resemble the neoplastic population seen in epithelioid sarcoma (choice D).

QCSP, **Epithelioid Sarcoma,** p 704.

116. **E.** **ALL OF THE ABOVE**

Epithelioid sarcoma is characterized by frequent recurrence and metastasis. Negative prognostic factors include large tumor size, proximal tumor location, male sex, and advanced age at diagnosis (choice E).

QCSP, **Epithelioid Sarcoma,** p 704.

20: Soft Tissue Answers

117. C. **THE CUT SURFACE EXHIBITS A SOLID, WELL-DEMARCATED, WHITE CUT SURFACE.**
Giant cell angiofibroma is a lesion that involves the eyelids of middle-aged adults (choice A). There is a male predominance (choice B). On gross examination, the lesion exhibits a hemorrhagic, cystic cut surface (choice C). Microscopic examination demonstrates bland spindle cells embedded in a collagenous or myxoid stroma with variable multinucleated giant cells lining vascular spaces. The spindle cells as well as the multinucleated giant cells express CD34 and CD99 (choice E). Local excision is curative (choice D).
QCSP, **Giant Cell Angiofibroma**, p 705-706.

118. D. **PROMINENT MYXOID MATRIX**
Hemangiopericytoma exhibits a proliferation of uniform peri- and intervascular cells with angulated nuclei that resemble endothelial cells admixed with spindle cells arranged in focal storiform growth (choices B, E). The lesion is typically surrounded by large, collapsed vessels with a staghorn appearance (choice A). Occasionally, there may be a significant component of mature adipose tissue, known as lipomatous hemangiopericytoma (choice C). Myxoid or hyalinized stroma is not a feature of this lesion (choice D).
QCSP, **Hemangiopericytoma**, p 706.

119. A. **CD31**
Hemangiopericytoma resembles solitary fibrous tumor immunohistochemically in that CD34 and CD99 are frequently positive (choices B, C). Factor XIIIa and vimentin are usually positive (choices D, E). Unlike normal endothelial cells, hemangiopericytoma does not stain for CD31 (choice A).
QCSP, **Hemangiopericytoma**, p 706.

120. E. **ALL OF THE ABOVE**
Malignant hemangiopericytoma is characterized by overtly malignant cytologic features, such as abnormal mitotic figures, tumor cell necrosis, and brisk mitotic activity (choices B, C, D). A tumor size of >5 cm is also suggestive of malignancy (choice A).
QCSP, **Hemangiopericytoma**, p 706.

121. D. **INTRADERMAL LOCATION**
Malignant extrarenal rhabdoid tumor is a neoplasm of childhood and typically presents as a unifocal, rapidly growing deep soft tissue mass (choices A, B, C, D). It is usually accompanied by pain (choice E).
QCSP, **Malignant Extrarenal Rhabdoid Tumor**, p 707.

122. C. **MULTIPLE SMALL INCONSPICUOUS NUCLEOLI**
Malignant extrarenal rhabdoid tumor is microscopically characterized by sheets of discohesive polygonal cells with eccentric round nuclei (choices A, D). There is typically a single prominent eosinophilic nucleolus (choice C). The dense eosinophilic inclusions present in the cytoplasm impart a rhabdoid appearance (choice B). Necrosis is frequently present (choice E).
QCSP, **Malignant Extrarenal Rhabdoid Tumor**, p 707-708.

123. B. **DESMIN**
Like rhabdoid tumors in other locations, malignant extrarenal rhabdoid tumor expresses vimentin, keratin, and EMA (choices A, C, D). CD99 is also positive (choice E). Since there is no true muscle differentiation, desmin is negative (choice B).
QCSP, **Malignant Extrarenal Rhabdoid Tumor**, p 708.

124.   C.   **Is discouraged in favor of itemizing differing lines of differentiation**
Malignant mesenchymoma refers to sarcomas with >2 lines of differentiation (choice A). Since there is marked variability in prognosis and treatment depending on the specific components of this lesion, this term is discouraged in favor of identifying and quantifying the individual lines making up the tumor (choice C). Malignant mesenchymoma in and of itself does not necessarily imply a worse prognosis (choice D) and is not a term restricted to metastatic sarcomas (choices D, E).
QCSP, **Malignant Mesenchymoma**, p 708,

125.   C.   **Knee**
Approximately 90% of cases of juxta-articular myxoma occur in association with the knee (choice C).
QCSP, **Myxoma**, p 709.

126.   B.   **Juxta-articular**
The intramuscular variant of myxoma is associated with Albright syndrome (fibrous dysplasia of bone, melanotic skin pigmentation, gastrointestinal polyps, osteomalacia, precocious puberty) and Mazabraud syndrome (skeletal fibrous dysplasia) (choice A). The cutaneous variant of myxoma is associated with Carney syndrome (lentiginosis, endocrine tumors, large-cell calcifying Sertoli cell tumor, psammomatous melanotic schwannoma) (choice C). There is no syndrome associated with juxta-articular myxoma (choice B).
QCSP, **Myxoma**, p 710.

127.   C.   **Extremities**
Ossifying fibromyxoid tumor typically involves the extremities, although it also occurs in the trunk, head and neck area, and mediastinum (choices A, B, C, E).
QCSP, **Ossifying Fibromyxoid Tumor**, p 710.

128.   E.   **Thrombotic vasculature**
Features suggestive of malignancy in ossifying fibromyxoid tumor include hypercellularity accompanied by brisk mitotic activity (choices A, B), as well as central ossification in association with large polygonal cells (choice D). Malignant lesions are frequently associated with an incomplete bony or fibrous capsule (choice C). The thrombotic vasculature of ossifying fibromyxoid tumor is also seen in benign tumors and is not a feature of malignancy (choice E).
QCSP, **Ossifying Fibromyxoid Tumor**, p 710-711.

129.   E.   **None of the above**
There is no recurrent molecular alteration associated with ossifying fibromyxoid tumor (choice E). The remaining choices presented represent alterations seen in well-differentiated liposarcoma (choice A), extraskeletal myxoid chondrosarcoma (choice B), deep fibromatosis (choice C), and infantile fibrosarcoma/congenital mesoblastic nephroma (choice D).
QCSP, **Ossifying Fibromyxoid Tumor**, p 711.

130.   E.   **Lower extremity**
The most common location of synovial sarcoma is the lower extremity, with 80% of cases involving the knee or the ankle (choice E). Despite its name, this lesion does not necessarily involve synovium and can occur in many different locations, including the remaining choices listed.
QCSP, **Synovial Sarcoma**, p 711.

20: Soft Tissue Answers

131. **B. CD34**

Synovial sarcoma typically expresses epithelial markers such as EMA and cytokeratin, although staining in monophasic variants may only be focal (choices A, D). The vast majority of cases also strongly express bcl-2 (choice E). CD99 staining is also present is many cases (choice C). CD34, however, is negative (choice B).
QCSP, **Synovial Sarcoma,** p 712.

132. **A. PRESENCE OF EXTENSIVE CALCIFICATIONS**

Favorable prognostic factors in synovial sarcoma include age <15 years, distal tumor location, low mitotic rate, minimal necrosis, lesions with >50% epithelioid morphology, and the presence of extensive calcifications (choices A, B, C, D). Negative prognostic factors include extensive necrosis, high mitotic rate, and the presence of rhabdoid cells (choice E).
QCSP, **Synovial Sarcoma,** p 712-713.

133. **C. ANGIOSARCOMA**

Long-standing lymphedema, frequently associated with mastectomy, has been associated with cutaneous angiosarcoma (choice C). This phenomenon is known as Stewart-Treves syndrome.
QCSP, **Angiosarcoma,** p 713.

134. **B. PSEUDOCAPSULE**

Angiosarcoma typically presents as an ill-defined lesion with diffusely infiltrative growth. A pseudocapsule is not a feature of this tumor (choice B). The lesion exhibits a spectrum of morphologic features ranging from those of a benign vascular lesion to those of an undifferentiated malignancy. The typical features include irregular, sinusoidal vascular channels lined by pleomorphic, atypical endothelial cells, some of which contain primitive vascular lumina (choices C, D, E). Necrosis is a variable feature (choice A).
QCSP, **Angiosarcoma,** p 713.

135. **C. HEMIDESMOSOMES**

The electron microscopy features of well-differentiated angiosarcoma resemble those of normal endothelium and include Weibel-Palade bodies, tight junctions, pinocytic vesicles, and prominent external basal lamina on the antiluminal border (choices A, B, D, E). Hemidesmosomes are seen in keratinocytes and are not a feature of endothelium (choice C).
QCSP, **Angiosarcoma,** p 714.

136. **D. SYMPLASTIC GLOMUS TUMOR**

The symplastic variant of glomus tumor exhibits prominent cytologic atypia, possibly as a result of degenerative changes (choice D). However, there are no concomitant findings of malignancy, such as necrosis or mitotic activity.
QCSP, **Glomus Tumor,** p 715.

137. **E. ALL OF THE ABOVE**

Glomangiosarcoma is clinically characterized by large tumor size, defined as >2 cm, and visceral or deep location (choices A, D). Microscopic features concerning for malignancy include brisk mitotic activity, atypical mitotic figures, cytologic atypia, and necrosis (choices B, C).
QCSP, **Glomus Tumor,** p 715.

20: Soft Tissue Answers

138. C. **It is characterized by vascular channels lined by markedly atypical cells with prominent nuclei that protrude into the lumina.**
Retiform hemangioendothelioma typically presents as a dermal mass involving the distal extremities (choice A). Microscopically, the lesion infiltrates the underlying subcutis (choice B). The lesion is typically composed of elongated vessels lined by bland cells with prominent nuclei that protrude into the lumina (choice C). Cytologic atypia and prominent mitotic activity are not features of this lesion (choice E). A lymphocytic infiltrate is commonly present (choice D).
QCSP, **Hemangioendothelioma,** p 716.

139. D. **It is negative for factor VIII-associated antigen.**
Malignant endovascular papillary angioendothelioma, also known as Dabska tumor, occurs predominantly in children (choices A, B). It presents as an indurated subcutaneous mass and is frequently associated with regional lymph node metastasis, although the overall prognosis is good (choice C). It is characterized by dilated vascular channels lined by papillary tufts of bland, hobnail endothelial cells, some of which contain intracytoplasmic lumina with erythrocytes. Immunohistochemical staining for factor VIII-associated antigen is typically positive (choice D). Electron microscopy features resemble those of benign endothelium and include Weibel-Palade bodies and pinocytic vesicles (choice E).
QCSP, **Hemangioendothelioma,** p 716-717.

140. B. **It is also known as Dabska tumor.**
Kaposiform hemangioendothelioma, like malignant papillary angioendothelioma, occurs predominantly in children, although young adults may be affected as well (choice A). It is the latter entity, however, that is known as Dabska tumor (choice B). Microscopic features of kaposiform hemangioendothelioma resemble those of capillary hemangioma and Kaposi sarcoma and include fascicles of bland spindle cells, hyaline globules, hemosiderin granules, and microthrombi (choice C). Unlike other variants of hemangioendothelioma, kaposiform hemangioendothelioma does not stain with factor VIII-associated antigen (choice D). Electron microscopy features resemble those of benign endothelium and include Weibel-Palade bodies and pinocytic vesicles (choice E).
QCSP, **Hemangioendothelioma,** p 716-717.

141. C. **Spindle cell hemangioma**
Maffucci syndrome (enchondromatosis and angiomas) is associated with spindle cell hemangioma (choice C). Other associations with this variant include Klippel-Trenaunay syndrome and congenital lymphedema.
QCSP, **Hemangioendothelioma,** p 717.

142. B. **Hemangioma**
The vast majority of tumors in infancy are hemangiomas (choice B).
QCSP, **Hemangioma,** p 718.

143. E. **Cavernous hemangioma: lower extremity of child**
Capillary, cavernous, synovial, and verrucous hemangiomas preferentially occur in childhood, while acquired tufted angioma, hobnail hemangioma, cherry angioma, arteriovenous hemangioma, venous hemangioma, intramuscular hemangioma and epithelioid hemangioma are more common in adults. The most common location of the capillary hemangioma is the head and neck, while the verrucous variant most commonly involves the lower extremity (choices A, B). Epithelioid hemangioma, also known as angiolymphoid hyperplasia with eosinophilia, preferentially involves the periauricular region (choice C). The intramuscular hemangioma occurs most commonly in the lower extremity (choice D). Cavernous hemangioma, however, usually involves the upper body and is capable of destructive local growth (choice E).
QCSP, **Hemangioma,** p 718-719.

20: Soft Tissue Answers

144. **D. PYOGENIC GRANULOMA**
Pyogenic granuloma, an unfortunate misnomer, is actually a type of capillary hemangioma resembling granulation tissue. While it can occur in patients of either sex during any age, it has a peculiar tendency to occur and recur during pregnancy, possibly due to hormonal influence (choice D).
QCSP, **Hemangioma,** p 719.

145. **C. IT IS ASSOCIATED WITH ANGIOSARCOMA.**
Angiomatosis typically affects infants and children and presents as a large, discolored area involving a limb or an organ (choice A). The treatment of choice is resection, although recurrence as high as 90% has been reported (choice B). The lesion may be fatal if vital structures become involved (choice E). It has been associated with Kasabach-Merritt syndrome in which vascular lesions result in thrombocytopenia, leading to a consumptive coagulopathy (choice D). An association with angiosarcoma, however, has not been described (choice C).
QCSP, **Hemangioma,** p 719.

146. **A. IT IS FREQUENTLY ASSOCIATED WITH AN UNDERLYING ANGIOSARCOMA.**
Papillary endothelial hyperplasia typically arises within a blood vessel in association with a vascular lesion, usually a benign hemangioma (choices A, C). It usually involves the superficial veins of the head and neck, although it may extend into the adjacent soft tissue (choices B, D). It is characterized by bland anastomosing vascular channels and fibrous or hyalinized papillae lined by bland, hyperchromatic, but benign endothelial cells (choice E). While it may histologically mimic angiosarcoma, there is no association between the 2 entities.
QCSP, **Hemangioma,** p 719.

147. **A. THE TYPICAL PATIENT IS HIV-INFECTED.**
Classic Kaposi sarcoma occurs predominantly in elderly Mediterranean men and is not associated with HIV (choice A). Lesions typically present as blue or red nodules involving the lower extremities, which eventually coalesce into plaques and ulcerate, although spontaneous regression has been reported (choices B, C, D). 1/3 of patients with chronic Kaposi sarcoma develop additional malignancies, most commonly hematopoietic (choice E).
QCSP, **Kaposi Sarcoma,** p 721-722.

148. **B. IN CHILDREN, THE INTERNAL ORGANS ARE COMMONLY INVOLVED.**
Lymphadenopathic Kaposi sarcoma occurs in African children and adults with differing clinical presentation. Adults typically present with lymphadenopathy and cutaneous lesions involving the lower extremities, while children commonly exhibit internal organ involvement (choice B). This lesion is not associated with HIV infection or transplantation (choices A, D). Lesions typically do not regress spontaneously, particularly when internal organ involvement is present (choice C). Like other variants of Kaposi sarcoma, immunohistochemical staining for HHV8 is positive (choice E).
QCSP, **Kaposi Sarcoma,** p 721-722.

149. **E. PROMINENT NUCLEAR ATYPIA**
Kaposi sarcoma is characterized by irregular anastomosing slit-like vascular channels lined by bland endothelium surrounded by fascicles of bland eosinophilic spindle cells, which become more prominent with the nodular stage of the disease (choices A, D). PAS-positive diastase-resistant intra- and extracellular hyaline globules are present, as well as stromal plasma cells and lymphocytes (choices B, C). While the endothelial lining of the vessels may be plump, nuclear atypia is not common and may be suggestive of angiosarcoma (choice E).
QCSP, **Kaposi Sarcoma,** p 722.

20: Soft Tissue Answers

150.   C.   **IT TYPICALLY PRESENTS AS A RAPIDLY ENLARGING LESION.**
Myopericytoma is an indolent lesion that may persist for years prior to presentation (choice C). It typically presents as a solitary mass in the distal extremities of adults (choices B, D, E). Males and females are equally affected (choice A).
QCSP, **Myopericytoma**, p 723.

151.   A AND E.   **S100; CYTOKERATIN**
Myopericytoma is positive for smooth muscle actin (choice D). It may also exhibit some staining for CD34 and desmin (choices B, C). S100 and cytokeratin are typically negative (choices A, E).
QCSP, **Myopericytoma**, p 723.

152.   A.   **PREFERENTIAL LOCALIZATION TO THE HEAD AND NECK AREA**
The lesion depicted in this image is an extraskeletal myxoid chondrosarcoma. Note the strands of hyperchromatic chondrocytes with minimal eosinophilic cytoplasm floating in a myxoid matrix. This variant is characterized by a slowly growing nodular mass frequently exhibiting a hemorrhagic and gelatinous cut surface (choices B, C, D). Unlike the mesenchymal variant of extraskeletal chondrosarcoma, which preferentially occurs in the head and neck area, the myxoid variant is more common in the extremities (choice A). There is a male predominance (choice E).
QCSP, **Extraskeletal Chondrosarcoma**, p 637.

153.   C.   **HIGH-DOSE ALKYLATING AGENTS**
The image is that of an extraskeletal osteosarcoma with prominent lacy osteoid matrix associated with large, atypical osteoblasts. Known associations of extraskeletal osteosarcoma include radiation therapy, administration of radioactive thorium dioxide, and trauma (choices A, B, D). An association with chemotherapeutics has not been described (choice C). Extraskeletal osteosarcoma occurs predominantly in older individuals and is rare in patients under the age of 40 years (choice E).
QCSP, **Extraskeletal Osteosarcoma**, p 638.

154.   A.   **HEAD AND NECK AREA**
The image shown demonstrates a highly atypical spindle cell lesion with several bizarre cells and mitotic figures consistent with atypical fibroxanthoma. Atypical fibroxanthoma typically occurs in older individuals on the sun-exposed areas of the head and neck area, including the nose, cheeks, and ears (choice A). While the lesion also occurs on the trunk and extremities, these are less common locations (choices B, C, D). The retroperitoneum does not give rise to atypical fibroxanthoma (choice E).
QCSP, **Atypical Fibroxanthoma**, p 640.

155.   D.   **NECROSIS**
Atypical fibroxanthoma, also known as superficial malignant fibrous histiocytoma, is microscopically characterized by a pleomorphic cell population with abundant mitotic activity centered in the dermis (choices A, B, E). The surrounding tissue frequently exhibits sun damage (choice C). Necrosis is only rarely seen (choice D).
QCSP, **Atypical Fibroxanthoma**, p 641.

156.   E.   **PRESENTATION IN THE 6TH DECADE**
Dermatofibrosarcoma protuberans typically presents as a firm nodule with a rim of discoloration located on the trunk and proximal extremities (choices B, C). On average, tumors measure >3 cm on presentation (choice D). There is a male predominance with peak presentation in the 2nd to 4th decades (choices A, E).
QCSP, **Dermatofibrosarcoma Protuberans**, p 641.

157. **E.** **MITOTIC FIGURES**

The image shown is an example of fibrous histiocytoma. Fibrous histiocytoma is a benign lesion composed of a bland fibroblastic proliferation accompanied by Touton giant cells, xanthoma cells, and lymphocytes (choices A, D). The background may exhibit extensive stromal hyalinization or hemorrhagic change (choices B, C). Frequent mitotic figures and cellular pleomorphism are not characteristic and should raise concern for a malignant process (choice E).

QCSP, **Fibrous Histiocytoma,** p 643.

158. **D.** **IT IS ASSOCIATED WITH UNDERLYING LIPID ABNORMALITIES.**

This image is an example of juvenile xanthogranuloma. Note the giant Touton cells and foamy histiocytes. Juvenile xanthogranuloma typically presents in infancy and may be present at birth (choice A). Such lesions frequently regress, unlike the ones presenting in older patients (choice C). The majority of lesions involve the head and neck area, although juvenile xanthogranuloma also occurs in deep soft tissue and internal organs (choices B, E). It is not associated with underlying lipid abnormalities (choice D); however, there is an increased incidence in patients with neurofibromatosis and urticaria pigmentosa.

QCSP, **Juvenile Xanthogranuloma,** p 645.

159. **E.** **NEUTROPHILIC INFILTRATE**

Juvenile xanthogranuloma is characterized by dermal sheets of histiocytes infiltrating the subcutis and adnexal structure with an overlying thinned epidermis and elongated rete ridges (choices A, B, D). Touton and Langerhans giant cells are typically present, along with an inflammatory infiltrate composed of lymphocytes, eosinophils, and plasma cells (choice C). Neutrophils are not a prominent feature of this lesion.

QCSP, **Juvenile Xanthogranuloma,** p 645.

160. **C.** **KNEE**

The most common location of tenosynovial giant cell tumor, diffuse type, is the knee in 80% of cases (choice C). In contrast, the localized type is common in the hand (choice E).

QCSP, **Tenosynovial Giant Cell Tumor, Diffuse Type,** p 648.

161. **E.** **RAPID GROWTH**

Elastofibroma is a lesion that classically arises superficial to the scapulae in older women (choice B). There is a higher incidence in the right scapular area, and tumors may occasionally be bilateral (choices A and D). There is frequently a history of repetitive manual labor involving the musculature of the back (choice C). The lesion typically enlarges slowly (choice E).

QCSP, **Elastofibroma,** p 652.

162. **A.** **HYPERCELLULARITY**

Aside from its infiltrative pattern of growth, fibromatosis microscopically exhibits few overtly malignant features (choice C). While scattered mitotic figures may be present, the lesion is not highly cellular, and the neoplastic population consists of bland, unremarkable fibroblasts (choices A, B, E). The vasculature is typically thin-walled (choice D).

QCSP, **Fibromatosis,** p 654.

163. **B.** **MOST CASES ARE LOCALIZED TO THE LUNGS.**

Inflammatory myofibroblastic tumor presents predominantly in the abdomen of infants and young children (choices A, B). The tumor may be associated with fever, night sweats, and weight loss as well as nonspecific laboratory findings, such as anemia, thrombocytosis, and hypergammaglobulinemia (choices C, D). While the lesion typically presents as a solitary mass, up to 1/3 of cases exhibit multiple masses (choice E).

QCSP, **Inflammatory Myofibroblastic Tumor,** p 658.

20: Soft Tissue Answers

164.   D.   **ATYPICAL MITOTIC FIGURES**

Inflammatory myofibroblastic tumors exhibit a spectrum of histologic patterns and may contain focal psammomatous calcifications, cellular atypia, and prominent nucleoli (choices A, B, C). Atypical mitotic figures should not be present (choice D). The stroma varies in appearance, ranging from myxoid to densely hyalinized (choice E).

QCSP, **Inflammatory Myofibroblastic Tumor,** p 658-659.

165.   E.   **ALL OF THE ABOVE**

All of the features listed are associated with more aggressive behavior in inflammatory myofibroblastic tumor (choice E).

QCSP, **Inflammatory Myofibroblastic Tumor,** p 659.

166.   C.   **WRIST**

Low-grade fibromyxoid sarcoma occurs predominantly in the proximal extremities or trunk (choices A, B). Less commonly, the lesion can be found in the head or retroperitoneum (choices D, E). The wrist is not a preferred location (choice C).

QCSP, **Low-Grade Fibromyxoid Sarcoma,** p 659.

167.   A.   **FASCICLES OF BLAND SPINDLE CELLS IN A BACKGROUND OF HYPOCELLULAR, COLLAGENIZED AREAS ADMIXED WITH MYXOID NODULES**

Low-grade fibromyxoid sarcoma is characterized histologically by foci of densely collagenized, hypocellular areas alternating with myxoid nodules. Fascicles of bland spindle cells comprise the neoplastic population (choice A). An inflammatory infiltrate is not common and raises the possibility of an inflammatory myofibroblastic tumor (choice B). Necrosis and sheets of pleomorphic cells suggest a high-grade process such as myxofibrosarcoma (choice C). The C-shaped bundles of fibroblasts in irregular stromal mucin pools describe nodular fasciitis (choice D), while infiltrative fascicles of spindle cells exhibiting pleomorphism and hyperchromatism are more characteristic of low-grade myofibroblastic sarcoma (choice E).

QCSP, **Low-Grade Fibromyxoid Sarcoma,** p 659.

168.   C.   **RADICAL EXCISION +/− ADJUVANT RADIATION**

Like many other sarcomas, low-grade fibromyxoid sarcoma requires radical excision as primary therapy and exhibits a negligible response to chemotherapy (choices B, E). Radiation therapy may be used for residual disease (choice C). Metastasis occurs hematogeneously; thus, lymph node dissections are not useful (choice D). Since the risk of local recurrence is not insignificant, local excision is typically insufficient (choice A).

QCSP, **Low-Grade Fibromyxoid Sarcoma,** p 660.

169.   B.   **HEAD AND NECK AREA**

While myofibroma can occur in all of the locations listed, the most common location for a solitary lesion is in the head and neck area (choice B). Kidney and liver involvement is more common in the presence of multicentric disease (choices D, E).

QCSP, **Myofibroma,** p 660.

170.   D.   **LESIONS GROW RAPIDLY AND MAY MEASURE UP TO 7 CM ON INITIAL PRESENTATION.**

Nodular fasciitis is a reactive process that occurs preferentially in the upper extremities and trunk and is occasionally associated with a history of trauma (choices C, E). It is only rarely encountered over the age of 60 years (choice A). Lesions present as rapidly growing masses measuring 2-3 cm on initial presentation and may be painful (choices B, D). Significantly larger lesions exhibiting such rapid growth are unusual and should raise concern for a sarcomatous process.

QCSP, **Nodular Fasciitis,** p 663.

20: Soft Tissue Answers

171. C. **FIBROBLASTIC NODULES LINED BY PLUMP MYOFIBROBLASTS**
Nodular fasciitis is characterized by an infiltrative growth of bland fibroblasts arranged in C-shaped bundles with admixed small thin-walled branching vessels (choices A, C). Extravasated red blood cells and thick, keloid-like collagen bands are frequently identified in the mucinous stroma (choices B, E). Fibroblastic nodules lined by plump myofibroblasts describe the microscopic appearance of myofibroma and are not a feature of nodular fasciitis (choice C).
QCSP, **Nodular Fasciitis,** p 663.

172. D. **PROLIFERATIVE FASCIITIS**
Proliferative fasciitis, unlike nodular fasciitis, occurs predominantly in the proximal extremities of older adults (choice D). The lesion is typically better defined than nodular fasciitis and exhibits characteristic large, eosinophilic ganglion-like cells within the stroma. Intravascular and cranial fasciitis are lesions of children and infants, respectively (choices A, B). Ossifying fasciitis involves the periosteum and exhibits ossification without the presence of ganglion-like cells (choice C).
QCSP, **Nodular Fasciitis,** p 663.

173. A. **25-YEAR-OLD MALE WITH A PAINLESS SHOULDER MASS**
Hibernomas are slowly growing tumors that typically arise in locations where brown fat cells are found in infants, such as the shoulders, mediastinum, and axilla. However, occasional cases do occur in the thigh. This tumor presents in young adults and is not usually accompanied by pain. Choice A best fits this description.
QCSP, **Hibernoma,** p 664.

174. C. **ABERRATION OF CHROMOSOME 11Q13**
Hibernoma has been associated with aberrations of chromosome 11q13 (choice C). Choices A, B, D, and E represent molecular alterations associated with myxoid liposarcoma, well-differentiated liposarcoma, lipoblastoma, and spindle/pleomorphic lipoma, respectively.
QCSP, **Hibernoma,** p 664.

175. B. **1-YEAR-OLD MALE INFANT WITH A LOWER EXTREMITY MASS**
Nearly all cases of lipoblastoma present in patients under the age of 3 years. The lesion demonstrates a significant male predominance and a predilection for the extremities. Choice B best fits this description.
QCSP, **Lipoblastoma,** p 665.

176. A. **SHEETS OF SMALL TUMOR CELLS WITH A HIGH NUCLEAR-CYTOPLASMIC RATIO; B. HIGH MITOTIC ACTIVITY; D. ABSENCE OF INTERVENING MYXOID STROMA**
Myxoid and round cell liposarcoma represent 2 ends of the same disease spectrum and exhibit the same molecular alteration, t(12;16)(q13;p11.2). Since the presence of a significant round cell component in an otherwise myxoid liposarcoma confers a worse prognosis, its identification is critical. Unfortunately, there is significant controversy over what constitutes a "significant" component, with 5% representing the lowest threshold. Round cell liposarcoma is characterized by sheets of small round tumor cells with high nuclear-cytoplasmic ratios, absence of intervening myxoid stroma, and significantly higher mitotic activity than is typically seen in myxoid liposarcoma (choices A, B). Lipoblasts and the classic "chicken-wire" vasculature seen in myxoid liposarcoma are much less distinct (choices C, E).
QCSP, **Liposarcoma,** p 668.

20: Soft Tissue Answers

177.   A.   **STEWART-TREVES SYNDROME**
The image is that of an angiosarcoma. Note the plethora of vascular channels lined by highly atypical endothelial cells, characteristic of this lesion. The eponym given to angiosarcoma arising in the breast or upper extremity following mastectomy with axillary dissection is Stewart-Treves syndrome (choice A). The prognosis is abysmal with the majority of patients succumbing to disease secondary to metastasis. While it is associated with chronic lymphedema, this tumor appears to arise from blood vessels and is thus better classified as an angiosarcoma. Gorlin syndrome is also known as nevoid basal cell carcinoma syndrome (choice B), while Denys-Drash syndrome refers to congenital nephropathy associated with Wilms tumor and intersex disorders (choice C). Mazabraud syndrome consists of polyostotic fibrous dysplasia in association with soft tissue myxomas (choice D). Bourneville disease is the eponym given to tuberous sclerosis (choice E).
QCSP, **Lymphangiosarcoma,** p 673.

178.   B.   **IT IS INHERITED IN AN AUTOSOMAL RECESSIVE FASHION.**
Cutaneous leiomyoma arises from a pilar erector muscle in young adults (choices A, C). Exposure to cold may result in pain, which can be treated by vasodilation with nitroglycerin (choice E). Unlike genital leiomyomas, cutaneous leiomyomas typically present as ill-defined lesions (choice D). An autosomal *dominant* inheritance pattern has been proposed (choice B).
QCSP, **Leiomyoma,** p 673-674.

179.   B.   **SPINDLE CELLS WITH WAVY NUCLEI**
The image shown is that of a leiomyosarcoma. Note the large atypical cells and easily identifiable mitotic figures. Although a more thorough count would have to be performed in the uterus, the mitotic activity in a soft tissue location is sufficient for a diagnosis of leiomyosarcoma. Leiomyosarcoma is characterized by a proliferation of spindle cells with blunt-ended nuclei arranged in a fascicular growth pattern (choices B, E). The neoplastic population exhibits prominent nuclear atypia and mitotic figures are usually easily identified (choices A, D). Necrosis may also be present (choice C). Spindle cells with wavy nuclei, while not completely specific, are suggestive of neural differentiation (choice B).
QCSP, **Leiomyosarcoma,** p 675.

180.   B.   **EMBRYONAL RHABDOMYOSARCOMA**
Adult rhabdomyoma exhibits lobules composed of large round cells with abundant eosinophilic cytoplasm, lipid, and glycogen. These features may be similar to those seen in granular cell tumor, paraganglioma, hibernoma, and oncocytoma (choices A, C, D, E). Embryonal rhabdomyosarcoma is typically composed of a primitive small blue rhabdomyoblasts exhibiting scant cytoplasm. Lobular growth is not a feature of embryonal rhabdomyosarcoma (choice B).
QCSP, **Rhabdomyoma,** p 678.

181.   D.   **ALVEOLAR RHABDOMYOSARCOMA**
The alveolar variant of rhabdomyosarcoma is clearly a distinct entity from the other types of rhabdomyosarcoma in that many cases contain the translocation t(2;13)(q35;q14) (choice D). The embryonal and pleomorphic types of rhabdomyosarcoma do not exhibit recurrent molecular alterations (choices A, B, C, E).
QCSP, **Rhabdomyosarcoma,** p 680.

182. **C.** **IT TYPICALLY PRESENTS AS A CUTANEOUS LESION INVOLVING THE HEAD AND NECK AREA.**
The image depicts clear cell sarcoma, characterized by nests of bland cells with clear cytoplasm and prominent nucleoli. Clear cell sarcoma, also known as malignant melanoma of soft parts, is a tumor of young adults and exhibits a female predominance (choices A, D). It typically presents as a deep-seated mass involving the tendons and aponeuroses of extremities (choice C). While the tumor is slow-growing, it exhibits relentless progression with 1/2 of cases exhibiting metastasis within 5 years, typically to the lungs and lymph nodes (choice E). Approximately 1/2 of cases are associated with trauma (choice B).
QCSP, **Clear Cell Sarcoma,** p 681-682.

183. **E.** **PROMINENT NUCLEAR PLEOMORPHISM WITH MULTIPLE INCONSPICUOUS NUCLEOLI**
Clear cell sarcoma exhibits nested growth and is composed of round cells containing abundant glycogen, which may contain clear or eosinophilic cytoplasm (choice A). Nuclear pleomorphism is not a feature of clear cell sarcoma; however, cells do typically contain a single prominent basophilic nucleolus, reminiscent of other melanocytic tumors (choice E). Multinucleated giant cells containing nuclei with similar characteristics are typically present (choice B). Intracytoplasmic melanin as well as abundant intra- and extracellular iron are commonly seen (choices C, D).
QCSP, **Clear Cell Sarcoma,** p 681.

184. **B.** **S100+HMB45+EMA−**
The immunohistochemical profile of clear cell sarcoma is similar to that of malignant melanoma with expression of S100 and HMB45 and lack of expression of EMA expression (choice B).
QCSP, **Clear Cell Sarcoma,** p 681.

185. **A.** **t(12;22)(q13;q12)**
The molecular alteration associated with clear cell sarcoma is t(12;22)(q13;q12), which creates the EWS-ATF-1 chimeric fusion protein (choice A). The other translocations presented are the alterations seen in primitive neuroectodermal tumor (choice B), desmoplastic small round cell tumor (choice C), infantile fibrosarcoma and congenital mesoblastic nephroma (choice D), and myxoid liposarcoma (choice E).
QCSP, **Clear Cell Sarcoma,** p 682.

186. **A.** **PSEUDOEPITHELIOMATOUS HYPERPLASIA**
Granular cell tumors have a distinct appearance, being composed predominantly of monomorphous large polygonal cells with granular eosinophilic cytoplasm. Malignant granular cell tumors are characterized by cellular pleomorphism, vesicular nuclei with prominent nucleoli, high nuclear-cytoplasmic ratio, >2 mitotic figures per 10 HPF, and necrosis (choices B, C, D, E). Pseudoepitheliomatous hyperplasia is seen in benign as well as malignant granular cell tumors (choice A).
QCSP, **Granular Cell Tumor,** p 684.

187. **D.** **GFAP**
Granular cell tumors contain abundant hydrolytic enzymes, which are strongly positive by Luxol fast blue (choice A). S100, NSE, and CD68 are typically positive (choices B, C, E). GFAP, which may be variable in schwannomas, is negative in granular cell tumor (choice D).
QCSP, **Granular Cell Tumor,** p 684.

188. **C.** **SCHWANN CELL**
Granular cell tumors are typically associated with peripheral nerves and may arise in many different locations. The lesion has a benign prognosis and only rarely recurs. The cell of origin is thought to be the Schwann cell (choice C).
QCSP, **Granular Cell Tumor,** p 684.

20: Soft Tissue Answers

189. **E.   PLEOMORPHIC MULTINUCLEATED GIANT CELLS**
Merkel cell carcinoma is a neuroendocrine carcinoma predominantly involving the skin of the head and neck area. Microscopically, the lesion resembles primitive neuroectodermal tumor in that it is densely populated by monotonous small round blue cells with brisk mitotic activity (choices A, B). Single cell necrosis is common (choice C). The stroma contains a high density of vascular spaces, which are lined by plump endothelial cells (choice D). Pleomorphic multinucleated giant cells are not a feature of Merkel cell carcinoma (choice E).
QCSP, **Merkel Cell Carcinoma,** p 688.

190. **C.   POSITIVE IN A PERINUCLEAR DISTRIBUTION**
It is worthwhile remembering that Merkel cell carcinoma exhibits dot-like perinuclear staining with cytokeratin 20 (choice C). This is a fairly specific finding.
QCSP, **Merkel Cell Carcinoma,** p 688.

191. **A.   MALIGNANT MELANOMA**
All of the choices presented are associated with Merkel cell carcinoma except for malignant melanoma (choice A).
QCSP, **Merkel Cell Carcinoma,** p 688.

192. **C.   TRUNK OF A CHILD**
Neurothekeoma commonly involves the head and neck area as well as the shoulders of children and young adults. In young adults, the fingers are another preferred location. (choice C). Mucosal surfaces are less commonly affected (choices A, B).
QCSP, **Neurothekeoma,** p 695.

193. **E.   NECROSIS**
Neurothekeoma is characterized by lobules composed of uniform round cells separated by thin collagen bands containing delicate blood vessels (choices B, D). There is typically prominent myxoid matrix (choice C). While not universal, benign giant cells are frequently present (choice A). Necrosis is not a feature of this lesion (choice E).
QCSP, **Neurothekeoma,** p 695.

194. **C.   ATYPICAL MITOTIC FIGURES**
Schwannomas are characterized by nuclear palisading and alternating cellular and hypocellular areas (Antoni A and Antoni B, respectively) (choices A, B). Some schwannomas undergo degenerative changes known as "ancient change," which may include necrosis, cellular pleomorphism and hyalinization (choice D). Atypical mitotic figures, however, should not be attributed to degenerative change (choice C). Thick hyalinized vessels are commonly seen in schwannoma (choice E).
QCSP, **Schwannoma,** p 699.

195. **B.   IT IS CHARACTERIZED BY RAPID GROWTH.**
Alveolar soft part sarcoma is a slowly growing, but relentless tumor (choice B). It most commonly occurs in the lower extremity of adolescents and young adults (choices A, D), although in children, the head and neck area is favored (choice C). Bony destruction is not uncommon (choice E).
QCSP, **Alveolar Soft Part Sarcoma,** p 700.

20: Soft Tissue Answers

196. **A.** **PAS WITH DIASTASE**

The neoplastic population in alveolar soft part sarcoma notably contains PAS-positive, diastase-resistant rhomboid or rod-shaped crystals in 80% of cases. While these can also be seen on an H&E stain, they are particularly pronounced on the PAS stain (choice A). PAS without diastase also confirms the presence of glycogen in these cells, but is less specific (choice B). Colloidal iron, Warthin-Starry, and GMS stains are not helpful in alveolar soft part sarcoma (choices C, D, E).

QCSP, **Alveolar Soft Part Sarcoma,** p 701.

197. **C.** **BRAIN**

Metastases involving the brain are more common in alveolar soft part sarcoma than any other soft tissue sarcoma (choice C). This lesion also commonly metastasizes to lungs and bone, as do many other sarcomas (choices A, D). The lymph nodes and liver are uncommon sites for alveolar soft part metastases (choices B, E).

QCSP, **Alveolar Soft Part Sarcoma,** p 701.

198. **E.** **IT IS CHARACTERIZED BY RAPID GROWTH.**

Angiomatoid fibrous histiocytoma is a slowly growing, painless mass, which typically involves the extremities of children and young adults (choices A, C, D, E). It can be associated with anemia, fever, and weight loss (choice B). Although this is a benign lesion, it does recur in a small percentage of cases.

QCSP, **Angiomatoid Fibrous Histiocytoma,** p 701.

199. **C.** **10-YEAR-OLD MALE WITH AN ABDOMINAL MASS**

Desmoplastic round cell tumor is a lesion of young adult males and typically involves the abdomen, although other sites have been described (choice C). The prognosis is poor, with only a 5% survival beyond 5 years.

QCSP, **Desmoplastic Small Round Cell Tumor,** p 702.

200. **B.** **CELLULAR PLEOMORPHISM**

The microscopic appearance of desmoplastic small round cell tumor is characterized by a monotonous population of small blue cells with no appreciable pleomorphism in a dense fibrous stroma (choice B). However, necrosis and abundant mitotic figures are common (choices C, D). Rhabdoid cells are present in 1/2 of cases, while epithelial differentiation such as gland or rosette formation is present in 1/3 of cases (choice E).

QCSP, **Desmoplastic Small Round Cell Tumor,** p 702.

201. **A.** **CK+EMA+DESMIN+**

The immunohistochemical profile of desmoplastic small round cell tumor is heterogeneous. The vast majority of cases are positive for cytokeratin, EMA, and desmin (choice A). Neuroendocrine markers are frequently positive as well, although synaptophysin reactivity is less common than NSE reactivity.

QCSP, **Desmoplastic Small Round Cell Tumor,** p 702.

202. **C.** **EPITHELIOID SARCOMA**

Epithelioid sarcoma is a malignancy of young adults, in whom it typically involves the distal upper extremities. In fact, it is the most common sarcoma affecting the wrist (choice C). Synovial sarcoma is seen in the same age group, but typically affects the lower extremities (choice A). Malignant peripheral nerve sheath tumor is an uncommon tumor, but preferentially involves the major nerve plexi (choice B). Extraskeletal chondrosarcoma and osteosarcoma occur in the lower extremities and limb girdles and do not commonly affect the wrist (choices D, E).

QCSP, **Epithelioid Sarcoma,** p 703.

203. E. **MOST CASES ARE DISCOVERED DURING THE FIRST 2 YEARS OF LIFE.**
Fibrous hamartoma of infancy is a benign tumor that occurs as a single mobile nodule in males within the first 2 years of life (choices A, C, E). The most common locations include the proximal upper and lower extremities, trunk, and inguinal regions. This lesion does not occur in the hands and feet (choice B). Malignant transformation is not a feature of this tumor (choice D).
QCSP, **Fibrous Hamartoma of Infancy,** p 704-705.

204. C. **MULTINUCLEATED GIANT CELLS**
Fibrous hamartoma of infancy is composed 3 3 cellular components arranged in an organoid growth pattern (choice E). These components include intersecting fascicles of spindle cells and collagen, areas composed of small stellate cells embedded in a mucoid matrix, and islands of mature adipose tissue (choices A, B, D). Multinucleated giant cells are not a feature of this lesion (choice C).
QCSP, **Fibrous Hamartoma of Infancy,** p 705.

205. D. **HYPOGLYCEMIA**
Hemangiopericytoma is occasionally associated with hypoglycemia (choice D) due to the elaboration of insulin-like growth factor (IGF)-II. This association is also seen in solitary fibrous tumor. The other laboratory findings listed are not associated with hemangiopericytoma (choices A, B, C, E).
QCSP, **Hemangiopericytoma,** p 706.

206. A. **INFILTRATIVE GROWTH**
Intramuscular myxoma is characterized by bland stellate fibroblast-like cells with inconspicuous, hyperchromatic nuclei in a prominent myxoid stroma. Nuclear atypia, pleomorphism, mitotic figures, and multinucleated giant cells should not be seen (choices B, C, D, E). The edge of the lesion typically exhibits an infiltrative growth pattern (choice A). Despite this latter feature, incomplete excision only rarely results in recurrence.
QCSP, **Myxoma,** p 709.

207. C. **FINGER**
The most common location of a glomus tumor is the subungual area of the finger (choice C). Other common locations include other areas of the extremities, the trachea, chest wall, and gastrointestinal tract.
QCSP, **Glomus Tumor,** p 714.

208. A. **THIS VARIANT OCCURS PREDOMINANTLY IN MEN.**
Epithelioid hemangioma exhibits no overall gender predilection, although parenchymal tumors occur more commonly in women (choice A). This variant usually affects young adults and presents either as a solitary mass in the distal extremities or as multifocal lesions in parenchymal organs (choices B, C). Microscopic features include bland cells with abundant cytoplasm and scattered intracellular cytoplasmic lumina containing erythrocytes, low mitotic activity, and a background of chondroid or myxoid stroma (choice D). 1/2 of cases are associated with vessel walls (choice E).
QCSP, **Hemangioendothelioma,** p 715-716.

209. D. **HHV8**
Kaposi sarcoma is associated with HHV8 (choice D).
QCSP, **Kaposi Sarcoma,** p 721.